AF792415

Occupational Therapy Interventions

Occupational Therapy Interventions

Editor: Oscar Alvarez

FOSTER
ACADEMICS
www.fosteracademics.com

www.fosteracademics.com

FOSTER ACADEMICS

Cataloging-in-Publication Data

Occupational therapy interventions / edited by Oscar Alvarez.
p. cm.
Includes bibliographical references and index.
ISBN 978-1-63242-672-7
1. Occupational therapy. 2. Medical rehabilitation. 3. Medicine, Physical.
4. Physical therapy. I. Alvarez, Oscar.
RM735 .O23 2019
615.8--dc23

© Foster Academics, 2019

Foster Academics,
118-35 Queens Blvd., Suite 400,
Forest Hills, NY 11375, USA

ISBN 978-1-63242-672-7 (Hardback)

This book contains information obtained from authentic and highly regarded sources. Copyright for all individual chapters remain with the respective authors as indicated. All chapters are published with permission under the Creative Commons Attribution License or equivalent. A wide variety of references are listed. Permission and sources are indicated; for detailed attributions, please refer to the permissions page and list of contributors. Reasonable efforts have been made to publish reliable data and information, but the authors, editors and publisher cannot assume any responsibility for the validity of all materials or the consequences of their use.

Trademark Notice: Registered trademark of products or corporate names are used only for explanation and identification without intent to infringe.

Printed and bound in China.

Contents

Preface

Occupational therapy is a type of therapy involving the use of assessment and intervention to recover, develop or maintain the occupations or meaningful activities of people. Occupational therapists usually deal with people having mental health problems, impairments or disabilities. They help individuals to achieve a fulfilled and satisfied state of life with the help of specially designed interventions. Injury rehabilitation, providing support to the elderly dealing with physical and cognitive changes, and assisting children with disabilities to enable them to participate properly in school and social situations, are some of the common examples of occupational therapy interventions. This book includes some of the vital pieces of work being conducted across the world, on various topics related to occupational therapy interventions. It presents researches and studies performed by experts across the globe. In this book, using case studies and examples, constant effort has been made to make the understanding of the difficult concepts of occupational therapy as easy and informative as possible, for the readers.

The information shared in this book is based on empirical researches made by veterans in this field of study. The elaborative information provided in this book will help the readers further their scope of knowledge leading to advancements in this field.

Finally, I would like to thank my fellow researchers who gave constructive feedback and my family members who supported me at every step of my research.

Editor

1

Perceptions about Authentic Leadership Development: South African Occupational Therapy Students' Camp Experience

Fatima Hendricks[1] and Susan Toth-Cohen[2]

[1]*OTASA, Vlaeberg, P.O. Box 15809, Cape Town 8018, South Africa*
[2]*Department of Occupational Therapy, Thomas Jefferson University, 130 S. 9th Street, 632 Edison, Philadelphia, PA 19107, USA*

Correspondence should be addressed to Fatima Hendricks; fatimahendricks@yahoo.com

Academic Editor: Lynette Mackenzie

Background. Twenty-three years into democracy, concern is deepening regarding the slow progress of Occupational Therapy (OT) in South Africa, especially with regard to diversity and inclusion within OT. *Methods.* This study explores authentic leadership development primarily among Black OT students attending a pilot Occupational Therapy Association of South Africa (OTASA) National Student Leadership Camp. It seeks to ascertain their perceptions on leadership and leadership development. This descriptive pilot study employs in-depth interviews and subsequent content analysis, with 12 OT students from six university OT programs in South Africa. *Findings.* Four categories of participant perceptions on authentic leadership development emerged from the analysis: (1) perceptions about oneself as a leader based on personal narrative, self-awareness, self-control, and psychological capital; (2) perceptions about others, specifically current leaders, with regard to their moral crisis, including continuing inequality, insincerity, greed, and selfishness; (3) goals and aspirations for leadership development via student camps; and (4) effects of leadership on the system. *Conclusions.* Recommendations for future practice include promotion of storytelling as a means of personal reflection for authentic leadership development and focused investment in camps for developing student leadership skills and building authentic leadership knowledge.

1. Introduction

The South African OT community continues to grapple with issues related to the slow pace of social transformation, particularly racial transformation, diversity, and inclusion [1]. Exploring emerging OT student leaders' perceptions of their leadership journeys and engagement with authentic leadership may provide insight into student leaders' implicit theories of leadership in a postcolonial context. This, in turn, may enable greater understanding of OT students' leadership development needs and lead to a more informed approach to developing transformational plans to enhance diversity within the OT profession in South Africa.

As per OTASA's vision for 2020, students are an important strategic driver in the OT community in South Africa for their potential contribution to societal transformation [2], and, as OTASA's future leadership pipeline at the branch and national level, they reflect diversity and inclusion. Table 1 represents the number of OT students registered with the Health Professions Council and their demographic profiles [3]. Approximately 12% of the students are members of OTASA, and there is significant opportunity for growth in student membership and participation [1].

The data in Table 1 reveal that the racial profile of the students relative to South Africa's demographics is skewed toward minority group overrepresentation, with 997 White students in OT programs compared with 773 Black African, 283 Colored, 167 Indian, and 2 Chinese students. At the same time, the number of Black students enrolling in OT programs is increasing, also illustrated in Table 1 [3]. Black African OT student admission has increased by 26.7% from 2013 to 2016 when compared to a 6.4% increase in White students during the same period. Diversity and inclusion to promote an Occupational Therapy community that reflects the demographics of the country is a key issue in the preliminary results of OTASA's National Listening & Dialogue Campaign,

TABLE 1: Demographic profile of OT students (OT S) and membership in OTASA.

REG_CODE	Race	Dec 2013	Dec 2014	Dec 2015	Apr 2016
OT S	African	610	673	678	773
	Chinese	1	1	2	2
	Colored	243	262	259	283
	Indian	136	148	152	167
	White	918	908	902	977
	(None)	80	87	88	99
OT S total		1,988	2,079	2,081	2,301
OTASA student membership		130	249	266	289
OTASA student membership%		6.54%	11.98%	12.78%	12.56%

Source. Health Professions Council of South Africa (2016); OTASA (2016).

a series of ongoing national consultative workshops [4]. From these discussions, it is evident that gaps exist in engaging emerging Black OT leaders among students, hence the strategic importance of the National Student Leadership Camp and its focus on authentic leadership development for Black emerging student leaders.

Another strategic drivers for transformation, diversity, and inclusion is the recent student protests, manifested by #feesmustfall and #rhodesmustfall, which have been accompanied by a vibrant student movement reemphasizing the role of students in leading change for accessible and relevant education [5]. In addition, there is the upcoming World Federation of OT (WFOT) Congress 2018, to be hosted in South Africa, titled "Connected in Diversity: Positioned for Impact" [6], which requires student engagement across the racial and social spectrum as a prerequisite for its success.

Hence, to engage emerging Black student leaders in leadership development, a pilot leadership camp was conducted to meet the strategic needs of the OT community and promote diversity within the profession. The residential student leadership camp drew primarily emerging Black student leaders from OT programs across the country. The research question for this pilot study focused on examining individual student perceptions of authentic leadership development during camp participation; hence, personal narrative in-depth interviews were conducted with OT student camp participants.

Authentic leadership [7–12] was chosen as the organizing framework for the pilot study, because it includes a developmental focus appropriate for emerging leadership in students [13]. At its core, authentic leadership contains key concepts related to the self—such as self- awareness, self-knowledge, self-regulation, and personal values—which can be controlled by students desiring to effect change. Walumba et al. [9] describe four dimensions of authentic leadership: self-awareness, balanced processing, relational transparency, and internalized moral perspective; these are significant in the context of constructing a life story narrative, as elucidated by Shamir and Eilam [8]. Self-awareness is the extent to which leaders know and understand their own true selves. Balanced processing refers to unbiased analysis of all relevant information and taking into account others' opinions and input before making a decision. Relational transparency involves openly sharing information and expressing one's true thoughts and emotions with others. Internalized moral perspective refers to the extent to which leaders' behaviors are guided by internal moral standards and values rather than by external pressures [14].

Shamir and Eilam [8] also define four characteristics of authentic leaders: they are (1) true to themselves (rather than conforming to the expectations of others); (2) motivated by personal convictions, rather than by status, honor, or other personal benefits; (3) original, leading from their own personal point of view; and (4) spurred to action based on their personal values and convictions.

The construction of a life story is a major element in the development of authentic leadership. Shamir and Eilam [8] further argue that authentic leadership "rests heavily on the self-relevant meanings the leader attaches to his or her life experiences, and these meanings are captured in the leader's life-story." They suggest that self-knowledge, self-concept clarity, and person-role merger are derived from the life story, making the construction of life story critical to the development of authentic leaders. This model provides a meaningful system of feeling, thinking, and acting [8], which is particularly relevant in the evolving sociopolitical, historical, and cultural contexts of South Africa. Hence, this pilot study aims to fill an important gap by focusing on authentic leadership development for primarily emerging Black OT student leaders by asking them how they perceive authentic leadership and its development. The descriptive findings from the study may contribute to theory development by revealing information about Black South African OT students' implicit theories of leadership. Greater understanding of these implicit theories of leadership may then inform development of strategies to help Black OT students in South Africa to further develop their leadership capacity and contribute their unique perspectives to leadership within the OT profession.

2. Materials and Methods

2.1. Aim of the Study. This descriptive pilot study explored the personal narratives of Black OT students attending the first OTASA National Student Leadership Camp designed to promote authentic leadership development, from September 23 to 25, in Limpopo, South Africa.

3. Method

The project was approved by the Institutional Review Board (IRB) of the authors' university and was part of a larger study using mixed methods to explore leadership development among South African OT students. Data were gathered from structured interviews based on key concepts of authentic leadership [7, 8, 10–12, 15].

Participants comprised 12 Occupational Therapy students from six university OT programs in South Africa. The purposive sample was drawn from first- to third-year OT students ($n = 34$), who attended the first pilot National Student Leadership Camp prior to commencement of the camp (see demographics in Table 2). Two students from each university were selected for the interviews, and six of the eight OT programs in South Africa were represented.

3.1. Data Collection and Analysis

Data Collection. A structured interview questionnaire was used, consisting of six questions based on the principles of authentic leadership according to Gardner et al. [11] and Shamir and Eilam [8]: life story and life purpose, positive psychological capital, positive moral perspective, self-regulation, self-awareness, and aspirations for the student leadership camp; these aspects were developed as a discussion guide. The questionnaire was developed from the principles of authentic leadership and formulated into a grid of key elements of authentic leadership, like positive psychological capital and other elements, to serve as a rubric. The rubric assessment for categorizing their responses as awareness, exploration/engagement, or generativity was then used after each response was recorded (see Table 3). Responses were captured in writing by the first author prior to student participation in the camp.

Data Analysis. Data analysis began with open coding of participants' survey responses using NVivo. Constant comparative analysis within and across survey data allowed the researchers to reduce categories and create a structured coding system through organizing and coding with nodes in trees in NVivo [16]. The investigators completed the coding processes separately and compared coded statements that demonstrated strong consensus, hence establishing intercoder reliability.

4. Results and Discussion

The findings of this study revealed participants' perceptions of leadership as reflective of their internalized beliefs and expectations of leaders (implicit leadership theories). The data in Figure 1 show that the primary themes can be divided into four main categories: (1) perceptions of authentic leadership in relation to self; (2) perceptions of key issues with current leaders; (3) goals and aspirations for authentic leadership development via camps; and (4) effects of leadership on the system.

Table 2: Participant demographics of personal narrative interviews.

Attribute	Description	$N = 12$
Gender	Male	5
	Female	7
Age	18–20	7
	21–23	3
	24–26	2
	27+	0
Race	Black	7
	Colored	2
	Indian	2
	White	1
Year of study	First	5
	Second	5
	Third	2
	Fourth	0
University	University of Cape Town	0
	University of Free State	0
	University of Kwa-Zulu Natal	2
	University of Pretoria	2
	Sefako Makgatho Health Sciences University	2
	University of Stellenbosch	2
	University of Western Cape	2
	University of Witwatersrand	2

4.1. Grading Rubric. The rubric outlined in Table 3 was based on the core elements of authentic leadership [8, 11]. This rubric was used to grade each participant according to the quality of their responses in terms of the awareness, exploration, or generativity levels for each of the five key questions asked, the sixth being a question on camp goals and aspirations.

For Question 1, 67% of the participants were found to be on the exploration level because they were able to briefly describe leadership components in relation to life goals or life story, whereas 33% were graded at the generativity level for their ability to engage in a thorough discussion of life goals or life story relating to the key components of leadership. In terms of the framework, authentic leaders are self-concordant individuals who pursue life goals expressing their authentic choices rather than following externally imposed duties or conventions and are motivated by internal commitment, which is a commitment to a self-concept [8].

Regarding Question 2, 83% were graded at the exploration level for demonstrating some understanding of the psychological competencies for becoming an authentic leader, whereas 17% were placed at the generativity level for demonstrating understanding that having confidence, a vision of success, perseverance, and resilience are key psychological competencies for becoming an authentic leader. According to Luthans et al. [17], an individual's positive psychological

TABLE 3: Grading rubric of the level of engagement with authentic leadership.

Question	Awareness	Exploration	Generativity	Percentage
(1) Life story and its relationship to leadership camp attendance	$N = 0$	$N = 8$	$N = 4$	Awareness: 0% Exploration: 66.66% Generativity: 33.33% 100% at exploration level or higher
(2) Psychological competencies for authentic leadership	$N = 0$	$N = 10$	$N = 2$	Awareness: 0% Exploration: 83.33% Generativity: 16.66 100% at exploration level or higher
(3) Ethical issues facing leadership today	$N = 1$	$N = 7$	$N = 4$	Awareness: 8.33% Exploration: 58.33% Generativity: 33.33% 91.66% at exploration level or higher
(4) Self-regulation and authentic leadership	$N = 1$	$N = 7$	$N = 4$	Awareness: 8.33% Exploration: 58.33% Generativity: 33.33% 91.66% at exploration or higher
(5) Self-awareness and personal examples	$N = 1$	$N = 8$	$N = 3$	Awareness: 8.33% Exploration: 66.66% Generativity: 25% 91.66% at exploration level or higher

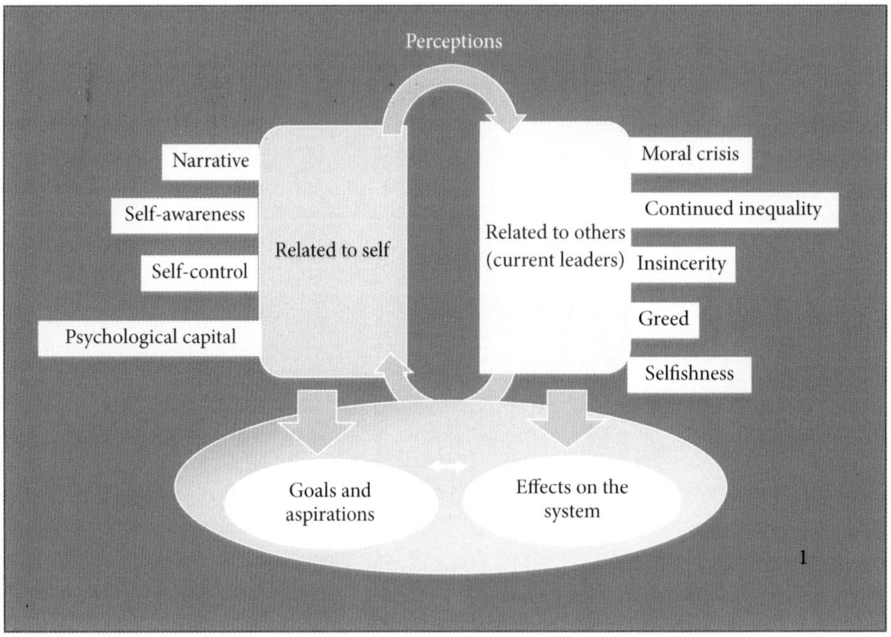

FIGURE 1: Student perceptions of authentic leadership.

state of development is characterized by (1) confidence, (2) being optimistic about succeeding, (3) perseverance toward goals and, when necessary, redirecting paths toward goals (i.e., showing hope) in order to succeed, and (4) when beset by problems and adversity, sustaining and bouncing back and even beyond (i.e., resilience) to attain success.

For Question 3, 8% of participants were graded at the awareness level for their ability to suggest some core ethical issues in relation to leadership and moral capacity, moral courage, and resiliency; 58% at the exploration level for discussing, in some detail, core ethical issues in relation to leadership and moral capacity, moral courage, and resiliency;

and 33% at generativity for their ability to analyze, with depth and clarity, core ethical issues in relation to leadership and moral capacity, moral courage, or resiliency. In terms of positive moral perspective, May et al. [18] provide an extensive discussion of this moral component, describing an ethical and transparent decision-making process whereby authentic leaders develop and draw upon reserves of moral capacity, efficacy, courage, and resiliency to address ethical issues and achieve authentic and sustained moral actions.

Among the participants for Question 4, 8% were graded at the awareness level for referring to certain details on the importance of self-control and the need to assess and manage alternate, divergent, or contradictory perspectives or ideas in comparison with internal standards. At the exploration level, 58% were graded for being able to highlight the importance of self-control and the need to assess and manage alternate, divergent, or contradictory perspectives or ideas in comparison with internal standards in an exploratory way, whereas 33% were graded at the generativity level. Self-regulation involves processes whereby people exert self-control by (1) setting internal (either existing or newly formulated) standards, (2) assessing discrepancies between these standards and actual or expected outcomes, and (3) identifying intended actions for reconciling these discrepancies [19].

George [20] describes self-awareness as an emerging process and not a destination point, in which individuals continually come to understand their unique talents, strengths, sense of purpose, core values, beliefs, and desires that include basic and fundamental awareness of their knowledge, experience, and capabilities. Gardner et al. [21] further describe four components: values, cognitions regarding identity, emotions, and motives/goals. Thus, among the participants for Question 5, 8% were graded at the awareness level for mentioning some strengths and weaknesses but with little connection to life goals or purpose, values, identity, and emotions, whereas 67% of participants were able to analyze personal strengths and weaknesses with some connection to life goals or purpose, values, identity, and emotions (exploration level), and 25% of the participants were able to effectively analyze strengths and weaknesses with a strong connection to life goals or purpose, values, identity, and emotions (generativity level).

Overall, for each of the questions, over 90% of the participants were graded at the exploration or generativity levels. The next section outlines the content of the in-depth interviews in terms of key themes that emerged.

4.2. Key Themes. Figure 1 illustrates the four categories of participant perceptions that emerged on authentic leadership development: (1) perceptions about self as a leader based on personal narrative, self-awareness, self-control, and psychological capital; (2) perceptions about others, specifically current leaders, relating to their moral crisis, continued inequality, insincerity, greed, and selfishness; (3) goals and aspirations for leadership development via camps; and (4) effect of leadership on the system.

Figure 1 outlines the subthemes in relation to perceptions of authentic leadership pertaining to leadership of the self as follows: (a) life narrative—the self as leader/role model, the influence of family and significant others on leadership development, and the relationship among leadership, OT, and life purpose; (b) self-awareness—being true to self, conscious of self, and accepting of self; (c) self-control—self-mastery, leading carefully through careful thinking, emotional control, and using a moral compass; and finally (d) positive psychological capital—perseverance/resilience, positivity, and openness. For example, relating to perceptions of authentic leadership pertaining to self in the subtheme of positive psychological capital, one student said,

> *I have a lot of zeal and persistence to press forward. I could have given up but I never gave up. I have to be positive, and I have to make a contribution. (Black, female)*

This statement is typical of the perceptions of the participants' highlighting their perseverance and resilience within the context of their personal life narratives.

Figure 1 also outlines the subthemes of critiquing current leaders in relation to their authentic leadership as follows: (a) moral crisis in leadership; (b) continued societal inequality as a serious leadership challenge; (c) insincerity of leadership; (d) greed and corruption; and (e) selfishness in looking out for one's own self-interests over the needs of the people. In a critique of current leaders on the subtheme of moral crisis, a student stated,

> *It is disconcerting with fraud, corruption and with misplaced values. I think it is because it is lonely at the top and they have become addicted to power and lost their moral compass. (Black, male)*

Finally, Figure 1 outlines camp goals and aspirations for authentic leadership development via camps, the subthemes being listed as follows: (a) pursuit of leadership knowledge and skills, (b) aspirations for becoming a leader, and (c) building confidence for leadership. Students perceived themselves as active agents of or catalysts for change in the OT profession because, by pursing their leadership goals and aspirations, they could effect positive change in the societal system. As an example of a statement representing camp goals and aspirations for authentic development as a leader through leadership camps, a student noted,

> *When I work with children, I look at them and say to myself—look at that dance, it's so imperfectly perfect. And that's what I want to be to the children—to sincerely help them, encourage them. It starts with the self—this commitment and desire I have to do good. We forget about ourselves in terms of pretending to care but rather the leadership must come from within. The way I lead will be different after this camp. I will spend time reflecting and evaluating myself, and then I want to go back and share my camp experience with the rest of the class. (Colored, female)*

In summary, the results indicate that over 90% of the participants were graded by the rubric at the exploration or generativity level in terms of exploring their authentic leadership development, and four themes emerged in terms

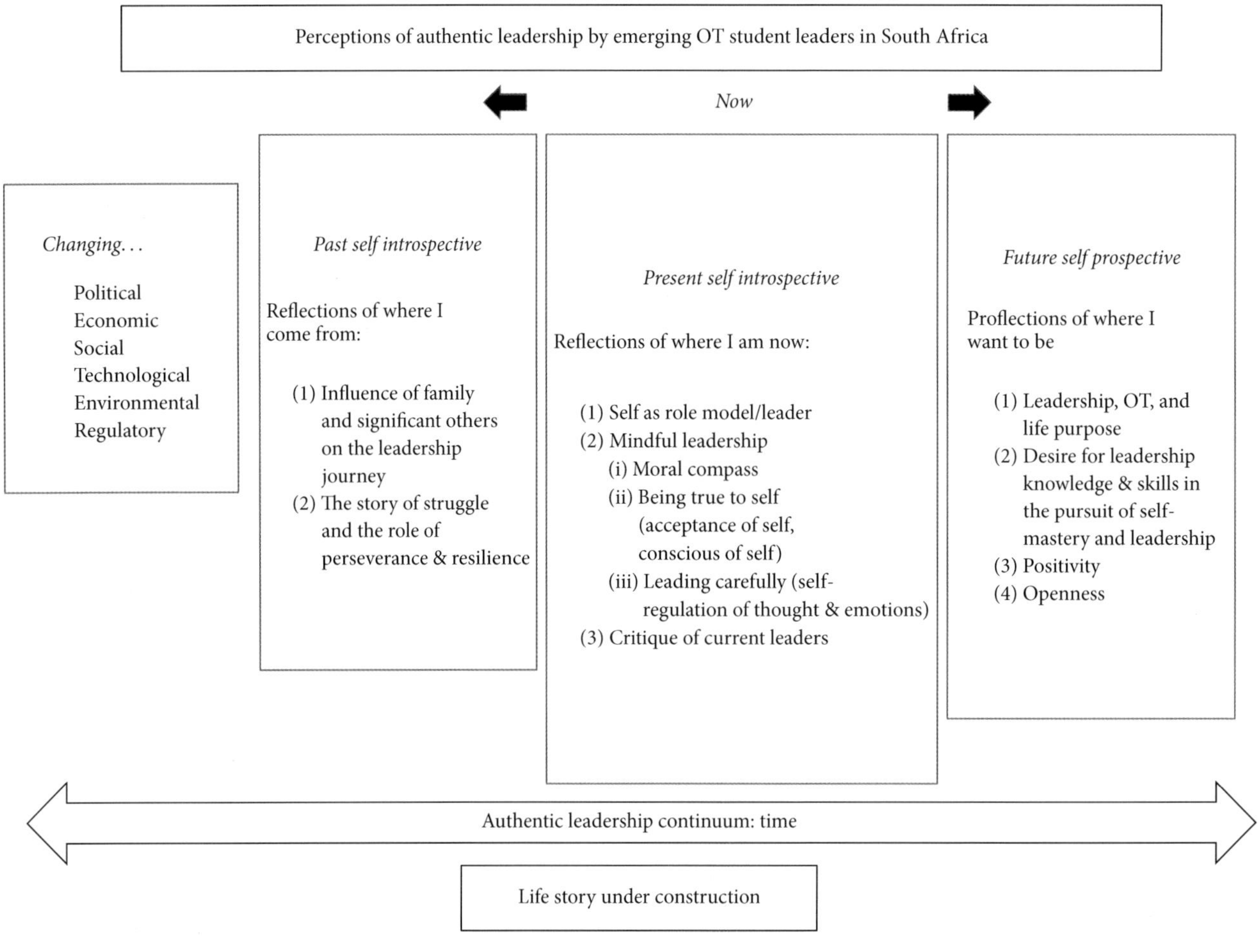

FIGURE 2: Working model of authentic leadership development for South African students.

of (a) perceptions of self as a leader, (b) perceptions of others, specifically current leaders, (c) goals and aspirations for leadership development using camps, and (d) effect of leadership on the system.

5. Discussion

A working model of the authentic leadership development model for students (Figure 2) is proposed based on the insights garnered from the results.

Preliminary findings from this pilot study indicate that the students are on a leadership continuum, given that they describe themselves retrospectively in terms of their "past self," such as where they come from; in subthemes like the important role of family and significant others in leadership development; the story of their struggle; and the role of perseverance and resilience in shaping their journeys. Students spent a significant amount of time describing themselves in terms of their "present self," such as in their reflections on role modeling, mindful leadership, and current leaders. The students "proflected"; that is, they began to consider the thoughts, feelings, and perceptions of their future, linking them to OT, life purpose, leadership, and a desire for leadership and self-mastery knowledge and skills, all the while valuing positivity and openness on the journey.

Interestingly, Erikson's developmental theory [22, 23] is not without its critics, especially in the area of identity formation and gender. Hoare [24] and Archer [25] describe the ages between 13 and 19, extending into the twenties, as the stage of fidelity in terms of identity versus role confusion in answering the questions, "Who am I, and what can I become?" It is characterized by an emerging sense of self through forging past experiences with anticipations of the future state with sufficient time for gaining clarity about values and convictions, exploring the role of leadership central to self-concept, developing self-resolution, and displaying self-expressive behavior with goals that are self-concordant [8].

Through a critical lens, this is where Shamir and Eilam's [8] proposition of authentic leadership development falters in presenting the notion of the life story as a "narrative" of leadership development. It is perhaps better considered as the life story "question" or "construction" rather than a "narrative" because, through a postcolonial lens, issues of contested identities exist [26], which have the potential to be in conflict with the concepts presented by both Shamir and Eilam [8] and Walumbwa et al. [14]: self-concept clarity, self-awareness, and self-knowledge for authentic leadership development. These concepts appear to be singular rather than hybrid or plural in nature. Postcolonial theories [26] present the notion that identities are multiple and evolving, whereas a self-concept is a combination of social categories comprising a set of social identities that is part of a collective of interwoven stories rather than an individual story—which in the South African context is called "Ubuntu." Ubuntu became prominent in mainstream discourse on race and identity during the transition from Apartheid into democracy and raises two important principles: the human being as being becoming (not static); and the importance of community. Whether Ubuntu can be claimed as the way South Africans experience their lived social realities and its relationships, order, and identities is debatable; however it can be described as a discursive South African social imaginary. Taylor [27] defines social imaginary as "common understanding that makes possible common practices and a widely shared sense of legitimacy." Ubuntu is important for the discussion of authentic leadership development in the context of the personal narrative of students' retrospective views of self in the past, introspective views of self in the present, and prospective views into the future shaping identities which are in a fluid state of construction and negotiation. This is consistent with the notion of authenticity of identity as contested at the intersection of racial and professional identities for OT students that was revealed in the narrative interviews.

Ubuntu is an African concept of philosophy according to which no one is self-sufficient, and all are interdependent: *umntu ngumntu ngabantu* means a person is a person because of others. Radically, Bujo [28] argues that an individual cannot be spoken about outside the notion of a community because "the human person in Africa is from the very beginning in a network of relationships that constitute his inalienable dignity," and that "African ethics does not define the person as self-realization or as ontological act; rather, it describes a person as a process of coming into existence in the reciprocal relatedness of individual and community, where the latter includes not only the deceased but also God" [28].

Hence, the proposed model of authentic leadership development includes students' *retrospective* views of self in the past, *introspective* views of self in the present, and *prospective* views into the future. These views of leadership are considered aspects of students' implicit theories of leadership and located within the macro context of the ever-changing social web of political, economic, social, technological, environmental, and regulatory environments in South Africa.

Within the historical context of a contested description of being "Born Frees" (i.e., born into Democratic South Africa), students face significant challenges from the macro environment in terms of socioeconomic-political struggles, requiring positive psychological capital. Furthermore, the need for positive psychological capital is amplified by the myriad of ethical and moral crises facing leaders today. Students described these challenges as having leaders who are corrupt and self-serving, power hungry, and morally decayed—leaders who lack discipline and respect for the rule of the law and are greedy.

In summary, the potential benefits of the proposed model of authentic leadership development are as follows: (1) leadership development is ongoing, a continuum, from youth till late adulthood; (2) leadership development is located in particular times and historical contexts that shape leadership, its formation, and expression and is therefore dynamic and responsive; (3) personal storytelling in camps is valuable in deconstructing and reconstructing life stories, individually or collectively, to facilitate leadership growth in self-knowledge, self-awareness, and other elements of mindful leadership; (4) leadership development requires follower development in a mutually symbiotic way, in consideration of the collective; (5) leadership development recognizes life purpose, values, morality, and God as elements of authenticity; (6) leadership development employs a scoring rubric designed for the youth.

The insights build a bridge between the conceptual understanding of authentic leadership and student perceptions of Occupational Therapy student leadership development through camping as a means of OT student leadership capacity building. It advocates for retrospective, introspective, and prospective views of leadership on a personal level as an enabler for Occupational Therapy students to engage in their own personal and professional leadership development through a diversity and inclusion approach of targeted student leadership development.

5.1. Limitations. The qualitative interviews were limited to 12 students from six of the eight universities of South Africa, of whom seven were Black African participants. Participation from all eight OT universities while maintaining the same racial demographics is a consideration for future work.

6. Conclusions

This exploratory pilot study provides insights into the potential for authentic leadership development for OT students based on four categories of authentic leadership: (1) perceptions about self as a leader based on personal narrative, self-awareness, self-control, and psychological capital; (2) perceptions about others, specifically current leaders, relating to moral crises, continued inequality, insincerity, greed, and selfishness; (3) goals and aspirations for leadership development via camps, and (4) the effect of leadership on the system. Although the sample size was relatively small, these findings provide insights into the potential for authentic leadership development and can be a springboard for further elaboration of student leadership development, particularly for emerging Black student leaders in OT. Findings may also contribute to further theory development in regard to students' own implicit theories of leadership.

Recommendations for future research and practice associated with authentic student leadership development include (1) the important role of storytelling in shaping leadership development narratives after 1994 for the so-called "Born Frees" as a means of sense-making and dreaming—in search of answers to the questions, "From where? To where?"; (2) the need for specific focused investment in the development of Black OT student leadership and the harnessing of all tools available in the context of the roles that family, educators, and the environment play in shaping leadership development; (3) authentic leadership and authentic leadership development from an African perspective, with particular consideration for postcolonial theorizing; and (4) enhancing camp experiences as a means of youth leadership development in the health professions sector, particularly OT, based on activity participation and experiential learning.

In conclusion, the proposed new model for authentic leadership development for OT students in South Africa has been built on OT students' perceptions of key issues with current leaders, perceptions about authentic leadership in relation to self, and student goals and aspirations for authentic leadership development via camps. This model can help the OT profession gain more understanding of the leadership development needs of emerging young Black leaders and may assist in theory development related to implicit theories of leadership. For example, as part of a mixed methods study, a survey could be designed to gather additional data on South African OT students' attitudes and perceptions of Occupational Therapy student leadership—with particular focus on diversity and inclusion. Together with a continued focus on storytelling and qualitative analysis of student narratives, results of the survey could provide insights for the formulation of transformational and leadership skills development plans for the OT profession in South Africa.

Acknowledgments

The pilot study was partly funded by the Occupational Therapy Association of South Africa (OTASA) and was completed in partial fulfillment of a post-professional doctorate in occupational therapy at Thomas Jefferson University in Philadelphia.

References

[1] OTASA Membership Office, "Membership demographics. Internal database," 2016.

[2] OTASA, "About, mission, vision & values," 2016, http://www.otasa.org.za/.

[3] Health Professions Council of South Africa (HPCSA), "Student register," 2016.

[4] OTASA Western Cape National Listening & Dialogue Campaign, "Preliminary results: internal report," 2015.

[5] S. Badat, "Deciphering the meanings, and explaining the South African higher education student protests of 2015-16," https://www.ru.ac.za/media/rhodesuniversity/content/uhuru/documents/Dr%20Saleem%20Badat%20-%20The%20Student%20Protests%20of%202015-16%20Final%20Draft-10March2016.pdf.

[6] World Federation of Occupational Therapy, "WFOT congress," http://www.wfotcongress.org.

[7] B. J. Avolio, F. Luthans, and F. O. Walumbwa, *Authentic Leadership: Theory Building for Veritable Sustained Performance*, The Gallup Leadership Institute, Lincoln, Neb, USA, 2004.

[8] B. Shamir and G. Eilam, "What's your story? A life- stories approach to authentic leadership development," *The Leadership Quarterly*, vol. 16, no. 3, pp. 395–417, 2005.

[9] F. Walumba, B. Avolio, W. Gardner, T. Wernsing, and S. Peterson, *Authentic Leadership: Development and Validation of a Theory-Based Measure*, Management Department Faculty Publications, 2008, http://digitalcommons.unl.edu/managementfacpub/24.

[10] B. J. Avolio, W. L. Gardner, F. O. Walumbwa, F. Luthans, and D. R. May, "Unlocking the mask: a look at the process by which authentic leaders impact follower attitudes and behaviors," *The Leadership Quarterly*, vol. 15, no. 6, pp. 801–823, 2004.

[11] W. L. Gardner, B. J. Avolio, B. J. Avolio, and F. O. Walumbwa, *Authentic Leadership Theory And Practice: Origins, Effects, and Development*, W. L. Gardner, B. J. Avolio, B. J. Avolio, and F. O. Walumbwa, Eds., Elsevier, San Diego, Calif, USA, 2005.

[12] B. J. Avolio and W. L. Gardner, "Authentic leadership development: getting to the root of positive forms of leadership," *The Leadership Quarterly*, vol. 16, no. 3, pp. 315–338, 2005.

[13] F. Luthans and B. J. Avolio, "Authentic leadership development," in *Positive Organizational Scholarship*, K. S. Cameron, J. E. Dutton, and R. E. Quinn, Eds., pp. 241–258, Berrett-Koehler, San Francisco, Calif, USA, 2003.

[14] F. O. Walumbwa, P. Wang, H. Wang, J. Schaubroeck, and B. J. Avolio, "Retracted: Psychological processes linking authentic leadership to follower behaviors," *The Leadership Quarterly*, vol. 21, no. 5, pp. 901–914, 2010.

[15] F. Luthans, C. M. Youssef-Morgan, and B. J. Avolio, *Psychological Capital and Beyond*, Oxford University Press, New York, NY, USA, 1st edition, 2015.

[16] P. Bazeley and P. Jackson, *Qualitative Data Analysis with Nvivo*, Sage, Los Angeles, Calif, USA, 2013.

[17] F. Luthans, C. M. Youssef, and B. J. Avolio, *Psychological Capital*, Oxford University Press, New York, NY, USA, 2007.

[18] D. R. May, A. Y. L. Chan, T. D. Hodges, and B. J. Avolio, "Developing the moral component of authentic leadership," *Organizational Dynamics*, vol. 32, no. 3, pp. 247–260, 2003.

[19] A. D. Stajkovic and F. Luthans, "Social cognitive theory and self-efficacy: going beyond traditional motivational and behavioral approaches," *Organizational Dynamics*, vol. 26, no. 4, pp. 62–74, 1998.

[20] W. George, *Authentic Leadership: Rediscovering The Secrets to Creating Lasting Value*, Jossey-Bass, San Francisco, Calif, USA, 2003.

[21] W. L. Gardner, B. J. Avolio, F. Luthans, D. R. May, and F. Walumbwa, "Can you see the real me? A self-based model of authentic leader and follower development," *The Leadership Quarterly*, vol. 16, no. 3, pp. 343–372, 2005.

[22] R. Stevens, *Erik Erikson: An Introduction*, St. Martin's Press, New York, NY, USA, 1983.

[23] E. H. Erikson, *The Life Cycle Completed: A Review*, W. W. Norton & Co, New York, NY, USA, 1985.

[24] C. H. Hoare, *Morality, Ethics, Spirituality, and Prejudice in The Writings of Erik H. Erikson*, Psychosocial Press, Madison, Conn, USA, 2000.

[25] S. L. Archer, "Commentary on 'Feminist perspectives on Erikson's theory: their relevance for contemporary identity development research'," *Identity*, vol. 2, no. 3, pp. 267–270, 2002.

[26] K. V. Korostelina, *Social Identity and Conflict: Structures, Dynamics and Implications*, Palgrave Macmillan, New York, NY, USA, 2007.

2

Correlation between Leisure Activity Time and Life Satisfaction: Based on KOSTAT Time use Survey Data

Yu-Jin Cha

Department of Occupational Therapy, Semyung University, Jecheon, Republic of Korea

Correspondence should be addressed to Yu-Jin Cha; occujin@naver.com

Academic Editor: Claudia Hilton

Rationale. This study aims to investigate the correlation between the available leisure activity time and life satisfaction of the healthy elderly and the factors affecting them. *Method.* For the analysis, data from the 2014 Time Use Survey (2014TUS) published by Statistics Korea (KOSTAT) was used. This study classified the detailed activities of 9228 subjects, based on the data in 2014TUS, and analyzed the differences in time use for occupation domains by age group. *Results.* It was found that a greater amount time used for outdoor leisure activities yielded a higher life satisfaction value. Differences were found in time use by occupation domains between younger and older groups. These showed higher life satisfaction for those with spouses, regular full-time jobs, higher education, and better health. *Conclusion.* Based on these results, in order to improve the quality of life (QoL) for older adults, it is necessary to develop various leisure programs that require dynamic physical activities and to prepare alternative policies at the national level to promote participation in leisure activities by older adults. This study will provide occupational therapists (OTs) with data they can use to help older adults who have difficulty in time usage through time management intervention to improve their life satisfaction and QoL.

1. Introduction

Unlike the time required for physiological needs or labor time, the quantity and nature of leisure time are not predetermined and may vary wildly depending on an individual's characteristics and tendencies. In particular, as the daily lives of older adults consist primarily of leisure time apart from the time required for physiological needs, their quality of life (QoL) can vary considerably depending on how they make use of their leisure time [1]. Besides having a lot of leisure time that they should manage somehow, the ways that older adults use their leisure time is fundamentally different from that of young people who use their leisure time for the purposes of reproducing and recovering from bodily and mental fatigue rather than for amusement [2].

For older adults, participation in leisure activities can help to provide solutions to the loneliness they have that results from loss of roles and can contribute to greater life satisfaction and happiness by providing chances for improving their self-esteem and self-realization. Life satisfaction values reflect the subjective level of individual satisfaction in achieving goals and expectations experienced in daily life [3]. Meaningful leisure activities are of critical importance because they are closely related to life satisfaction and quality of life for older adults in the contemporary era [4]. As the period spent in old age is getting longer, there is increasing concern regarding strategies for successful old age and improvement in the QoL for older adults [5]. Numerous studies regarding QoL for older adults have reported that participation in leisure activities contributes to maintaining and improving their physical health as well as their psychological and mental health and helps to maintain and increase their QoL by providing them with good opportunities for positive interaction with their families and others in society [6, 7].

Kelly argues that leisure activities are a more important factor than other experiences or activities, with regard to QoL [8]. Adams et al. asserted that a higher frequency of participation in leisure activities brings a higher QoL for older adults and allows them to live more happily [9]. That is, in order to maintain or improve older adults' QoL, it is most important to increase their opportunities to participate in leisure activities that can bring improvements in their physical, psychological, and social health [10].

Older adults should maintain a good balance in how they spend their time for various activities including self-care, leisure, rest, and social participation in order to improve their life satisfaction and health [11]. As the elderly population is increasing due to global demographic changes, it has become important to investigate older adults' time usage, that is, how they spend their days, in order to find ways to improve their QoL [12].

Occupational therapists (OTs) are experts in extending concern and encouraging participation by older adults in leisure activities, one of the fields of occupational therapy (OT) [4]. These global demographic changes will increase the number of older adults among OT clients, and consequently the contribution of OT to the lives of older adults will grow more and more important. In order for OTs to improve QoL for older adults, it is very important to investigate older adults' time usage, that is, how they spend their days [12]. If the status of older adults' time usage can be effectively analyzed, OTs will be able to suggest how older adults can participate actively in meaningful activities [1]. As daily life, which is closely related to temporal flow, proceeds in repeated cycles, one statistical source that can show the experiences and problems in daily living is time use survey data [13].

The investigation of time usage is necessary to evaluate the occupational balance that indicates how people subjectively choose mandatory and nonmandatory activities depending on personal values [14, 15]. Time management should be planned to provide an effective balance of private living, work, leisure, and rest to improve satisfaction and health [16]. The study of 24/7 living time usage enables us to investigate individual daily life and daily living within the social structure that surrounds individuals. In particular, such a temporally based approach is appropriate in dealing with older adults' daily living habits, which are difficult to study through official and economic approaches [13], as efficient time usage affects people's successful pursuit of meaningful activities and is an important criterion in deciding living modes, living aspects, and QoL [17]. In OT, studies regarding the time usage of individual persons such as those based on living time usage surveys are currently a primary concern and interest [18].

The *Occupational Therapy Practice Framework: Domain and Process (OTPF)* published by the American Occupational Therapy Association (AOTA) classifies various occupations in which a person or group participates into eight categories, namely, activities of daily living (ADL), instrumental activities of daily living (IADL), rest and sleep, education, work, play, leisure, and social participation, which are referred to as "occupation domains" [19]. For human beings, occupations are very critical elements, and each time a person participates in an occupation, an inevitable relation between occupation and time arises [20].

Looking into the causal relationship between the participation of the elderly population of South Korean in leisure activities and their life satisfaction mediated by leisure satisfaction that can be found in previous relevant literature, it is shown that the more older adults participated in leisure activities and were satisfied with them, the higher their life satisfaction [21]. Most of the studies analyzed the frequency of leisure activities by type or the subjective level of participation using a Likert scale. However, these research results have limitations in explaining precisely the relationship between increases in leisure activities and increases in the QoL and life satisfaction in the elderly of South Korea. Previous studies about life satisfaction in South Korea have focused on determining sociological and demographic variables affecting QoL, and there have been few studies analyzing the usage of leisure activity time as a variable. In addition, most of the previous studies have utilized limited sampling methods; therefore, their results were too limited to apply generally to the South Korean elderly population.

Even though South Korea entered the ranks of aged societies later than Europe or Japan, it is expected that by 2050, South Korea may become the most superaged society, as the portion of the population over 65 will increase dramatically [22]. Therefore, concern and interest regarding the comprehensive life satisfaction of older adults are likely to increase. This study investigated the correlation between the current status of leisure activity time use and life satisfaction of the healthy elderly in South Korea, factors affecting them, and the time usage of older adults as categorized according to the eight occupation domains suggested by OTPF-3 (OTPF 3rd Ed) and the aims at providing OTs with data so that they can help older adults who have difficulty in utilizing their time effectively through time management intervention aimed at improving their life satisfaction and QoL.

2. Method

2.1. Collecting Data. The 2014 Time Use Survey (2014TUS) used in this study was conducted by Statistics Korea (KOSTAT) in order to provide basic data for determining the 24-hour daily living modes and QoL of South Koreans, establishing policies related to labor, welfare, and transportation and conducting studies. A time use survey has been made every 5 years since 1999, and this study used the raw data collected in 2014 that measured South Koreans' lifestyles and QoL. For the analysis in this study, data regarding 9229 persons, the portion of the population aged 65 and over, was extracted from that of the 26,988 total subjects included in KOSTAT's 2014 Time Use Survey.

2.2. Overview of the Survey. The 2014 Time Use Survey (2014TUS) consists of a two-day diary record with respondents recording their primary activities and coactivities every 10 minutes. This analysis in this study included only the respondents' main activities. The respondents filled out the time diary with a record of activities based on classifications of activities (as of 2014: 9 major classifications, 42 medium classifications, and 138 minor classifications) covering their own activities as well as those of their companions, the location of the activities, and means of transportation involved, making an entry every 10 minutes for two days [23].

2.3. Subjects for the Analysis. The subjects for analysis were classified into a younger elderly group aged between 65 and 74 and an older elderly group aged 75 and over. Recently, as the life expectancy has increased, attempts have been made to subcategorize the age groups in studies on older adults. Neugarten et al. classified older adults into the younger elderly under 75 and the older elderly at 75 and older [24]. Compared to the younger elderly, the older elderly are more dependent on others due to their decreasing ability to conduct their daily life activities independently and have more difficulties in life due to the deaths of spouses and friends, economic hardship, deteriorating physical ability and health, and an increase in grave experiences in life [25]. The younger and the older elderly groups also differ in their respective health situations, which are affected by activities of daily living, family or social support, and health status. Therefore, when conducting studies and interventions related to them, different approaches should be taken for each group [26].

2.4. Classifications of Occupation Domains. Time use measuring instruments vary depending on research goals; therefore, activities were classified using a variety of methods. For this study, the subactivities included in the raw data of "2014 Time Use Survey" were categorized into a total of eight occupation domains (Appendix 1) [27]. Among these, leisure activities were classified into four subcategories, namely, indoor activities, outdoor activities, internet use, and other leisure activities (Table 1).

2.5. Analysis Method and Main Variables. For leisure time use in both elderly groups, frequency analysis was conducted, and in order to verify differences in the amount of time spent for leisure according to demographic characteristics, cross tabulation analysis (χ^2 test) and an F test using one-way ANOVA were conducted. In addition, for the differences in time usage by occupation domain in the South Korean elderly by age, Pearson's correlation coefficient test was conducted; for the correlation between leisure time spent and life satisfaction, analysis by averages was conducted; and for the correlation between leisure time spent, types of leisure activities, and life satisfaction, ordinary least squares (OLS) analysis was applied.

3. Results

Among the total of 9228 subjects, the younger elderly (at age 65–74) were 5436 (58.91%) and the older elderly (over 75 years) were 3792 (41.09%). For leisure activities, gender, educational attainment level, economic activity status, rural residence status, outdoor activities according to size of residential area, indoor activities, internet use, and other leisure activities showed significant differences ($p < 0.05$). Male older adults, those with higher educational attainment, those with nonworking status, those not living in rural areas, and those with urban/communal residence showed a significantly longer time usage in outdoor activities, indoor activities, internet use, and other leisure activities when their time spent on leisure activities was analyzed. For those with a spouse, the time for indoor activities and internet use was longer, while in the case of those with no spouse, the time for outdoor activities was longer (Table 1).

In a review of differences in time usage by the South Korean elderly population by age in occupation domains including leisure and the seven domains other than education, that is, activities of daily living (ADL), instrumental activities of daily living (IADL), rest and sleep, work, play, leisure, and social participation, showed significant differences ($p < 0.001$). The younger elderly group showed higher time usage in the domains of ADL, IADL, and work, while the older elderly group showed higher time usage in the domains of rest and sleep, play, leisure, and social participation. Among the eight occupation domains, leisure ranked highest in both the younger and the older elderly groups, followed by indoor activities (Table 2, Figure 1).

The analysis of time use by the South Korean elderly showed that as their use of time for leisure activities increased, their life satisfaction was higher, and all controlled variables except for economic activity status exerted significant influences on life satisfaction. The subjects showed higher life satisfaction if they had spouses, regular full-time jobs, higher education, and better health. They had significantly longer time usage for outdoor activities, indoor activities, internet use, and other leisure activities if they were male, or had higher education, nonworking status, or residence in urban (communal) housing not in agricultural and rural areas (Table 3).

The correlation between leisure time use and life satisfaction are shown in Table 4 and Figure 2. There is a general positive correlation between total time used for leisure and life satisfaction. For distribution of leisure time length according to a five-phase scale of life satisfaction level, in the case of very high life satisfaction, the average time spent for leisure activities was 325.24 minutes, while in the case of very low life satisfaction, the average daily time use for leisure activities was 291.28 minutes. Outdoor activities also showed a positive correlation, with longer leisure time used for outdoor activities corresponding to higher life satisfaction. However, in the case of indoor activities, an inverse correlation was shown, with longer time spent on indoor leisure activities corresponding to a lower life satisfaction.

4. Discussion

South Korean society has become a superaged society due to a rapid increase in the number of older adults, and concern for their comprehensive QoL is increasing. In this study, the usage of time by older adults over eight occupation domains suggested by OTPF-3 was studied, and correlations between leisure activity time use and life satisfaction were investigated to identify the satisfaction factors related to use of leisure time, and these factors were analyzed.

As a result of this study, it has been shown that there are differences in leisure activities related to gender, educational attainment, marital status, economic activities, residency in agricultural area all affecting outdoor activities according to size of residential area, indoor activities, internet use, and

Table 1: Differences of leisure activities in the Korean elderly according to demographic characteristics.

Items	Classifications	N (%)	Outdoor activities M	Outdoor activities SD	Outdoor activities $\frac{t}{F}$	Indoor activities M	Indoor activities SD	Indoor activities $\frac{t}{F}$	Internet use M	Internet use SD	Internet use $\frac{t}{F}$	Other M	Other SD	Other $\frac{t}{F}$
Age	Younger elderly (aged 65–74)	5436 (58.91)	50.53	70.22	23.89 $p \leq 0.001$	220.69	140.88	221.16 $p \leq 0.001$	2.99	17.58	30.20 $p \leq 0.001$	3.42	17.22	1.11 $p = 0.293$
	Older elderly (aged 75 and over)	3792 (41.09)	43.57	62.90		265.96	148.02		1.21	11.32		3.86	23.09	
Gender	Male	3800 (41.18)	65.35	77.86	466.79 $p \leq 0.001$	270.04	153.19	*297.50* $p \leq 0.001$	4.90	22.86	*195.66* $p \leq 0.001$	6.23	26.99	*114.28* $p \leq 0.001$
	Female	5428 (58.82)	35.30	55.73		217.77	135.91		0.41	5.13		1.77	12.31	
Educational attainment	No educational attainment	1900 (20.59)	30.49	51.17		242.41	145.08		0.06	1.47		1.88	10.94	
	Elementary school	3498 (37.91)	40.77	62.34		237.25	142.64		0.25	5.08		2.07	11.57	
	Middle school	1500 (16.25)	51.24	68.72	111.35 $p \leq 0.001$	230.01	144.82	4.70 $p = 0.001$	1.75	13.76	121.30 $p \leq 0.001$	3.11	15.13	41.27 $p \leq 0.001$
	High school	1520 (16.47)	66.49	77.79		240.21	152.21		5.06	22.67		5.99	24.49	
	Postsecondary education	810 (8.78)	75.90	79.69		256.30	146.54		11.75	33.46		10.72	44.73	
Marital status	Not married	3604 (28.11)	244.99	146.06	*9.07* $p = 0.003$	39.94	60.04	*78.55* $p \leq 0.001$	0.52	6.91	*76.02* $p \leq 0.001$	2.76	15.32	*10.67* $p = 0.001$
	Married	5624 (43.87)	235.64	145.14		52.63	71.27		3.37	18.78		4.14	22.25	
Reason for needing care	Care not needed	8654 (93.78)	47.97	67.92		233.87	142.93		2.34	15.49		3.69	20.29	
	Dementia	62 (0.67)	51.77	61.18		327.42	142.54		0.00	0.00		2.10	12.43	
	Stroke	40 (0.43)	59.50	75.38	1.68 $p = 0.153$	392.00	176.64	52.43 $p \leq 0.001$	1.50	9.49	1.21 $p = 0.305$	2.25	14.23	0.83 $p = 0.508$
	Disability	102 (1.11)	42.75	70.19		327.84	173.16		0.78	7.92		0.78	5.57	
	Other reasons	370 (4.01)	40.22	52.27		310.54	155.43		1.08	15.33		2.84	11.35	
Economic activity status	Working	2.87 (31.19)	29.86	55.33	301.84 $p \leq 0.001$	172.62	124.69	969.57 $p \leq 0.001$	1.61	11.27	7.48 $p = 0.006$	2.68	14.64	9.01 $p = 0.003$
	Not working	6350 (68.81)	55.75	70.74		269.51	144.29		2.55	16.86		4.02	21.79	
Average monthly household income	Less than 1 million KRW	7080 (76.70)	45.60	65.53		240.20	145.44		1.77	13.89		3.54	19.73	
	One million KRW–less than 2 million KRW	1420 (15.40)	51.76	70.82	*16.90* $p \leq 0.001$	233.60	150.40	*0.94* $p = 0.420$	4.12	19.26	*12.36* $p \leq 0.001$	4.22	21.70	*1.11* $p = 0.346$
	2 million KRW–less than 3 million KRW	422 (4.60)	61.59	74.66		243.44	134.28		4.29	20.89		4.02	20.26	
	Over 3 million KRW	306 (3.30)	67.75	84.21		233.60	142.17		4.46	22.45		1.90	11.90	
Classifications of agricultural residence	Agricultural residence	1694 (18.36)	26.71	54.45	*205.19* $p \leq 0.001$	198.71	131.90	*164.16* $p \leq 0.001$	0.83	8.66	*17.92* $p \leq 0.001$	1.68	11.18	*19.48* $p \leq 0.001$
	Nonagricultural residence	7534 (81.64)	52.39	69.10		248.42	146.94		2.58	16.46		4.04	21.29	
Size of residential area*	County/eup	2774 (30.06)	54.45	1.32	205.19 $p \leq 0.001$	131.90	3.20	164.16 $p \leq 0.001$	8.66	0.21	17.92 $p \leq 0.001$	11.18	0.27	19.48 $p \leq 0.001$
	Urban/dong	6454 (69.94)	69.10	0.80		146.94	1.69		16.46	0.19		21.29	0.25	
Period covered by research data	Weekdays	5464 (59.21)	47.06	67.05	1.10 $p = 0.294$	236.98	144.75	3.40 $p = 0.065$	2.18	14.74	0.34 $p = 0.559$	3.78	20.03	1.01 $p = 0.314$
	Weekend	3764 (40.79)	48.56	67.87		242.66	146.70		2.37	16.19		3.35	19.57	
Cohabitant status	Living alone	2330 (25.25)	232.16	143.83	7.49 $p = 0.006$	40.39	61.70	36.59 $p \leq 0.001$	0.90	9.12	24.40 $p \leq 0.001$	3.58	20.59	0.01 $p = 0.937$
	Having cohabitants	6898 (74.75)	241.70	146.08		50.13	69.04		2.72	16.92		3.61	19.58	

*Based on KOSTAT criteria, "county/eup" is a designation use in agricultural and rural areas and "urban/dong" in urban areas.

TABLE 2: Differences in time use in occupation domains by the Korean elderly population by age (min).

Occupations	Age: Over 65 years old M	SD	Younger elderly people (aged 65–74) M	SD	Older elderly people (aged 75 and over) M	SD	t-test
ADL	185.47	59.32	187.97	59.93	181.89	58.25	5.84***
IADL	245.13	156.46	257.40	159.87	227.53	149.71	9.65***
Rest and sleep	532.82	110.44	514.19	101.51	559.53	117.05	−17.67***
Work	87.83	27.42	111.90	184.29	53.32	118.62	14.59***
Education	3.36	20.29	3.39	20.59	3.32	19.85	1.16
Play	15.16	43.2	13.25	40.60	17.91	46.56	−4.77***
Leisure							
Total leisure time	292.83	166.76	277.64	167.28	314.60	163.61	−8.68***
Outdoor activities	47.67	67.39	50.53	70.22	43.57	62.90	
Indoor activities	239.29	145.57	220.69	140.88	265.96	148.02	
Internet use	2.26	15.35	2.99	17.58	1.21	11.32	
Others	3.60	19.84	3.42	17.22	3.86	23.09	
Social participation	55.41	65.04	52.28	62.71	59.89	67.99	−7.01***
N	9228		5436		3792		

Note: $^{***}p < 0.001$.

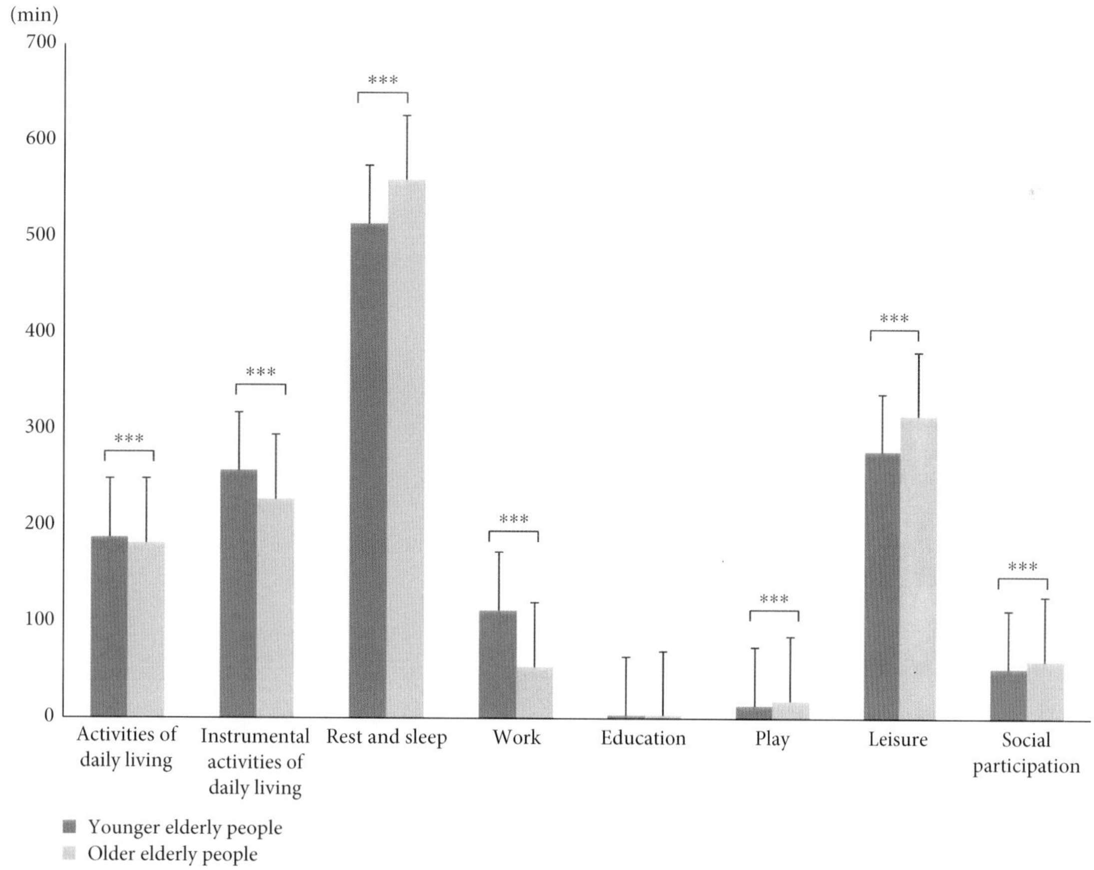

FIGURE 1: Differences of occupation domain time use between younger and older elderly groups ($^{***}p < 0.001$).

Table 3: The influences of leisure time on life satisfaction.

Model	Nonstandardization coefficient B	Nonstandardization coefficient Standard deviation	Standardization coefficient Beta	t	Probability of significance	VIF
(Constant)	3.393	.137		24.750	.000	
Leisure time	.000	.000	.027	2.320	.020	1.32
Age	−.007	.002	−.051	−4.578	.000	1.25
Gender	−.148	.023	−.080	−6.382	.000	1.58
Educational attainment	−.106	.008	−.166	−13.334	.000	1.56
Marital status	.074	.019	.044	3.934	.000	1.28
Reason for needing care	.177	.011	.165	16.123	.000	1.05
Economic activity status	−.002	.013	−.002	−.128	.898	1.69
Average monthly income	−.063	.006	−.126	−10.669	.000	1.40
Living in agricultural residence	.108	.031	.046	3.547	.000	1.69
Rural/urban residences	−.006	.004	−.017	−1.648	.099	1.03
Study conducted on weekdays	.068	.024	.034	2.865	.004	1.42
Elderly household code	.005	.004	.012	1.185	.236	1.00

$F = 69.808$ ($p = 0.000$).

Table 4: Level of life satisfaction in relation to the amount of leisure activity time and type of leisure activity.

	Very dissatisfied		Somewhat dissatisfied		Neutral		Somewhat satisfied		Very satisfied	
	M	SD	M	SD	M	SD	M	SD	M	SD
Total leisure time	291.28	169.16	284.74	163.91	289.89	164.02	299.42	169.62	325.24	183.29
Outdoor activities	222.65	140.25	224.38	140.59	237.90	141.87	250.47	150.64	280.36	168.86
Indoor activities	56.60	70.72	52.74	71.49	46.66	66.67	44.93	62.78	40.02	68.55
Internet use	4.91	23.64	2.71	15.60	2.48	16.60	1.00	9.60	0.56	6.10
Others	7.12	38.05	4.90	22.85	2.85	15.02	3.04	20.51	4.29	19.14

other leisure activities. It was shown that males and those with higher education, nonworking status, no residency in agricultural and rural areas, and urban (communal) residence recorded longer time usage in outdoor activities, indoor activities, internet use, and other leisure activities. In Noh's study, the female elderly in South Korea had the lowest perception of any demographic among the population regarding the use of leisure time, and their values and attitudes on leisure activities were negative [28]. Therefore, it is necessary to provide proper leisure education programs for the female elderly. On the other hand, Lee et al.'s study revealed that the female elderly spent more time than the male elderly in social leisure, voluntary works, and social activities [1]. The study noted that this was largely due to the fact that the female elderly spend comparatively more time participating in religious activities than the male elderly. Since religious activities are categorized as to IADL rather than leisure, the balance of the research outcome was affected by this categorization.

As a result of reviewing differences in time usage by occupation domains between the younger elderly and older elderly populations in South Korea, the seven domains other than education—ADL, IADL, rest and sleep, work, play, leisure, and social participation—showed significant differences. In addition, the younger elderly group showed higher time usage in ADL, IADL, and work, while the older elderly group showed higher time usage in rest and sleep, play, leisure, and social participation. Therefore, this study found out that methodologies for intervention in time management for older adults should differ according to age.

Among the eight occupation domains, leisure was the highest in both the younger and older elderly groups, and indoor activities were the highest among leisure activities. For these results, according to KOSTAT data as of 2008, the average retirement age in South Korea was 53, and life after retirement transitioned from a focus on work to one on leisure [29]. Regarding time used for rest and sleep by older adults, there was no change, with older adults using more time in rest and sleep than children and younger adults [15].

The South Korean elderly engage primarily in passive and static leisure activities, and this is borne out by the KOSTAT data [30]. The highest leisure activity for older adults was watching TV, followed by religion, cultural activities, and sports activities in that order. This result was also consistent with the previous studies [27, 31]. If older adults' leisure activities consist primarily of static ones such as watching TV, they are not activities with high meaning

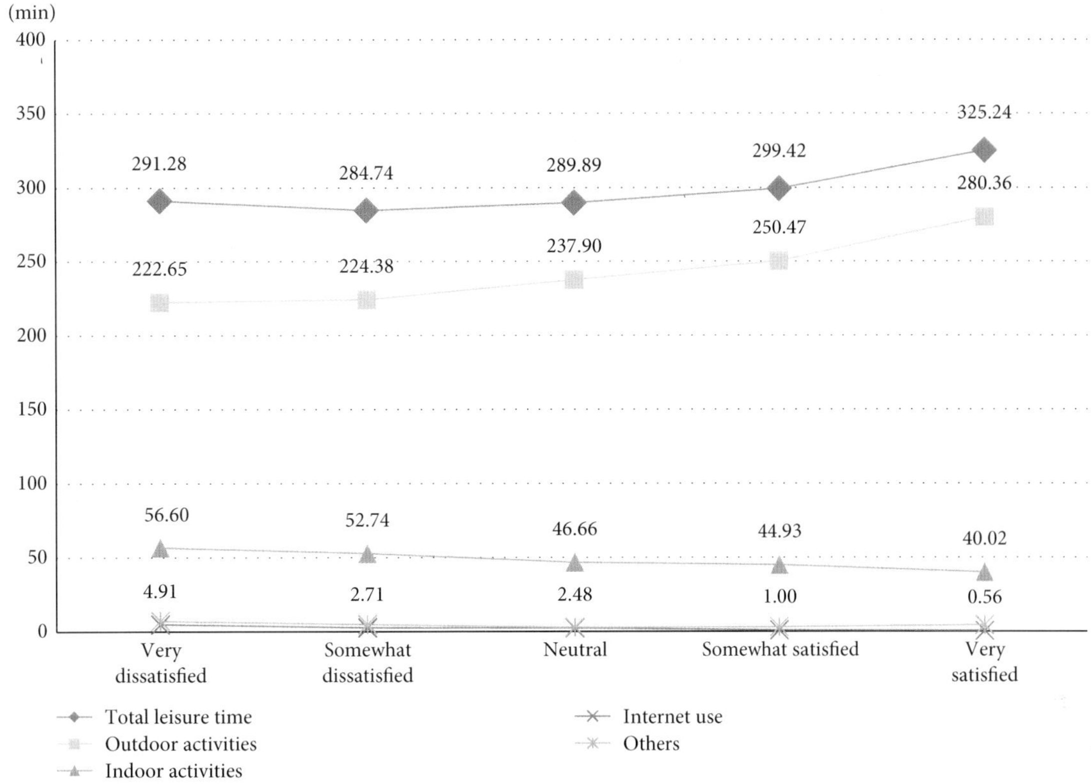

FIGURE 2: Life satisfaction in relation to length of leisure activity time and types of leisure activities.

value. In order to improve older adults' QoL, it is necessary to develop various leisure programs that require dynamic physical activities, because this can relieve older adults of anxiety, help them regain their self-esteem, and help them maintain interpersonal relationships with those who participate together [32]. It is also necessary to implement alternative policies at national level in order to promote the participation of older adults' in leisure activities. Older adults in the western world including the USA, Canada, and the UK showed cultural differences from older adults in South Korea as they spend extensive time engaged in various sports activities such as golf, jogging, and swimming for their leisure [33, 34].

For the South Korean elderly, the longer their leisure time, the higher their life satisfaction. In addition, except for economic activity status, all control variables exert significant influence on life satisfaction. Study subjects showed higher life satisfaction if they had spouses, regular full-time jobs, higher education, and better health. They had significantly longer time usage for outdoor activities, indoor activities, internet use, and other leisure activities if they were male, or had higher education, nonworking status, and urban (communal) housing not in agricultural and rural areas. These results are consistent with previous studies and with ordinary expectations related to life satisfaction for older adults [35, 36].

This study did not show a significant influence on life satisfaction due to the status of economic activities, a finding which supports the previous studies that indicated cultural factors such as educational attainment or individual environment including area of residences could affect leisure activities more than economic factors including income and occupation. The reason for this is that education contributes to the ability to maintain a higher level of stimuli, cultures, or insights required for utilizing leisure time effectively [37]. In the capitalist social system, individual economic capability is required to maintain one's life, but it is appropriate to view it as an instrument rather than a requirement.

For the limitations of this study, first, differences in living time usage depending on individual characteristics or socioeconomic position were not considered since the statistical analysis was made by classifying the groups according to age. Second, the occupation domains cited by OTPF-3 were created in the US context; therefore, they may contain cultural differences from the actual domains of living time usage by the South Korean elderly. In future studies, it is necessary to compare the time usage of older adults who have health issues with that of healthy older adults in order to prepare a foundation for intervening with regard to time usage and also to further investigate the current status of space and facilities available for leisure activities.

It is expected that this study, which has analyzed KOSTAT's 2014TUS, will provide basic data for the academic community and staff persons charged with the care of the elderly to help improve older adults' life satisfaction and QoL by helping them to make optimal meaningful use of their time, as physical, social, psychological, and mental problems are bound to occur with increasing frequency due to the longer average life expectancy.

5. Conclusions and Implications for Occupational Therapy Practice

Although time is a resource identically distributed to everyone, depending on how it is utilized by a person, their individual performances and QoL can vary. In this study, we investigated the status of time usage of the healthy South Korean elderly through classification by eight occupation domains suggested by OTPF-3, along with the correlations between the status of leisure activity time use and life satisfaction, in order to identify characteristics of leisure activities and factors affecting them. As a result, it was shown that the South Korean elderly showed higher life satisfaction as the amount of time they spend in leisure activities is increased. In addition, while longer time for outdoor activities of leisure brought a higher life satisfaction, the opposite was true in the case of indoor activities. Differences were found in the distribution of time over occupation domains between the younger group and the older group of the South Korean elderly. This study has a significance in having analyzed a national time use data based on the 2014TUS by KOSTAT from an occupational perspective and suggests evidence for developing various leisure programs incorporating dynamic physical activities in order to improve older adults' QoL. Older adults should have the opportunity to increase their health and emotional support through various physical leisure activities such as hobbies, sports activities, and social gatherings, which means that programs requiring more dynamic physical activities should be developed. OTs are experts who can organize high-quality programs reflecting the physical abilities and needs of older adults and can help those in need of assistance to achieve a balanced life and participate as fully as possible in everyday tasks. OTs should develop leisure education programs for individuals that take into account the physical abilities of older adults, finding an optimal active attitude for older adults so that they can enjoy high-quality leisure life. This study will provide OTs with data they can use to assist older adults who have difficulty in time usage through time management intervention in order to improve their life satisfaction and QoL.

Additional Points

Concise Description. For this study, subactivities found in the raw data of "2014 Time Use Survey" were categorized into a total of eight occupation domains (activities of daily living, instrumental activities of daily living, rest and sleep, work, education, play, leisure, and social participation). This was based on eight "occupation domains" suggested by OTPF-3.

Acknowledgments

This paper was supported by Semyung University Research Grant of 2017. The data used to support the findings of this study was provided by Statistics Korea (KOSTAT) under license.

References

[1] J. H. Lee, S. H. Park, E. Y. Yoo, M. Y. Jung, and D. Y. Cho, "Characteristics of time use and types of activities of daily living in non-disabled urban elderly," *The Journal of Korean Society of Occupational Therapy*, vol. 20, no. 2, pp. 85–98, 2012.

[2] J. D. Kwon and J. Y. Cho, "A study of factors influencing the life satisfaction of the aged," *Korean Journal of Research in Gerontology*, vol. 20, no. 3, pp. 61–76, 2000.

[3] B. J. Lee and S. W. Hong, "The effect of older people's leisure activities on their self-esteem and life satisfaction," *Journal of Tourism Institute of Northeast Asia*, vol. 8, no. 2, pp. 139–156, 2012.

[4] H. J. Lee and Y. A. Yeong, "A correlation between leisure activities and life satisfactions of the old adults," *Journal of Occupational Therapy for the Aged and Dementia*, vol. 6, no. 2, pp. 47–53, 2012.

[5] S. L. Dupuis and M. Alzheimer, "Leisure and ageing well," *World Leisure Journal*, vol. 50, no. 2, pp. 91–107, 2008.

[6] L. M. Chiang, K. Casebolt, J. Tan, S. V. Lankford, and J. Wilson, "A pilot study of an instrument measuring leisure satisfaction and life satisfaction in an outpatient leisure activity program," *Therapeutic Recreation Journal*, vol. 45, no. 3, pp. 234–255, 2011.

[7] P. M. Simone and A. L. Haas, "Frailty, leisure activity and functional status in older adults: relationship with subjective well being," *Clinical Gerontologist*, vol. 36, no. 4, pp. 275–293, 2013.

[8] J. R. Kelly, *Leisure (3rd)*, Allyn and Becon, Boston, MA, USA, 1996.

[9] K. B. Adams, S. Leibbrandt, and H. Moon, "A critical review of the literature on social and leisure activity and wellbeing in later life," *Ageing and Society*, vol. 31, no. 4, pp. 683–712, 2011.

[10] Y.-S. Yi and K.-R. Park, "A study of leisure constraints, leisure activities participation and life satisfaction of the elderly," *Korean Journal of Human Ecology*, vol. 18, no. 1, pp. 1–12, 2009.

[11] American Journal of Occupational Therapy, "Uniform terminology for occupational therapy," *American Journal of Occupational Therapy*, vol. 48, pp. 1047–1054, 1994.

[12] J. W. Kim, "A study on the time of the elderly in Korea: analysing their use of time upon work, family and leisure," *Journal of Welfare for the Aged*, vol. 32, pp. 149–177, 2006.

[13] J. P. Robinson and G. A. Godbey, *Time for Life: The Surprising Ways Americans Use their Time*, University Park, Pennsylvania State University Press, 1997.

[14] C. L. Backman, "Occupational balance: exploring the relationships among daily occupations and their influence on well-being," *Canadian Journal of Occupational Therapy*, vol. 71, no. 4, pp. 202–209, 2004.

[15] S. P. Hong and J. Y. Lee, "Time use of areas of occupation according to the periods of life in Koreans," *Journal of Korean Society of Occupational Therapy*, vol. 18, no. 1, pp. 95–106, 2010.

[16] M. J. Youngstrom, S. J. Brayman, P. Anthony et al., "Occupational therapy practice framework: domain and process," *American Journal of Occupational Therapy*, vol. 56, pp. 609–639, 2002.

[17] Y. G. Kim, "The analysis study of life- style for efficient occupational performance," *The Journal of Korean Society of Occupational Therapy*, vol. 13, no. 2, pp. 51–61, 2005.

[18] E. A. McKay and E. Hunt, "A scoping review of time-use research in occupational therapy and occupational science," *Scandinavian Journal of Occupational Therapy*, vol. 22, no. 1, pp. 1–12, 2015.

[19] American Journal of Occupational Therapy, "Occupational therapy practice framework: domain & process 2nd edition," *American Journal of Occupational Therapy*, vol. 62, no. 6, pp. 625–683, 2008.

[20] American Journal of Occupational Therapy, "Occupational therapy practice framework: domain and process (3rd edition)," *American Journal of Occupational Therapy*, vol. 68, Supplement 1, pp. S1–S48, 2014.

[21] S. H. Hong, "The effects of leisure participation and leisure satisfaction on life satisfaction of elderly," *Journal of Korean Home Management Association*, vol. 16, no. 1, pp. 107–124, 1998.

[22] Statistics Korea, *Aged Person Statistics in 2013*, Statistics Korea, Sejong, 2013.

[23] Y. K. Lee, "The effect of father's socio-economic characteristics on time use of the undergraduate student children," *Social Sciences Research Institute*, vol. 31, no. 1, pp. 159–190, 2016.

[24] B. L. Neugarten, J. W. Moore, and J. C. Lowe, "Age constraints and adult socialization," *American Journal of Sociology*, vol. 70, no. 6, pp. 710–717, 1995.

[25] I. J. Lee, "A study on the differences between the younger old and the older old: comparison of the effects of stressful life events and social support on their health," *Journal of the Korean Gerontological Society*, vol. 19, no. 3, pp. 35–50, 1999.

[26] K.-C. Lim and S. Kim, "Prevalence and correlates of depression in older Koreans: comparison of young-old and old-old," *Journal of Korean Academy of Psychiatric and Mental Health Nursing*, vol. 21, no. 1, p. 1, 2012.

[27] Y.-J. Kim, Dept. of Occupational therapy, Seoul National University Hospital, S.-P. Hong, and H. Y. Park, "Analysing Korean occupational time changing trend based on ages using 2004, 2009, 2014 time use survey," *The Journal of Korean Society of Occupational Therapy*, vol. 25, no. 3, pp. 13–25, 2017.

[28] Y. K. Noh, "The effects of a leisure education on leisure attitude and leisure satisfaction for Korean older adults," *Journal of Sport and Leisure Studies*, vol. 13, pp. 351–361, 2000.

[29] Korea National Statistical Office, *Korean Demographic Profile*, Korea National Statistical Office, Sejong, 2008.

[30] Korea National Statistical Office, *Korean Demographic Profile*, Korea National Statistical Office, Sejong, 2014.

[31] R. Chilvers, S. Corr, and H. Singlehurst, "Investigation into the occupational lives of healthy older people through their use of time," *Australian Occupational Therapy Journal*, vol. 57, no. 1, pp. 24–33, 2010.

[32] I. J. Kwak, "Study on use style and satisfaction for welfare facilities and physical activity program in elderly people," KonKuk University, Seoul, 2007.

[33] J.-W. Kang, Dept. of Occupational Therapy, Graduate School of Yonsei University, J.-H. Park, and H. Y. Park, "Analysis of time use in healthy elderly: a systematic review," *Journal of Korean Society of Occupational Therapy*, vol. 25, no. 2, pp. 87–102, 2017.

[34] S. S. Lee, "A study on the time usage of the retired elderly," *Korean Journal of Human Ecology*, vol. 20, no. 2, pp. 311–325, 2011.

[35] E. Diener and S. Oishi, "Money and happiness: income and subjective well-being across nations," The MIT Press, Cambridge, 2000.

[36] F. Jonathan, "The effect of leisure activity on depression in the elderly," *Occupational Therapy in Health Care*, vol. 13, no. 1, pp. 45–51, 2000.

[37] E. S. Joo, "Work, care or leisure?- the effects of gender and education on time allocation of full-time working parents," *Korean Journal of Social Welfare Studies*, vol. 45, no. 3, pp. 5–34, 2014.

3

Awareness and Knowledge about Occupational Therapy in Jordan

Wesam Barakat Darawsheh

Department of Occupational Therapy, School of Rehabilitation Sciences, The University of Jordan, Amman, Jordan

Correspondence should be addressed to Wesam Barakat Darawsheh; w.darawsheh@gmail.com

Academic Editor: Jodie A. Copley

Knowledge and awareness about occupational therapy (OT) are essential for the delivery of quality care to all clients and for occupational therapists' (OTRs) job satisfaction. OT has been a poorly understood profession in Jordan. The current study reports on the assessment of Jordanians' awareness and knowledge of occupational therapy. Convenience sampling was used. There were 829 participants (474 males, 355 females), with mean age of 32 ± 11.6 yrs. They were recruited from the three main geographical areas of Jordan (northern, central, and southern) and from all educational levels. The sample included 222 (26.8%) healthcare personnel, 146 (17.6%) clients, and 461 (55.6%) lay persons. Participants completed questionnaires, and the results revealed that 48% of the sample had poor or no knowledge about OT, while 28.3% were unaware of it. Also, OT was commonly (50%) perceived to be exclusively targeting people with disabilities (PWDs) and neurological and physical conditions (58% and 53%, resp.) in addition to exclusively providing services for the rehabilitation of the upper extremity (48%). Common misconceptions associated with OT were that OTRs prescribe medication (43%) and OTRs are physiotherapists (44%). These preliminary findings suggest that efforts need to be directed by OTRs, the Jordanian Society of Occupational Therapy (JSOT), and the Ministry of Health to preserve the OT identity and value and promote knowledge about OT in the public and among members of interdisciplinary teams. More interprofessional learning needs to be incorporated within the curricula and placements of all healthcare personnels.

1. Introduction

Occupational therapy (OT) is one of the components of a multidisciplinary team approach that focuses on enabling participation in meaningful occupations as an essential element of healthcare [1–3]. Generally, the conceptualization of OT has been vague among the public [4] and even among healthcare professionals [5]. This becomes more evident in some countries with low and lower middle-income economies, such as Jordan and Nigeria [6, 7], and in some clinical settings such as mental health and school-based settings [4, 8].

Knowledge about OT among healthcare professionals is essential to guarantee the delivery of comprehensive, holistic, and quality care services [3, 6]. Healthcare professionals need to understand other team members' roles so that appropriate referrals can be made and to prevent role confusion [9]. Clients can sometimes be deprived of OT services because healthcare professionals lack knowledge about the services provided by registered occupational therapists (OTRs) [6, 9]. In addition, other healthcare professionals' knowledge about OT affects the status of the profession and the level of job satisfaction among OTRs [10].

Carrier et al. [11] and Kristensen et al. [12] found that decision making about suitable methods for implementing evidence-based practices is affected by the cultural knowledge of the therapists and the way culture influences healthcare practices. Shafaroodi et al. [13] found that public knowledge about OT affects the process of clinical reasoning among OTRs. They found that managers have erroneous expectations concerning the role of OTRs which, in return, affects the process of treatment planning and decreases the quality of outcomes of OT intervention [13]. The lack of knowledge of healthcare professionals about OT reduces the opportunities of engaging in mutual planning and reasoning with OTRs which reflects negatively on the quality of care [13]. The level of knowledge of clients about OT affects their expectations and acceptance of OT services [13]. OTRs often find themselves iteratively altering their treatment plans to enable clients to overcome issues related to denial, over or under expectations, or lack of acceptance of OT services. Thus, OTRs have to face issues related to confidence where they continuously question their abilities and skills to meet the clients' demands [13].

Vincent et al. [14] explored the perceptions of four primary school teachers in South Australia concerning OT. OT was perceived to be useful and needed. However, teachers expressed a need to develop further channels of collaboration and interaction between educators and OTRs to maximize educational outcomes. Benson et al. [15] surveyed 47 public school teachers (37 special education and 10 regular education teachers) concerning OT in Pennsylvania. Teachers taught children from preschool age to 12th grade and had experience working with OTRs before. They expressed the valuable contribution of OT in the educational setting, but that it needed to be further supported by the educational system as more collaboration between educators and OTRs was required. In these studies, participants acknowledged the value of OT in multidisciplinary teams, but they could not identify or define the role of OTRs. Participants perceived OT as an extra pair of hands for care provision when there was an excessive caseload, and the value of OT was not based on a genuine understanding of the uniqueness of the role and services provided.

Smith and Mackenzie [16] investigated the knowledge of nurses about OT. Participants expressed that they had to work with OTRs by guessing their role due to a lack of information, interprofessional communication, and collaboration. Olaoye et al. [6] investigated the knowledge and awareness of OT in 581 Nigerian undergraduate healthcare students (medicine, dentistry, nursing, and rehabilitation). They found that even though 80% of the students were aware of OT, 62.3% of them had poor to moderate actual knowledge about the OT role. Factors such as specialization and level of education were found to influence the level of knowledge and awareness about OT. Such studies did not consider public knowledge or the knowledge of healthcare professionals from all healthcare backgrounds such as para healthcare professionals (e.g., social work and counseling professionals and medical laboratory professionals) and associate healthcare professionals (e.g., medical and pharmaceutical technicians and nursing and midwifery associate professionals). Research to date indicates that further information is required about public and healthcare professionals' knowledge about OT and factors that may influence knowledge and awareness about OT in each unique cultural context.

OT in the Middle East was first introduced in Jordan in 1986 [17] and is therefore a relatively young profession especially when compared to other healthcare professions [17, 18]. Only two studies have been conducted to explore the knowledge about OT in Jordan. Abu Tariah et al. [18] investigated the knowledge of 556 healthcare professionals, who were nurses, physicians, and physiotherapists, about OT. AlHeresh and Nikopoulos [17] investigated the knowledge of 153 participants (physicians, nurses, and rehabilitation specialists) about OT. In both studies, the same hospitals located in the capital city of Amman were targeted. They were general hospitals offering OT services for clients from all age ranges and for physical and neurological conditions. Although the results of both studies reflected a limited knowledge about OT in Jordan, they could not be generalized to all geographical areas in Jordan, to the general public, or even to all categories of healthcare professions. It has been over five years since these investigations were conducted, and there is a need for current studies to determine any changes in the level of knowledge about OT. Therefore, the aim of the current investigation was to explore the level of knowledge and awareness about OT in the general public and among clients who had/were receiving OT services in all areas of Jordan. Another purpose was to investigate the level of awareness and knowledge of healthcare professionals from the various healthcare fields that make up the rehabilitation team.

2. Methods

2.1. Participants. Participants were adults (age $\geq$ 18 yrs) from the three areas of Jordan (northern, central, and southern). Participants from all educational levels and occupations according to the International Standard Classification of Occupations (ISOC) [19] were included in the study. Healthcare professionals and workers in the healthcare field were included. OTRs/OT assistants were excluded to meet the aims of this study, which was to investigate the knowledge and perception of members of the community, who did not study the field of OT, about this profession, whether they were lay people, clients, or from other healthcare professions. Clients who received occupational therapy services were included. Lay people who had never received OT services and who were not healthcare professionals nor working in the healthcare field were also included.

2.2. Procedures and Recruitment. Ethical approval was granted by the Board of the Occupational Therapy Department and the Board of the Rehabilitation Sciences Faculty at the University of Jordan. Participants were approached in all of the three areas in Jordan in public and private institutions and settings. The lay people were approached in crowded areas such as stores, offices, schools, malls, and universities. The principal researcher used her personal and professional networks in clinics, healthcare centers, and hospitals to connect with healthcare professionals, most of whom assisted in approaching clients and inviting them to participate in the study. All participants were invited to complete a questionnaire after the aims of the study had been explained and participants had been encouraged to ask questions.

2.3. Assessment Tool/Instrumentation. The questionnaire was specifically developed for this study based on prior questionnaires that had been previously constructed in similar and pertinent studies conducted in Jordan, such as Abu Tariah et al. [18] and AlHeresh and Nikopolous [17], and in other countries, such as Benson et al. [15] and Olaoye et al. [6]. A draft of the questionnaire was reviewed by a group of nine occupational therapists working in the field. Their comments, suggestions, and feedback were taken into account to finalize the questionnaire.

The survey comprised seven sections: (1) background information (age, gender, occupation educational level, and area of living), (2) sources of knowledge of OT, (3) awareness and general evaluation of self and public knowledge/awareness about OT, (4) general knowledge about the aims and services of OT, (5) knowledge about OT domains and places of service provision, (6) misconceptions about OT, and (7) means to promote knowledge and awareness about OT. Questions in sections 1, 2, 3, 7, and 8 included options from which participants could make a selection, and an option of "other" was listed in case none of the listed options met their answer. Sections 4, 5, and 6 were the main sections of the survey. They comprised 40 questions/statements against which the knowledge of OT was scored out of 80. Statements in sections 4 and 5 included actual facts about OT while statements in section 6 included statements that examined the common misconceptions about OT. Answers in sections 4, 5, and 6 were closed ended where participants were required to choose one answer from three options (Yes, I do not know, No) against each statement. Each answer was scored from 0 to 2 where Yes = 2, Do not know = 1, and No = 0, except for the misconception section (section 6) where answers were scored as Yes = 0, Do not know = 1, and No = 2. This method of scoring was followed so that the better the knowledge about OT, the higher the total score.

2.4. Data Analysis. Statistical analysis was performed using SPSS Version 22.0 (2016, IBM Corporation, New York). Descriptive statistical analysis was employed to report on the frequency of categorical variables. The comparisons of the scores in sections 4–6 between groups classified by age, gender, educational level, area (northern, central, and southern), and status (lay, client, or healthcare personnel (HP)) were performed by the multivariate analysis of variance MANOVA. The Tukey post hoc test was utilized to identify the subgroup comparisons that caused significant differences.

Educational level was subcategorized into five subcategories: primary and elementary school levels (Sch), high school (HS), associate degrees (Asso), bachelor degrees (Bch), and master and doctoral degrees (MA+). This classification follows the common classification of academic degrees [20]. Participant age ranges were subcategorized into five subcategories as per the most common standardized method of classification used in surveys: 18–24 yrs (A), 25–34 yrs (B), 35–44 yrs (C), 45–54 yrs (D), and 55+ yrs (E) [21, 22].

The reliability assessment of the developed survey in this study was implemented by calculating the value of the internal consistency reliability coefficient (Cronbach's alpha reliability coefficient). A conventional benchmark value of Cronbach's α value of ≥0.7 is commonly used to indicate that relatively most of the items measure the same construct [23]. In addition, the receiver operating characteristic (ROC) curve analysis of the SPSS software was used to identify and compare the sensitivity and specificity of the questions of the survey [24, 25]. The value of the area under the ROC curve (AUC), calculated through the ROC analysis, is an effective measure that reflects the accuracy of the test where the greater the value, the more reliable the test [26, 27]. The interpretation of the following values of AUC was used in this study: 1.00–0.9 = excellent test of a perfect sensitivity and specificity; 0.89–0.8 = accurate; 0.79–0.7 = not that accurate; 0.69–0.6 = rare to use; and 0.59 or below = worthless test that does not predict outcomes very well [24–28]. Furthermore, the ROC analysis was conducted to determine the total cut-off score where the state of having knowledge about OT can be identified and the range of scores where the level of knowledge can be described as average, poor (below average), and excellent (above average) [28].

3. Results

The total number of participants was 829 with a mean age of 32 ± 11.6 yrs (age range 18–80 yrs). The mean total score of participants in the survey was 53.1 ± 10.4, and the total scores of the sample ranged 19–78 out of 80. Numbers, percentages, and mean total scores of participants as arranged by subgroups are displayed in Table 1. The sample included 222 (26.8%) personnel who have background knowledge in healthcare (i.e., physicians, nurses, pharmacists and pharmacologists, rehabilitation specialists, dentists, and paraprofessionals). There were 146 (17.6%) clients who had received or were receiving OT services at the time of conducting the study. Lay people from all other disciplines, and who had never received OT services, constituted 55.6% ($n = 461$) of the sample. Through the subsequent sections, the 40 statements/questions of the main sections 4, 5, and 6 of the questionnaire will be presented along with a focus on presenting the highest percentage of three responses (Yes, No, and I do not know) against each statement/question.

3.1. Reliability and Accuracy of the Survey Questions and Cut-Off Score. The results showed that all of the main subscales of the survey were characterized by high values of Cronbach's alpha, which confirmed the reliability of the survey in all of its three main subscales. *Cronbach's* α values were 0.845, 0.831, and 0.765 for sections 4, 5, and 6, respectively.

The AUC of the questions of the survey was AUC = 0.8 which meant that the survey presented an accurate tool in measuring the level of knowledge and awareness about OT. The calculated cut-off score using the ROC analysis was 49.5. Thus, all participants who scored <50 ($n = 313$) were considered not to know or to be aware about OT. The levels of knowledge were determined using the calculated cut-off score of 50 and the overall sample mean and SD scores of 53.1 ± 10.4. The 95% confidence interval was correspondent with the scores ranging 32–74. Accordingly, the categorization of the levels of knowledge was as follows: no knowledge (≤49), poor knowledge (50–52), average knowledge (53–64), above average (65–74), and distinctive knowledge (75–80). As shown in Figure 1, 48% of the sample had poor or no knowledge about OT.

3.2. Awareness and Sources of Knowledge about OT. Forty-five and a half percent (45.5%) of participants reported not to have any prior knowledge about OT, and 28.3% of participants stated that this was their first time hearing about OT. Sources of knowledge about OT as reported by participants were as follows: working in healthcare, receiving OT services,

Table 1: Mean scores and SD of subgroups and p values.

	Significance (p value)	Number & (percentage)	Code	Age μ and SD	Score μ and SD
Gender	**0.16**				
Males		474 (57.2%)	M	33.2 ± 12.3	52.3 ± 10.4
Females		355 (42.8%)	F	30.4 ± 10.4	54.2 ± 10.4
Age groups	**0.004***				
18–24		284 (34.4%)	A	21.6 ± 2	51.5 ± 9.9
25–34		266 (32.1%)	B	28.9 ± 3.1	54.4 ± 10.6
35–44		145 (17.5%)	C	38.7 ± 2.9	53.1 ± 10.4
45–54		94 (11.3%)	D	49.4 ± 3.5	51.9 ± 10.2
55+		40 (4.8%)	E	61.9 ± 6.1	58.1 ± 11.9
Educational level	**0.021***				
School (primary & elementary)		56 (6.8%)	Sch	36.6 ± 15.5	50.1 ± 10.2
High school		160 (19.3%)	HS	33.9 ± 13.2	49.6 ± 9.9
Associate degrees		119 (14.4%)	Asso	37.9 ± 11.6	52.4 ± 10.4
Bachelor degrees		459 (55.4%)	Bch	28.8 ± 9.3	54.6 ± 10.2
Master and doctoral degrees		35 (4.2%)	MA+	37.7 ± 9.3	56 ± 11.3
Status	**0.007***				
Clients		146 (17.6%)	Client	37.3 ± 13.9	55.5 ± 8.2
Lay people		461 (55.6%)	Lay	31.5 ± 11.4	49.8 ± 9.9
Healthcare background		222 (26.8%)	HP	29.7 ± 9	58.4 ± 10.3
Physicians		*43 (19.4%)*			
Nurses		*46 (20.7%)*			
Rehabilitation specialists		*38 (17.1%)*			
Dentists		*17 (7.7%)*			
Pharmacists & pharmacologists		*23 (10.4%)*			
Paraprofessionals		*55 (24.8%)*			
Area	**0.544**				
Northern		221 (26.7%)	North	31.9 ± 10.9	52 ± 10
Central		436 (52.6%)	Cen	32.5 ± 11.6	54.5 ± 10.6
Southern		93 (11.2%)	South	32.3 ± 13.8	51.1 ± 10.8
Unspecified		79 (9.5%)	Unsp	29.4 ± 10.5	51 ± 10

Note. n = number; μ = mean; SD = standard deviation. Age groups in years. *Significant on the 0.05 level.

a relative or a friend working or studying in healthcare, social media and the internet, TV or radio, and books (Figure 2).

3.3. Knowledge about Aims and Services Provided in OT. Most participants (63%–68%) knew that OT aims at maximizing the level of participation in meaningful occupations by maintaining and/or developing performance skills that assist clients to adapt to the new health condition and that it is a comprehensive profession that targets social, psychosocial, motor, and mental aspects of health. Participants defined OT as one of the rehabilitation professions that employs a client-centered approach to treatment and that targets all age groups.

The majority of participants (53%) indicated that OTRs work at a preventative level of care and that assessment, measurement, and alteration of wheelchairs and other mobility aids were part of the services provided in OT. The prescription of equipment for the facilitation of performance of daily life activities was perceived to be one of the services provided in OT by 48% of participants while 45% perceived that the organization and running of group therapy sessions were part of OT services.

Most of the participants did not know whether the fabrication of splints was an OT service (48%). The same was true of environmental adaptations, where 50% of participants' answers fell under the category "I do not know."

3.4. Knowledge concerning Fields of OT and Places of Service Provision. Over half (55%) of the sample did not have any knowledge concerning places that provided OT services. Most participants (77%) believed that OT services were mainly provided in hospitals, then community-based rehabilitation (CBR) centers (67%), followed by centers for special education (60%), nursing homes (55%), and mental health institutions (48%). However, only 32% of the participants reported that OT services could be provided in schools.

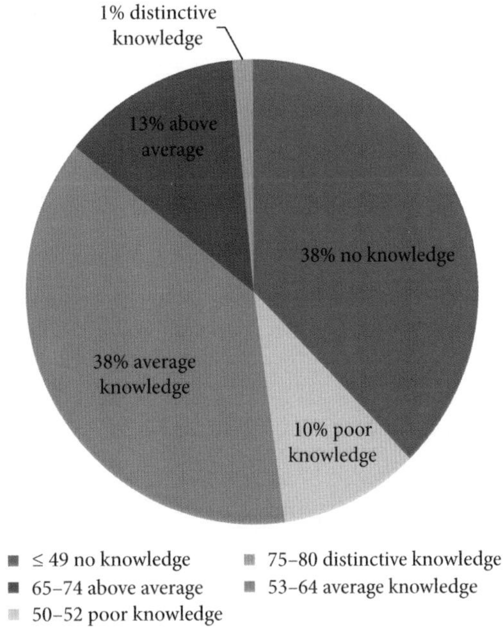

Figure 1: Level of knowledge and awareness of OT.

Most participants reported that OT was a profession that was concerned with pediatric conditions, then teenagers, and lastly older people with percentages of 73%, 70%, and 69%, respectively.

Over half (58% and 53%) of the participants believed that OT was mainly concerned with the treatment of neurological and physical conditions, respectively. However, the majority of participants' answers (44%) were "No" concerning the statement: OT is concerned with the provision of services for mental and psychological health conditions.

3.5. Common Misconceptions about OT. The common misconceptions about OT were that OTRs are solely concerned with people with disabilities (50%), OT is merely focused on the treatment of the conditions of the upper extremity (48%), OTRs are physiotherapists (44%), the prescription of medications is one of the services provided by OTRs (43%), OT is a profession that is concerned with the provision of recruitment and staffing services (38%), an OTR is certified from the school of educational studies (34%), OT is one of the professions related to humanities and social sciences (34%), an OTR is the same as an orthotics and prosthetics specialist (32%), and a physiotherapist can perform/substitute for the role of an OTR (27%) (Figure 3).

Most responses were positive in identifying the following statements as misconceptions about OT which were that OT is a medical profession (78%), an OTR is mainly a masseuse who provides professional massage treatment (47%), and an OTR diagnoses the client's condition prior to provision of services (44%) (Figure 3).

3.6. Significance of the Effect of Gender, Age, Educational Level, Area, and Status on the Total Score. The results of the MANOVA revealed significant differences in scores attributed to the effect of independent variables of age, educational level, and status. However, there were no significant differences between subgroup scores as arranged by gender and area (Table 1).

Looking closely at the cross tabulation between the age subgroups and the status subgroups, the majority of participants ($n = 178$, 63%) of the A age subgroup were from the lay subgroup. A similar pattern was revealed for the D age subgroup where the majority were from the lay subgroup ($n = 61$, 65%). The highest percentage of HP participants was concentrated in the B age subgroup ($n = 98$, 44%), and the B age subgroup also contained the largest percentage of clients ($n = 43$, 29%). Thus, the status (clients, lay, and HP) variables were the main factors in causing the significant difference between the mean scores of the age subgroups.

3.7. Effect of Background in Healthcare on the Total Score. The demographics of subgroups included in the HP group are displayed in Table 1. Less than a third of the HP group ($n = 70$, 31.5%) reported not to have any prior knowledge about OT, while 34 (15.3%) of them stated that it was the first time for them to hear about OT and thus were not aware of OT. The percentages of misconceptions about OT in the HP subgroup were reflective of the percentages of misconceptions about OT in the whole sample (Figure 3).

The MANOVA revealed a significant difference between the scores of subgroups of healthcare backgrounds ($p \leq 0.001$). The Tukey post hoc test revealed that there were significant differences between the score of the rehab subgroup and all other subgroups where the p values were $p \leq 0.001$. There was also a significant difference between the scores of the physicians and paraprofessionals subgroups ($p \leq 0.001$), where the mean score of the physicians' subgroup was higher Figure 4.

4. Discussion

This study has shown that the role of occupational therapists is still not well recognized in Jordan, which resonates with the results of previous studies [17, 18]. The following subsections will present further interpretations of the sources and implications of this main result in light of the literature.

4.1. Role of Professional Bodies in Preserving OT Identity and Prevent Role Confusion. This study found that there was confusion concerning the role of OTRs among the public and even among clients and other healthcare professionals, which resonated with the findings of Abu Tariah et al. [18] and Katz et al. [29]. In Jordan, some special education specialists pursue the role of OTRs and in some healthcare facilities, the role of an OTR is carried out by physiotherapists. Anecdotal evidence from practicing OTRs in Jordan suggests that OTRs may even face several situations where they have to compromise their professional identity to preserve their jobs. For example, in some institutions in Jordan, OTRs have been asked to pursue the role of physiotherapists, special education specialists, or teachers in addition to their duties as OTRs to reduce the amount of paid wages. Thus, the clinical reasoning skills of the OTRs could be directed at implementing practices far from the original philosophy of OT in order to meet the cultural expectations and conceptualization of

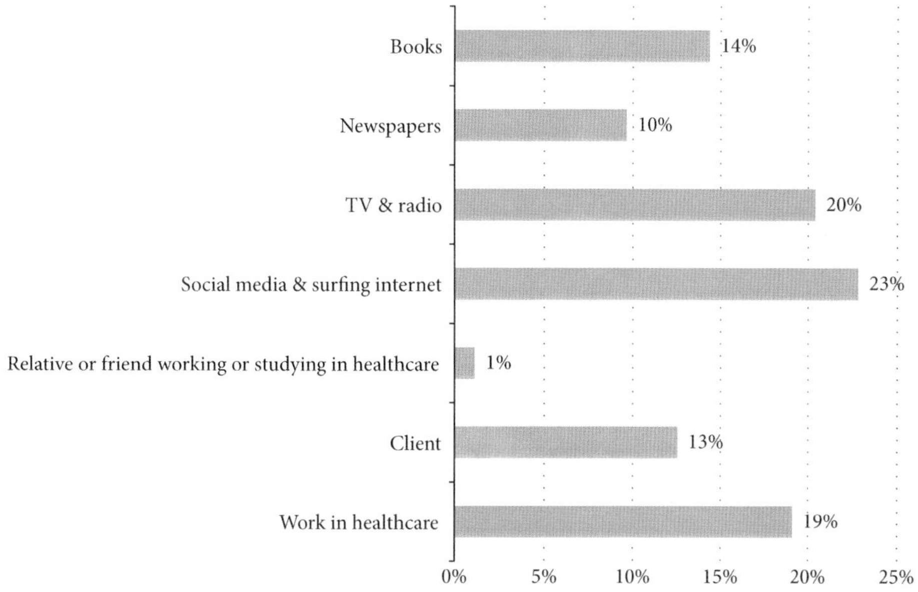

FIGURE 2: Sources of knowledge and awareness of OT.

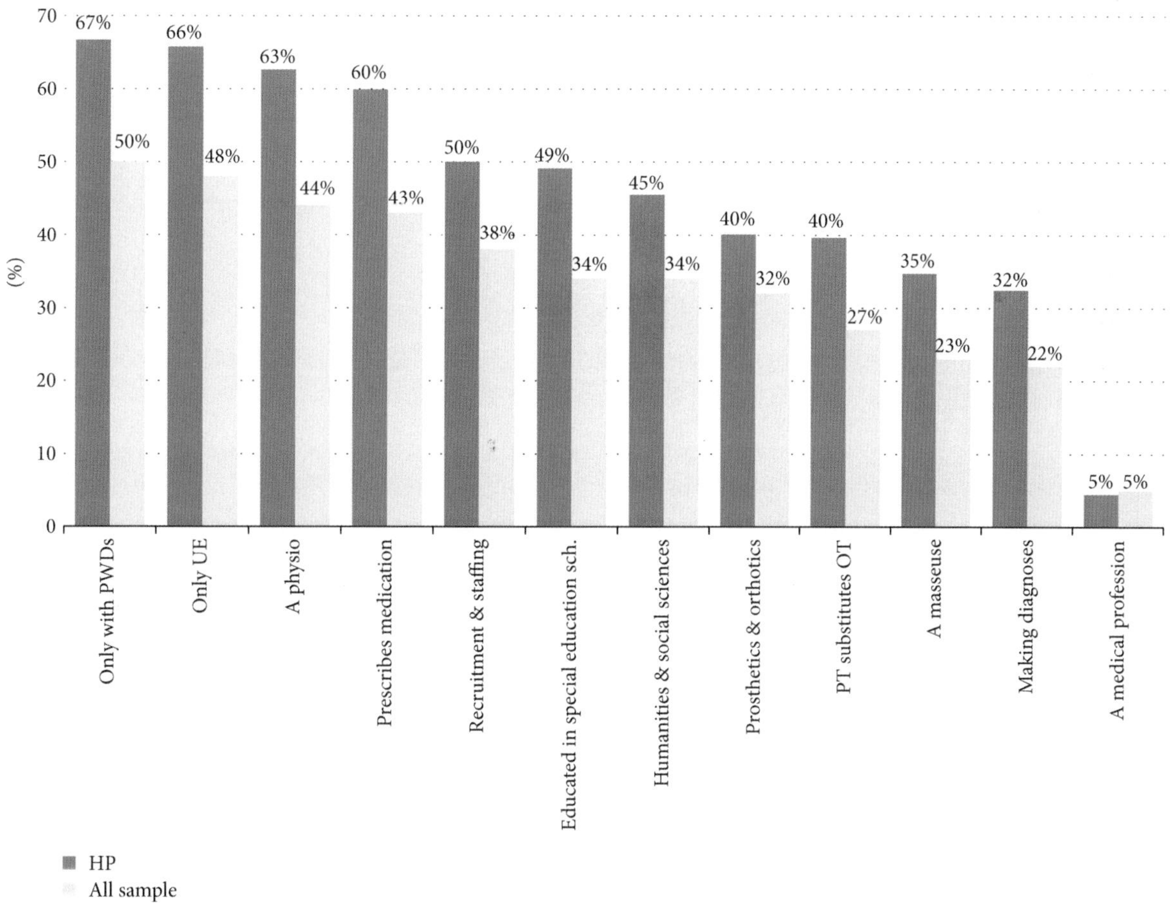

FIGURE 3: Misconceptions about OT in healthcare personnel subgroup (HP) and the whole sample.

OT [11–13]. Responses such as this could promote confusion about OT and moves OT practice away from its original underpinnings where a new distorted definition becomes a self-fulfilling prophecy [17, 30]. This, in return, promotes a lack of awareness and knowledge about OT and feeds a cycle that further devalues the OT role [31].

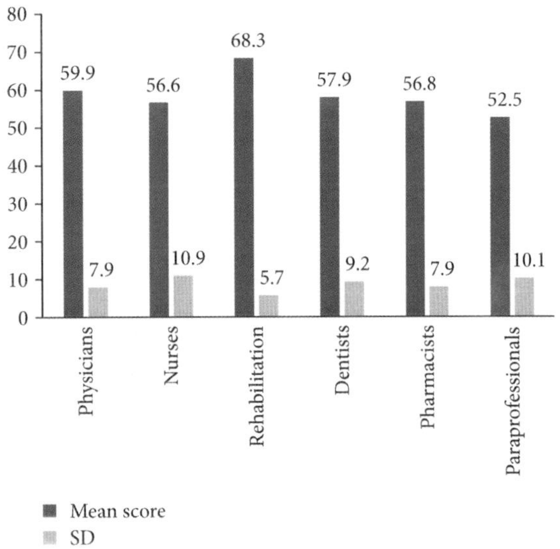

FIGURE 4: Mean scores and standard deviations of healthcare personnel subgroups.

The Ministry of Health (MOH) is the overarching body of issuing certification for all healthcare professionals in Jordan. Currently, the regulation number (84) for governing occupational therapy practice, issued by the MOH [32], does not clearly delineate the role of OTRs nor does support the autonomy of OT practice. The boundaries between practices of healthcare professions need to be delineated [18, 33]. The lack of an active role of OT representative bodies is one of the causes of the lack of public awareness and knowledge about OT [6]. There is a need for legislative standards to be established by professional bodies to define and preserve the OT scope of practice and the rights of OTRs [6, 33].

This study showed that participants' main source of knowledge about OT was the media (social media, TV, and radio) which was also the case in the studies conducted by Olaoye et al. [6] and Patel and Shriber [34] who also found prevailing misconceptions about OT. In Jordan, the Jordanian Society of Occupational Therapy (JSOT) is the relevant body that set plans and implement activities directed at promoting the awareness of the definition and concepts of the OT profession as defined by the World Federation of Occupational Therapists (WFOT). The JSOT may need to consider working on the culturalization of certain concepts. For example, occupational therapy is usually misconceived as aimed at providing jobs because of linguistics ambiguity/confusion associated with the word "occupation" in Arabic. Media panels, social media in particular, could be creatively and intensively used to market and promote an accurate image of OT [18].

4.2. Creating Channels of Communication and Collaboration. The knowledge of rehabilitation professionals about OT was the highest among all healthcare subgroups in the current investigation. This result resonated with the results of Abu Tariah et al. [18] who found physiotherapists to have a higher level of knowledge about OT than nurses and physicians. However, it was not expected in this study that the level of knowledge and awareness of other healthcare professional subgroups were similar to the knowledge level of clients. Abu Tariah et al. [18] and AlHeresh and Nikpoulos [17] described the level of knowledge of Jordanian healthcare professionals to be limited. It has been over five years since those studies have been conducted, and it was unexpected to find that the level of knowledge of Jordanian healthcare professionals has not developed much regarding OT. Such a result reflects a lack of communication channels between OTRs and other healthcare professionals [18]. This can restrict interdisciplinary work which would affect the quality and comprehensiveness of services provided for clients [4, 6, 18].

In this study, the value of OT was unacknowledged in school-based settings and this mirrors the results found by Vincent et al. [14] and Benson et al. [15]. Jackman and Stagnitti [4] found that students who needed OT intervention did not receive the required intervention due to the lack of school teachers' knowledge about OT. In contrast, Olaoye et al. [6] also found little knowledge among healthcare undergraduate students but in this study, participants perceived OT services to be exclusively provided in schools and rehabilitation homes. Another finding of this study was that there was a limited awareness of the role of OTRs in mental and psychiatric health settings, in particular. This result resonated with what was found by Fossey [8], who attributed this reduced awareness to the lack of shared education and dialogue opportunities among members of the multidisciplinary team. OTRs have a duty and an obligation to set goals and intervention plans in collaboration with other members of the healthcare team (including family members, clients, teachers, and other healthcare professionals) [2, 15]. This is part of the professional obligations of OT for the delivery of holistic, equal, and client-centered care [2, 3].

Clients in this study were found to have a significantly higher level of knowledge about OT compared to the public though their level of knowledge remained average. This result was unexpected as clients are in direct touch and communicate the most with OTRs who should work with clients using a client-centered approach [3]. Fiss et al. [35] found a discrepancy between the perceptions of the OTRs and those of the clients concerning the focus of treatment. According to Fiss et al. [35], this was attributed to a lack of communication between therapists and clients and an alienation from the approach of client-centeredness. Clients constitute one of the main means of promoting knowledge and awareness about OT, and they can be described as "OT ambassadors" ([33]: p. 17). In their study, Belik et al. [33] found that 70% of the participants knew about OT through receiving direct OT services or through a family member who did. Thus, clients need to be treated as an invaluable source to counteract the public lack of knowledge about OT.

4.3. Curricula Reevaluation and Interprofessional Education. The finding that rehabilitation specialists had better knowledge about OT can be explained by the fact that they study in the same school as OTRs and have shared lectures and courses together [18]. In training and even work settings, rehabilitation students and specialists work and train together in the overarching divisions of rehabilitation [18]. Thus, the curricula of other healthcare professions (e.g., medicine, nursing, counseling, and para-professions) need to include courses directed to familiarize students with rehabilitation specialties and interdisciplinary work [2, 5, 17, 18]. Patel and Shriber [34] suggest that direct contact with OTRs can be the best method for promoting knowledge about OT. Rotational clinical placements constitute another interprofessional mechanism of teaching [6]. In addition, promoting awareness about misconceptions about OT that were found in the current investigation, for example, will promote accurate knowledge about OT and its standards among other healthcare professionals [5, 8].

4.4. Directing Future Effort and Research to Promote Knowledge about OT. The results of this study suggest that it is the responsibility of OTRs and the JSOT to promote their profession, in order to counteract the lack of knowledge about OT in the public and among members of the multidisciplinary team. This study did not target OTRs' perception and knowledge of OT and how OTRs define OT in Jordan, which would be an essential topic to be targeted in future research.

References

[1] A. Atwal, K. Tattersall, K. Caldwell, and C. Craik, "Multidisciplinary perceptions of the role of nurses and healthcare assistants in rehabilitation of older adults in acute health care," *Journal of Clinical Nursing*, vol. 15, no. 11, pp. 1418–1425, 2006.

[2] M. Lidskog, A. Löfmark, and G. Ahlström, "Interprofessional education on a training ward for older people: students' conceptions of nurses, occupational therapists and social workers," *Journal of Interprofessional Care*, vol. 21, no. 4, pp. 387–399, 2009.

[3] College of Occupational Therapists (COT), *College of Occupational Therapists Code of Ethics and Professional Conduct*, College of Occupational therapists, London, 2015.

[4] M. Jackman and K. Stagnitti, "Fine motor difficulties: the need for advocating for the role of occupational therapy in schools," *Australian Occupational Therapy Journal*, vol. 54, no. 3, pp. 168–173, 2007.

[5] B. Jamnadas, J. Burns, and S. Paul, "Understanding occupational therapy: nursing and physician assistant students' knowledge about occupational therapy," *Occupational Therapy In Health Care*, vol. 14, no. 1, pp. 13–25, 2009.

[6] O. A. Olaoye, A. A. I. Emechete, A. T. Onigbinde, and C. E. Mbada, "Awareness and knowledge of occupational therapy among Nigerian medical and health sciences undergraduates," *Hong Kong Journal of Occupational Therapy*, vol. 27, pp. 1–6, 2016.

[7] The World Bank Group, "World Bank country and lending groups," November 2017https://datahelpdesk.worldbank.org/knowledgebase/articles/906519.

[8] E. Fossey, "Effective interdisciplinary teamwork: an occupational therapy perspective," *Australasian Psychiatry*, vol. 9, no. 3, pp. 232–234, 2001.

[9] C. Dunford, E. Street, H. O'Connell, J. Kelly, and J. R. Sibert, "Are referrals to occupational therapy for developmental coordination disorder appropriate?," *Archives of Disease in Childhood*, vol. 89, no. 2, pp. 143–147, 2004.

[10] K. Moore, M. Cruickshank, and M. Haas, "Job satisfaction in occupational therapy: a qualitative investigation in urban Australia," *Australian Occupational Therapy Journal*, vol. 53, no. 1, pp. 18–26, 2006.

[11] A. Carrier, M. Levasseur, A. Freeman et al., "Influence of societal and practice contexts on health professionals' clinical reasoning: a scoping study protocol," *BMJ Open*, vol. 3, no. 4, article e002887, 2013.

[12] H. K. Kristensen, T. Borg, and L. Hounsgaard, "Aspects affecting occupational therapists' reasoning when implementing research-based evidence in stroke rehabilitation," *Scandinavian Journal of Occupational Therapy*, vol. 19, no. 2, pp. 118–131, 2012.

[13] N. Shafaroodi, M. Kamali, S. Parvizy, A. Mehraban, and G. O'Toole, "Factors affecting clinical reasoning of occupational therapists: a qualitative study," *Medical journal of the Islamic Republic of Iran*, vol. 28, p. 8, 2014.

[14] R. Vincent, H. Stewart, and J. Harrison, "South Australian school teachers' perceptions of occupational therapy reports," *Australian Occupational Therapy Journal*, vol. 55, no. 3, pp. 163–171, 2008.

[15] J. D. Benson, K. A. Szucs, and J. J. Mejasic, "Teachers' perceptions of the role of occupational therapist in schools," *Journal of Occupational Therapy, Schools, & Early Intervention*, vol. 9, no. 3, pp. 290–301, 2016.

[16] E. Smith and L. Mackenzie, "How occupational therapists are perceived within inpatient mental health settings: the perceptions of seven Australian nurses," *Australian Occupational Therapy Journal*, vol. 58, no. 4, pp. 251–260, 2011.

[17] R. AlHeresh and C. K. Nikopoulos, "The role of the occupational therapist in Jordan: a survey of the members of the healthcare team exploring their knowledge about occupational therapy in rehabilitation hospitals," *Disability and Rehabilitation*, vol. 33, no. 9, pp. 778–786, 2011.

[18] H. S. A. Tariah, K. Abulfeilat, and A. Khawaldeh, "Health professionals' knowledge of occupational therapy in Jordan," *Occupational Therapy In Health Care*, vol. 26, no. 1, pp. 74–87, 2012.

[19] International Labor Organization (ILO). International Standard Classification of Occupations, *(ISCO-08) – Draft Structure*, International Labour Office, NewYork, 2008.

[20] Wikipedia the Free Encyclopedia, "Classification of academic degrees," November 2017 https://en.wikipedia.org/wiki/Classification_of_Academic_Degrees.

[21] PGA Group Consulting Psychologists, "Standardized survey classifications – individuals," November 2017 http://www.pgagroup.com/standardized-survey-classifications.html.

[22] H. Tolonen, K. Kuulasmaa, and E. Ruokokoski, "MONICA population survey data book," November 2017 http://www.thl.fi/publications/monica/surveydb/section5.htm.

[23] J. Nunnaly, *Psychometric Theory*, McGraw-Hill, New York, 1987.

[24] T. Dendumrongsup, A. A. Plumb, S. Halligan, T. R. Fanshawe, D. G. Altman, and S. Mallett, "Multi-reader multi-case studies using the area under the receiver operator characteristic curve as a measure of diagnostic accuracy: systematic review with a

focus on quality of data reporting," *PLoS One*, vol. 9, no. 12, article e116018, 2014.

[25] K. Hajian-Tilaki, "Receiver operating characteristic (ROC) curve analysis for medical diagnostic test evaluation," *Caspian Journal of Internal Medicine*, vol. 4, no. 2, pp. 627–635, 2013.

[26] N. A. Obuchowski, "ROC analysis," *American Journal of Roentgenology*, vol. 184, no. 2, pp. 364–372, 2005.

[27] E. K. Schultz, "Multivariate receiver-operating characteristic curve analysis: prostate cancer screening as an example," *Clinical Chemistry*, vol. 41, no. 8, pp. 1248–1255, 1995.

[28] B. Sharma and R. Jain, "Right choice of a method for determination of cut-off values: a statistical tool for a diagnostic test," *Asian Journal of Medical Sciences*, vol. 5, no. 3, 2014.

[29] J. S. Katz, V. M. Titiloye, and J. A. Balogun, "Physical and occupational therapy undergraduates' stereotypes of one another," *Perceptual and Motor Skills*, vol. 92, no. 3, pp. 843–851, 2001.

[30] A. G. Fisher, "Why is it so hard to practise as an occupational therapist?," *Australian Occupational Therapy Journal*, vol. 50, no. 4, pp. 193-194, 2003.

[31] A. Bowling and S. Ebrahim, *Handbook of Health Research Methods: Investigation, Measurement and Analysis*, Open University Press, Buckingham, 2002.

[32] Ministry of Health (MOH), "Regulations of governing the scope of practice of occupational therapy profession," November 2017 http://www.moh.gov.jo/Echobusv3.0/SystemAssets/a999f153-cfef-4af9-82f3-33719712fa5b.pdf.

[33] J. Belik, K. Bratten, T. Bui et al., "Brief investigation of east central Illinoisans' awareness of occupational therapy," *Communiqué*, vol. 2, pp. 16-17, 2014.

[34] A. Patel and L. Shriber, "Nurse practitioners' knowledge of occupational therapy," *Occupational Therapy In Health Care*, vol. 13, no. 2, pp. 53–71, 2001.

[35] A. C. LaForme, F. Sarah, W. McCoy, L. A. Chiarello, and Move & PLAY Study Team, "Comparison of family and therapist perceptions of physical and occupational therapy services provided to young children with cerebral palsy," *Physical & Occupational Therapy in Pediatrics*, vol. 32, no. 2, pp. 210–226, 2012.

4

Occupational Therapy in Complex Patients: A Pilot Randomized Controlled Trial

Martina Pellegrini,[1] Debora Formisano,[2] Veronica Bucciarelli,[1] Margherita Schiavi,[3] Stefania Fugazzaro,[1] and Stefania Costi[4,5]

[1]*Department of Physical and Rehabilitation Medicine, Arcispedale Santa Maria Nuova-IRCCS, Azienda Unità Sanitaria Locale, 42100 Reggio Emilia, Italy*
[2]*Scientific Directorate, Arcispedale Santa Maria Nuova-IRCCS, Azienda Unità Sanitaria Locale, 42100 Reggio Emilia, Italy*
[3]*BSc in Occupational Therapy, Azienda Unità Sanitaria Locale, 42100 Reggio Emilia, Italy*
[4]*Children Rehabilitation Special Unit, Arcispedale Santa Maria Nuova-IRCCS, Azienda Unità Sanitaria Locale, 42100 Reggio Emilia, Italy*
[5]*Surgical, Medical and Dental Department of Morphological Sciences related to Transplant, Oncology and Regenerative Medicine, Università degli Studi di Modena e Reggio Emilia, 41100 Modena, Italy*

Correspondence should be addressed to Stefania Fugazzaro; stefania.fugazzaro@ausl.re.it

Academic Editor: Lynette Mackenzie

Introduction. To determine effect size and feasibility of experimental occupational therapy (OT) intervention in addition to standard care in a population of complex patients undergoing rehabilitation in a hospital-home-based setting. *Method.* 40 complex patients admitted to the rehabilitation ward of the Local Health Authority-Research Institute of Reggio Emilia (Italy) were randomized in a parallel-group, open-label controlled trial. Experimental OT targeting occupational needs in the areas of self-care, productivity, and leisure was delivered by occupational therapists. Standard care consisted of task-oriented rehabilitation delivered by a multiprofessional team. *Results.* The experimental OT intervention was completed by 75% of patients assigned to this group. The average changes in the Canadian Occupational Performance Measure (COPM) performance score significantly and clinically favored experimental OT [−3,06 (−4.50; −1.61); delta > 2 points, resp.]. Similar trends were detected for COPM satisfaction and independence in instrumental activities of daily living (ADL). At follow-up, level of social participation was higher for patients treated with experimental OT ($p = 0.043$) than for controls. *Conclusions.* Experimental OT was feasible in complex patients in a hospital-home-based setting. It ameliorated both patients' performance and satisfaction in carrying out relevant activities and improved independence in instrumental ADL. The trial is registered with ClinicalTrials.gov NCT02677766.

1. Introduction

Since the introduction of the International Classification of Functioning, Disability and Health (ICF) in 2001, the World Health Organization has been promoting the implementation of a client-centered, biopsychosocial approach in healthcare programs and rehabilitation services [1]. This conceptual framework focuses on individual functioning more than on disease and contemplates the health condition as a dynamic status resulting from a comprehensive view of biological, individual, and social perspectives [1].

The ICF approach is particularly appropriate for patients during rehabilitation, as the latter relies on the interaction between functions, activities, participation, and contextual factors [2, 3]. Indeed, regardless of the underlying pathology, patients undergoing rehabilitation habitually manifest similar basic needs, while their level of functioning and advanced needs, namely, those related to leisure, productivity, and social role, may be different [4]. This was brought to light also by Phipps and Richardson's work [5], which showed that when rehabilitation focuses on individual significant activities, gains in performance and satisfaction are noticeable both in patients with traumatic brain injury and in those with stroke. Similarly, occupational therapy (OT) has proven to be beneficial in patients with different types of cancer when based on patient requests [6].

In line with this approach, an assessment tool based on the complexity of patients' care needs has been validated to classify individuals who require rehabilitation interventions [7, 8]. This classification makes it possible to create homogeneous populations according to the complexity of their care needs, not to their diagnosis. Moreover, this approach may facilitate conducting valid rehabilitative studies, whose results may be highly generalizable.

A complex patient suffers from a disease that affects clinical stability and functional autonomy. This patient is dependent on others when carrying out daily activities and manifests regular need for medical monitoring, for specialized nursing care and for two or more specialized interventions, for example, occupational therapy, physiotherapy, or speech therapy. Frequently, complex patients need special aids to carry out tasks. Thus, complex patients benefit from multiprofessional rehabilitation, which may include client-centered OT interventions.

Our research group recently conducted an observational study aimed at identifying the needs of complex inpatients in a rehabilitation ward to develop a client-centered OT intervention targeted at this population [9]. To our knowledge, no well-designed randomized clinical trial on the efficacy of OT in the rehabilitation process of complex patients has yet been published.

We thus decided to conduct this ICF concept-based pilot randomized controlled trial (RCT) in order to detect the effect size of an experimental, client-centered OT intervention in a population of complex patients in their rehabilitation phase.

2. Materials and Methods

This single-center, open-label RCT with two parallel groups was designed in accordance with the CONSORT statement and the Helsinki declaration. The study was approved by the local Ethics Committee (19/03/2014, number 325).

2.1. Study Objectives. The primary aim of this exploratory study was to estimate the effects of experimental OT on complex patients' perception of occupational performance during relevant activities. If the experimental OT proved beneficial, its effect size estimate would be used to plan a powered randomized controlled trial.

The secondary aim was to verify the feasibility of the OT experimental intervention in a mixed hospital-home-based setting for a population of complex patients undergoing rehabilitation.

Further objectives were to estimate the effects of experimental OT on (a) complex patients' self-perception of occupational satisfaction with the way they perform their relevant occupational activities, (b) mood disturbances, (c) independence in basic and instrumental activity of daily living (ADL), and (d) reintegration to normal social activities and quality of life (QoL).

2.2. Participants. All adult patients admitted to the Physical and Rehabilitation Medicine (PRM) ward of the Local Health Authority-Research Institute (AUSL-IRCCS) of Reggio Emilia, Italy, and deemed complex on the basis of the Rehabilitation Complexity Scale-Extended (RCS-E) were screened for eligibility. The RCS-E score ranges from zero to 22, with the cut-off value for complexity set at nine [7].

Exclusion criteria were the presence of severe cognitive impairment, verified by the physiatrist through direct observation and an exploratory interview (evaluating memory, orientation in time and space, adequacy to the context, absence of disinhibition or frontal disorders, and risk evaluation), primary psychiatric disorders, communication disability, and language barriers that, in the opinion of the healthcare team, would prevent the patient from participating in the experimental OT program. Furthermore, to allow assessment of the feasibility of the experimental intervention, patients living over 30 km from the hospital and patients for whom it was known a priori that they would be discharged to a retirement home were excluded.

We also excluded complex patients already recruited in a competing clinical trial (ISRCTN75290225).

Informed consent was obtained from all participants by physicians during the admission process.

2.3. Outcomes. The primary outcome measure for this study was the performance score of the Canadian Occupational Performance Measure (COPM) [10]. The COPM is a standardized client-centered measure designed to detect changes in occupational performance and satisfaction over time, based on patient perception. The COPM is administered by a semistructured interview resulting in a list of up to five priority occupational activities, suited to satisfy relevant needs in three areas: self-care, productivity, and leisure.

The feasibility of the experimental OT intervention was assessed by calculating the ratio between the number of patients who completed it according to the predefined posology and the total number of patients enrolled in the intervention group (IG). We established a priori that the study would be judged feasible if 75% of patients randomized to the intervention group completed the experimental OT. Given the complex nature of these patients, we also collected information on the appropriateness of estimates made a priori regarding the timing of achievement of treatment goals and the level of independence achieved by any participant enrolled in the IG.

Further outcome measures applied to verify the effects of experimental OT in complex patients were the satisfaction score of the COPM [10], the Hospital Anxiety and Depression Scale (HADS) [11], the modified Barthel Index (MBI) [12], the Instrumental Activity Daily Living (IADL) scale [13], the Reintegration to Normal Living Index (RNLI) [14], and the Short-Form 12 (SF-12) [15].

2.4. Assessments. Study participants were assessed at baseline (T0), upon discharge (T1), and at follow-up (T2) (Table 1).

Baseline assessment (T0) was carried out within 1 week from admission to the PRM ward and before randomization. At T0, the degree of comorbidity was assessed using the Charlson Comorbidity Index (CCI), which is also a measure of burden of disease [16]. T0 also included the assessments of occupational performance and satisfaction, mood disturbances, B-ADL, and I-ADL.

T1 took place within three days before discharge from the PRM ward. Except for comorbidity assessment, it included all the above-mentioned measurements plus the RNLI and QoL assessments.

The follow-up (T2) took place at the patient's domicile 45 ± 15 days from discharge and included all the assessments administered at T1.

T2 assessments and all the COPM interviews were collected by the occupational therapists. Given the aim of this study, the rehabilitation team was integrated with two occupational therapists working specifically on this trial. T0 and T1 assessments were collected by members of the rehabilitation health care team (physiatrists, physiotherapists, occupational therapists, and nurses), as per habit of the ward.

Data regarding the feasibility of the experimental OT intervention in this specific hospital-home-based setting were collected by researchers throughout the trial and were unified at T2.

2.5. Randomization. Shortly after T0, patients were randomly assigned to the control group (CG) or to the IG, with a 1 : 1 allocation ratio. The Research and Statistics unit of the AUSL-IRCCS generated the computerized random allocation lists and proceeded with the concealed allocation of patients to groups, once the patients had been enrolled by clinicians and after T0 assessment.

Patients assigned to CG were provided with the standard care already in place in the PRM ward. Patients assigned to IG followed the experimental OT intervention delivered in addition to standard care.

2.6. Control Group. The CG underwent standard care, which consisted of task-oriented rehabilitation targeted at the recovery of autonomy in B-ADL (basic activity of daily life). Patients were cared for by an interdisciplinary multiprofessional rehabilitation team composed of physiatrists, nurses, physiotherapists, and speech therapists, as well as by a psychologist and social worker when necessary.

During the postacute phase, standard care was carried out daily, six days a week, during hospitalization. Standard care also included some (one to three) therapeutic authorizations to go home for the weekend in the predischarge phase. On the basis of predischarge assessment, rehabilitation was continued postdischarge on an outpatient basis when deemed necessary by the rehabilitation team.

2.7. Intervention Group. The experimental OT intervention was provided by the occupational therapists in addition to standard care and was based on the Canadian Model of Occupational Performance and Engagement [17]. Experimental OT is aimed at satisfying the occupational needs in the areas of self-care, productivity, and leisure that emerged through the COPM assessment at baseline.

During the postacute phase, experimental OT was delivered daily, five days a week, during hospitalization. In this setting, experimental OT was targeted at the accomplishment of occupational needs in the self-care area and, when needed, in the productivity and leisure areas.

After discharge from the PRM ward, experimental OT was delivered at the patient's domicile for up to ten sessions over a period of one to two months. In this setting, experimental OT was targeted at the accomplishment of occupational needs related to productivity and leisure areas and to any residual goals of the self-care area.

The experimental OT intervention was planned by the occupational therapists, was tailored to each patient, and was carried out according to the following phases:

(1) Identification of three to five subjective priority occupational needs, which become the focus of the experimental OT intervention

(2) Observation of patient while performing the activities related to the occupational needs in the hospital or at home after discharge

(3) Setting the treatment goals (accomplishment of occupational activity) for each occupational need

Plus, for each goal set:

(4) Definition of the implementation time

(5) Definition of the level of independence expected at the end of the treatment

(6) Planning the appropriate OT intervention (i.e., content and modalities) according to a specific planning checklist (Table 2)

2.8. Withdrawal from Trial. Participants were withdrawn from the study for any of the following reasons:

(a) Serious adverse events or death

(b) Patient referred to other wards for clinical reasons

(c) Patient discharged to a nursing home after in-hospital rehabilitation

(d) Patient lost to follow-up

(e) Patient withdrawal of consent to participate

All withdrawals with specific reason were recorded. Data collected up to the patient's discontinuation of the study were analyzed with the intention-to-treat approach.

2.9. Data Analysis. The analyses were carried out by the Research and Statistics units of the AUSL-IRCCS of Reggio Emilia. This was an exploratory study as there was no information to set the sample size based on statistical criteria. Thus, it was considered appropriate to randomly recruit 40

TABLE 1: Clinical outcome measures and study assessments.

	T0 Baseline (within one week from admission to PRM ward)		T1 Discharge (within 3 days up to discharge)	T2 Follow up (45 ± 15 days from discharge)
Comorbidities (CCI)	X			
Performance in carrying out occupational activities (COPM)	X		X	X
Satisfaction in carrying out occupational activities (COPM)	X		X	X
Mood disturbances (HADS)	X	Randomization	X	X
B-ADL (MBI)	X		X	X
I-ADL (IADL)	X		X	X
Reintegration to Normal Living Index (RNLI)			X	X
Quality of life (SF-12)			X	X

PRM: physical and rehabilitation medicine; CCI: Charlson Comorbidity Index; COPM: Canadian Occupational Performance Measure; HADS: Hospital Anxiety and Depression Scale; B-ADL: basic activities of daily living; MBI: modified Barthel Index; I-ADL: instrumental activities of daily living; IADL: instrumental activities of daily living; RNLI: Reintegration to Normal Living Index; SF-12: Short Form-12.

TABLE 2: Planning checklist of OT intervention for each goal set.

Phase	Activity	Options	
A	Definition of the OT rehabilitative approach	Restorative	Compensative
B	Definition of treatment posology	Number of sessions Frequency of sessions Duration of each session	
C	Definition of any supports and/or facilitation strategies to be used during sessions (e.g., aids, caregivers, and facilities)		
D	Definition of the intervention setting/s		
E	Group sessions	Yes	No

subjects to estimate the average effect size of experimental OT measured by the performance score of the COPM. To compute the effect size, we compared the changes in COPM performance score between IG and CG in the T2-T0 time frame. Furthermore, to evaluate the clinical relevance of this finding, we matched it with the minimal clinically important difference of the COPM performance score, which was estimated equal to two points [18].

In addition, to estimate the effects of experimental OT in this population, the mean variations of all the outcome measures were compared between groups at the T1-T0, T2-T1, and T2-T0 time frames.

Descriptive statistics were performed to investigate the sample characteristics; mean and standard deviation were chosen to summarize continuous variables, while absolute and relative frequencies (n, %) were used for categorical variables.

The assumption of normality for continuous variables was verified statistically using the Shapiro-Wilk test.

To test differences between the groups, numerical data were compared using the Student t-test and Mann–Whitney U test, and categorical data were compared using Pearson's chi-squared test or Fisher's exact test. The threshold for statistical significance was set at $p < 0.05$. IBM SPSS Statistics 23 for Windows (SPSS, Chicago, IL) was used for statistical analyses.

3. Results

The Consolidated Standards of Reporting Trials (CONSORT) flow diagram of the RCT is shown in Figure 1. From February 2016 to June 2017, 414 patients were admitted to the PRM ward, 151 of whom were deemed complex. After screening for eligibility, 40 patients were recruited and randomized to experimental intervention or standard care. Eight patients withdrew from the trial and were not reassessed at follow-up (T2), five in the IG, and three in the CG. Two patients verbally withdrew their consent to continue the experimental OT after discharge to their domicile. One participant was discharged to a nursing home, so the home-based phase of experimental OT could not be implemented. One patient dropped out due to clinical worsening during the in-hospital phase, and four participants died.

The baseline demographics and clinical data of the sample are shown in Table 3.

The mean age of all participants was 64 years (range 26–85). Most patients were men (23; 57%). The mean complexity

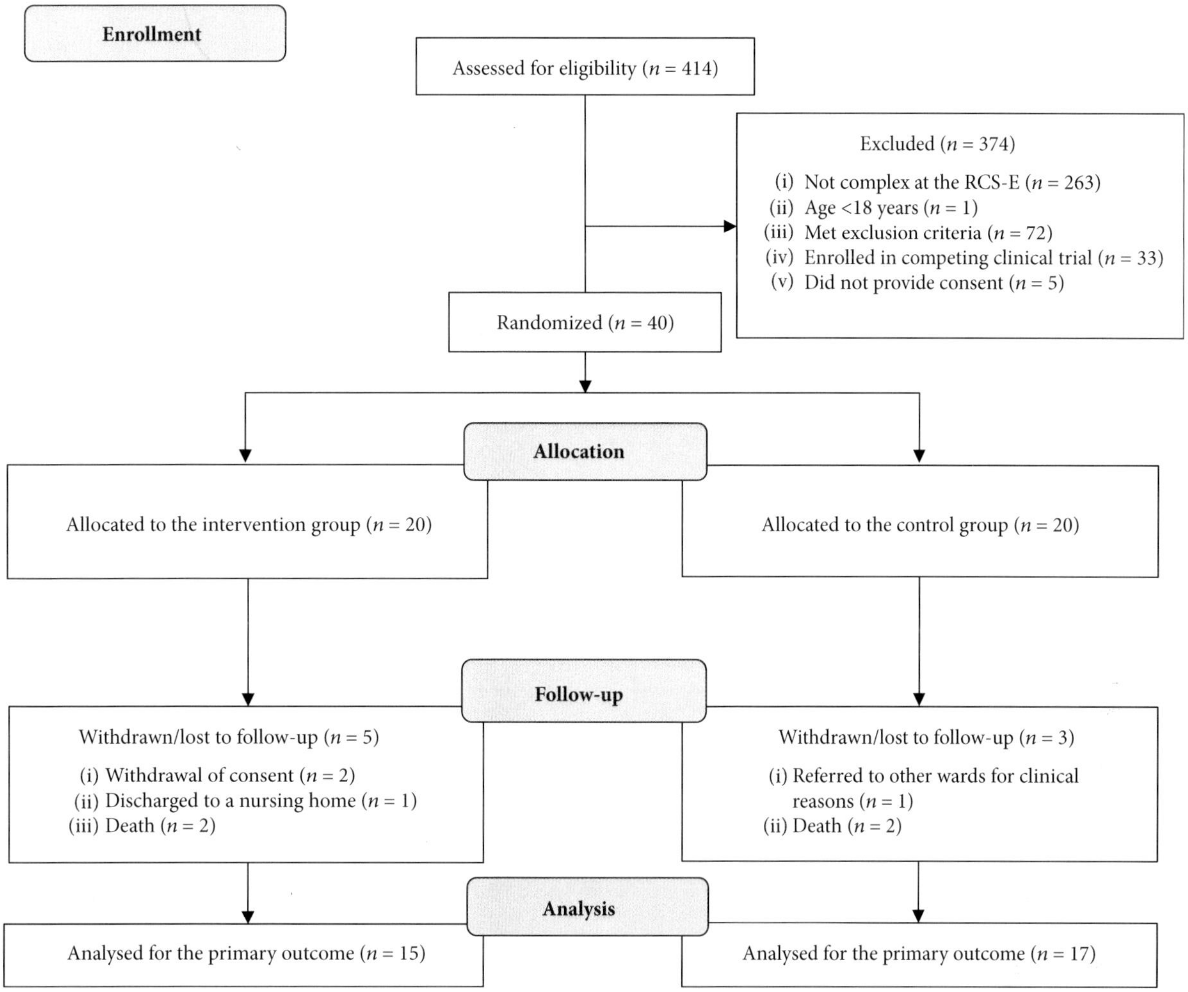

FIGURE 1: CONSORT 2010 flow diagram of the study.

TABLE 3: Baseline characteristics of the study participants.

Characteristics	IG ($n = 20$)	CG ($n = 20$)	p value
Age (mean ± SD)	66.35 (±14.67)	62.75 (±10.99)	0.38[a]
Gender, F/M (%)	8/12 (40/60%)	9/11 (45/55%)	0.74[b]
RCS-E (mean ± SD)	10.75 (±0.96)	10.75 (±0.91)	1.00[a]
CCI (mean ± SD)	5.20 (±2.41)	5.15 (±2.18)	0.94[a]
Main diagnosis of access for rehabilitation (%)			0.853[b]
Acute polyneuropathy	6 (30%)	5 (25%)	
Stroke	5 (25%)	4 (20%)	
Cancer	4 (20%)	3 (15%)	
Hemiparesis due to acute neurological syndrome	2 (10%)	2 (10%)	
Lower limb amputation	1 (5%)	3 (15%)	
Orthopedic diseases or musculoskeletal trauma	1 (5%)	2 (10%)	
Paraplegia	1 (5%)	1 (5%)	

IG: intervention group; CG: control group; SD: standard deviation; [a]Student's t-test; F/M: female versus male ratio; [b]Pearson's chi-square test or Fisher's exact test; RCS-E: Rehabilitation Complexity Scale-Extended; CCI: Charlson Comorbidity Index.

of care needs for the sample was 10.75 (range 9–13), and the average comorbidity index was 5.18 (SD 2.27). At T0, the groups were balanced in terms of the main demographic and clinical characteristics recorded. The diagnoses of access to rehabilitation were acute polyneuropathy ($n = 11$), stroke ($n = 9$), cancer ($n = 7$), hemiparesis due to acute neurological syndrome ($n = 4$), lower limb amputation ($n = 4$), orthopedic diseases or musculoskeletal trauma ($n = 3$), and paraplegia ($n = 2$). The average duration of hospitalization was 48.84 (SD 27.59) days in IG and 40.61 (SD 24.88) days in CG ($p = 0.34$).

Figure 2 shows the distribution of relevant occupational activities chosen by study participants to satisfy their priority occupational needs and corresponding to the goals of the experimental OT intervention. As expected, most of these activities regarded the self-care area, with particular attention to personal care (32.5%) and functional mobility issues (12%). Within the productivity and leisure areas, household management and dynamic recreation activities were chosen by 14.5% and 14% of participants, respectively.

Regarding the main objective of this study, 32 patients were included in the primary outcome analysis of COPM performance because both baseline and follow-up data were available. The difference between follow-up and baseline scores was, on average, 5.62 (±2.10) for the IG and 2.56 (±1.89) for the CG. Thus, the gain obtained by the experimental OT intervention was significantly higher than by standard care ($p < 0.001$; CI = −4.50 to −1.61) and amply exceeded the MCID established for the COPM performance score (Table 4).

This result was consistent with that of COPM satisfaction: in the same time frame, this difference was on average 5.52 (±2.10) for the IG and 2.70 (±1.88) for the CG. Once again, the gain obtained with the experimental OT intervention was significantly higher than with standard care ($p < 0.001$; CI = −4.25 to −1.37), and again, it was clinically relevant.

To note, the advantage in favor of the intervention group was already evident for COPM performance and satisfaction scores in the T1-T0 comparison.

Figures 3 and 4 show the proportion of patients in the two groups whose gain in COPM performance and satisfaction exceeded the MCID; of note, this proportion was statistically significant for both measures in the comparisons versus baseline. Gain in satisfaction was also significant in the follow-up versus discharge (T2-T1) comparison. Furthermore, at the end of the study, all patients in the IG reached clinically relevant gains in their performance and satisfaction.

Additionally, the change in the IADL score followed a trend consistent with that showed by the COPM.

Concerning the other secondary outcome measures, no other statistically significant between-group differences were demonstrated, although the change in the MBI at the T2-T0 comparison and the change in the RNLI at the T1-T0 comparison were on the verge of statistical significance, in favor of the IG (HADS and SF-12 values are not represented in Table 4).

For completeness of results, Table 5 shows the between-group comparisons of the average scores for each of the clinical outcomes measured at each point in time.

The groups were balanced at baseline, although for the main outcome measure IG scores were clearly less favorable. Despite this, and in line with the results shown in Table 4, the IG demonstrated significantly higher average values for COPM performance and satisfaction at T1 and, above all, at T2. No other significant differences were registered, with the exception of a higher reintegration to normal living scores for the IG at T2.

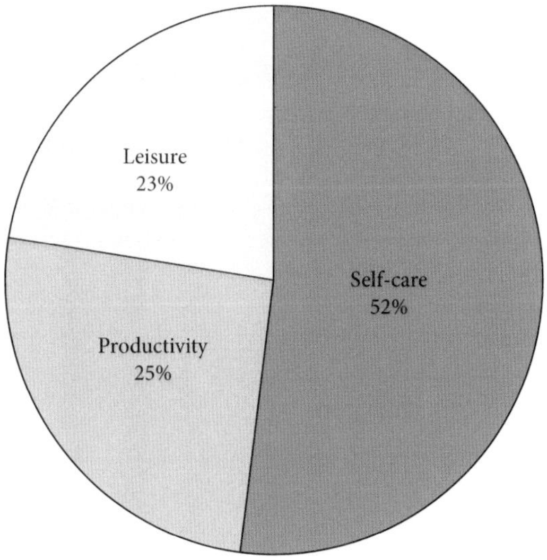

Figure 2: Distribution of relevant occupational activities chosen by participants in this study.

3.1. Feasibility of the OT Experimental Intervention. Fifteen of the 20 complex patients enrolled in the IG (75%) completed the experimental intervention according to the predefined posology. The experimental OT was therefore deemed feasible in the context of application. Furthermore, 70% of participants enrolled in IG achieved at least four treatment goals within the a priori estimated time of implementation and the same percentage reached the goals with the estimated level of independence.

4. Discussion

One of the key findings of this pilot study was that the experimental OT intervention, implemented in a mixed hospital-home-based setting, was feasible in complex patients undergoing rehabilitation. Of note, although we did not define a priori harms (e.g., accidental falls) or unintended effects of experimental treatment, none occurred during the course of the study. The results of this study can therefore be generalized in highly complex patients, which are increasingly present in clinical settings.

Moreover, the experimental OT improved patients' performance and satisfaction during the implementation of relevant activities, as perceived by participants. The estimated size effect is undoubtedly clinically relevant, and it may be used in the near future to plan methodologically sound clinical trials.

Further, the experimental OT improved the patients' independence in IADL and enhanced their level of reintegration to normal social activities.

Although current guidelines already state the effects of OT in specific populations [19], this pilot study is the first to confirm that a client-centered OT program based on sound methodology [17] may benefit a population of complex patients, regardless of their underlying disease.

Table 4: Between-group differences of average changes during the study course for the main clinical outcome measures.

	ΔIG (mean ± SD)	ΔCG (mean ± SD)	p value	Mean difference (95% CI)
COPM perf.				
T1-T0	3.18 ± 1.89	1.21 ± 1.13	0.001	−1.97 (−3.03; −0.91)
T1-T2	1.98 ± 1.98	1.26 ± 2.16	0.336	−0.72 (−2.22; 0.78)
T2-T0	5.62 ± 2.10	2.56 ± 1.89	0.001	−3.06 (−4.50; −1.61)
COPM satisf.				
T1-T0	3.01 ± 2.25	1.26 ± 1.15	0.006	−1.75 (−2.96; −0.53)
T1-T2	1.97 ± 2.53	1.35 ± 2.05	0.454	−0.61 (−2.27; 1.04)
T2-T0	5.52 ± 2.10	2.70 ± 1.88	0.001	−2.81 (−4.25; −1.37)
MBI				
T1-T0	41.77 ± 20.34	30.16 ± 22.37	0.113	−11.61 (−26.10; 2.88)
T1-T2	6.00 ± 6.34	4.52 ± 10.98	0.652	−1.47 (−8.06; 5.12)
T2-T0	49.33 ± 20.14	37.00 ± 18.58	0.082	−12.33 (−26.31; 1.64)
IADL				
T1-T0	−1.15 ± 0.81	−0.51 ± 0.46	0.007	0.64 (0.18; 1.09)
T1-T2	−0.55 ± 0.62	−0.53 ± 0.79	0.938	0.02 (−0.50; 0.54)
T2-T0	−1.83 ± 0.88	−1.06 ± 0.78	0.014	0.76 (0.16; 1.36)
RNLI				
T2-T1	24.46 ± 20.28	10.47 ± 21.39	0.068	−13.98 (−29.05; 1.07)

Δ = within-group change; IG: intervention group; CG: control group; SD: standard deviation; CI: confidence interval; COPM: Canadian Occupational Performance Measure; perf.: performance; satisf.: satisfaction; MBI: modified Barthel Index; IADL: instrumental activities of daily living; RNLI: Reintegration to Normal Living Index.

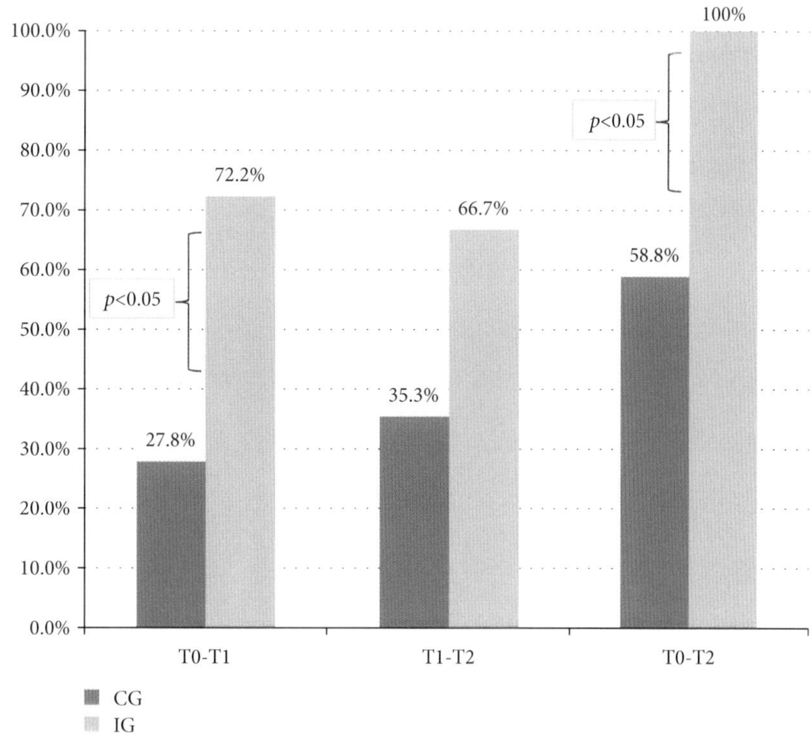

Figure 3: Proportion of patients whose gain in COPM performance score exceeded the minimal clinically important difference set for the COPM.

This study also highlights that complex patients would like to be able to satisfy a broad range of needs related to their well-being right from the beginning of rehabilitation, shortly after the onset of an acute illness. These needs range from basic personal-care needs, which many in the population of interest expressed, to more "advanced" needs, which

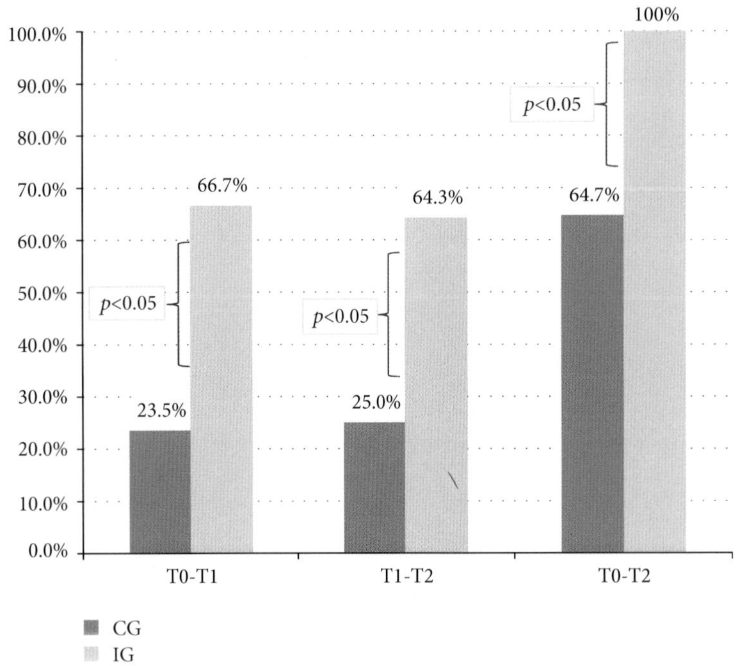

FIGURE 4: Proportion of patients whose gain in COPM satisfaction score exceeded the minimal clinically important difference set for the COPM.

reflected various necessities expressed by only few patients. Therefore, this research also focused on the patients' perspective, oriented towards the return to the community and to social participation right from the beginning of the rehabilitation process, even in the presence of limitations and priority clinical needs. Thus, this study's results encourage the implementation of client-centered OT interventions focused on ameliorating the transition between rehabilitation programs and the community, as also suggested by individuals with long-term physical disabilities [20]. Accordingly, the experimental intervention setting of this study was hospital plus home-based. It is known that the provision of timely home-based rehabilitation facilitates hospital discharge, reduces the risk of readmission, improves functional independence, and helps people with stroke recover social participation [21–23]. Moreover, home-based OT has been proven to improve occupational performance in older adults [24, 25]. Consistent with previous evidence, this study showed an average higher reintegration to normal living of patients treated with experimental OT, compared to the control group, although this advantage was barely significant, and this significance was not confirmed in the between-group differences of average changes for this measure. This might be explained by the fact that reintegration to normal living was addressed in the home-based phase of the intervention, which might not have been of sufficient intensity or duration to maintain the pace of improvement shown in the hospital [21, 24]. In fact, it is evident that the greater gains in all outcomes measured were not obtained in the home-based phase of the study (Table 4), although the experimental OT allowed for slight improvement at follow-up of the positive achievements already obtained at hospital discharge.

A possible limitation of this study is that we excluded patients with cognitive impairment as determined through clinical evaluation. However, we excluded only those patients with severe cognitive impairment, and the intervention performed, which requires good patient compliance, was feasible in the population of interest. It is unlikely that differences in the cognitive level of the patients may have biased the results of the study, since the two groups were balanced for average age and diagnoses represented. However, future studies aimed at verifying the OT effectiveness in a complex and heterogeneous population should also include an objective assessment of the patients' cognitive level.

This study failed to demonstrate a positive effect of OT in important clinical outcome measures such as HADS, QoL, and MBI. Some of these unsuccessful results are consistent with those already shown in patients with stroke, brain tumor, or trauma, where individualized rehabilitation interventions have failed to reduce mood symptoms [26, 27] and QoL [26, 28, 29]. This failure could be due to the limited sample recruited; looking at the results, it should be noted that at baseline, the IG scores were worse than those of the CG in all the outcomes measured, though not statistically significantly so. As during the study the gain obtained by the IG was definitely greater than that obtained by the CG, it is plausible that a larger sample would have had the power to highlight this difference even in statistical terms. However, it should not be forgotten that the study was designed with the main objective of detecting the effect size of OT on the performance score of the COPM, and this aim was completely achieved. Nevertheless, when interpreting the size of the estimated OT effect, the fact that the COPM was administered by an occupational therapist not blinded to the allocation group of patients and involved in the experimental

Table 5: Between-group comparisons of average scores for all clinical outcome measures.

	T0			T1			T2		
	IG ($n = 20$)	CG ($n = 20$)	p value	IG ($n = 18$)	CG ($n = 18$)	p value	IG ($n = 15$)	CG ($n = 17$)	p value
COPM perf. (mean ± SD)	1.73 ± 0.78	2.21 ± 0.81	0.064	4.89 ± 1.73	3.44 ± 1.41	0.009	7.28 ± 1.67	4.77 ± 1.89	0.001
COPM satisf. (mean ± SD)	1.86 ± 0.69	2.22 ± 1.05	0.21	4.86 ± 2.0	3.55 ± 1.44	0.031	7.33 ± 1.89	4.98 ± 1.81	0.001
HADS anx. (mean ± SD)	6.90 ± 3.74	6.80 ± 3.79	0.93	5.78 ± 3.93	5.56 ± 4.20	0.87	4.13 ± 3.29	6.77 ± 4.67	0.08
HADS depr. (mean ± SD)	7.40 ± 4.26	6.35 ± 3.94	0.42	6.44 ± 4.33	6.17 ± 4.20	0.85	5.53 ± 3.16	6.65 ± 5.04	0.47
MBI (mean ± SD)	37.85 ± 20.32	49.60 ± 25.11	0.11	77.11 ± 23.29	80.50 ± 20.17	0.64	88.00 ± 14.40	88.18 ± 13.20	0.97
IADL (mean ± SD)	5.09 ± 1.15	4.55 ± 1.12	0.14	3.99 ± 1.26	4.01 ± 0.97	0.95	2.98 ± 1.13	3.42 ± 1.06	0.26
RNLI (mean ± SD)				46.86 ± 17.11	46.81 ± 16.79	0.99	72.57 ± 15.56	58.11 ± 22.04	0.043
SF-12 PCS (mean ± SD)				32.80 ± 5.39	33.89 ± 7.89	0.63	34.84 ± 7.19	31.68 ± 7.49	0.23
SF-12 MCS (mean ± SD)				42.59 ± 11.05	43.21 ± 17.09	0.90	46.32 ± 11.87	42.90 ± 13.41	0.45

IG: intervention group; CG: control group; COPM: Canadian Occupational Performance Measure; perf.: performance; SD: standard deviation; satisf.: satisfaction; HADS: Hospital Anxiety and Depression Scale; anx.: anxiety; depr.: depression; MBI: modified Barthel Index; IADL: instrumental activities of daily living; RNLI: Reintegration to Normal Living Index; SF-12: Short Form-12; PCS: Physical Health Composite Score; MCS: Mental Health Composite Score.

treatment must be borne in mind. This limit may thus have biased the results of this study. The choice of administering the COPM open label was dictated by local constraints in professional and environmental resources, which themselves would have prevented the blindness of the assessments. However, to the best of our knowledge, the COPM is not usually administered blindly because, by its nature, it entails the building of a partnership between patient and assessor that constitutes the foundation for OT interventions. We suggest that future studies combine COPM with blinded measures of relevant outcomes.

5. Conclusions

To conclude, this pilot study allowed the detection of the effect size of experimental OT implemented in complex patients in a hospital-home-based setting. This effect size was markedly greater than the MCID detected for the COPM, a client-centered outcome measure widely used in clinical and research settings. Thus, this study strongly supports the application of client-centered rehabilitation programs supplemented by OT right from the early stages of rehabilitation of patients with high clinical complexity levels. Moreover, the effect size detected in this research study will help scientists design future powered randomized controlled trials aimed at confirming the effectiveness of client-centered OT in similar populations and heterogeneous settings.

Acknowledgments

This work was entirely supported by Arcispedale Santa Maria Nuova-IRCCS, Azienda Unità Sanitaria Locale, Reggio Emilia, 42100, Italy. The authors thank Jacqueline M. Costa for the English language editing.

References

[1] World Health Organization, *International Classification of Functioning, Disability and Health: ICF*, WHO, Geneva, 2001.

[2] G. Stucki, T. Ewert, and A. Cieza, "Value and application of the ICF in rehabilitation medicine," *Disability and Rehabilitation* vol. 24, no. 17, pp. 932–938, 2002.

[3] D. Wade, "Rehabilitation - a new approach. Part two: the underlying theories," *Clinical Rehabilitation*, vol. 29, no. 12, pp. 1145–1154, 2015.

[4] M. Müller, E. Grill, M. Stier-Jarmer et al., "Validation of the comprehensive ICF core sets for patients receiving rehabilitation interventions in the acute care setting," *Journal of rehabilitation medicine*, vol. 43, no. 2, pp. 92–101, 2011.

[5] S. Phipps and P. Richardson, "Occupational therapy outcomes for clients with traumatic brain injury and stroke using the Canadian Occupational Performance Measure," *American Journal of Occupational Therapy*, vol. 61, no. 3, pp. 328–334, 2007.

[6] College of Occupational Therapists, *Occupational Therapy Intervention in Cancer: Guidance for Professionals, Managers and Decision-Makers*, COT, London, 2004.

[7] L. Turner-Stokes, H. Scott, H. Williams, and R. Siegert, "The rehabilitation complexity scale–extended version: detection of patients with highly complex needs," *Disability and Rehabilitation*, vol. 34, no. 9, pp. 715–720, 2012.

[8] F. Rodà, M. Agosti, E. Corradini, F. Lombardi, M. Maini, and R. Brianti, "Cross-cultural adaptation and preliminary test-retest reliability of the Italian version of the Complexity Rehabilitation Scale-Extended (13th Version)," *European Journal of Physical and Rehabilitation Medicine*, vol. 51, no. 4, pp. 439–446, 2014.

[9] M. Schiavi, S. Costi, M. Pellegrini, D. Formisano, S. Borghi, and S. Fugazzaro, "Occupational therapy for complex inpatients with stroke: identification of occupational needs in post-acute rehabilitation setting," *Disability and Rehabilitation*, vol. 40, no. 9, pp. 1026–1032, 2017.

[10] M. Law, S. Baptiste, A. Carswell, M. A. McColl, H. Polatajko, and N. Pollock, *Canadian Occupational Performance Measure (COPM)*, CAOT Publications ACE, 2014.

[11] A. S. Zigmond and R. P. Snaith, "The hospital anxiety and depression scale," *Acta Psychiatrica Scandinavica*, vol. 67, no. 6, pp. 361–370, 1983.

[12] S. Shah, B. Cooper, and F. Maas, "The Barthel Index and ADL evaluation in stroke rehabilitation in Australia, Japan, the UK and the USA," *Australian Occupational Therapy Journal*, vol. 39, no. 1, pp. 5–13, 1992.

[13] M. P. Lawton and E. M. Brody, "Assessment of older people: self-maintaining and instrumental activities of daily living," *The Gerontologist*, vol. 9, 3, Part 1, pp. 179–186, 1969.

[14] S. L. Wood-Dauphinee, M. A. Opzoomer, J. I. Williams, B. Marchand, and W. O. Spitzer, "Assessment of global function: the reintegration to normal living index," *Archives of Physical Medicine and Rehabilitation*, vol. 69, no. 8, pp. 583–590, 1988.

[15] G. Apolone, P. Mosconi, L. Quattrociocchi, E. A. L. Gianicolo, N. Groth, and J. E. Ware, *Questionario sullo stato di salute Sf-12*, Guerini e Associati, 2005, Versione Italiana.

[16] M. Charlson, T. P. Szatrowski, J. Peterson, and J. Gold, "Validation of a combined comorbidity index," *Journal of Clinical Epidemiology*, vol. 47, no. 11, pp. 1245–1251, 1994.

[17] H. J. Polatajko, E. A. Townsend, and J. Craik, "Canadian model of occupational performance and engagement (CMOP-E)," in *Enabling Occupation II: Advancing an Occupational Therapy Vision of Health, Well-Being & Justice Through Occupation*, E. A. Townsend and H. J. Polatajko, Eds., vol. 23, pp. 22–36, CAOT Publications ACE, Ottawa, ON, 2007.

[18] M. Law, S. Baptiste, A. Carswell-Opzoomer, M. A. McColl, H. Polatajko, and N. Pollock, *Canadian Occupational Performance Measure*, CAOT Publications ACE, Toronto, 1991.

[19] AOTA, "Practice guidelines," April 2018, https://www.aota.org/Practice/Researchers/practice-guidelines.aspx.

[20] C. Cott, "Client-centred rehabilitation: client perspectives," *Disability and rehabilitation*, vol. 26, no. 24, pp. 1411–1422, 2004.

[21] C. Langstaff, C. Martin, G. Brown et al., "Enhancing community-based rehabilitation for stroke survivors: creating a discharge link," *Topics in stroke rehabilitation*, vol. 21, no. 6, pp. 510–519, 2014.

[22] A. Ávila, M. Durán, M. Peralbo, G. Torres, M. Saavedra, and I. M. Viana, "Effectiveness of an occupational therapy home programme in Spain for people affected by stroke," *Occupational Therapy International*, vol. 22, no. 1, 9 pages, 2015.

[23] L. Allen, M. Richardson, A. McIntyre et al., "Community stroke rehabilitation teams: providing home-based stroke rehabilitation in Ontario, Canada," *Canadian Journal of Neurological Sciences*, vol. 41, no. 06, pp. 697–703, 2004.

[24] T. L. Nielsen, N. T. Andersen, K. S. Petersen, H. Polatajko, and C. V. Nielsen, "Intensive client-centred occupational therapy in the home improves older adults' occupational performance. Results from a Danish randomized controlled trial," *Scandinavian Journal of Occupational Therapy*, pp. 1–17, 2018.

[25] S. Stark, A. Landsbaum, J. L. Palmer et al., "Client-centred home modifications improve daily activity performance of older adults," *Canadian Journal of Occupational Therapy*, vol. 76, Supplement 1, pp. 235–245, 2009.

[26] J. Wu, S. G. Faux, J. Estell et al., "Early rehabilitation after hospital admission for road trauma using an in-reach multidisciplinary team: a randomised controlled trial," *Clinical Rehabilitation*, vol. 31, no. 9, pp. 1189–1200, 2017.

[27] F. Khan, B. Amatya, B. Physio, K. Drummond, and M. Galea, "Effectiveness of integrated multidisciplinary rehabilitation in primary brain cancer survivors in an Australian community cohort: a controlled clinical trial," *Journal of rehabilitation medicine*, vol. 46, no. 8, pp. 754–760, 2014.

[28] B. Brouwer, D. Bryant, and S. J. Garland, "Effectiveness of client-centered "tune-ups" on community reintegration, mobility, and quality of life after stroke: a randomized controlled trial," *Archives of physical medicine and rehabilitation*, vol. 99, no. 7, pp. 1325–1332, 2018.

[29] S. Rotenberg-Shpigelman, A. B. H. Erez, I. Nahaloni, and A. Maeir, "Neurofunctional treatment targeting participation among chronic stroke survivors: a pilot randomised controlled study," *Neuropsychological rehabilitation*, vol. 22, no. 4, pp. 532–549, 2012.

5

Play, Playfulness, and Self-Efficacy: Parental Experiences with Children on the Autism Spectrum

Rosa Román-Oyola, Verónica Figueroa-Feliciano, Yoliannie Torres-Martínez, Jorge Torres-Vélez, Keyshla Encarnación-Pizarro, Samariz Fragoso-Pagán, and Luis Torres-Colón

University of Puerto Rico, Medical Sciences Campus, School of Health Professions, Occupational Therapy Program, PO Box 365067, San Juan, PR 00936-5067, USA

Correspondence should be addressed to Rosa Román-Oyola; rosa.roman2@upr.edu

Academic Editor: Karen Stagnitti

Background. Play serves as an essential medium for parent-child interaction; however, engaging children with ASD through play can be a challenge for parents. *Purpose.* The purpose of this phenomenological study was to explore the perspectives of parents with children on the autism spectrum regarding play experiences and self-efficacy during play encounters. *Method.* Semistructured interviews were administered to 8 parents of children 3–7 years of age with ASD. The analysis was guided by the constant comparison method. *Findings.* Parental narratives denoted playful experiences reflecting components of Skard and Bundy's model of playfulness. The facilitation of framing and suspension of reality were generally more challenging than facilitating intrinsic motivation and internal control. Participants associated self-efficacy during play with their perceived ability to interact with their child and with positive emotions experienced during play. Fathers generally derived a greater sense of self-efficacy from play encounters than mothers, and this was explained by differences in fathers' and mothers' motivations for playing. Mothers were motivated to play for outcome-oriented reasons (e.g., promote the child's progress) whereas fathers' motivations depicted greater emotional emphasis, reflecting a better match between motivation and perceived indicators of efficacy during play. *Conclusion.* The results suggest that a good match between motivation for playing and perceived indicators of efficacy during play is important for a parental sense of self-efficacy. Occupational therapists should utilize coaching strategies to increase parents' understanding of play and playfulness and how they can affect a sense of parental self-efficacy.

1. Introduction

Playing has an important and primary role in childhood. As a child's primary occupation [1], play is as natural as breathing [2]. Play involves a child's active participation in an activity or time spent with peers and involves agency and the ownership of ideas [3]. During play, children learn important motor, cognitive, and social skills as well as creativity and self-confidence, which are skills that are required throughout life [1, 4, 5].

Children approach play in different ways based on different motivations and dispositions. These motivations and dispositions form the subject's attitude during play, also known as playfulness. Skard and Bundy [6] proposed a model of playfulness that identifies four primary characteristics of play. The first characteristic is *framing*, which refers to behaviors used during play that identify the nature of the activity as play. Players give framing cues to others, and good players must be able to give and read cues. The second characteristic of play is that it is *intrinsically motivated*. This means that players engage in the play activity because they enjoy the activity and experience benefits as a result. The third characteristic of play is *internal control*; this characteristic allows players to decide what they want to play, who they want to play with, and how and when the play should end. The fourth and final characteristic is *freedom to suspend reality*, which determines how closely a play transaction resembles the objective reality. Different strategies are employed to facilitate the suspension of reality. A player can pretend that he is someone else or that an object is something other than what it really is (e.g., pretends to be a chef; pretends that a box is an airplane). Players can also suspend reality by teasing or telling jokes [6, 7].

According to Skard and Bundy's model [6], a child's level of playfulness is determined by the summation of all the aforementioned characteristics. Evidence indicates that playfulness can differ among children with various developmental challenges. Playfulness in children with autism spectrum disorders (ASD) is affected by behaviors inherently related to their condition; children with ASD tend to be less playful than their typically developing counterparts [8, 9]. Behavioral challenges for play in children with ASD include fixed interests, lack of flexibility, impaired social skills, engagement in ritual repetitive behaviors, low levels of pretend play, anger or frustration, hyper- or hyposensitivities, and difficulty understanding nonverbal cues [10, 11].

Evidence suggests that the inability of some children with ASD to fully engage in play has negative effects on parents' as well as the child's well-being and sense of self-efficacy [12, 13]. Bandura [14] defined self-efficacy as an individual's belief in their ability to achieve a goal or outcome. Parental self-efficacy refers to the confidence and expectations of a parent regarding their ability to perform the parental role competently and effectively [15]. Compared to parents of typically developing children, parents of children with ASD experience higher levels of stress, depression, and hopelessness [16–18]. Participation in and enjoyment of play have important benefits for both parents and children, especially in families of children with ASD. Adult playfulness is a significant predictor of emotional parental self-efficacy among parents raising children with ASD, more so than the degree of sensory processing impairment inherently related to the child's diagnosis [19].

Playfulness is a relationship-based phenomenon and an important factor for the development of social relationships between children and their main caregivers [2, 20, 21]. Given social and communication difficulties in children with ASD, their parents may feel incompetent in their ability to establish an emotional connection with them. Additionally, the quality of involvement of the parents is an important variable for the ability of children with ASD to participate in play [22–24] and can also benefit the parents. Parents of young children with ASD that actively participate in coaching processes or guided educational treatments based on the use of strategies to maximize engagement opportunities with their child exhibit increased competence and higher levels of effect [13, 25].

Available evidence supports a potential relationship between play, playfulness, and parental self-efficacy, especially in families raising young children on the autism spectrum. Yet few studies have examined the experiential components underlying this relationship. The purpose of this phenomenological study was to explore the perspectives of parents with children on the autism spectrum regarding play experiences and self-efficacy during play encounters. The study addressed two research questions: (1) How do parents' narratives about play encounters reflect the elements of a playful experience for their child (based on the model of Skard and Bundy)? (2) How efficient do fathers and mothers feel when playing with their child with ASD?

2. Methods

2.1. Study Design. This study was guided by a phenomenological design with an interpretative approach. Interpretative approaches within phenomenology allow ample examination of relationships and the significance of knowledge and contexts [26]. Interpretative approaches are philosophically associated with social constructivism, which emphasizes the subjective meaning of an individual's experiences [27]. Phenomenology studies these subjective meanings to explicate the structure or essence of the lived experience in search of the unity of meanings [28]. Our research involved a detailed examination of the significance of participant play experiences with their children with ASD, which we defined as the phenomenon under study.

2.2. Participants. All study procedures were reviewed and approved by the Institutional Review Board of the University of Puerto Rico, Medical Sciences Campus. Four couples of parents of children with ASD from different parts of Puerto Rico consented to participate in semistructured in-depth interviews. The inclusion criteria were as follows: (a) availability of both parents for participation, (b) parents ≥ 21 years of age, and (c) children 3–7 years of age with a diagnosis of ASD. Age range selections were made based on previous investigations of the importance of reciprocal interactions between parents and children [29]. Table 1 describes some characteristics of participant parental couples.

2.3. Recruitment. Participants were recruited through direct contact or by referral from occupational therapists of children with ASD. In cases of recruitment by referral, occupational therapists were asked to make the first contact with parents regardless of whether the children were currently receiving therapy. After parents communicated interest in the study, we personally delivered a participation package including two consent forms (one for each parent), a sociodemographic information data form and an instruction sheet. Interviews with participants were scheduled at the participants' convenience. To minimize the possibility of bias associated with social desirability and interviewers' gender in participant narratives [30, 31], fathers were interviewed by male researchers and mothers were interviewed by female researchers.

2.4. Data Collection and Analysis. Data were collected via in-depth semistructured interviews. Open-ended questions were employed to allow participants to interpret the meaning of the question and respond based on their personal feelings and perceptions. Probe questions were included as part of the protocol and used to enrich the discussion as needed. Examples are as follows:

Table 1: Description of participants.

Participants	Age	Gender and age of the child with ASD	Couple living together/apart	Additional members of the family
Mother 1	25	Female, 7	Together	2 sisters (5 and 3 y/o, respectively)
Father 1	31			
Mother 2	38	Female, 4	Together	No additional members
Father 2	43			
Mother 3	27	Male, 5	Apart	Child lives with mother but stays with father frequently. Has a brother (14 y/o) on his father's side, who lives with the father
Father 3	43			
Mother 4	40	Male, 5	Together	No additional members
Father 4	45			

Main question: how do you feel when playing with your son/daughter?

Possible probes: how satisfied do you feel with the way you play? Do you think that you interact effectively while playing? What makes you think that way? Is there anything you would change about those playing moments?

Interviewing researchers were trained in qualitative methods and use of the interview protocol. Prior to the study data collection, all researchers performed practice interviews with volunteer mothers and fathers of typically developing children using the study protocol. Mothers and fathers were interviewed separately. The length of each study interview varied by participant in accordance with their comments and experiences but generally lasted approximately 45 minutes to an hour. Interviews were audio-taped with the participants' consent for later transcription in Spanish. All identifying information was removed from transcripts, and the names mentioned during the interview were replaced with pseudonyms to protect the identities of the participants. Each parent received $15.00 as compensation for their time.

The process of data analysis was guided by the principles of the constant comparison method [32], which allowed structural corroborations among members of the research team. The analysis steps included two cycles of coding as described by Saldaña [33]. For the purposes of the first coding cycle, each researcher was assigned to 1 of 2 analysis teams. The principal researcher and 2 other researchers participated in both teams. First, researchers thoroughly read the transcripts assigned to their respective team and individually identified initial categories. Then, individual researchers met with their respective teams to read transcripts as a group and discuss/agree upon emergent categories.

In the second coding cycle, portions of transcripts were organized into tables presenting mothers' and fathers' responses to the same questions side by side for intracouple comparisons of responses. Then, couples' responses were examined side by side for intercouple comparisons. During this cycle, researchers met several times to revise codes, share analytic memos, and reconfigure codes from the first cycle by linking interview chunks and/or initial codes. A total of four major patterns/themes were identified from the data: (1) general context of the playing experience; (2) playfulness in the context of parent-child interactions; (3) self-efficacy during play; and (4) motivations vs. benefits.

In qualitative studies, rigor is determined by the criteria of credibility, dependability, confirmability, and transferability [26]. Broad descriptions of the data collection and analysis process serve to reinforce credibility and dependability. Confirmability is achieved by showing that results are derived from a well-documented research process and through informants (e.g., participants' direct quotes) that support the results [34]. Transferability of the findings is demonstrated when practical implications derived from the findings are pertinent to other contexts [34].

3. Results

The following results include verbatim excerpts of participant narratives selected to exemplify the underlying themes. Identifying information has been removed from quotations. The verbatim texts were translated into English by the Translation Center, College of Humanities (University of PR), for the sole purpose of this article. Preservation of essential meaning, content, and, insofar as possible, general tone were the main goals of the translation. To enhance clarity and preserve the parents' anonymity, participants are identified with numbers 1 to 4 (e.g., mother number 1 and father number 1 form a parental couple). Each participant's number is shown at the beginning of each quotation.

3.1. General Context of the Play Experience. Prior to in-depth examination of the excerpts as they relate to the research questions, it is pertinent to contextualize participants' perspectives about play experiences with their children. In general, parents' play experiences were defined by codes related to emotions regarding play, relevance of play as part of a routine, and awareness of the child's diagnosis. All participants expressed positive emotions related to play experiences with their children. Satisfaction, happiness, and trust were among the most frequently expressed emotions. Participants also commented about the importance of playing with their children; their narratives reflected that moments for playing are specified as parts of the family routine. Generally, fathers indicated that they played with their children after arriving home from work.

In contrast, mothers more frequently commented about how they integrate play into household chores and child-care activities:

Mother 1: *We are playing from the moment we wake up, from the moment we are brushing our teeth we are already playing because it's a brushing teeth game, it's another one to get dressed, and that's how we move forward ...*

Father 1: *(We play) When I get home from work, before going to sleep... Like almost all of the time I am home, I try to spend it with my daughters and we are always playing*

Mother 3: *Look, I can be cooking, and he comes to the kitchen because he helps me a lot... He's very collaborative and he comes to the kitchen and wants to add sauce very carefully, right [... And while ...] the food is getting ready, we have a tickle or kiss game...*

Mother 4: *[...] When we get home, dad and I get turns. Dad makes dinner and mom helps with homework. I start playing with him while dinner is ready. After dinner, I make the next day's lunch and dad plays with him, that is to say, we switch.*

Narratives about the difficulty of incorporating play encounters into ordinary routines were also very common among the participants. Main reasons for this challenge were related to the time demands of complex daily routines as well as to the inherent social-emotional challenges faced by children with ASD:

Mother 1: *Sometimes it's complicated because she's not always in the mood to play or learn or to do things or every day activities such as getting dressed or whatever. But, that's why it's simpler with play, because there are moments in which [we lose control and] we start yelling and we see how agitated she is and truth is nothing will be solved that way. We have learned... we'll take it slowly, we'll take a breath, and we'll do it a different way, and playing, well, makes it simpler...*

Mother 4: *Well, we are not at home most of the day; we work from 8 (am) to 7 at night. So, he is in activities most of the day, but when we get home, dad and I take turns [to play].*

Father 4: *Obligations... like you have to do the laundry, you have to cook ... Here we both do the chores; my wife does some and I do some others. Sometimes my wife may be there (points to the dining room) working and I am over here making dinner for him and sometimes that moment, well, I am not dedicating it to him... Well, I do dedicate it to him because it's for him, but I am not playing with him. You get me?*

Mother 3: *Well look, in some aspect it is (easy for the boy to play), what happens is that there are moments where he wants to play and [...] I am a mom and I do not stop working and I still have responsibilities and, the truth is that, as a person, I get exhausted ...*

Participant narratives also denoted awareness of the challenges associated with their child's diagnosis. In the case of Mother 2, it was possible to perceive some frustration about the ways in which she was able or unable to play with her daughter:

Mother 2: *[...] When I notice we start playing (while moving a toy she's holding and acting like paying) "hi, how are you?" she hates that... when I grab a toy and [try imaginary play], she hates it. And the anxiety of not being able to accomplish it... It freezes me [...]. Because I get so anxious that "I must do it, and I have to do it" and that [anxiety] I need to control. It's something that "kills" me (laughs).*

Another way in which participants denoted consciousness about the child's diagnosis was by highlighting the importance of play interactions as a mean to promote and follow their child's progress:

Father 1: *Well, the moments I enjoy the most, sometimes are when, when she does something that surprises me. In other words, let us say, well, that she does not pay attention to some things or she's very reluctant to do so and so activity and in that moment, you are doing something, and she comes and starts doing what you are doing and we are getting along. (...) It's said that children [on the spectrum], do not let people hug them, that [they avoid] visual contact, that they do not let... And you can hug that girl! You can be with her, she comes to me when I get home, she jumps at me! I enjoy those things because I thought they would not happen.*

Mother 2: *Yes, (play has its benefits) because I can tell you that six months ago, we could not [play]. Then, as a mom and human being who has been there, I was very frustrated, right, over the diagnosis ... [But play] helps me to feel that we are moving forward, that it's worth the effort and it makes me feel that we are doing it right because we are seeing progress.*

3.2. Playfulness in the Context of Parent-Child Interactions. Analysis of participant narratives revealed the elements of playfulness embedded in parents' experiences. It was clear that play was often shaped by the child's preferences, indicating that parents sought interactions that were *intrinsically motivating* for their child. Most parents explained that the best way to play with their child was by immersing themselves in the type of play the child had already established, thus reflecting the element of motivation proposed in Skard and Bundy's model [6]. From parents' perspectives, parent-child interactions were more effective and enjoyable when play was intrinsically motivated rather than when the child's play preference was disrupted or when parents tried to impose their own choices on children during the play interaction:

Mother 2: *I try to play by her rules, and to not impose on her my way of playing. I can deal with her a little better when we play by her rules.*

Father 1: *... if you want to force the game she'll get difficult, but difficult as in she'll want to hit you and everything because she's doing something and you cannot interrupt what she's doing; because she'll start kicking at you and [yell] "I don't want to" and there will not be any break.*

Mother 4: *I try to play the same games he likes to encourage him.*

Father 2: *It's easy [to play]... The only thing I have to do is show her something she likes, and it's over. I show her the water bomb, and that's it, we start playing.*

Internal control was another element apparent in the narratives. Parents indicated that parent-child interactions were mainly arbitrated by the child, meaning that the child maintained overall control within play encounters. Although parents had some influence over some activities, they were mostly regulated by the child's preferences and feedback during the parent-child interaction. Parents indicated that children enjoyed play encounters and that interactions were reciprocal and occurred for longer periods of time when the child was in control. Both, mothers and fathers, denoted that when play preferences were forced, children tended to avoid play by displaying tantrums or trying to change play activities. This corresponds to Skard and Bundy's model [6]. When children feel in control and feel no constraints during play encounters, the outcomes of interactions are more effective, especially during parent-child interactions.

Father 4: ... *it's easy [to play] as long as he likes the kind of play, it's easy. It's going to be very difficult if it's something he does not like...*

Father 2: *The hardest part, well, when the play is guided, you know there is free play and guided play [...] if it's a guided game, well, it is harder because setting a pattern with a structure is not so easy with her, but if it's a free activity you can spend the whole day playing.*

The element of *framing* was also noted in the narratives. Often, mothers and fathers indicated a desire to prolong play encounters. When the child's preference or interest during an activity was interrupted, parents resorted to framing or cueing the child to continue the play process. Main framing strategies included the presentation of preferred toys or games that the child would enjoy and the initiation of cues (or responses to child cues) for playing. These strategies prolonged attention and participation during play encounters.

Father 1: *I get one of her favorite toys or I take her blanket away from her to make her come after me because she loves blankets and she takes with her 4 or 6 blankets wherever she goes [...] Well, since I know she likes them, I take it away from her and I run to the bedroom and she comes looking for it. So, that's the moment I take to start playing. It's the same as with the little dolls [or other toys she love]... those are the little tricks I use [to play with her] (laughs)."*

Father 2: *She does not give up. When I get home, she tells me, "Seated" and then grabs me, pulls me by my arm, and takes me to the room and sits me on the floor (smiles) [saying:]. "Seated, let's play" and from there we start playing with anything that's available.*

Mother 2: *We are always having to create playtime in a way that gets her attention, whether cheering: "Yeah, Betsy, that's it, very good, we're going to play!" (lifting her arms in a cheering motion)... Very energetic, so it like grabs her attention and then she comes. That's what gets her.*

Furthermore, parents' descriptions of play encounters with their children reflected the element of *freedom to suspend reality*. It was relatively easy to observe simple forms of reality suspension such as teasing or rule stretching, especially among fathers. For example, Father 1 talked about play-wrestling with his daughter *("She knows the mood I have. She knows my attitude [...] Sometimes, she even knows what I want to do. You know if I pick her up and take her to bed, she knows that we're going to play wrestle or something like that... Then she gets excited, she gets motivated.")*. This brief excerpt from Father 1 denotes, not only the suspension of reality by stretching the rules (fathers do not typically wrestle with their daughters) but also the importance of his playful attitude ("*She knows the mood I have. She knows my attitude...*") to cue the daughter and frame the play experience. Another strategy for reality suspension was pretending to be an object (e.g., a doll or action figure); however, this was not effective for all participants. While Father 1 indicated the use of little dolls to maintain his daughter's attention during play, Mother 2 confessed that she would love to engage in more imaginary play with her daughter and suggested that this affected her sense of self-efficacy during play activities:

Mother 2 ... *I would like to make her playtime last longer. That's why, I do not feel a hundred percent satisfied, even though I feel happy that I am able to play with her... but it's really frustrating because you have to pull off this cooperative game and... I am like, "Here goes the car: beep beep." (Moving her hands like she's driving a car), but she does not like that. She does not like it to the point that she will even get rid of the toys, and take them away from me... She'll play with me; but it has to be dolling me up, putting makeup on me, doing my nails, but anything that has to do with grabbing toys or having conversations, she does not like it. That's where I am frustrated, I would love to be able to do that a little.*

3.3. Self-Efficacy during Play: Motivations vs. Benefits. All participants communicated feelings of efficacy and satisfaction regarding play experiences with their children. Perceived ability to interact with their child was the main aspect that made parents feel competent. Playing provided parents with an opportunity to relate to their children and strengthen parent-child bonds. Additionally, parents connected play efficacy with positive feelings experienced during play moments, such as the emotion of seeing a child participating in, completing, and enjoying a play activity:

Father 1: *I mean, I consider myself pretty effective. Any person can come along, even her mother, and tries to do what I do, and it will not work ... I mean, I have my way, my tricks... because it's a matter of motivating her to play, to take her the things she likes. If she likes dolls, or if you see on this day she woke up wanting her blanket or on that day she woke up wanting dolls... you already know which way to go to motivate her to play with you.*

Mother 1: ...*For example, we were playing um ... bowling, and then, it happened that she knocked down the pins, and you see her joy... it's like "I did it!", like she feels successful.*

Overall, fathers verbalized feelings of better efficacy during play experiences with their children than did mothers. This observation is exemplified by the excerpt from Father 1 shown above. Indeed, mothers were more likely to identify aspects of the play process that they wanted to improve or change:

Mother 1: *[I would like to get better] as far more improvisation [...] and... I do not know maybe a little more athleticism, running harder.*

Mother 2: *I still need to learn a little more, how to get through to her, how to get her a little more interested, uh, work a little more in that area.*

Mother 3: *[How effective I feel] depends really on the game. There are games where like ... for example PlayStation: [He invites me] "Mommy come play with me." Now, there are other games, for example, painting... Surprisingly, that does not really get his attention. So, since I have to struggle a little bit for him to sit with me [...] it's a little challenging to get him interested and it's like (sighs) let me see what else I can do to get his attention.*

The analysis also identified different *motivations for playing* between fathers and mothers. It was notable that fathers' spontaneous responses about motivations for playing reflected a greater emphasis on emotional aspects such as seeing their children laughing, smiling, and happy, while mothers were motivated to play to promote progress and enhance their child's necessary skills. This difference is shown in the excerpts below, presented by a parental couple (e.g., Mother 1 followed by Father 1):

Mother 1: *[It motivates me] to see that you can accomplish a lot of things through playtime [for] example, writing, reading, colors, everything... Playing ... is the easiest way of teaching these children.*

Father 1: *Seeing her laugh, seeing that she's having a good time; also, we can learn too...*

Mother 4: *...Helping him, more than anything, to socialize, that when he sees the neighbors or his friends outside, he can be sociable [...] and that he spends time with them, that he does not become a shy person and above all, share with people.*

Father 4: *The first thing is the love I have towards him, as my son... that motivates me.*

Interestingly, when asked about the perceived *benefits* of playing experiences, an opposite trend was observed. Mothers' spontaneous responses tended to emphasize more emotional benefits of play (e.g., trust and bonding) while fathers were likely to identify aspects related to the child's progress or skill development.

Mother 3: *Aside from working on what we call quality time for both [...] Playing develops trust. He feels how we speak during playtime. So, he gets aware that: "Oh, I can speak with mommy", or "I can tell things to mommy", and since he's young now, it's important to develop this confidence and this communication with him... Playtime helps a lot with this. In addition, we have fun and we laugh together. So, when he gets older he's going to say: "I remember when mommy played that with me..."*

Father 3: *[...] Oh, yes, it [play]soothes him, it helps him to go to bed more relaxed.*

Mother 1: *Yes [play is beneficial]. As it pertains to confidence, I think my daughter pretty much trusts me ...*

Father 1: *Yes, because [in addition to strengthens the attachment], she develops a lot better, she accepts physical contact. If I had never played with her, if I had never become interested in playing with her, well, she would not want contact with anybody [...Also,] I think movement [coordination] is developed, I mean, before, she would trip over herself a lot. Sometimes, she did not even want to play. But now, not anymore. Now she's well-coordinated, very agile, and she has great equilibrium!*

4. Discussion

The purpose of this phenomenological study was to explore the play experiences of parents with children on the autism spectrum. First, we focused on parents' narratives reflecting playfulness while playing with their child. Consistent with previous research, there were characteristic differences in the contexts and types of play used by mothers and fathers [35–37]. Mothers tended to insert play moments into daily routines while fathers had opportunities for playing that were not necessarily embedded within other daily tasks.

We were able to identify elements of Skard and Bundy's model of playfulness [6] in participant comments. Mothers and fathers assigned importance to facilitating their child's *intrinsic motivation* and *internal control* and recognized that, by doing so, they were better able to engage the child in play. Skard and Bundy [6] stated that internal control requires that all participants in the play experience can make decisions regarding the details of the play encounter, thus implying a certain degree of negotiation. Yet we found that when parents, specifically fathers, wished to see the child's enjoyment during play moments, they opted to relinquish internal control to a substantial extent.

Parents' comments indicative of *framing* were generally efforts to offer "play cues" to children. The message "this is play" was deliberately linked to things that intrinsically motivated the child. The observed relationship between intrinsic motivation and framing is not surprising. Rather, we were interested in the "tangible quality" of the framing cues used by parents (or the child; e.g., the use of specific objects or a very energetic attitude). Although these types of cues can be used by any parent with any child, it is possible that tangible qualities have particular importance in families with children on the autism spectrum. Framing and scaffolding, although not equivalent, are conceptually related to one another. Various terms that refer to scaffolding strategies (e.g., prompting, modeling) can also be used as cues to portray a play situation to the child [38–40]. Social participation difficulties are thought to interfere with the development of complex play skills in children with ASD and might make it more difficult for parents to scaffold play [39]. Further, evidence suggests that children with ASD rely on others to generate novel ideas about how to play to a greater degree than do typically developing children [41].

Pretend play is the most common form of *suspension of reality* [7]. Children with ASD have a reduced preference for this type of play [42–44]. Experiences of participants in this study corroborated this idea and generally recounted less obvious suspensions of reality such as teasing (e.g., the father running with his daughter's blanket) or stretching the rules (e.g., the father play-wrestling with his daughter), especially in the narratives of fathers. We also recognized challenges related to engaging the child in pretend play situations. One mother verbalized significant frustration about not being able to actively engage her daughter in pretend play. This is consistent with previous evidence; in a cross-sectional study, Case-Smith and Kuhaneck [45] found that children with developmental delays tended to prefer rough-and-tumble play and object exploration and presented lower preferences for drawing and coloring, construction, and doll and action figurine play.

Our results indicated that, in terms of playfulness, facilitating the elements of framing and suspension of reality was more challenging than facilitating child's intrinsic motivation and internal control. This is in line with previous research stating that the number of imitated actions and amount of elaborate pretend play (both areas of difficulty for children with ASD) are positively associated with the suspension of reality and framing dimensions of playfulness, respectively [41]. Despite the difficulty of certain elements, it was perceived that participants assumed an important role in facilitating playful experiences with their children and that the playful attitude of parents was an important facilitator or barrier in this context.

The second question guiding our analysis in this study was how competent do fathers and mothers feel when playing with their child with ASD? Perceived ability to interact with the child and positive emotions experienced during play moments were among the main aspects that participants associated with self-efficacy during play. Fathers derived a greater sense of self-efficacy from play encounters while mothers were more likely to identify areas of their own performance that they wanted to improve. A key factor explaining differences in the perceived efficacy of mothers and fathers during play is their perceptions about the motivations for playing and the benefits associated with the play experience.

As stated, an ability to interact with children and the derivation of positive emotions from play interactions were identified by all participants as indicators of efficacy. The analysis of fathers' narratives reflected a better match between motivators for playing and the aforementioned indicators of efficacy. While fathers' motivations depicted a greater emotional emphasis (e.g., *"seeing her smiling"*), mothers' motivators were more outcome-oriented (i.e., more focused on promoting the child's development of skills; e.g., *"help him to socialize better"*). Interestingly, the opposite was observed when analyzing the benefits that parents derived from play moments. Fathers identified benefits that were more outcome- or task-oriented (e.g., ability to move more efficiently; a more relaxed state at sleeping time) while mothers identified more emotionally oriented benefits (e.g., own enjoyment and enhancement of the child's trust in them). Considering that fathers were more inclined to judge themselves as competent during play than mothers, the findings of this study suggest that a better match between motivators for playing and perceived indicators of efficacy during play are relevant to a parental sense of self-efficacy.

The present findings have several important implications. First, it may be useful to help parents to better understand the difference between play or playfulness and the elements of playfulness. A comprehensive understanding of the elements of playfulness can guide parents in equalizing the importance attributed to play as a means as well as an end. Too often, parents (in the case of this study, especially mothers) of children with ASD and other disabilities are so overwhelmed by delays in their child's development that they forget the importance of *playing playfully* and making play encounters a pleasurable experience for everyone involved. The enjoyment of these encounters not only addresses the child's challenges in social participation but also enhances parental self-efficacy [19].

Participants in this study cared about having opportunities to relate to and play with their children, but some (mothers more than fathers) were unable to derive a sensation of self-efficacy from playing. Education-based treatments may help parents like these to adjust their perceptions to improve consistency between definitions of efficacy during play and motivations to play, resulting in the enhanced perception of parental self-efficacy. Occupational performance coaching (OPC) can be an alternative. OPC is an educational treatment that uses collaborative problem-solving within a coaching relationship in which parents are guided to identify and apply effective solutions to occupational performance problems with their children [46].

This is particularly significant in the context of occupational therapists' family-centered interventions, since role competence is an important desired intervention outcome [47]. Occupational therapists have the opportunity to use coaching, especially when working with families with children in early childhood [48, 49]. In terms of play, important reflections include the following: How are we focusing coaching processes? Are we balancing teaching families about play as a means and as an end? Evidence indicates that there is still a long way to go; a study by Kuhaneck et al. [50] found that only 4% of 198 pediatric occupational therapists reported the use of play as an intervention outcome.

On the other hand, differences between parents in motivators for playing might be attributed to parents' perceptions about what is expected from them based on traditional gender roles [51]. Research suggests that gender roles are critical for defining the implicit objectives of parent-child interactions [52]. Further, evidence suggests that playfulness is a trait with likely ties to environmental and interactional characteristics [53]. Thus, it is pertinent to help parents to visualize playfulness not only simply as a personality trait but also as an environmental and interactional component. Parents themselves are a key part of the child's environment. Additionally, traditional gender roles are, to some extent, part of the parents' environment and can influence parents' expectancies about play encounters with their children. This concept merits further exploration in future studies. In summary, the results of this study suggest that parents' expectancies and attitudes affect not only the way in which they approach play encounters but also the way in which their children approach the play experience; this in turn has effects on parents' sense of self-efficacy during play.

4.1. Limitations. This study contributes to a body of knowledge about play and playfulness in families of children with ASD and the potential relevance of these constructs for parental self-efficacy. The profiles of couples that participated in this study were relatively diverse. This allowed the collection of information covering a broad spectrum of family contexts (e.g., parents living together with more than one child; parents living together with only one daughter with ASD; parents with one son with ASD not living together; and parents living together with very demanding workloads). While this can be considered a strength, it must be recognized that this was a phenomenological study with a limited number of participants (4 parental couples and therefore 8 participants). We understand that having a limited quantity of participant couples along with such diverse profiles entailed the main limitation of this study, because it impeded reaching saturation. For example, the narratives of Mother 2 (who had an only daughter) depicted substantial frustration regarding play interactions with her daughter with ASD (e.g., *when I grab a toy and [try imaginary play]... she hates it. And the anxiety of not being able to accomplish it... It freezes me [...]. Because I get so anxious...).* On the opposite, Mother 1 (who had two additional typically developing daughters) did not describe comparable frustrations with her daughter with ASD. Having additional participant mothers with similar family context (e.g., more mothers with an only daughter with ASD and mothers with additional neurotypical daughters) would have allowed us to verify if their experiences and perceptions were similar.

The abovementioned issues give rise to areas deserving additional exploration in future studies, such as play styles of parents of children with ASD in the context of families with multiple children, between dyads of mothers/fathers-daughters with ASD, among mothers/fathers-sons with ASD, and in the context of families in which parents do not live together or in which children are under the care of family members other than the parents. Additionally, it would be worthwhile to evaluate our findings against the narratives of parents with neurotypical children to verify whether the ability to sustain and enjoy play encounters with their children is linked in any way to their sense of self-efficacy. Finally, we recommended that future studies examining areas explored in this study utilize more comprehensive qualitative designs such as grounded theory.

5. Conclusion

The purpose of this study was to explore the perspectives of parents of children on the autism spectrum regarding play experiences and self-efficacy during play encounters with their children. Specific attention was given to elements of playfulness and parents' sense of self-efficacy during play encounters with their children. Participants' narratives indicated that facilitating framing and suspension of reality was more challenging than facilitating the child's intrinsic motivation and internal control during play. Finally, the results suggest that a better match between motivators for playing and perceived indicators of efficacy during play has a significant relevance for parental self-efficacy. Occupational therapists should employ coaching strategies to help parents increase their understanding of play and playfulness and how these elements can affect their sense of self-efficacy.

Disclosure

The authors alone are responsible for the content and writing of the paper.

Acknowledgments

The preparation and publication of this article were partially funded by the Hispanic in Research Capability Endowment (HiREC), Universidad de Puerto Rico, Medical Sciences Campus.

References

[1] L. D. Parham and L. Fazio, *Play in Occupational Therapy for Children*, Mosby, St. Louis, MO, USA, 2nd edition, 2008.

[2] C. E. Schaefer and A. A. Drewes, "The therapeutic power of play and play therapy," in *Foundations of Play Therapy*, C. E. Schaefer, Ed., pp. 15–23, Wiley, Hoboken, NJ, USA, 2011.

[3] M. Theobald, S. Danby, J. Einarsdóttir et al., "Children's perspectives of play and learning for educational practice," *Education Sciences*, vol. 5, no. 4, pp. 345–362, 2015.

[4] E. P. Fisher, "The impact of play on development: a meta-analysis," *Play & Culture*, vol. 5, pp. 159–181, 1992.

[5] L. A. Barnett, "Characterizing playfulness: correlates with individual attributes and personality traits," *Play & Culture*, vol. 4, pp. 371–393, 1991.

[6] G. Skard and A. C. Bundy, "Test of playfulness," in *Play in Occupational Therapy for Children*, L. D. Parham and L. S. Fazio, Eds., pp. 71–93, Mosby, St. Louis, MO, USA, 2008.

[7] A. C. Bundy, "Children and play: can I play, too?," in *Kids Can Be Kids: A Childhood Occupation Approach*, S. J. Lane and A. C. Bundy, Eds., pp. 28–43, F. A. Davis, Philadelphia, PA, USA, 2012.

[8] R. P. Hobson, A. Lee, and J. A. Hobson, "Qualities of symbolic play among children with autism: a social-developmental perspective," *Journal of Autism and Developmental Disorders*, vol. 39, no. 1, pp. 12–22, 2009.

[9] N. Skaines, S. Rodger, and A. Bundy, "Playfulness in children with autistic disorder and their typically developing peers," *British Journal of Occupational Therapy*, vol. 69, no. 11, pp. 505–512, 2006.

[10] R. MacDonald, S. Sacramone, R. Mansfield, K. Wiltz, and W. H. Ahearn, "Using video modeling to teach reciprocal pretend play to children with autism," *Journal of Applied Behavior Analysis*, vol. 42, no. 1, pp. 43–55, 2009.

[11] J. Howard and K. McInnes, "The impact of children's perception of an activity as play rather than not play on emotional well-being," *Child: Care, Health and Development*, vol. 39, no. 5, pp. 737–742, 2013.

[12] T. W. Vernon, R. L. Koegel, H. Dauterman, and K. Stolen, "An early social engagement intervention for young children with autism and their parents," *Journal of Autism and Developmental Disorders*, vol. 42, no. 12, pp. 2702–2717, 2012.

[13] D. Keen, D. Couzens, S. Muspratt, and S. Rodger, "The effects of a parent-focused intervention for children with a recent diagnosis of autism spectrum disorder on parenting stress

and competence," *Research in Autism Spectrum Disorders*, vol. 4, no. 2, pp. 229–241, 2010.

[14] A. Bandura, "Self-efficacy: toward a unifying theory of behavioral change," *Psychological Review*, vol. 84, no. 2, pp. 191–215, 1977.

[15] D. M. Teti and D. M. Gelfand, "Behavioral competence among mothers of infants in the first year: the mediational role of maternal self-efficacy," *Child Development*, vol. 62, no. 5, pp. 918–929, 1991.

[16] P. R. Benson and K. L. Karlof, "Anger, stress proliferation, and depressed mood among parents of children with ASD: a longitudinal replication," *Journal of Autism and Developmental Disorders*, vol. 39, no. 2, pp. 350–362, 2009.

[17] R. P. Hastings and T. Brown, "Behavior problems of children with autism, parental self-efficacy, and mental health," *American Journal on Mental Retardation*, vol. 107, no. 3, pp. 222–232, 2002.

[18] V. Totsika, R. P. Hastings, E. Emerson, D. M. Berridge, and G. A. Lancaster, "Prosocial skills in young children with autism, and their mothers' psychological well-being: longitudinal relationships," *Research in Autism Spectrum Disorders*, vol. 13-14, pp. 25–31, 2015.

[19] R. Román-Oyola, S. Reynolds, I. Soto-Feliciano, L. Cabrera-Mercader, and J. Vega-Santana, "Child's sensory profile and adult playfulness as predictors of parental self-efficacy," *American Journal of Occupational Therapy*, vol. 71, no. 2, 2017.

[20] G. L. Landreth, "Play therapy in elementary school settings," in *Handbook of Play Therapy*, C. E. Schaefer and K. J. O'Connor, Eds., pp. 202–212, Wiley, New York, NY, USA, 1983.

[21] B. Youell, "The importance of play and playfulness," *European Journal of Psychotherapy & Counselling*, vol. 10, no. 2, pp. 121–129, 2008.

[22] M. Flippin and L. R. Watson, "Fathers' and mothers' verbal responsiveness and the language skills of young children with autism spectrum disorder," *American Journal of Speech-Language Pathology*, vol. 24, no. 3, pp. 400–410, 2015.

[23] S. Y. Shire, A. Gulsrud, and C. Kasari, "Increasing responsive parent-child interactions and joint engagement: comparing the influence of parent-mediated intervention and parent psychoeducation," *Journal of Autism and Developmental Disorders*, vol. 46, no. 5, pp. 1737–1747, 2016.

[24] C. Kasari, A. C. Gulsrud, C. Wong, S. Kwon, and J. Locke, "Randomized controlled caregiver mediated joint engagement intervention for toddlers with autism," *Journal of Autism and Developmental Disorders*, vol. 40, no. 9, pp. 1045–1056, 2010.

[25] R. L. Koegel, A. Bimbela, and L. Schreibman, "Collateral effects of parent training on family interactions," *Journal of Autism and Developmental Disorders*, vol. 26, no. 3, pp. 347–359, 1996.

[26] Y. S. Lincoln and E. G. Guba, *Naturalistic Inquiry*, Sage Publications, Beverly Hills, CA, USA, 1985.

[27] J. Creswell, *Qualitative Inquiry and Research Design*, Sage Publications, Los Angeles, CA, USA, 2013.

[28] P. Rose, J. Beeby, and D. Parker, "Academic rigour in the lived experience of researchers using phenomenological methods in nursing," *Journal of Advanced Nursing*, vol. 21, no. 6, pp. 1123–1129, 1995.

[29] T. Keller, J. Ramisch, and M. Carolan, "Relationships of children with autism spectrum disorders and their fathers," *The Qualitative Report*, vol. 19, no. 33, pp. 1–15, 2014.

[30] B. Pini, "Interviewing men: gender and the collection and interpretation of qualitative data," *Journal of Sociology*, vol. 41, no. 2, pp. 201–216, 2005.

[31] A. Broom, K. Hand, and P. Tovey, "The role of gender, environment and individual biography in shaping qualitative interview data," *International Journal of Social Research Methodology*, vol. 12, no. 1, pp. 51–65, 2009.

[32] M. B. Miles, A. M. Huberman, and J. Saldaña, *Qualitative Data Analysis: A Methods Sourcebook*, Sage Publications, Thousand Oaks, CA, USA, 3rd edition, 2014.

[33] J. Saldaña, *The Coding Manual for Qualitative Researchers*, Sage Publications, Los Angeles, CA, USA, 2013.

[34] H. J. Streubert and D. R. Carpenter, *Qualitative Research in Nursing*, Wolters Kluwer Health, Philadelphia, PA, USA, 2011.

[35] R. Fletcher, J. StGeorge, and E. Freeman, "Rough and tumble play quality: theoretical foundations for a new measure of father–child interaction," *Early Child Development and Care*, vol. 183, no. 6, pp. 746–759, 2013.

[36] L. A. Newland, H. H. Chen, D. D. Coyl-Shepherd et al., "Parent and child perspectives on mothering and fathering: the influence of ecocultural niches," *Early Child Development and Care*, vol. 183, no. 3-4, pp. 534–552, 2013.

[37] D. Paquette, "Theorizing the father-child relationship: mechanisms and developmental outcomes," *Human Development*, vol. 47, no. 4, pp. 193–219, 2004.

[38] L. Fava, K. Strauss, G. Valeri, L. D'Elia, S. Arima, and S. Vicari, "The effectiveness of a cross-setting complementary staff- and parent-mediated early intensive behavioral intervention for young children with ASD," *Research in Autism Spectrum Disorders*, vol. 5, no. 4, pp. 1479–1492, 2011.

[39] J. M. Pierucci, "Mothers' scaffolding techniques used during play in toddlers with autism spectrum disorder," *Journal of Developmental and Physical Disabilities*, vol. 28, no. 2, pp. 217–235, 2016.

[40] L. A. Vismara, C. Colombi, and S. J. Rogers, "Can one hour per week of therapy lead to lasting changes in young children with autism," *Autism*, vol. 13, no. 1, pp. 93–115, 2009.

[41] Y. C. Lee, P. C. Chan, S. K. Lin, C. T. Chen, C. Y. Huang, and K. L. Chen, "Correlation patterns between pretend play and playfulness in children with autism spectrum disorder, developmental delay, and typical development," *Research in Autism Spectrum Disorders*, vol. 24, pp. 29–38, 2016.

[42] C. Jarrold, "A review of research into pretend play in autism," *Autism*, vol. 7, no. 4, pp. 379–390, 2003.

[43] K. Stagnitti and C. Unsworth, "The importance of pretend play in child development: an occupational therapy perspective," *British Journal of Occupational Therapy*, vol. 63, no. 3, pp. 121–127, 2000.

[44] K. Stagnitti, "Play therapy for school-age children with high-functioning autism," in *Play Therapy in Middle Childhood*, A. A. Drewes and C. E. Schaefer, Eds., pp. 237–255, American Psychological Association, Washington, DC, USA, 2016.

[45] J. Case-Smith and H. M. Kuhaneck, "Play preferences of typically developing children and children with developmental delays between ages 3 and 7 years," *Occupational Therapy Journal of Research*, vol. 28, no. 1, pp. 19–29, 2008.

[46] F. Graham, S. Rodger, and J. Ziviani, "Coaching parents to enable children's participation: an approach for working with parents and their children," *Australian Occupational Therapy Journal*, vol. 56, no. 1, pp. 16–23, 2009.

[47] American Occupational Therapy Association, "Occupational therapy practice framework: domain and process (3rd edition)," *American Journal of Occupational Therapy*, vol. 68, pp. S1–S48, 2017.

[48] C. T. Myers, J. Case-Smith, and J. Cason, "Early intervention," in *Occupational Therapy for Children and Adolescents*, J. Case-Smith and J. C. O'Brien, Eds., pp. 636–663, Elsevier, St. Louis, MO, USA, 2015.

[49] D. Simpson, "Coaching as a family-centred, occupational therapy intervention for autism: a literature review," *Journal of Occupational Therapy, Schools, & Early Intervention*, vol. 8, no. 2, pp. 109–125, 2015.

[50] H. M. Kuhaneck, K. J. Tanta, A. K. Coombs, and H. Pannone, "A survey of pediatric occupational therapists' use of play," *Journal of Occupational Therapy, Schools, & Early Intervention*, vol. 6, no. 3, pp. 213–227, 2013.

[51] K. Suwada, "Being a traditional dad or being more like a mum? Clashing models of fatherhood according to Swedish and Polish fathers," *Journal of Comparative Family Studies*, vol. 46, no. 4, pp. 467–481, 2015.

[52] J. M. StGeorge, J. C. Goodwin, and R. J. Fletcher, "Parents' views of father–child rough-and-tumble play," *Journal of Child and Family Studies*, vol. 27, no. 5, pp. 1502–1512, 2018.

[53] S. Pinchover, C. Shulman, and A. Bundy, "A comparison of playfulness of young children with and without autism spectrum disorder in interactions with their mothers and teachers," *Early Child Development and Care*, vol. 186, no. 12, pp. 1893–1906, 2016.

6

Relationships between Caregiving Stress, Depression, and Self-Esteem in Family Caregivers of Adults with a Disability

DeokJu Kim

Department of Occupational Therapy, Health Science College, Cheongju University, Cheongju, Republic of Korea

Correspondence should be addressed to DeokJu Kim; dj7407@hanmail.net

Academic Editor: Kathleen M. Matuska

This study aimed to examine the relationships between caregiving stress, depression, and self-esteem of family caregivers of an adult person with a disability and to identify their effects on their caregiving burden. The study was performed with 108 care providers of adult people with a disability who visited hospital rehabilitation centers. Caregiving stress showed a significant positive correlation with depression and with economic and psychological stress, and it showed a significant negative correlation with self-esteem. When the care provider was aged, female, and without a job and the caregiving cost and time were higher, the caregiving stress was high. When the care provider was female and had a lower income, the depression index was high. When the person with a disability was male and in the forties and the level of disability was higher, the caregiving stress was high. When the disability was related to spinal cord damage, the care provider's depression index was the highest. To reduce caregiving stress and depression in the family caregivers and to improve their self-esteem, continuous support and help from specialists are necessary. Additionally, a variety of intervention programs need to be designed to motivate them to participate regularly at the community level.

1. Introduction

According to surveys, the disabled population has continued to grow, with 3.09% in 2000, 4.59% in 2005, and 5.61% in 2011 [1]. A person with a disability often has no choice but to rely on his/her family. Supporting a family member with a disability is one of the most challenging experiences. Many preceding studies have reported that family caregivers of a person with a disability experience deterioration in mental and physical health due to stress [2, 3]. Addressing familial burdens arising from an increasing population of the elderly and of patients with chronic diseases, Goodman and Punoos [4] called family caregivers who care for a patient for a long period a "second victim" and the family of a person with a chronic disease a "potential patient." Issues around the presence of disability within a family are not just limited to the person with the disability, but they concern the whole family as the mental and financial burden are shared and care is provided as per the level of severity of the disability [5].

Some families build a closer relationship and successfully look after the member with a disability using a variety of resources, while other families experience more tensions, conflicts, and frustrations between members [6]. Families who experience growing conflicts also experience sorrow, desperation, anger, and lowered self-esteem internally, and, on the outside, they experience physical burden, lack of time owing to work and caregiving, and financial challenges [7]. If these feelings and emotions are left unresolved, familial tensions and conflicts become chronic and extreme, which occasionally leads the family to fall apart [5]. At varying degrees, majority of the families with a member with a disability show depression symptoms and feel stress over their caregiving responsibilities. Caregiving stress is, in other words, expressed in the form of familial tensions and pressure, which is inevitably experienced owing to the imbalances between the caregiving responsibility and actual capability [8]. Families are put in a situation that is overwhelming and they experience mental and psychological confusion, which acts as a threat to their physical and mental health. Therefore, it is critical that the family members measure their level of stress and maintain their health.

Depression influences one's behavior, cognition, and emotions, and it significantly brings down the quality of care [9]. Depression is caused by the negative evaluation of oneself, which makes it difficult to carry out daily routines as one feels fatigued and loses motivation. It may also lead to physical pain and even suicidal behavior [10]. Hence, it is important to seek solutions to relieve such symptoms and to improve the health of family caregivers of a person with a disability to protect their mental health and to ensure that they lead a healthy family life.

Self-esteem is one of the characteristics that enable individuals to cope with hardships. Rosenberg [11] defined self-esteem as a subjective evaluation of oneself, and he proposed that a strong self-esteem indicates that one accepts and respects oneself and believes that he/she is a valuable human being. Coopersmith [12] defined self-esteem as a level of self-evaluation that is created and maintained by oneself, which is expressed either positively or negatively. It makes the individual see oneself as capable, important, successful, and valuable. He argued that self-esteem serves as a critical component in building a healthy mindset and personality, leading the individuals to self-realization. In other words, self-esteem, as a factor of self-concept, pertains to recognizing oneself as a valuable person. Self-esteem also mediates a variety of stressors experienced in daily life and serves as a social resource for a person with depression and as an internal resource that protects one from negative influences in a stressful environment [13]. In reality, however, families who support a member with a disability experience the lowering of self-esteem due to the difficulties they face. Low self-esteem creates a vicious cycle in which one is reluctant to ask for help and narrows one's social network, which in turn aggravate the burden of care. A person with a strong self-esteem, on the other hand, experiences less stress as he/she can protect himself/herself from psychological challenges and is able to respond to situations more positively [7]. Therefore, it is very important that we find ways to help the families improve self-esteem.

The studies that have been conducted on supporting a family member with a disability have largely focused on the difficulties and stress experienced by parents of a child with a disability. Very few studies have examined the stress, depression, and self-esteem of family caregivers of an adult with a disability. Therefore, this study aimed to examine the above, to analyze the correlations between the factors, and to find ways to improve the quality of life of family members caring for an adult with a disability. This study also sought to provide basic data necessary for designing interventions to mitigate depression and stress and to improve self-esteem.

2. Methods

2.1. Participants. The study subjects were family members of adult persons with a disability who visited rehabilitation centers at hospital S and A in S city, from June 1, 2016, to July 5, 2016. I briefed the subjects on the purpose and procedures of this study and requested their consent. The 115 family members who consented to participation in the study were questioned regarding the level of caregiving-related stress, depression, and self-esteem, and 108 questionnaires, excluding 7 invalid ones, were used for analysis. The unit and currency applied to the expression of the participants' monthly caregiving expenses and their average monthly income were Korean won.

2.2. Instruments

2.2.1. Caregiving-Related Stress. We used the tools used by Kim (2010) to assess the burden of caregiving experienced by the family members, which was based on the Caregiver Burden Inventory developed by Novak and Guest [14] to measure the level of caregiving stress. The tool contains 20 questions across the following 4 areas: 5 questions on financial stress, 5 on physical stress, 5 on psychological stress, and 5 on social stress. Financial stress refers to the stress pertaining to the expenditure related to treatment. Physical stress included the experience of chronic fatigue and physical conditions. Psychological stress pertains to the negative feelings experienced related to caregiving. Social stress concerns the stress arising from conflicting social roles. A 5-point Likert scale is used, with 1 representing "not at all" and 5 indicating "very much so." Total scores range from 25 to 125 points, with a higher score indicating a higher level of stress. Cronbach's α of this tool reported in previous studies was 0.86 [15].

2.2.2. Depression. The level of depression was assessed using the Korean Depression Scale (KDS) developed by M. S. Lee and M. K. Lee [16]. This scale comprises 30 questions, with 5 questions for each of the following 6 areas: negative thoughts about the future, negative thoughts about oneself, anxiety, restlessness, depressive feelings, physical symptoms, and loss of motivation. Each question is rated on a 5-point Likert scale, with 0 representing "not at all" and 4 indicating "very much so." The gross score ranges from 0 to 120, with a higher score indicating a higher level of depression. The tool's Cronbach α was 0.88 [16]. I evaluated the total score of KDS in this study.

2.2.3. Self-Esteem. Rosenberg's Self-Esteem Scale (1985) was used. This scale is a self-report tool that includes 10 questions, with 5 positive and 5 negative statements. Responses are made on a 4-point Likert scale, with 1 representing "generally not" and 4 indicating "always." Negative statements are reverse scored and the total scores range from 10 to 40, with a higher score indicating a higher level of self-esteem. The tool's Cronbach α was 0.83 [17]. I evaluated the total score of Rosenberg's Self-Esteem Scale in this study.

2.3. Analysis Methods. This study used the SPSS 18.0 statistics program for the analysis. t-test and ANOVA were carried out to evaluate associations of caregiving stress, depression, and self-esteem levels with demographic and personal characteristics of the subjects, and the Duncan group categorization was used as a post hoc test. Correlations between caregiving stress, depression, and self-esteem were examined using the Pearson correlation coefficient and the variables affecting caregiving stress were examined using a multiple regression analysis. The significance level is $\alpha = 0.05$.

3. Results

3.1. General Characteristics of the Subjects

3.1.1. General Characteristics of the Family Caregivers. The family caregivers showed the following characteristics: the female group (65.8%) was larger than the male group was (34.2%); the distribution across age groups was as follows: 60 years or older (38.1%), 50 to 59 years (33.3%), and 40 to 49 years (15.7%); the most commonly observed relationship with the person with a disability was spouse (62.1%); the largest group had no occupation (66.7%); the distribution according to academic qualifications was as follows: Bachelor's degree (37.9%), high school graduate (37.0%), and middle school graduate or lower (18.5%); 81.5% of them were married; the distribution of monthly expenses incurred on supporting the person with a disability was as follows: 500,000₩ to 1,000,000₩ (36.1%) and 1,500,000₩ to 2,000,000₩ (26.4%); 64.9% of the participants spent 10 hours or longer each day on caregiving; and their monthly income distribution was as follows: 2,000,000₩ to 3,000,000₩ (25.9%), 4,000,000₩ or more (24.1%), and 1,000,000₩ to 2,000,000₩ (22.2%) (Table 1).

3.1.2. General Characteristics of the Persons with a Disability. The general characteristics of the adults with a disability were as follows: the 70 years or older age group was the largest (35.9%); the most common type of disability was brain stroke (63.3%), followed by spinal cord injury (17.3%), traumatic brain injury (10.2%), and other bodily injuries (9.2%); the distribution as per the grade of the disability was as follows: Grade 1 (50.0%), Grade 3 or higher (29.6%), and Grade 2 (20.4%) (in the disability grades, Grade 1 indicates the severest degree of disability, and the degree of disability decreases towards Grade 3); and the distribution as per duration of disability was as follows: less than 1 year (44.9%), 1 to 3 years (26.9%), and 10 years or longer (14.3%) (Table 2).

3.2. Correlation among Caregiving Stress, Depression, and Self-Esteem. The correlation between the caregiving stress, depression, and self-esteem experienced by the family caregivers was as follows: there was a significant correlation between the total score on caregiving stress and depression ($p < 0.01$). Additionally, a significant correlation was observed with the subareas of stress: financial stress ($p < 0.01$), physical stress ($p < 0.01$), and psychological stress ($p < 0.01$). No significance was observed for the correlation with social stress ($p > 0.01$). Financial stress ($p < 0.01$) and psychological stress ($p < 0.01$) showed a significant negative correlation with self-esteem. Finally, a significant negative correlation was observed between depression and self-esteem ($p < 0.01$) (Table 3).

3.3. Caregiving Stress, Depression, and Self-Esteem by the General Characteristics of the Subjects

3.3.1. Associations of Demographic Characteristics with Study Measures for Caregivers. Associations of caregiving stress, depression, and self-esteem varied according to the general characteristics of the family caregivers. Specifically, significant differences were observed in the level of caregiving stress experienced according to sex ($p < 0.01$), age ($p < 0.01$), relationship with the patient ($p < 0.01$), marital status ($p < 0.05$), presence of occupation ($p < 0.01$), highest academic degree ($p < 0.01$), support expense ($p < 0.05$), caregiving hours ($p < 0.01$), and monthly income ($p < 0.05$). Further, significant differences were shown in the level of depression based on sex ($p < 0.05$), support expense ($p < 0.01$), and monthly income ($p < 0.01$). With reference to self-esteem, age ($p < 0.01$), highest education ($p < 0.01$), and

Table 1: General characteristics of family caregivers ($N = 108$).

Classification	Number (N)	Percent (%)
Sex		
Male	37	34.2
Female	71	65.8
Age		
30~39	14	12.9
40~49	17	15.7
50~59	36	33.3
60 or older	41	38.1
Relationship with patient		
Spouse	67	62.1
Child	32	29.6
Others	9	8.3
Whether they are currently employed		
Yes	36	33.3
No	72	66.7
Highest academic education		
Midschool graduated or lower	20	18.5
High school graduate	40	37.0
Bachelor's degree	41	37.9
Master's or higher	7	6.6
Marital status		
Married	88	81.5
Single	20	18.5
Caregiving expense (₩ 10,000)		
Less than 50	5	4.6
50 to 100	39	36.1
100 to 150	23	21.3
150 to 200	30	26.4
200 or more	11	11.6
Time spent on caregiving (per days)		
Less than 5 hrs	24	22.2
5 to 10 hrs	14	12.9
10 or more hrs	70	64.9
Monthly income (₩ 10,000)		
Less than 100	13	12.1
100 to 200	24	22.2
200 to 300	28	25.9
300 to 400	17	15.7
400 or more	26	24.1

TABLE 2: General characteristics of adults with a disability (N = 108).

Classification	Number (N)	Percent (%)
Sex		
Male	51	47.2
Female	57	52.7
Age		
40 or younger	16	14.8
40~49	14	12.9
50~59	16	14.8
60~69	25	23.1
70 or older	37	34.4
Highest academic education		
Midschool graduated or lower	12	11.1
High school graduate	51	47.2
Bachelor's degree	36	33.3
Master's or higher	9	8.4
Marital status		
Married	77	71.2
Single	13	12.1
Divorced/separated/widowed	18	16.7
Type of disability		
Stroke	65	60.2
Traumatic brain injury	13	12.0
Spinal cord injury	20	18.5
Other bodily injuries	10	9.3
Grade of disability		
Grade 1	52	48.1
Grade 2	23	21.3
Grade 3 or higher	33	30.6
Period of disability		
Less than a year	46	42.5
1 to 3 years	28	25.9
3 to 6 years	6	5.5
6 to 10 years	12	11.1
10 years or longer	16	15.0

monthly income ($p < 0.01$) resulted in significant differences. Thus, caregivers who were female, were aged 60 years or higher, were the care recipient's spouse, were single, had no occupation, were responsible for a high level of support expense, or spent more time on caregiving showed a higher level of caregiving stress. Similarly, among the female group, those who incurred higher support expenses or had a lower monthly income showed a higher level of depression. Finally, those who were younger, had a higher educational level, or had a higher monthly income showed a higher level of self-esteem (Table 4).

3.3.2. Associations of Demographic Characteristics with Study Measures for Patients with a Disability. Associations of caregiving stress, depression, and self-esteem experienced by the family caregivers varied according to the general characteristics of the person they cared for. Specifically, caregiving stress differed significantly in terms of sex ($p < 0.01$), age ($p < 0.01$), grade of disability ($p < 0.05$), and duration of disability ($p < 0.05$). In terms of depression, age ($p < 0.01$), type of disability ($p < 0.01$), grade of disability ($p < 0.01$), and duration of disability ($p < 0.01$) resulted in significant differences. With reference to self-esteem, grade of disability ($p < 0.01$) and duration of disability ($p < 0.01$) led to significant differences. This indicated that, among the caregivers who catered to a male care recipient, a higher level of stress was shown when the latter was aged 40 to 49 years, when the grade of disability was higher, and when the duration of disability was longer. A higher level of depression was displayed among family caregivers when the care recipient was 40 to 49 years, the type of disability was stroke or spinal cord injury, the grade of disability was higher, or the duration of disability is less than a year. When the grade of disability was higher or the duration of disability was longer, the family members' self-esteem was lower (Table 5).

3.4. Factors That Influence Caregiving Stress. To identify the factors that influence caregiving stress, we conducted a multiple regression analysis with caregiving stress as the dependent variable (using the total caregiving stress score) and the total depression and self-esteem as the independent variables. In addition, I conducted a multiple regression analysis with "age, gender, whether they are currently employed, caregiving expenses, time spent on caregiving, and monthly income," which can represent the general characteristics of caregivers, as independent variables.

Testing for multicollinearity between the independent variables showed that none of the Variance Inflation Factors crossed 2.5, indicating no multicollinearity. The variable that exerts the greatest influence on caregiving stress was the total depression score ($\beta = 0.445$) followed by self-esteem ($\beta = -0.293$), age among general characteristics ($\beta = 0.515$), time spent on caregiving ($\beta = 0.401$), and caregiving expenses ($\beta = 0.303$) (Table 6).

4. Discussion

This study was designed to examine the relationships between the caregiving stress, depression, and self-esteem experienced by family caregivers of an adult patient with a disability and to understand the factors influencing caregiving stress to help relieve the burden on the caregivers.

The analysis of the correlations between caregiving stress, depression, and self-esteem revealed that caregiving stress had a positive correlation with depression and that financial and psychological stress (subitems of caregiving stress) showed a significant negative correlation with self-esteem. Further, depression and self-esteem were negatively correlated. This indicates that though family caregivers may have accepted the presence of a disability to a certain degree, they continued to experience severe stress owing to the irrecoverable state of the disability and the care recipient's continuous need for care. This psychological burden led to loss of self-esteem, finally resulting in depression [18]. Thus, caregivers need to seek professional help to handle their stress, but there are few programs or professionals who can help relieve

Table 3: Correlation between caregiving stress, depression, and self-esteem ($N = 108$).

	Total caregiving stress	Financial stress	Physical stress	Psychological stress	Social stress	Depression	Self-esteem
Total caregivingstress	1	0.786**	0.883**	0.719**	0.589**	0.445**	−0.136
Financialstress		1	0.699**	0.297**	0.153	0.362**	−0.336**
Physical stress			1	0.473**	0.367**	0.382**	−0.171
Psychologicalstress				1	0.512**	0.349**	−0.473**
Social stress					1	0.220	−0.100
Depression						1	−0.570**
Self-esteem							1

** $p < 0.01$.

such stress. Therefore, it is necessary that local community centers implement intervention programs for families, to help them reduce such stress. Of most common interventional activities for caregiving stress, a group consultation program, which had been found to be widely effective, can address the caregivers' emotional needs, can be used to teach behavioral and relaxation techniques, and can act as a source of social support. Such a program can help the caregivers talk about their feelings with others and feel less isolated, which will help reduce the stress and will help participants separate themselves from stress [19, 20]. Regular participation in such programs will improve caregivers' self-esteem and reduce depression.

The varying degrees of caregiving stress, depression, and self-esteem with reference to the general characteristics of the subjects showed that female caregivers, who are older, are the care recipient's spouse, have no occupation, and spend more time and money on caregiving showed a higher level of stress. Additionally, female caregivers who spent more on caregiving and earned a lower income showed a higher level of depression, while caregivers who were younger, had a higher educational level, and had higher income showed a higher level of self-esteem. Sim and An's study [21] results also showed that a caregiver who incurs higher expenditure on caregiving and has a lower income showed a lower level of caregiving stress, which is in line with this study's findings. If a caregiver is financially vulnerable, one has to spend most of the income on caregiving and cannot afford to save for the future or enjoy leisure, and his/her quality of life will be hampered. A female caregiver who has no occupation naturally experiences more difficulties because of having to make ends meet, which could lead to depressive feelings. These findings show that an aged spousal caregiver finds caregiving more stressful than others do. As medical advances have continued to extend the life span of people with disabilities, the strongest fear for a caregiver who becomes aged is that he/she herself is getting older [22]. Additionally, an elderly caregiver would fear that when he/she dies, there will be no one left to take care of the person with a disability [23]. Spousal conflict with a care recipient who is the caregiver's husband is one of the factors that aggravates caregiving stress or depression. The wife feels that her stress over caregiving is not appreciated by the other family members and becomes depressed; she considers divorce but soon gives up because she is not financially independent; and she goes back to caregiving. This leads to a vicious cycle, and the relationship deteriorates with no communication between the couple [24]. Such deepened divides between couples worsen the family atmosphere.

With reference to the general characteristics of the care recipient, caregiving stress was strong when the care recipient was male, was aged 40 to 49 years, or had a higher grade of disability. When the patient is aged 40 to 49 years, a higher grade of disability led to a higher level of depression in the caregiver, and having a disability owing to a spinal cord injury was related to a higher level of depression. The more severe the disability was, the stronger the caregiving stress was. This may be because a person with a severe disability would have to rely more on the caregiver, meaning that the caregiver will have less time to spend on oneself and would face more difficulties and stress. Any family member with a relative who had a physical disability may experience depression, but it is notable that the caregivers of persons with spinal cord injury showed a high level of depression. In a study on patients with spinal cord injury, Tatiana [25] found that 50.6% of the respondents reported that their spousal relationship deteriorated after the disability occurred, indicating that the injury has a serious effect on the spousal relationship. In particular, loss of sexual functionality greatly undermines satisfaction with life, and 60% of the persons with spinal cord injury said they had issues with sex life and that the sexual dysfunction may have caused high stress in their spouse [3]. Those who experienced spinal cord injury at a young age and those who suddenly lost a source of income with no time for preparation experienced great pressure both financially and mentally.

Support programs for people with disabilities in Korea are largely focused on individual support and services for people with a disability, and no support is provided to their family [26]. It is important that measures are taken to provide specific and realistic assistance to family members who are financially vulnerable. Additionally, community service institutions for those with a disability should develop programs that invite people with a disability and their spouses together, to help them build a good relationship. However, such programs should not be temporary, and they need to be provided in a systematic manner, offering psychological and social support.

Depression was found to be a factor affecting caregiving stress. Depression causes caregivers to lose the will to live, tire easily, and feel physically heavy accompanied by physical pain [27]. Caregivers who take care of family members with

TABLE 4: Caregiving stress, depression, and self-esteem according to the general characteristics of the subjects ($N = 108$).

Variables	Caregiving stress		Depression		Self-esteem	
	[a]M ± SD	p	M ± SD	p	M ± SD	p
Sex						
Male	62.69 ± 12.63	0.009**	44.76 ± 15.79	0.041*	27.76 ± 4.31	0.988
Female	71.55 ± 14.33		54.25 ± 30.10		27.78 ± 5.49	
Age						
30~39	54.75 ± 16.51	0.001**	46.00 ± 21.81	0.782	32.20 ± 6.61	0.002**
40~49	67.80 ± 7.92		53.00 ± 29.63		29.03 ± 2.47	
50~59	65.86 ± 14.47		51.93 ± 27.71		24.25 ± 2.31	
60 or older	75.00 ± 12.19		45.96 ± 25.61		26.22 ± 5.87	
Relationship with patient						
Spouse	71.98 ± 15.11	0.008**	51.63 ± 26.52	0.176	28.05 ± 5.34	0.576
Child	64.44 ± 10.83		48.88 ± 29.60		27.77 ± 5.54	
Other	56.60 ± 11.06		49.08 ± 26.28		26.00 ± 5.10	
Marital status						
Married	67.37 ± 14.61	0.041*	47.34 ± 25.67	0.172	27.80 ± 5.21	0.306
Single	75.33 ± 10.88		58.66 ± 28.67		27.66 ± 4.69	
Whether they are currently employed						
Yes	63.21 ± 13.15	0.001**	47.74 ± 22.01	0.082	27.81 ± 14.10	0.924
No	81.47 ± 16.87		57.08 ± 133.06		27.69 ± 17.06	
Highest education						
Midschool or lower	83.28 ± 9.77	0.001**	58.07 ± 34.59	0.053	25.64 ± 7.04	0.008**
High school graduate	61.58 ± 11.49		46.89 ± 21.85		26.24 ± 4.32	
Bachelor's degrees	70.61 ± 12.69		50.25 ± 25.61		30.03 ± 4.23	
Master's or higher	52.50 ± 12.12		24.50 ± 16.74		29.00 ± 1.15	
Caregiving expense (₩ 10,000)						
Less than 50	57.00 ± 16.06	0.015*	58.64 ± 14.06	0.001**	20.00 ± 4.12	0.089
50 to 100	65.55 ± 14.42		52.62 ± 24.13		28.41 ± 4.46	
100 to 150	64.88 ± 10.19		44.63 ± 14.82		29.35 ± 5.14	
150 to 200	71.86 ± 16.31		47.13 ± 23.06		26.60 ± 5.67	
200 or more	82.85 ± 12.67		82.00 ± 33.67		27.42 ± 4.27	
Time spent on caregiving						
Less than 5 hrs	56.50 ± 16.00	0.005**	51.06 ± 22.86	0.815	28.86 ± 5.33	0.663
5 to 10 hrs	63.73 ± 9.52		43.75 ± 24.28		27.50 ± 4.17	
10 or more hrs	71.69 ± 14.08		49.32 ± 27.69		27.52 ± 5.20	
Monthly income (₩ 10,000)						
Less than 100	81.82 ± 11.90	0.012*	67.53 ± 21.01	0.001**	29.00 ± 5.74	0.002**
100 to 200	71.80 ± 10.97		36.44 ± 19.43		23.46 ± 5.55	
200 to 300	67.90 ± 15.60		49.90 ± 27.01		27.66 ± 5.07	
300 to 400	68.00 ± 18.61		54.83 ± 23.49		28.41 ± 3.44	
400 or more	61.85 ± 9.49		31.52 ± 7.19		30.09 ± 3.57	

$^{*}p < 0.05$, $^{**}p < 0.01$, and [a]M ± SD are the comprehensive points of evaluation tool.

disabilities frequently complain of constant pain in limbs and back as they do not have time to take care of themselves [21]. The physical pain triggers psychological burden and the symptom of depression, leading to demotivation. Depression of caregivers eventually aggravates caregiving stress.

Self-esteem was also identified as a factor that influences caregiving stress. A caregiver with strong self-esteem, that is, one who sees oneself as valuable and positive, is able to face the painful and challenging burden arising from caring for a person with a disability in a positive way, which will lead to a lower level of stress. Therefore, family caregivers need to be provided with psychological support to help them accept themselves as valuable and to help them deal with issues positively. It is necessary to facilitate the realization of positive experiences that can be derived from caregiving in addition to the negative experiences [28]. This may lessen the burden of support and help them accept the responsibility while having a positive image of themselves and feeling awarded as

Table 5: Caregiving stress, depression, and self-esteem according to the general characteristics of the person with a disability ($N = 108$).

Variables	Caregiving stress		Depression		Self-esteem	
	^{a}M ± SD	p	M ± SD	p	M ± SD	p
Sex						
Male	74.19 ± 12.84	0.001**	47.08 ± 24.95	0.536	28.02 ± 5.65	0.679
Female	63.80 ± 13.94		50.80 ± 27.54		27.57 ± 4.63	
Age						
40 or younger	65.66 ± 13.94		58.33 ± 37.41		25.33 ± 8.94	
40~49	82.50 ± 5.19		85.00 ± 31.17		30.50 ± 6.35	
50~59	80.40 ± 10.78	0.002**	28.40 ± 10.84	0.003**	30.60 ± 2.95	0.072
60~69	70.10 ± 12.67		48.68 ± 18.54		28.00 ± 6.05	
70 or older	63.54 ± 14.15		47.87 ± 23.11		27.45 ± 4.46	
Type of disability						
Stroke	68.08 ± 13.45		52.28 ± 15.07		27.61 ± 4.80	
Traumatic brain injury	75.14 ± 12.68	0.061	25.50 ± 10.15	0.005**	29.00 ± 4.56	0.056
Spinal cord injury	76.00 ± 11.75		55.73 ± 28.42		26.42 ± 5.38	
Other bodily injuries	74.71 ± 16.92		37.71 ± 8.87		27.92 ± 4.28	
Grade of disability						
Grade 1	76.60 ± 14.24		72.60 ± 19.71		18.80 ± 3.83	
Grade 2	67.07 ± 14.10	0.045*	54.42 ± 26.34	0.001**	27.50 ± 4.34	0.001**
Grade 3 or higher	67.37 ± 13.63		49.00 ± 22.23		27.87 ± 4.27	
Period of disability						
Less than a year	64.78 ± 13.51		67.33 ± 31.32		29.06 ± 5.32	
1 to 3 years	68.76 ± 17.07		38.12 ± 24.23		27.04 ± 4.45	
3 to 6 years	76.00 ± 12.06	0.019*	63.00 ± 20.06	0.001**	26.00 ± 3.26	0.001**
6 to 10 years	77.06 ± 12.78		55.55 ± 19.62		16.33 ± 2.64	
10 years or longer	76.50 ± 6.86		50.00 ± 8.73		25.53 ± 3.14	

$^{*}p < 0.05$, $^{**}p < 0.01$, and ^{a}M ± SD are the comprehensive points of evaluation tool.

Table 6: Factors that influence caregiving stress ($N = 108$).

Independentvariable	Nonstandardized coefficient		Standardized coefficient	t	p	95% confidence interval
	B	S.E	β			
Depression	0.243	0.056	0.445	4.332	0.001**	0.146–0.340
Self-esteem	−1.251	0.322	−0.293	2.996	0.003**	0.503–0.612
Age	8.773	1.449	0.515	9.054	0.001**	3.001–8.337
Gender	4.341	2.679	0.124	1.224	0.136	0.593–5.411
Whether they are currently employed	4.719	4.401	0.140	1.072	0.287	0.300–1.258
Caregiving expense	4.535	1.023	0.303	4.432	0.001**	2.005–7.038
Time spent on caregiving	8.437	1.988	0.401	4.243	0.001**	1.366–8.086
Monthly income	4.401	3.554	0.136	1.238	0.219	0.297–2.423

Dependent variable: total score on caregiving stress. $R^2 = .710$, adjusted $R^2 = .688$, $F = 32.209$, and $^{**}p < 0.01$.

a more mature person [29]. The factors exerting the greatest influence in caregiving stress out of general characteristics were age, time spent on caregiving, and caregiving expenses, in that order. Older people are more prone to muscular skeletal disease. Symptom severity is likely to be worse for caregivers who provide physical care for family members with disabilities and could work as a factor aggravating caregiving stress. The higher the proportion of caregiving expenses to total income is and the longer the time of caregiving is, the harder it is to invest time and money in leisure for rest and recreation (Sim, 2013). Leisure enhances the level of satisfaction with life and ability to deal with stress, thereby playing an important role in self-realization and decent quality of life. If leisure activities that are highly correlated with quality of life are cut off from the lives of caregivers because of the burden of caregiving expenses and increase in the time spent on caregiving, it would result in more caregiving stress [30].

South Koreans are strongly family oriented and the responsibility of looking after a patient with a disability often falls upon the family. In this sense, a family can only be happy when they are considered physically and psychologically stable for providing care. For healthy families and the society, practical policies need to be prepared to lend financial and emotional help not only to those with a disability but also to their family caregivers.

The limitation of this study was that the subjects were visitors of particular hospitals located in Seoul, and therefore they do not reflect the overall characteristics of family caregivers across all regions. Future studies should ensure that subjects cover a wider area and the findings are more representative of the general public.

5. Conclusions

This study sought to examine the relations between caregiving stress, depression, and self-esteem experienced by the family members of an adult patient with a disability and to identify the factors influencing caregiving stress. Caregiving-related stress showed a significant correlation with depression, and financial and psychological stress, subitems of caregiving stress, had a significant negative correlation with self-esteem. Caregiving stress was stronger among caregivers who were female, older, and the spouse of the care recipient; had no occupation; and spent more time and money on caregiving. Depression level was higher in those who were female and had a lower income.

Caregiving stress was higher among those whose care recipient was male and aged 40 to 49 years, while depression levels were higher among those whose care recipient suffered from spinal cord injury. In order to reduce the levels of caregivers' stress and depression and to improve their self-esteem, continued and consistent support and help from professionals are needed. A variety of intervention programs need to be planned and implemented for family caregivers at the national and municipal levels.

References

[1] Ministry of Health and Welfare, "2011, Survey of the Disability. Korea: Ministry of Health and Welfare".

[2] C. S. Aneshensel, L. I. Pearlin, J. T. Mullan, and C. J. Whitlatch, *Profiles in Caregiving: The Unexpected Carrer*, Academic Press, San Diego, CA, USA.

[3] L. I. Pearlin, J. T. Mullan, S. J. Semple, and M. M. Skaff, "Caregiving and the stress process: an overview of concepts and their measures," *The Gerontologist*, vol. 30, no. 5, pp. 583–594, 1990.

[4] C. C. Goodman and J. Punoos, "A model telephone information and support program for caregivers of Alzheimer's patients," *The Gerontologist*, vol. 30, no. 3, pp. 399–404, 1990.

[5] S. K. Oh, "A study on a model for families adapting to disability," *Ewha Social Welfare Review*, vol. 1, no. 1, pp. 1–20, 2002.

[6] Y. H. An, "Family resilience: Implications for nursing practice," *Journal of Nursing*, vol. 15, no. 1, pp. 5–24, 2006.

[7] J. H. Lim and E. P. Lee, "The influence of parenting stress on the parenting attitude and moderating effect analysis of depression in multi-cultural family mother," *Journal of Future Early Childhood Education*, vol. 17, no. 2, pp. 49–70, 2010.

[8] H. I. McCubbin and M. A. McCubbin, "Typologies of Resilient Families: Emerging Roles of Social Class and Ethnicity," *Family Relations*, vol. 37, no. 3, p. 247, 1988.

[9] S. Tanaka, E. Ishikawa, A. Mochida, K. Kawano, and M. Kobayashi, "Effects of Early-Stage Group Psychoeducation Programme for Patients with Depression," *Occupational Therapy International*, vol. 22, no. 4, pp. 195–205, 2015.

[10] A. T. Beck, *DeprEssion: Clinical, Experimental And Theoretical Aspects*, Haper and Row, NY, New York, USA, 1986.

[11] M. Rogenberg, *Self-Concept and Psychological Well-Being in Adolescence*, Academic Press, Orlando, Fla, USA, 1985.

[12] S. Coopersmith, *The Antecedents of Self-Esteem*, W. H. Freeman and Company, San Francisco, SF, USA, 1967.

[13] L. A. Hall, J. B. Kotch, D. Browne, and M. K. Rayens, "Self-Esteem as a Mediator of the Effects of Stressors and Social Resources on Depressive Symptoms in Postpartum Mothers," *Nursing Research* , vol. 45, no. 4, pp. 231–238, 1996.

[14] M. Novak and C. Guest, "Application of a multidimensional caregiver burden inventory," *The Gerontologist*, vol. 29, no. 6, pp. 798–803, 1989.

[15] K. H. Kim, *Study of child support burden and life satisfaction of parents of children with disability [M.S. thesis]*, Seoul Christian University, Seoul, South Korea, 2012.

[16] M. S. Lee and M. K. Lee, Korean Depression Scale (KDS-30). Seoul: Hakjisa.

[17] J. Choi, "Mediating Effects of Self-Concealment in the Associations between Social Support, Self-Esteem, and Depression among College Students in Daegu and Gyeongbuk Areas," *The Journal of the Korea Contents Association*, vol. 15, no. 10, pp. 236–252, 2015.

[18] J. H. Lee and H. Y. Kim, "A Study on maternal stress in rearing children with disabilities and maternal quality of life," *Child Health Nursing Research*, vol. 13, no. 1, pp. 5–12, 2007.

[19] S. H. Zarit, C. R. Anthony, and M. Boutselis, "Interventions with care givers of dementia patients: comparison of two approaches.," *Psychology and Aging*, vol. 2, no. 3, pp. 225–232, 1987.

[20] I. Yalom, *Theory and practice of group psychotherapy*, Basic Book, New York, NY, USA, 3rd edition, 1985.

[21] M. Y. Sim and S. A. An, "A Study on the influences of family stress on family adaptation of disabled families," *Journal of Rehabilitation Research*, vol. 17, no. 3, pp. 135–157, 2013.

[22] R. A. Pruchno and S. Meeks, "Health-related stress, affect, and depressive symptoms experienced by caregiving mothers of adults with a developmental disability," *Psychology and Aging*, vol. 19, no. 3, pp. 394–401, 2004.

[23] P. Minnes, L. Woodford, and J. Passey, "Mediators of well-being in ageing family carers of adults with intellectual disabilities," *Journal of Applied Research in Intellectual Disabilities*, vol. 20, no. 6, pp. 539–552, 2007.

[24] H. K. Park, "A narrative inquiry about a family life experienced by mothers of an adult-child with mental disorder," *Korean Journal of Family Social Work*, vol. 52, pp. 241–275, 2016.

[25] M. Tatiana, "Pain in patients with spinal cord injury: An A to Z approach," *Anesthesia and Pain Management*, vol. 16, no. 4, pp. 180–183, 2012.

[26] M. J. Kwon, "A study on the experience of spouses care giving their husband with spinal cord injuries," *Social Science Research Institute*, vol. 39, no. 2, pp. 145–178, 2015.

7

Developing and Sustaining Recovery-Orientation in Mental Health Practice: Experiences of Occupational Therapists

Alexandra Nugent, Nicola Hancock, and Anne Honey

The University of Sydney, Cumberland Campus, 74 East St., Lidcombe, NSW 2141, Australia

Correspondence should be addressed to Nicola Hancock; nicola.hancock@sydney.edu.au

Academic Editor: Claudia Hilton

Background/Aim. Internationally, mental health policy requires clinicians to shift from a medical to a recovery-oriented approach. However, there is a significant lag in the translation of policy into practice. Occupational therapists have been identified as ideally situated to be recovery-oriented yet limited research exploring how they do this exists. This study aimed to explore Australian occupational therapists' experiences of developing and sustaining recovery-orientation in mental health practice. *Methods.* Semistructured, in-depth interviews were conducted with twelve occupational therapists working across different mental health service types. Participants identified themselves as being recovery-oriented. Data were analysed using constant comparative analysis. *Results.* Occupational therapists described recovery-oriented practice as an active, ongoing, and intentional process of seeking out knowledge, finding fit between understandings of recovery-oriented practice and their professional identity, holding hope, and developing confidence through clinical reasoning. Human and systemic aspects of therapists' workplace environment influenced this process. *Conclusions.* Being a recovery-oriented occupational therapist requires more than merely accepting a specific framework. It requires commitment and ongoing work to develop and sustain recovery-orientation. Occupational therapists are called to extend current leadership activity beyond their workplace and to advocate for broader systemic change.

1. Introduction

In contrast to a medical understanding of mental health recovery as "cure," recovery as defined by people with lived experience of mental illness refers to an individual's ongoing and nonlinear journey towards creating and living "a meaningful and contributing life in a community of choice with or without the presence of mental health issues" [1]. With this definition of recovery, people using mental health services, or "consumers," are necessarily active and leading agents in their own recovery [2, 3]. Therefore, recovery cannot be done to, or for, consumers by service providers [4]. Rather, services are called on to adopt recovery-oriented practice to better support consumers as they take the lead in their unique recovery journeys [5–7].

Recovery-oriented practice involves being consumer-focused, facilitating choice and opportunity, and holding and promoting hope for each consumer's future [8]. Recovery journeys are driven by the consumers and their choices, goals, and rights [9]. This requires movement away from medically oriented care in which absence of symptoms is the primary outcome measured and medication is the focus of treatment [9]. Recovery-oriented practice instead strives to enable consumers to reclaim and develop new meaning in their lives [8, 10].

Occupational therapists have repeatedly been identified as ideally placed to facilitate a shift towards recovery-oriented practice due to the congruence between occupational therapy theory and recovery-oriented principles [11–14]. Autonomy, choice, strong therapeutic partnerships, and enablement are central components of both client-centred occupational therapy [15] and recovery-oriented practice.

Current policies and guidelines across the English-speaking world, including Australia, require the adoption of recovery-oriented practice in mental health service delivery [16–20]. Further, recent outcome studies indicate that recovery-oriented practice may lead to better consumer engagement in treatment and quality of life [21] and that aspects of recovery-oriented practice such as choice and therapeutic alliance are strongly linked to positive recovery outcomes [22]. Yet, commentators in the field have consistently identified a lag in the implementation of recovery-oriented practice in mental health services (e.g., [23]). In fact, services have been described as "simply repackaging old wine in the new bottle of recovery language" [24].

Research that, with the exception of nursing, does not distinguish between professional backgrounds has identified a range of challenges in operationalising recovery-oriented practice (e.g., [25, 26]). These include a lack of clarity regarding what recovery-oriented practice entails [7, 8, 27], staff scepticism [27, 28], and incongruence between recovery and workplace priorities [7, 25–27]. Facilitators of recovery-oriented practice are less commonly reported but include developing a workplace culture that values innovation and clinicians having a willingness to test the boundaries set by restrictive organisations [25, 27, 29]. Various guidelines are available which explain what recovery-orientation looks like in practice (e.g., [9]). However, missing from the literature are (1) a nuanced understanding of how recovery-oriented clinicians actually go about sustaining their recovery-orientation within the context of the identified barriers and facilitators and (2) a specific investigation of recovery-orientation amongst occupational therapists despite assertions that they are uniquely placed to be recovery-oriented.

The aim of the current study was to explore Australian occupational therapists' experiences of developing and sustaining recovery-orientation in mental health practice.

2. Methods

2.1. Study Design. A detailed and contextualised understanding of the experiences of occupational therapists is required to aid in the operationalisation of recovery-oriented approaches. Therefore, a qualitative design was needed [30]. Grounded theory data collection and analysis techniques were used to ensure methodological rigour and inductively explore and understand participants' experiences. The techniques used were purposive and theoretical sampling, concurrent data collection and analysis, and constant comparative analysis [31]. These are described below. Ethical approval for this research was obtained from the University of Sydney Human Research Ethics Committee.

2.2. Initial Sampling and Recruitment. Participants were purposively sampled based on their direct experience with, and thus insight into, the research topic. Australian occupational therapists working in any mental health service who identified themselves as adopting recovery-oriented practice were eligible to participate. Participants were recruited through an email sent to members by the Mental Health Interest Group in the NSW Division of Occupational Therapy Australia. All participants provided written informed consent.

2.3. Data Collection and Analysis. Data collection and analysis were conducted concurrently to allow the researchers to pursue lines of inquiry informed by their ongoing analyses [30]. Data were collected through in-depth, semistructured interviews to foster a deep understanding of participants' unique experiences [30]. An interview guide was designed to encourage participants to raise important issues within the research topic and allow the interviewer to flexibly follow up on these issues [32]. Participants were asked about what being recovery-oriented meant for their own practice and how they sustained their recovery-orientation in their unique context. Because preliminary analysis of each interview occurred before engaging with the next participant [31], questions could be modified in response to emerging ideas. For example, after four interviews, risk management was identified as an important concept. Risk was discussed with subsequent participants to deepen the researchers' understanding. Interviews lasted 40–60 minutes and were audio recorded and transcribed verbatim.

Constant comparative analysis was used throughout the study [31]. Each section of data was coded with one or more words or phrases that described its underlying meaning. For example, the statements "not all managers have an understanding of what recovery-oriented practice might look like" and "it's hard if you have to be the one to convince your boss" were coded "lack of understanding from seniors." These initial codes were compared with each other and with new data as they were collected. Conceptually similar codes were grouped to form categories [31]. The broad category "workplace attitudes and culture," for example, was created by comparing the initial code "lack of understanding from seniors" with other initial codes such as "negative team attitudes." Methodological rigour was enhanced through frequent reflective discussions between authors about the codes and their relationships. This enabled consensus to be reached on the interpretation of data.

After analysis of twelve interviews, it became apparent that while no new codes were emerging, two potentially important concepts were underdeveloped: the fit between occupational therapy and recovery-oriented principles and the ongoing development (as opposed to simply maintenance) of recovery-orientation. Therefore, in accordance with theoretical sampling, further data collection was required. Examination of transcripts revealed that some participants had not been asked to expand on these issues as they had emerged in later interviews. Thus, follow-up interviews were conducted with a purposively selected subset of existing participants using a new interview guide designed to address these topics. Participants whose interviews had not covered these topics in detail were selected to obtain coverage of the topic across different service settings and levels of seniority [33]. After five follow-up interviews, new data were no longer revealing new concepts and all categories were well covered. Data collection therefore ceased, with no recruitment of new participants being required [30]. Participant characteristics are provided in Table 1.

In the final stage of constant comparative analysis, the relationships between categories were confirmed, and a framework was developed to explain the experiences of occupational therapists developing and sustaining recovery-orientation in mental health practice.

Table 1: Participant demographics.

Participant	Years since graduation	Current role			Current setting				
		OT-specific	Generic	Clinical supervisor	Acute/inpatient	Community	Forensic	Youth/early psychosis	NGO[†]
Addison[‡]	6	x				x		x	
Anna	14	x			x		x		
Jessica	16	x		x		x			
Chloe[‡]	<1		x						x
Ava[‡]	<1	x				x			
Chris[‡]	10		x	x					
Pat	22		x	x		x		x	
Amelia[‡]	19		x	x		x		x	
Jordan	13	x		x	x		x		
Charlotte	11		x	x		x			
Jamie	<1	x			x	x		x	
Casey	8	x		x	x		x		

[†]Nongovernmental Organisation.
‡ denotes those who participated in follow-up interviews.

3. Results

Participants described developing and sustaining recovery-oriented practice as an active and ongoing process. It was not a static, singular decision to be recovery-oriented or not. Neither was it a destination that participants had reached or hoped to reach. Rather, participants relayed stories of continued growth and a process or journey of striving towards recovery-oriented practice. This journey was shaped by participants' environments and they described both working within and attempting to modify or change their environments to enhance their capacity to work in a more recovery-oriented manner.

3.1. A Journey of Actively Striving towards Recovery-Oriented Practice. Participants described a need to continuously develop and strengthen their recovery-orientation. In order to do this, they detailed an active and ongoing process consisting of four components: intentionally seeking out knowledge, working to find fit or synergy between recovery-oriented practice principles and their professional identity and roles, maintaining hope, and developing confidence in defending recovery-oriented practices by strengthening their clinical reasoning skills.

3.1.1. Seeking Out Knowledge. All participants emphasised the importance of having a clear conceptualisation of recovery and recovery-oriented practice. Cultivating this was an intentional and active process. Participant understandings were constantly developing in response to new experiences and knowledge. They all highlighted a need to seek out opportunities to develop their knowledge, including learning directly from people with lived experience of mental illness. Casey highlighted the importance of taking time to "actually hear first-hand people's perspectives." In addition, participants described seeking out and reading recovery-based literature and personal narratives, attending recovery-focused training and conferences, and seeking advice from other recovery-oriented clinicians. Charlotte advised: "Do the course! Start doing workshops... things that are recovery-focused... you've got to have an understanding of what it means... It took me a lot of conscious effort."

3.1.2. Finding Fit. As participants learnt more and more about recovery and recovery-oriented practice, they described simultaneously integrating their developing conceptualisations with their personal and professional identities. All participants described a strong compatibility or synergy between recovery-oriented principles and occupational therapy philosophies. They talked about aspects such as person-centredness, supporting engagement in meaningful activity, empowerment of the individual, and taking a holistic and contextualised approach as being key and common facets of both recovery-oriented practice and occupational therapy. For example, Pat said, "I think naturally [occupational therapists are] attuned to being... holistic in our approach... the importance of meaningful activity ... how the environment plays a part in people's recovery... people developing meaningful roles... It's ingrained in us in our training." Similarly, Jamie felt that recovery-oriented practice "ties in really well with OT... finding out what is meaningful to them and framing our engagement with them around that," while Chris described the core business of occupational therapy as being "to facilitate them to have the life that they want, where they want."

Four participants suggested that recovery-orientation was more compatible with occupational therapy than other health professions. For example, Chris believed that occupational therapy was "a lot more about a person's roles and their overall functioning and how their entire life is, rather than 'you have this exact symptom, this is how you fix it.'" Because of this synergy, some participants saw the shift to recovery-oriented practice as an opportunity for the profession: "What's exciting about... recovery-orientated practice [is that it] supports a lot of what occupational therapists do... It might get to a point where... OTs find it easier to practice [and other professions] value the role of OT more" (Casey).

While two participants saw the alignment between occupational therapy and recovery as a straightforward "marriage made in heaven" (Charlotte), most also identified areas of potential misfit or challenge: "I still find 'recovery' a hard concept... trying to figure out what it means for me personally [and] professionally... What service it is that I want to be involved in providing... That was the first battle" (Ava).

Therapists described grappling to find fit between recovery and elements of their occupational therapy learning and identity. At times they needed to actively change their ways of thinking and "unlearn" old, medically oriented understandings and practices. Charlotte explained, "It took me a while... to move away from [a] deficit focus... When I went to uni it... looked at people's deficits... A lot of the assessments we still use are deficit-focused." Participants also wrestled with relinquishing the role of expert clinician to offer choice and hand control over to the consumer. For example, Chris thought that health professionals were trained to use their clinical expertise and to expect consumers to "kneel at the feet of clinicians." Likewise, Addison described her struggle with "trying to drop the therapist and the 'solving problems' part," adding that "sometimes it's not about solving the problem... it's about walking the journey."

Finally, while being not identified by participants as a challenge, a number appeared to define recovery through an occupational therapy or clinically based framework, emphasising independence and function as desired outcomes. For example, Amelia described recovery as being about consumers becoming "independent and able to look after themselves... in the community," and Chloe stated that having "that end goal of independence where possible is probably the tick we [OTs] have in our box compared to others."

3.1.3. Maintaining Hope. Having knowledge of recovery and recovery-oriented practice and being able to find fit between emerging recovery knowledge and occupational therapy were not enough for participants to practice in a recovery-oriented manner. They also stressed the importance of having and maintaining hope and holding a genuine belief in recovery.

Casey explained, "You have to [have] hope that… recovery is possible… It would become an awful place to work if you thought that was as good as it gets for people."

A belief that people can recover drove participants' recovery-orientation. Jessica, for example, described needing to have "a really strong belief that, [for] every single consumer that I work with… this is not your life. It will get better than this." Being witness to people recovering and seeing consumers benefiting from a recovery-oriented approach helped to ignite participants' hope and encouraged them to further pursue this approach to practice.

> *I was [initially] a bit nervous… these people have been through the mental health service for such a long period of time, so how much change are we going to be able to achieve? It really has amazed me… If you're working under a recovery model it is possible to make change. (Pat)*

In order to actively nurture this hope, some therapists sought connections with people recovering from mental illness outside of their immediate workplaces. For example, because Jessica's work primarily involved contact with people in acute phases of illness, she volunteered at the Hearing Voices Network in order to "spend time with people who are recovered and that maintains my hope." Casey also described observing people living their lives beyond the immediate workplace as critical because "if you look at the bigger picture, you can be… more hopeful."

3.1.4. Developing Confidence through Clinical Reasoning. To apply their knowledge and adopt practices they believed in, participants also described needing to develop confidence in their ability to make sound clinical decisions and to justify recovery-oriented practices when they conflicted with practice-as-normal. They particularly highlighted the practices around positive risk taking, a central mantra of recovery-oriented practice. Participants repeatedly talked about the confidence they needed to support and advocate for each consumer's right to choose to take positive risks. For example, Chris noted that being able to help consumers to take risks with treatments that might benefit their recovery "only comes with the confidence that your clinical skills and your clinical reasoning and decision making… are all good enough." Similarly, Jessica explained that because "the support network isn't really there yet to help us make those 'risky decisions'… you have to have really, really strong clinical reasoning and understanding of recovery to be able to justify why you made those decisions."

As they gained more experience and developed sound clinical reasoning skills, clinicians described becoming more comfortable and confident with advocating for recovery-oriented practice. Chris summed this up by saying that "the more of a new grad you are, the less comfortable you feel implementing recovery practices because it involves risk… The less experienced you are, the more frightening that is."

3.2. Working on and Working within the Environment. The journey of striving towards recovery-oriented practice was inextricably linked to and influenced by participants' work environments. Participants reported navigating, utilising, and, at times, struggling with both human and structural aspects of their environments in order to develop and sustain their recovery-orientation to practice.

3.2.1. Human Aspects. The human environment of the workplace, consisting of coworkers, supervisors or leaders, and peer workers, both positively and negatively influenced participants' ability to develop and sustain recovery-orientation. Most participants reported currently or previously experiencing negative coworker attitudes towards recovery. Medical orientation, poor communication, and a general lack of hope thwarted participants' recovery-oriented growth and discouraged their belief in recovery-oriented practice. Ava, describing a previous workplace, said the following:

> *[Negative attitudes] can really give you a negative point of view of your professional development and your career. Like… there's no point in trying to improve or change things because these people have been around longer than you and have kind of been damaged by being burnt out or not knowing the latest evidence or concepts.*

Casey explained how some staff attitudes in a forensic context made it difficult to be recovery-oriented: "they still want to see people punished and that can be really awful… they want to contain these people in these settings. That's a real challenge."

In contrast, working with a team of like-minded, recovery-oriented coworkers was perceived as highly beneficial. "You need to be strongly supported by a really good and caring team of people… in an environment where you never feel afraid to ask a question or… to get people to check that your reasoning is sound" (Chris). In these supportive environments, participants described pursuing and using the advice and support of recovery-oriented colleagues, more senior clinicians, and supervisors. Amelia described how her recovery-oriented colleagues helped and inspired her: "Sharing of that knowledge and supporting each other… That's what makes you come in and try, even though you've been butting your head." Addison used her sessions with her recovery-focused supervisor to "chat through… how I best could approach some situations."

While colleagues were an important part of the human environment, decision-makers or "people at the top" who supported recovery-oriented initiatives were seen as central to a supportive workplace. Describing the benefit of recovery-focused management or decision-makers, Jordan explained that their "support flows down into the frontline staff… It's reassuring and supportive." Casey concurred:

> *There is a hierarchy and if your consultant is recovery-orientated it makes a world of difference… they still direct treatments and they can push for recovery-orientated practices and have more authority than any other clinician… So, having them on board with recovery is the biggest enabler of all.*

Participants also repeatedly highlighted the benefit of having people with lived experience working in their service. Peer workers were viewed as valuable assets. In Chris's workplace, for example, peer workers "are getting more involved with actually improving the [recovery focus of the] service." Participants actively used their peer workers as sounding boards for their ideas and peer workers sometimes challenged clinicians' decision-making, prompting participants to critically reflect on their recovery-oriented principles and take action accordingly. Participants described peer workers as inspiring hope in consumers and clinicians alike. As Chloe reported, their presence "really helps with that understanding and that recovery-base and providing people hope that you can recover."

Importantly, participants did not see their relationship with the human environment of their workplace as a one-way transaction. Therapists also described taking action to enrich their workplace culture through leadership and example. As a supervisor, Casey said that "you have to be recovery-orientated yourself... be aware of what recovery is and bring that into the conversation... be aware of what tools are available... [to] guide people to be recovery-orientated."

Amelia suggested that, to influence the human environment, "you can use the language, you can talk about the frameworks, you can lead by example." She saw this leadership as an obligation for occupational therapists because of the synergy between the profession's philosophies and recovery-oriented approaches: "We are the ones that need to be leading the recovery-orientated approach within health services and if we're not there is something that is really wrong."

3.2.2. Structural Aspects. The structural elements of participants' work environments presented challenges to their journey of striving towards recovery-orientation. These structural aspects were both workplace specific and generic to the mental health system more broadly. Structural challenges included the biomedical outcome-driven and risk-averse nature of the mental health system, restrictive environments, and time limitations.

First, participants described a clinical outcome-driven system that did not recognise or place value on recovery-based practices or outcomes. As Ava said, "Meeting your KPIs [key performance indicators] as an OT does not necessarily mean giving them holistic care. But if you don't meet your KPIs then to your employer you're not doing your job."

Second, legislative and policy requirements, such as the Mental Health Act 2007 (NSW), lead to practices that restrict consumers' choice such as involuntary admission to hospital and compulsory treatment under community treatment orders (CTOs). Participants viewed these as restrictive, coercive, risk-averse, and therefore incompatible with recovery-oriented practice. Chris highlighted the challenge:

> *How do we actually implement [recovery-oriented practice] when we are dealing with CTOs and scheduling people... [and] having to dictate to people that they have to do these things under their forensic order... How do we... marry all those things up?*

Some environments, such as acute inpatient and forensic services, were described as particularly restrictive as they reduced opportunities for consumer choice and created greater power differentials between consumers and hospital staff. Jordan, for example, described the built environment of the hospital and its swipe-card access and exit for staff as reinforcing a "don't mess with authority" message.

Finally, participants across all service settings highlighted time limitations impacting negatively their ability to sustain recovery-orientation. For community-based participants, time restraints related to caseload size. Pat explained how care coordinators with "extraordinary numbers of consumers" had difficulty getting beyond "putting out fires." This made it difficult for them to focus on recovery. Anna described how, in acute settings, rapid consumer turnover created time constraints: "You really have no time to build up that [rapport]. They load up the patient with tablets and off [they] go." In contrast, participants in forensic settings described the difficulty of maintaining hope and progress towards recovery goals with patients who remained in inpatient settings for many years: "People want to set recovery goals and work towards them but then feel let down by the system, so we're not actually supporting their recovery. The length of time is too much" (Casey).

Despite these challenges, all participants continued to strive towards recovery-oriented practice because "engagement with [consumers] becomes much more meaningful" (Jamie), and as Jessica said, "for me, it's pleasurable to work in a recovery-orientated way."

4. Discussion

This study is, to our knowledge, the first to explore the ways in which occupational therapists go about developing and sustaining recovery-orientation in mental health practice. While it confirms previous findings on challenges and facilitators to recovery-oriented practice, it adds to the existing literature by outlining the ongoing, active, and intentional journey of striving to be recovery-oriented. Rather than simply putting their recovery-oriented beliefs into action, all participants, irrespective of workplace setting, described this as a process or journey that involved a combination of actively seeking out knowledge, finding fit, maintaining hope, developing confidence through clinical reasoning, and working on and within the environment.

A number of parallels can be drawn between the occupational therapists' ongoing journey of developing and sustaining recovery-orientation and some aspects of the mental health recovery journey described by consumers. First, both are individually driven [2]. Second, rather than being a singular event, both are characterised as a continual process with no fixed end-point or final destination [3]. Third, each process can be facilitated or hindered by the human and structural elements within the environment [6]. For example, just as participants in this study highlighted the importance of the support and guidance they gave to and received from colleagues, consumers have repeatedly identified the value of giving and receiving peer support from others travelling a similar journey [5]. Fourth, for therapists, strengthening their knowledge, hope, and confidence was essential in cultivating their recovery-oriented practice. Similarly, consumers have described an ongoing need to learn about themselves and make sense of their experiences in order to progress along their recovery journey [2]. Both describe needing hope and a belief that recovery can occur to inspire their ongoing efforts [3]. While consumers describe benefiting from the support of recovery-focused professionals, our participants valued the contributions of recovery-focused consumers to their practice. Perhaps recognition by both occupational therapists and consumers of the parallel journeys being undertaken could facilitate a consciously reciprocal alliance, each mutually supporting the other in their continual efforts and progress.

Participants in this study all described good synergy between principles of recovery-orientation and their occupational therapy professional identity. In this regard, clinicians' experiences are in keeping with perspectives previously expressed by occupational therapy scholars [11, 12, 14], adding credence to this argument. The overwhelming majority of participants in this study, however, described a need to actively find fit, suggesting that the common perception of occupational therapy and recovery-oriented practice as unproblematically synergistic may be an oversimplification. Participants described needing to unlearn aspects of their training and struggling to relinquish their expert role to better embrace principles such as choice and dignity of risk. Indeed, Lal [34] has warned against an oversimplistic assumption that there is perfect symmetry between occupational therapy philosophies and recovery-oriented practice.

Interestingly, while participants' conceptualisations of recovery were mostly consistent with consumer definitions [1], a number included an additional element: independent functioning. This is somewhat in contrast to consumer definitions of recovery in which independence may or may not be an individual's goal. Further, previous research has identified that sense of self and connecting with others, rather than independent functioning, were aspects of occupational engagement that consumers described as most meaningful [35]. The discrepancy is likely due to participants viewing recovery-oriented practice through a traditional occupational therapy lens that prioritises independent function. Similarly, it is meaningful engagement in activities that has been described as critical for recovery rather than the outcomes or products of activities which occupational therapists may be inclined to focus on [13]. Recognising these discipline based values and being wary of inadvertently superimposing them on consumers are important for occupational therapists in developing and sustaining their recovery-oriented practice [13, 34, 36].

Despite the perceived congruence between occupational therapy and recovery compared to other disciplines, participants experienced environmental barriers to and facilitators of recovery-oriented practice that were consistent with findings in previous multidisciplinary research. These included human aspects such as coworker attitudes towards recovery [8, 27, 28] and structural elements such as restrictive contexts [25] and dominance of systemic priorities [26]. Most participants in this study, however, did not merely recognise the environmental influences on their practice; they also described working to exert influence by doing things like using recovery-oriented language and leading by example, defending their practices with strong clinical reasoning, and supporting recovery-orientation in their supervision of others.

However, it is clear that changes at a systemic level are also needed. For example, health services should consider review and modification of KPIs to better align with recovery-oriented principles. Examples of recovery-oriented KPIs might include the percentage of consumers with a wellness or recovery action plan, scores of consumer satisfaction with service, measures of hopefulness, or percentage of consumers with self-identified goals. Health services can also better support therapists to use strategies they have identified to enhance their recovery-orientation. Our research supports the inclusion of peer workers in services and the creation of opportunities for therapists, particularly those working in restrictive or acute environments, to meet and learn from consumers who are further along their recovery journeys. For example, provision of consumer-facilitated training or rotating work positions that enable all therapists to experience working with consumers at varying stages of recovery might facilitate therapists' belief in and hope for recovery and thus their recovery-oriented practice. Because our results suggest that different practice contexts may present unique challenges, a one-size-fits-all, whole of system approach alone may be inadequate in supporting the realisation of recovery-oriented reform. Rather, engagement and troubleshooting at a context-specific level may prove essential to facilitating practice change.

Occupational therapists have been criticised for being "complicit in perpetrating oppressive institutional practices" and falling victim to organisational red tape rather than advocating for consumers [36]. The active strategies described by our participants suggest that occupational therapists may be beginning to take on a leadership role in helping shift mental health practice towards a more recovery-oriented approach as they have been called to do [12–14]. However, participants' spheres of influence appeared to remain at the immediate workplace level. They tried to work creatively within the existing systemic constraints rather than describing advocacy for change at this broader level. The next step for occupational therapy as a profession is to extend our leadership beyond our immediate workplaces and facilitate systemic transformation towards a more recovery-oriented mental health system. This can occur at all levels within the profession. Occupational therapists working directly with consumers can, for example, pursue opportunities to sit in on decision-making committees or panels with influence as well as advocating for consumers to be included on these. University educators can enhance the capacity of new graduates by focusing upon intervention at a systemic, rather than just an individual, level. Occupational therapy associations can also play a role through their advocacy and policy-based activities and provision of continuing professional education focused on facilitating system change.

4.1. Limitations. As with any qualitative research, the findings of this study are not universally applicable and should be interpreted with reference to the sample characteristics. All participants worked in New South Wales or Victoria, Australia. While the process of developing and sustaining recovery-oriented practice is likely to be relevant for occupational therapists in other geographical locations, as evidenced by the congruence of the findings with international literature, systemic and cultural differences warrant further research. Additionally, participants' experiences were diverse, and participants themselves identified contextual issues such as training, experience, practice context, and roles as influencing these. Research on larger samples would allow a more robust comparison of therapists' experiences and identification of issues that might be especially pertinent to particular groups. The aim to examine how occupational therapists develop and sustain recovery-orientation required targeted recruitment of therapists who identified themselves as being recovery-oriented. Future research exploring the experiences of those who feel unable or are unwilling to adopt recovery-oriented practice will be beneficial in further understanding the lag between policy and practice.

5. Conclusion

This small exploratory study describes how occupational therapists consciously and actively develop and sustain recovery-orientation in their mental health practice. It adds to previous multidisciplinary research by (a) illuminating active strategies, which may well be similarly relevant to other health professionals, and (b) highlighting specific tensions between occupational therapy and recovery-oriented practice frameworks and philosophies. This work provides guidance for therapists regarding the ongoing work needed to realise and maintain their own recovery-oriented practice, as well as challenging occupational therapists to extend their influence to broader system-level reform.

Competing Interests

The authors declare that there are no competing interests regarding the publication of this paper.

References

[1] Australian Health Ministers' Advisory Council, *A National Framework for Recovery-Oriented Mental Health Services: Guide for Practitioners and Providers*, Department of Health and Ageing, Canberra, Australia, 2013.

[2] J. Repper and R. Perkins, *Social Inclusion and Recovery: A Model for Mental Health Practice*, Baillière Tindall, Edinburgh, UK, 2003.

[3] M. Leamy, V. Bird, C. Le Boutillier, J. Williams, and M. Slade, "Conceptual framework for personal recovery in mental health: systematic review and narrative synthesis," *British Journal of Psychiatry*, vol. 199, no. 6, pp. 445–452, 2011.

[4] J. Williams, M. Leamy, V. Bird et al., "Measures of the recovery orientation of mental health services: systematic review," *Social Psychiatry and Psychiatric Epidemiology*, vol. 47, no. 11, pp. 1827–1835, 2012.

[5] M. A. Mancini, E. R. Hardiman, and H. A. Lawson, "Making sense of it all: consumer providers' theories about factors facilitating and impeding recovery from psychiatric disabilities," *Psychiatric Rehabilitation Journal*, vol. 29, no. 1, pp. 48–55, 2005.

[6] B. Happell, "Determining the effectiveness of mental health services from a consumer perspective: part 1: enhancing recovery," *International Journal of Mental Health Nursing*, vol. 17, no. 2, pp. 116–122, 2008.

[7] C. Le Boutillier, A. Chevalier, V. Lawrence et al., "Staff understanding of recovery-orientated mental health practice: a systematic review and narrative synthesis," *Implementation Science*, vol. 10, no. 1, article no. 87, 2015.

[8] C. Le Boutillier, M. Leamy, V. J. Bird, L. Davidson, J. Williams, and M. Slade, "What does recovery mean in practice? A qualitative analysis of international recovery-oriented practice guidance," *Psychiatric Services*, vol. 62, no. 12, pp. 1470–1476, 2011.

[9] M. Slade, *100 Ways to Support Recovery: A Guide for Mental Health Professionals*, Rethink, London, UK, 2009.

[10] Australian Health Ministers' Advisory Council, *A National Framework for Recovery-Oriented Mental Health Services: Policy and Theory*, Department of Health and Ageing, Canberra, Australia, 2013.

[11] M. Kelly, S. Lamont, and S. Brunero, "An occupational perspective of the recovery journey in mental health," *British Journal of Occupational Therapy*, vol. 73, no. 3, pp. 129–135, 2010.

[12] K. L. Rebeiro Gruhl, "Reflections on ... the recovery paradigm: should occupational-therapists be interested?" *The Canadian Journal of Occupational Therapy*, vol. 72, no. 2, pp. 96–102, 2005.

[13] D. J. Sutton, C. S. Hocking, and L. A. Smythe, "A phenomenological study of occupational engagement in recovery from mental illness," *Canadian Journal of Occupational Therapy*, vol. 79, no. 3, pp. 142–150, 2012.

[14] C. Lloyd, S. Tse, and H. Bassett, "Mental health recovery and occupational therapy in Australia and New Zealand," *International Journal of Therapy & Rehabilitation*, vol. 11, no. 2, pp. 64–70, 2004.

[15] M. Law, S. Baptiste, and J. Mills, "Client-centred practice: what does it mean and does it make a difference?" *Canadian Journal of Occupational Therapy*, vol. 62, no. 5, pp. 250–257, 1995.

[16] New Freedom Commission on Mental Health, *Achieving the Promise: Transforming Mental Health Care in America. Executive Summary*, New Freedom Commission on Mental Health, Rockville, Md, USA, 2003.

[17] Her Majesty's Government, *No Health without Mental Health: A Cross-Government Mental Health Outcomes Strategy for People of All Ages*, Department of Health, London, UK, 2011.

[18] Council of Australian Governments, *The Roadmap for National Mental Health Reform 2012–2022*, Council of Australian Governments, Canberra, Australia, 2012.

[19] Department of Health and Ageing, *Fourth National Mental Health Plan: An Agenda for Collaborative Government Action in Mental Health 2009–14*, Commonwealth Department of Health and Aged Care, Canberra, Australia, 2009.

[20] World Health Organization, *Comprehensive Mental Health Action Plan 2013–2020*, World Health Organisation, Geneva, Switzerland, 2013.

[21] G. H. Gudjonsson, C. S. V. Savona, T. Green, and R. Terry, "The recovery approach to the care of mentally disordered patients. Does it predict treatment engagement and positive social behaviour beyond quality of life?" *Personality and Individual Differences*, vol. 51, no. 8, pp. 899–903, 2011.

[22] V. Stanhope, S. Barrenger, M. Salzer, and S. Marcus, "Examining the relationship between choice, therapeutic alliance and outcomes in mental health services," *Journal of Personalized Medicine*, vol. 3, no. 3, pp. 191–202, 2013.

[23] M. Slade, N. Adams, and M. O'Hagan, "Recovery: past progress and future challenges," *International Review of Psychiatry*, vol. 24, no. 1, pp. 1–4, 2012.

[24] L. Davidson, M. J. O'Connell, J. Tondora, M. Lawless, and A. C. Evans, "Recovery in serious mental illness: a new wine or just a new bottle?" *Professional Psychology: Research & Practice*, vol. 36, no. 5, pp. 480–487, 2005.

[25] S.-P. Chen, T. Krupa, R. Lysaght, E. McCay, and M. Piat, "The development of recovery competencies for in-patient mental health providers working with people with serious mental Illness," *Administration and Policy in Mental Health and Mental Health Services Research*, vol. 40, no. 2, pp. 96–116, 2013.

[26] C. Le Boutillier, M. Slade, V. Lawrence et al., "Competing priorities: staff perspectives on supporting recovery," *Administration and Policy in Mental Health and Mental Health Services Research*, vol. 42, no. 4, pp. 429–438, 2015.

[27] M. Piat and S. Lal, "Service providers' experiences and perspectives on recovery-oriented mental health system reform," *Psychiatric rehabilitation journal*, vol. 35, no. 4, pp. 289–296, 2012.

[28] S. A. Kidd, K. J. McKenzie, and G. Virdee, "Mental health reform at a systems level: widening the lens on recovery-oriented care," *Canadian Journal of Psychiatry*, vol. 59, no. 5, pp. 243–249, 2014.

[29] M. Slade, M. Amering, M. Farkas et al., "Uses and abuses of recovery: implementing recovery-oriented practices in mental health systems," *World Psychiatry*, vol. 13, no. 1, pp. 12–20, 2014.

[30] S. J. Tracy, *Qualitative Research Methods: Collecting Evidence, Crafting Analysis, Communicating Impact*, Wiley, Hoboken, NJ, USA, 2012.

[31] K. Charmaz, *Constructing Grounded Theory*, SAGE, London, UK, 2014.

[32] B. DiCicco-Bloom and B. F. Crabtree, "The qualitative research interview," *Medical Education*, vol. 40, no. 4, pp. 314–321, 2006.

[33] T. Harris, "Grounded theory," *Nursing Standard*, vol. 29, no. 35, pp. 32–39, 2015.

[34] S. Lal, "Prescribing recovery as the new mantra for mental health: does one prescription serve all?" *The Canadian Journal of Occupational Therapy*, vol. 77, no. 2, pp. 82–89, 2010.

[35] N. Hancock, A. Honey, and A. C. Bundy, "Sources of meaning derived from occupational engagement for people recovering from mental illness," *British Journal of Occupational Therapy*, vol. 78, no. 8, pp. 508–515, 2015.

[36] K. W. Hammell, "Client-centred practice: ethical obligation or professional obfuscation?" *British Journal of Occupational Therapy*, vol. 70, no. 6, pp. 264–266, 2007.

8

Deep, Surface, or Both? A Study of Occupational Therapy Students' Learning Concepts

Tore Bonsaksen[1,2]

[1]Department of Occupational Therapy, Prosthetics and Orthotics, Faculty of Health Sciences, OsloMet-Oslo Metropolitan University, Oslo, Norway
[2]Faculty of Health Studies, VID Specialized University, Sandnes, Norway

Correspondence should be addressed to Tore Bonsaksen; tore.bonsaksen@hioa.no

Academic Editor: Jodie A. Copley

Background. Students' conceptualization of learning has been associated with their approaches to studying. However, whether students' learning concepts are associated with their personal characteristics is unknown. *Aim.* To investigate whether sociodemographic, education-related, and personal factors were associated with the learning concepts of Norwegian occupational therapy students. *Methods.* One hundred and forty-nine students (mean age 23.9 years, 79.2% women) participated in the study. The employed self-report questionnaires included the Approaches and Study Skills Inventory for Students, the Rosenberg Self-Esteem Scale, and the General Self-Efficacy Scale. Differences between student cohorts were analyzed with one-way analyses of variance and χ^2 tests, whereas factors associated with the students' learning concepts were analyzed with bivariate correlation and linear regression models. *Results.* The students' mean scores on the deep and surface learning concept scales were similar. Spending more time on the independent study was associated with having higher scores on the unidimensional learning concept measure. *Conclusions.* The students' learning concept appears to encompass a surface concept as well as a deep concept of learning, and the two ways of conceptualizing learning were positively related to each other. Over time, a mature deep concept may add to, rather than replace, a basic surface concept of learning.

1. Introduction

According to Biggs [1], the factors important for students' learning in higher education can be organized according to the presage, process, and product of learning—the three P model. The presage factors are those that constitute the student's readiness for the tertiary educational experience, emphasizing intellectual inquiry, logical reasoning, and the development of a comprehensive understanding of the phenomena under scrutiny. These factors include the student's background characteristics but also the situational context within which learning takes place [1]. The process factors are concerned with how the student engages with the study materials. A substantial amount of educational research has built on the concepts of deep, strategic, and surface approaches to studying, denoting a typology of different attitudes and behaviors when engaged in studying [2, 3]. Finally, the product or outcome of learning is considered to be a blend of theoretical knowledge, practical skills, and generic competence [4]. For practical purposes, much research has operationalized "learning outcome" as exam grades, although for students of occupational therapy and other healthcare professions, professional skill acquisition should be considered of equal importance [5].

A substantial amount of educational research suggests a relationship between the learning process and the subsequent learning product. Students' approaches to studying have been shown to play a significant part in determining learning outcomes, as frequently measured by their academic performance results. Specifically, researchers have found a relatively consistent pattern of associations between employing deep and strategic study approaches and achieving good academic grades [5–10]. Conversely, using a surface approach to studying has been associated with poorer academic grades.

In view of the detected relationships between productive study approaches and subsequent learning outcomes, researchers have also examined how the presage factors may have an impact on the students' learning process, often conceptualized as their approaches to studying. Among the individual student factors, higher age has been found to be associated with the deep and strategic study approaches [11–13], whereas the impact of gender has been ambiguous [11]. Other personal factors, like general self-efficacy [13] and intrinsic motivation [14], have also been shown to be associated with productive study approaches among undergraduate students of occupational therapy and psychology, respectively. Much research attention has been devoted to exploring relationships between the learning environment and the students' approaches to studying (e.g., [15–17]). An illustrating example was provided by Sun and Richardson [18] in their study of British business candidates. Their results showed that all subscales of a course experience questionnaire (e.g., appropriate assessment and workload, clarity of goals and standards, and good teaching) were positively associated with deep and strategic approaches to studying and negatively associated with a surface approach.

Notwithstanding the demonstrated impact of the learning environment, Richardson [19] argued that a substantial variance proportion related to approaches to studying was still left unexplained, even after adjusting for perceptions of the learning environment. Considering other factors that might contribute to explain students' variations in study approaches, he pointed towards another presage factor—the students' own conceptions of learning. In support of this reasoning, early research demonstrated relationships between "reproductive" conceptions of learning (i.e., the belief that learning is mainly concerned with the ability to remember facts) and a surface approach to studying and conversely, between a "reconstructive" concept of learning (i.e., the belief that learning is concerned with understanding things differently) and a deep approach to studying [20]. Dart and coworkers [21] similarly found that students who conceived learning as understanding, perceiving something in a different way, personal fulfilment, and developing social competence were more inclined to use a deep approach to studying. Conversely, students who conceived learning predominantly as increase in knowledge, remembering, and reproducing were more inclined to use a surface approach to studying. Sharma [22] found that the majority of his sample of accounting students conceived learning to be about acquiring knowledge rather than developing their understanding and expressed concern in the anticipation of what could be called "robotic" accountants.

However, there is reason to suggest that students' conceptions of knowledge are not either deep or surface but that they evolve into more sophisticated forms over time. Building on the ideas of William Perry, Entwistle and Peterson [23] described a typical course of learning concept development. Starting out from dualism, the student is inclined to think that something is right or wrong. The next phase, multiplicity, indicates that the student accepts there exist several views on an issue. Entering the relativism phase indicates that the student has arrived at an understanding of the different views as depending on the person's interpretation of evidence. Commitment within relativism, the final phase in the model, involves making a personal stand, while accepting other views to be concurrently valid. In support of such a view, the recent study of occupational therapy students found that those with broader conceptions of learning also had higher scores on the deep and strategic study approach scales, compared to their counterparts with narrower conceptions of learning [24].

Applying this model to occupational therapy education, a student may for example initially feel certain that group-based activities are good for persons with depression (dualism): depressed persons need to break out from isolation. He or she may then accept that others have different opinions on the matter (multiplicity): group activities can be overwhelming and may stimulate feelings of inferiority in relation to others. Later, the student may realize that the assessment of potential benefits and risks of group activities for depression depend on the employed perspective (relativism) and may choose to become more involved in one such perspective while still acknowledging the perspective of others (commitment within relativism).

To summarize, a long line of education research has taken the students' approaches to learning (SAL) tradition as the point of departure. There is a need for research oriented towards relevant outcomes but also research that explores how the different elements of the educational setting—presage, process, and product—work together [25]. In this study, Richardson's [19] view that students' learning conceptions are of importance for both the process and the outcomes of learning is pursued further. To date, it appears that no such study of learning conceptions has been conducted with occupational therapy students. Given the importance of students' learning concepts, an inquiry into their associated factors would allow for a more comprehensive understanding of their role in occupational therapy students' learning. The research question guiding the current study is the following: What are the relationships between occupational therapy students' sociodemographic, personal, and education-related characteristics and their concepts of learning?

2. Methods

2.1. Design and Setting of the Study. A cross-sectional design was used. The study was conducted in the context of a cross-cultural study, which included four different countries [26]. In the current study, only the data from the Norwegian students were used.

2.2. Participants and Recruitment. For inclusion in the study, the students needed to be enrolled in the university's undergraduate occupational therapy education program and provide informed consent to participate. Students from all three-year cohorts participated in the study. The questionnaires were distributed to the students during breaks in classes in January 2015.

2.3. Measurement

2.3.1. Sociodemographic Factors. Data regarding age (years) and gender (male = 0, female = 1) were collected by questionnaire.

2.3.2. Personal Factors. The *Rosenberg Self-Esteem Scale* (RSES; [27]) was used to assess self-esteem. The original RSES has ten items, with responses ranging 1–4 ("strongly agree" to "strongly disagree"). One example item is "I take a positive attitude toward myself." A Norwegian version with four items (RSES-4) was used in this study, and the scale consisting of the four extracted items was strongly correlated ($r = 0.95$) with the full 10-item version [28, 29]. The RSES-4 sum score ranges 4–16, with higher score representing higher self-esteem. In the Norwegian sample, Cronbach's α was 0.67 [30], which is lower than the internal consistency shown in other Norwegian studies [31, 32].

The *General Self-Efficacy Scale* (GSE) [33] measures optimistic self-beliefs about coping with a variety of challenges and demands in life. The scale's 10 items are each rated 1–4 ("not at all true" to "exactly true"), and a sum score is calculated by adding the scores on the ten items. The GSE score range is therefore 10–40, with higher scores indicating higher general self-efficacy. One example item is "I can solve most problems if I invest the necessary effort." Psychometric studies of the GSE have consistently produced a one-factor solution [34, 35], and internal consistency (Cronbach's α) of the GSE scale was 0.86 [30], which is considered very good [36, 37].

2.3.3. Education-Related Factors. Data related to the students' learning concepts were obtained from the Approaches and Study Skills Inventory for Students (ASSIST; [2, 38]). In this study, we used a Norwegian instrument translation [39] that has been psychometrically examined within the same sample [40].

The first part of the ASSIST, concerned with the conceptions of learning, consists of six statements. To each of these statements, the respondent rates his or her level of agreement on a 1–5 scale. A rating of "1" means the statement content is "very different" from the student's own thinking, whereas a rating of "5" means it is "very close" to the student's own thinking. The conceptions of learning were originally considered to be of two different kinds [2, 41]: learning conceived as a process of reproducing information (surface concept) and as a process of constructing personal understanding and meaning (deep concept). However, a recent study of the psychometric properties of the learning concepts reflected in these items concluded that the six items might preferably constitute a unidimensional scale, with all six items reflecting aspects of one higher-order concept of learning [40]. Factor loadings for the one-factor measure, tentatively labeled "collected efforts," ranged between 0.42 and 0.76, and internal consistency of the scale items was $\alpha = 0.70$. For the deep learning concept, factor loadings ranged between 0.54 and 0.81 and internal consistency was $\alpha = 0.61$. For the surface learning concept, factor loadings ranged between 0.67 and 0.78 and internal consistency was $\alpha = 0.61$. The collected efforts' measures, in addition to the deep and surface concept measures, were used as dependent variables in the current study.

One last item of the ASSIST [2, 38] asks the students to think of the grades they have obtained and then perform an overall self-assessment in terms of how well they have been doing in the course so far. Students rated themselves on a 1–9 scale, where 1 indicated "rather badly", 3 "not so well", 5 "about average", 7 "quite well", and 9 "very well."

Each participant was registered as belonging to one of the three-year cohorts. Previous higher education experience was dichotomized into two categories: having prior education from university or college (coded 1) versus not having any prior education from university or college (coded 0). The average number of weekly hours spent on the independent study was registered as a continuous variable.

2.4. Data Analysis. All data were entered into the computer program IBM SPSS version 24 [42]. Descriptive analyses were performed on all variables using means (M), standard deviations (SD), frequencies, and percentages as appropriate. Differences between students in different study cohorts were examined with chi-squared tests (for categorical variables) and with one-way analyses of variance (for continuous variables). When conducting multiple comparisons between student cohorts, the Tukey honest significant difference (HSD) correction was applied to adjust for inflating error rates.

Bivariate associations between variables were assessed with Pearson's correlation coefficient r. To assess the extent to which the three learning concept measures could be explained by the independent variables, three subsequent hierarchical linear regression analyses were performed. These analyses also assessed the strength of the independent associations between each of the independent variables and the participants' learning concept. The hierarchy of each of the regression models adhered to Bonsaksen's previous modeling [43]: (1) age and gender, (2) self-esteem and general self-efficacy, and (3) cohort, prior higher education, average time per week spent on the independent study, and self-assessment of study performance. Effect sizes (ES, r, and β) were interpreted according to Cohen [44]: small ES = 0.10, medium E S = 0.30, and large ES = 0.50. The level of statistical significance was set at $p < 0.05$.

2.5. Ethics. Approval for conducting the study was obtained from the Norwegian Centre for Research Data (project number 40314). The students were informed that completion of the questionnaires was voluntary, that their responses would be kept confidential, and that there would be no negative consequences from opting not to participate in the study.

3. Results

3.1. Participants. One hundred and sixty students opted to participate in the study. Of these, 149 students had valid scores on all variables used in the current study, and these students constitute the sample. The study sample is described in Table 1. All three-year levels were included (first year students $n = 51$, second year $n = 49$, and third year $n = 49$). The students' mean age was 23.9 years (SD = 4.4 years), and there was a majority of female students ($n = 118$, 79.2%). The sample as a whole had similar scores on the deep learning concept ($M = 12.8$, SD = 1.5), compared to their scores on the surface learning concept ($M = 12.8$, SD = 1.4). There were statistically significant differences between study cohorts

TABLE 1: Characteristics of the study sample ($n = 149$).

Variables	Total sample ($n = 149$)	1st year ($n = 51$)	2nd year ($n = 49$)	3rd year ($n = 49$)	p
Sociodemographic factors					
Age, *M* (SD)	23.9 (4.4)	22.9 (4.4)	23.0 (2.4)	25.7 (5.2)	0.001
Female gender, *n* (%)	118 (79.2)	42 (82.4)	36 (73.5)	40 (81.6)	0.48
Personal factors					
Self-esteem, *M* (SD)	12.3 (1.9)	12.1 (1.9)	12.5 (1.8)	12.5 (1.9)	0.38
General self-efficacy, *M* (SD)	28.4 (5.0)	27.6 (5.0)	28.8 (4.9)	28.9 (5.3)	0.37
Education factors					
Prior higher education, *n* (%)	65 (43.6)	22 (43.1)	22 (44.9)	21 (42.9)	0.98
Average time per week on the independent study, *M* (SD)	9.3 (5.0)	11.0 (4.1)	6.7 (3.6)	10.2 (6.7)	<0.001
Self-assessment of study performance, *M* (SD)	6.2 (1.3)	5.7 (1.5)	6.3 (1.2)	6.5 (1.2)	<0.01
Learning concepts					
Deep concept, *M* (SD)	12.8 (1.5)	12.7 (1.5)	12.9 (1.3)	12.9 (1.6)	0.85
Surface concept, *M* (SD)	12.8 (1.4)	13.1 (1.5)	12.4 (1.5)	12.9 (1.3)	0.08
Collected efforts' concept, *M* (SD)	25.6 (2.3)	25.8 (2.4)	25.3 (2.3)	25.6 (2.3)	0.50

Note. Statistical tests are chi-squared test and one-way ANOVA.

regarding age, average time spent on the independent study, and self-assessment of study performance.

3.2. Unadjusted Associations with the Learning Concepts. The unadjusted associations between the study variables are shown in Table 2. Being of higher age, having higher general self-efficacy, spending more time on the independent study, and having higher self-assessment of own study performance were associated with higher scores on the deep learning concept. Spending more time on the independent study was also associated with higher scores on the surface learning concept and with higher scores on the combined, unidimensional measure ("collected efforts"). The positive association between the deep and the surface learning concepts was statistically significant and of medium size.

3.3. Adjusted Associations with the Learning Concepts. The adjusted associations between the independent study variables and the three learning concepts are shown in Table 3. The deep concept regression model was statistically significant, accounting for 13.7% of the data variance. However, none of the independent variables was significantly associated with scores on the deep concept, while controlling for all variables. The surface concept regression model was not statistically significant, accounted for 6.0% of the variance, and no direct associations were detected. The collected efforts' regression model accounted for 10.0% of the variance. It was not statistically significant, but spending more time on the independent study was directly associated with higher scores on the concept.

4. Discussion

The aim of the current study was to examine associations between sociodemographic factors, personal factors, education-related factors, and learning concepts among Norwegian occupational therapy students. Four variables—higher age, higher general self-efficacy, more time spent on the independent study, and higher self-assessment of study performance—showed bivariate associations with the deep concept. Time spent on the independent study showed bivariate associations with all three learning concepts. However, most of the associations vanished when controlling for all variables in the multivariate analyses.

The bivariate analyses of factors associated with the deep learning concept showed the same pattern as shown in previous studies, in which the deep approach to studying [24] and a measure of preferences for teaching "supporting understanding" [43] were used as outcomes (Table 2). The shared pattern of associations lend support to the notion that these aspects of learning are interrelated. Entwistle and Peterson [23], for example, suggested the occurrence of two-way relationships between learning conceptions and study approaches. Conceptions might be developed from experiences of teaching and studying and may then influence subsequent ways of studying. An unpublished factor analysis, including learning concept items and study approach items together, similarly linked a deep concept of learning with study behaviors that reflect a deep approach to studying [45]. Thus, the unadjusted analysis suggest that some of the same factors that contribute to shape a deep approach to studying [13, 24] and a matching preference for courses and teaching [43] may also contribute to explain variations in the deep concept of learning.

However, the associations with the deep concept scores vanished when statistically controlling for all variables in the multivariate regression analysis. This is in contrast to the study of factors associated with teaching preferences [43]. In that study, age, general self-efficacy, and time spent on the independent study were significantly associated with the teaching preference "supporting understanding," while controlling for the exact same set of variables as in the current study. The different results may indicate that while some factors stand out as individually associated with a deep-

TABLE 2: Bivariate associations between the study variables ($n = 149$).

Variables	Deep concept		Surface concept		Collected effort concept	
	r	p	r	p	r	p
Age	0.18	<0.05	−0.03	0.76	0.10	0.25
Gender	0.14	0.10	0.12	0.16	0.15	0.06
Self-esteem	0.12	0.14	−0.00	0.98	0.08	0.36
General self-efficacy	0.19	<0.05	−0.06	0.45	0.08	0.32
Cohort	0.04	0.60	−0.07	0.39	−0.02	0.84
Prior higher education	−0.05	0.54	0.09	0.27	0.02	0.77
Average time per week on the independent study	0.24	<0.01	0.17	<0.05	0.25	<0.01
Self-assessment of study performance	0.17	<0.05	0.05	0.54	0.14	0.10
Surface concept	0.29	<0.001				

Note. Statistical test is Pearson correlation coefficient r. Coding of categorical variables: male = 0; female = 1. No prior higher education = 0; prior higher education = 1. For all other variables, higher scores indicate higher levels.

TABLE 3: Hierarchical linear regression analyses showing direct associations with the students' learning concepts ($n = 149$).

Independent variables	Deep concept		Surface concept		Collected effort concept	
	β	p	β	p	β	p
Sociodemographic factors						
Age	0.14	0.11	−0.08	0.41	0.04	0.66
Gender	0.17	0.06	0.08	0.36	0.16	0.08
Explained variance	**4.5%**	**0.03**	**1.4%**	**0.35**	**3.1%**	**0.10**
Personal factors						
Self-esteem	0.05	0.61	0.07	0.53	0.08	0.48
General self-efficacy	0.15	0.15	−0.11	0.32	0.03	0.80
R^2 change	**5.2%**	**0.02**	**0.6%**	**0.65**	**2.1%**	**0.21**
Explained variance	**9.7%**	**<0.01**	**2.0%**	**0.56**	**5.1**	**0.11**
Education factors						
Cohort	−0.03	0.73	−0.06	0.54	−0.05	0.55
Prior higher education	−0.10	0.24	0.09	0.31	−0.01	0.93
Average time per week on the independent study	0.15	0.09	0.16	0.08	0.19	<0.05
Self-assessment of study performance	0.11	0.20	0.08	0.39	0.12	0.18
R^2 change	**4.0%**	**0.17**	**3.9%**	**0.22**	**4.8%**	**0.12**
Explained variance	**13.7%**	**<0.01**	**6.0%**	**0.36**	**10.0%**	**0.06**

Note. Table content is standardized beta weights and corresponding p values. Coding of categorical variables: male = 0; female = 1. No prior higher education = 0; prior higher education = 1. For all other variables, higher scores indicate higher levels.

related teaching preference, a more complex pattern of interrelationships between several factors may cancel each other out when attempting to relate the scores to a deep learning concept. Further studies may investigate other variables of interest, as well as combinations of variables, that may contribute to explain variations in deep learning concept scores.

More time spent on the independent study remained associated with higher scores on the unidimensional learning concept measure, "collected efforts," after adjusting for the effect of all variables. The meaning of this finding is that more persistent study behaviors occurred among students who had a broader view of learning, that is, among those who agreed more strongly to more of the items on the learning concept measure. Students with a narrower view of learning spent less time studying. Previous research has shown that time spent on independent studying is important for subsequent academic performance among occupational therapy students, regardless of their study approaches [5]. However, the recent study also showed that a broader learning concept was significantly associated with higher scores on both deep and strategic approaches to studying [24]. Taken together, these variables may be related in a cyclical pattern. More time spent on the independent study appears to be related to a broader view of what learning is (Table 3) and also to using productive approaches to studying [13]. Conversely, a broader view of learning has been shown to be associated with productive study approaches [24] and may also make spending time on studies more attractive to students. However, the cross-sectional design of the current study precludes us from being conclusive about the direction of these relationships. Further studies should preferably investigate learning concepts, preferences for teaching, and approaches to studying prospectively and in a longitudinal perspective. That way, researchers will be better positioned to clarify the nature of associations and to predict outcomes at subsequent time points.

Considering the scale range (3–15) for both of the deep and the surface learning concepts, the students had high and similar scores on both concept measures (Table 1). Moreover, the two scales for measuring learning concepts were positively correlated (Table 2). The positive association was unexpected, as theory tends to emphasize their differences and not their possible similarities [2, 23, 41]. On the other hand, we notice that Buckley and coworkers [46] found an even stronger positive association ($r = 0.60$, $p < 0.01$) between the deep and surface concept measures used in their study. Further, a recent factor analysis found that a one-factor structure, comprised by all learning concept items together, was a better fit to the data than the two-factor solution [40].

According to the above, the deep and surface learning concepts may not be as different from one another as theory might suggest. In view of William Perry's work, as described by Entwistle and Peterson [23], we may rather think of them both as constituents of a learning concept that develops over time. In the first two developmental phases (dualism and multiplicity), the student may be strongly rooted in a surface concept of learning. This is the phase where he or she wants to get the facts straight and be sure to remember the right answer. In the next two phases (relativism and commitment within relativism), the student needs to incorporate a view that knowledge depends on interpretations. Taking into consideration the results of this study, this development may not imply abandoning the surface concept of learning. However, incorporating a view of learning as something that extends the mere acquisition of facts is required in higher education. Thus, we may assume a line of development starting with a surface-based learning concept, which then gradually incorporates a "deeper" concept according to a growing awareness of the difference between empirical facts and theoretical understanding. In line with critique relating to an overly simplistic dichotomy between deep and surface approaches to studying [47], we may apply a similar critique on the issue of students' ways of conceptualizing learning. Such differences appear to be a matter of nuance rather than a clear-cut dichotomy.

Last, a few comments go beyond the immediate scope of the current study. The study is situated in a context where more research related to occupational therapy education is explicitly called for. The call is not just related to establishing evidence for instructional methods but also to learn more broadly about who occupational therapy students are and how and why they learn [25, 48, 49]. The current study goes beyond these questions in its investigation of the even more fundamental question: the students' idea of what learning is all about. Following Hooper's [50] idea of merging AOTA's research agenda [51] with their education research agenda [52], the study could be classified as basic research concerned with learner characteristics and competencies. Although basic research is based on a long-standing tradition, as it is concerned with describing, clarifying, and testing concepts relevant for the profession, basic research concerned with occupational therapy students seems to be less well developed. Consequently, this study adds to the state of knowledge related to the learning concepts among the students in our own profession.

5. Study Limitations

The study is limited by a relatively small sample. The participants were recruited by convenience, and they all came from one particular education program at one particular university in Norway. Thus, generalizations should be performed with much caution. Further, the cross-sectional design of the study prohibits inferring cause and effect relationships; thus, the directions of the detected associations are uncertain and may also be cyclical in their nature. A number of statistical tests were performed, and with an increasing number of tests, the probability of obtaining false results also increase (type I error; [53]).

All data were collected using self-report questionnaires, which is frequently used in this field of research. However, one should also be aware that study approach questionnaires provide data that may or may not fit well with the students' own narrative. For example, one mixed-method study found that the study process questionnaire data from teaching students in Spain suggested that they had a largely deep, nonsurface approach to learning [54]. However, judging from the students' own narratives (data derived from the responses to one open-ended question about how they learned), their study approach was instead surface-based. Such inconsistencies between findings derived from quantitative and qualitative data also suggest caution when interpreting the results of this and similar studies.

6. Conclusion and Implications

This study found similar levels of deep and surface conceptions of learning among the Norwegian occupational therapy students. The two theoretically derived concepts were positively associated, suggesting that some of their characteristics are shared rather than different from one another. A clear-cut dichotomy between the deep and the surface learning concepts appears not to be appropriate, rather a gradual development, where the deep concept over time adds to and expands the more basic surface concept, is suggested. Students who spent more time on independent studies had a more broadly composed learning concept, compared to their counterparts. In the future, studies of occupational therapy students' learning concepts should be conducted in a longitudinal perspective.

For occupational therapy educators, the study has several implications. First, understanding the background for students' learning concepts is not a straightforward task. Several sociodemographic, personal, and education-related variables were included as explanatory factors in this study, but only a small proportion of the outcome variance was accounted for. Thus, educators should not worry if they feel they do not fully understand what makes their students think about learning the way they do—a state of mild confusion in this area may seem to reflect the state of the art. Second, students may sustain the idea that learning is about acquiring facts and pieces of information, and obviously, being able to remember facts is not a problem in itself. Problems arise if and when students believe that learning is synonymous to memorizing and comprises nothing else. Thus, educators may try to develop a patience toward students they believe is too hung up on memorizing, and rather aim to assist them in widening their perspective of what learning is—not necessarily try to make them abandon their original ideas. This study suggests that the wider perspective of learning builds on the narrower view but does not replace it. Lastly, a broader view of learning appears to be related to spending more time on the independent study. Educators may therefore guide and motivate students to engage in independent studies. In turn, engaging in independent learning activities may add to the students' ideas of what learning is altogether.

Acknowledgments

The author would like to acknowledge the participants who volunteered to take part in this study.

References

[1] J. B. Biggs, *Student Approaches to Learning and Studying*, Australian Council for Educational Research, Hawthorn, Victoria, 1987.

[2] H. Tait, N. J. Entwistle, and V. McCune, "ASSIST: a reconceptualisation of the Approaches to Studying Inventory," in *Improving Students as Learners*, C. Rust, Ed., pp. 262–271, Oxford Brookes University, Oxford, England, 1998.

[3] F. Marton and R. Säljö, "On qualitative differences in learning: I - outcome and process," *British Journal of Educational Psychology*, vol. 46, no. 1, pp. 4–11, 1976.

[4] Department of Knowledge, *National Framework for Qualifications for Lifelong Learning*, Department of Knowledge, Oslo, 2011.

[5] T. Bonsaksen, T. Brown, H. B. Lim, and K. Fong, "Approaches to studying predict academic performance in undergraduate occupational therapy students: a cross-cultural study," *BMC Medical Education*, vol. 17, no. 1, p. 76, 2017.

[6] W. May, E. K. Chung, D. Elliott, and D. Fisher, "The relationship between medical students' learning approaches and performance on a summative high-stakes clinical performance examination," *Medical Teacher*, vol. 34, no. 4, pp. e236–e241, 2012.

[7] W. A. Reid, P. Evans, and E. Duvall, "Medical students' approaches to learning over a full degree programme," *Medical Education Online*, vol. 17, no. 1, article 17205, p. 1, 2012.

[8] P. J. Ward, "First year medical students' approaches to study and their outcomes in a gross anatomy course," *Clinical Anatomy*, vol. 24, no. 1, pp. 120–127, 2011.

[9] P. J. Ward, "Influence of study approaches on academic outcomes during pre-clinical medical education," *Medical Teacher*, vol. 33, no. 12, pp. e651–e662, 2012.

[10] Y. Salamonson, R. Weaver, S. Chang et al., "Learning approaches as predictors of academic performance in first year health and science students," *Nurse Education Today*, vol. 33, no. 7, pp. 729–733, 2013.

[11] P. Zeegers, "Approaches to learning in science: a longitudinal study," *British Journal of Educational Psychology*, vol. 71, no. 1, pp. 115–132, 2001.

[12] L. Beccaria, M. Kek, H. Huijser, J. Rose, and L. Kimmins, "The interrelationships between student approaches to learning and group work," *Nurse Education Today*, vol. 34, no. 7, pp. 1094–1103, 2014.

[13] T. Bonsaksen, T. Sadeghi, and M. M. Thørrisen, "Associations between self-esteem, general self-efficacy, and approaches to studying in occupational therapy students: a cross-sectional study," *Occupational Therapy in Mental Health*, vol. 33, no. 4, pp. 326–341, 2017.

[14] M. Prat-Sala and P. Redford, "The interplay between motivation, self-efficacy, and approaches to studying," *British Journal of Educational Psychology*, vol. 80, no. 2, pp. 283–305, 2010.

[15] M. Baeten, E. Kyndt, K. Struyven, and F. Dochy, "Using student-centred learning environments to stimulate deep approaches to learning: factors encouraging or discouraging their effectiveness," *Educational Research Review*, vol. 5, no. 3, pp. 243–260, 2010.

[16] C. Kreber, "The relationship between students' course perception and their approaches to studying in undergraduate science courses: a Canadian experience," *Higher Education Research & Development*, vol. 22, no. 1, pp. 57–75, 2003.

[17] A. Lizzio, K. Wilson, and R. Simons, "University students' perceptions of the learning environment and academic outcomes: implications for theory and practice," *Studies in Higher Education*, vol. 27, no. 1, pp. 27–52, 2002.

[18] H. Sun and J. T. E. Richardson, "Students' perceptions of the academic environment and approaches to studying in British postgraduate business education," *Assessment & Evaluation in Higher Education*, vol. 41, no. 3, pp. 384–399, 2016.

[19] J. T. E. Richardson, "Approaches to studying, conceptions of learning and learning styles in higher education," *Learning and Individual Differences*, vol. 21, no. 3, pp. 288–293, 2011.

[20] E. J. van Rossum and S. M. Schenk, "The relationship between learning conception, study strategy and learning outcome," *British Journal of Educational Psychology*, vol. 54, no. 1, pp. 73–83, 1984.

[21] B. C. Dart, P. C. Burnett, N. Purdie, G. Boulton-Lewis, J. Campbell, and D. Smith, "Students' conceptions of learning, the classroom environment, and approaches to learning," *The Journal of Educational Research*, vol. 93, no. 4, pp. 262–270, 2000.

[22] D. S. Sharma, "Accounting students' learning conceptions, approaches to learning, and the influence of the learning - teaching context on approaches to learning," *Accounting Education*, vol. 6, no. 2, pp. 125–146, 1997.

[23] N. J. Entwistle and E. R. Peterson, "Conceptions of learning and knowledge in higher education: relationships with study behaviour and influences of learning environments," *International Journal of Educational Research*, vol. 41, no. 6, pp. 407–428, 2004.

[24] T. Carstensen, N. B. Ødegaard, and T. Bonsaksen, "Approaches to studying: associations with learning conceptions and preferences for teaching," *Cogent Education*, vol. 5, no. 1, pp. 1–11, 2018.

[25] B. Hooper, J. Gupta, A. Bilics, and S. D. Taff, "Balancing efficacy and effectiveness with philosophy, history, and theory-building in occupational therapy education research," *The Open Journal of Occupational Therapy*, vol. 6, no. 1, p. 11, 2018.

[26] T. Brown, K. N. K. Fong, T. Bonsaksen et al., "Approaches to learning among occupational therapy undergraduate students: a cross-cultural study," *Scandinavian Journal of Occupational Therapy*, vol. 24, no. 4, pp. 299–310, 2016.

[27] M. Rosenberg, *Society and the Adolescent Self-Image*, Princeton University Press, Princeton, NJ, USA, 1965.

[28] M. Ystgaard, *Vulnerable Youth and Social Support [Sårbar ungdom og sosial støtte], Report no. 1/93*, Center for social networks and health [Senter for sosialt nettverk og helse], Oslo, 1993.

[29] K. Tambs and E. Røysamb, "Selection of questions to short-form versions of original psychometric instruments in MoBa," *Norsk Epidemiologi*, vol. 24, no. 1-2, pp. 195–201, 2014.

[30] T. Bonsaksen, "Predictors of general self-efficacy and self-esteem in occupational therapy students: a cross-sectional study," *Occupational Therapy in Mental Health*, vol. 31, no. 3, pp. 298–310, 2015.

[31] K. Tambs, "Moderate effects of hearing loss on mental health and subjective well-being: results from the Nord-Trøndelag Hearing Loss Study," *Psychosomatic Medicine*, vol. 66, no. 5, pp. 776–782, 2004.

[32] T. Bonsaksen, M. S. Fagermoen, and A. Lerdal, "Factors associated with self-esteem in persons with morbid obesity and in persons with chronic obstructive pulmonary disease: a cross-sectional study," *Psychology, Health & Medicine*, vol. 20, no. 4, pp. 431–442, 2015.

[33] R. Schwarzer and M. Jerusalem, "Generalized self-efficacy scale," in *Measures in Health Psychology: A User's Portfolio*, J. Weinman, S. Wright, and M. Johnston, Eds., pp. 35–37, Nfer-Nelson, Winsor, England, 1995.

[34] A. Leganger, P. Kraft, and E. Roysamb, "General and task specific self-efficacy in health behaviour research: conceptualization, measurement and correlates," *Psychology & Health*, vol. 15, no. 1, pp. 51–69, 2000.

[35] T. Bonsaksen, A. Kottorp, C. Gay, M. Fagermoen, and A. Lerdal, "Rasch analysis of the General Self-Efficacy scale in a sample of persons with morbid obesity," *Health and Quality of Life Outcomes*, vol. 11, no. 1, pp. 202–202, 2013.

[36] P. M. Fayers and D. Machin, *Quality of Life. The Assessment, Analysis, and Interpretation of Patient-Reported Outcomes*, Wiley, West Sussex, 2 edition, 2007.

[37] D. L. Streiner and G. R. Norman, *Health Measurement Scales - A Practical Guide to Their Development and Use*, Oxford University Press, Oxford, 4 edition, 2008.

[38] N. Entwistle, V. McCune, and H. Tait, *ASSIST: Approaches and Study Skills Inventory for Students*, University of Edinburgh, Edinburgh, 2006.

[39] Å. Diseth, "Validation of a Norwegian version of the approaches and study skills inventory for students (ASSIST): application of structural equation modelling," *Scandinavian Journal of Educational Research*, vol. 45, no. 4, pp. 381–394, 2001.

[40] T. Bonsaksen and M. M. Thørrisen, "Psychometric properties of two interrelated measures: 'conceptions of learning' and 'preferences for different types of courses and teaching'," *Ergoterapeuten*, vol. 60, no. 4, pp. 32–45, 2017.

[41] N. Entwistle, "Motivation and approaches to learning," in *Motivating Students*, S. Brown, G. Thompson, and S. Armstrong, Eds., pp. 15–24, Routledge, London, 1998.

[42] IBM Corporation, *SPSS for Windows, Version 24*, IBM Corporation, Armonk, NY, USA, 2016.

[43] T. Bonsaksen, "Factors associated with occupational therapy students' preferences for courses and teaching," *Cogent Education*, vol. 5, no. 1, pp. 1–10, 2018.

[44] J. Cohen, "A power primer," *Psychological Bulletin*, vol. 112, no. 1, pp. 155–159, 1992.

[45] N. Entwistle, *E-mail correspondence*, 2017.

[46] C. A. Buckley, E. Pitt, B. Norton, and T. Owens, "Students' approaches to study, conceptions of learning and judgements about the value of networked technologies," *Active Learning in Higher Education*, vol. 11, no. 1, pp. 55–65, 2010.

[47] V. Beattie IV, B. Collins, and B. McInnes, "Deep and surface learning: a simple or simplistic dichotomy?," *Accounting Education*, vol. 6, no. 1, pp. 1–12, 1997.

[48] J. P. Burke and N. Harvison, "A systematic focus on occupational therapy education," *American Journal of Occupational Therapy*, vol. 68, Supplement 2, pp. S1–S2, 2014.

[49] J. Gupta and A. Bilics, "Scholarship and research in occupational therapy education," *American Journal of Occupational Therapy*, vol. 68, Supplement 2, pp. S87–S92, 2014.

[50] B. Hooper, "Broadening the scope and impact of occupational therapy education research by merging two research agendas: a new research agenda matrix," *The Open Journal of Occupational Therapy*, vol. 4, no. 3, p. 1, 2016.

[51] American Occupational Therapy Association, "Occupational therapy research agenda," *American Journal of Occupational Therapy*, vol. 65, Supplement 6, pp. S4–S7, 2011.

[52] American Occupational Therapy Association, "Occupational therapy education research agenda," *The American Journal of Occupational Therapy*, vol. 68, Supplement 2, pp. S83–S86, 2014.

[53] A. Field, *Discovering Statistics Using SPSS*, Sage, London, 2 edition, 2005.

[54] F. Monroy and J. L. González-Geraldo, "Measuring learning: discrepancies between conceptions of and approaches to learning," *Educational Studies*, vol. 44, no. 1, pp. 81–98, 2018.

9

The Construct of the Schizophrenia Quality of Life Scale Revision 4 for the Population of Taiwan

Chia-Ting Su,[1] Ai-Lun Yang,[2] and Chung-Ying Lin[3]

[1]*Department of Occupational Therapy, College of Medicine, Fu Jen Catholic University, New Taipei City, Taiwan*
[2]*Department of Sports Sciences, University of Taipei, Taipei, Taiwan*
[3]*Department of Rehabilitation Sciences, Faculty of Health and Social Sciences, The Hong Kong Polytechnic University, 11 Yuk Choi Road, Hung Hom, Hong Kong*

Correspondence should be addressed to Chung-Ying Lin; cylin36933@gmail.com

Academic Editor: Erna I. Blanche

This study examines the factor structure of the Schizophrenia Quality of Life Scale Revision 4 (SQLS-R4) for inpatients with schizophrenia in a psychiatric hospital in southern Taiwan. All the participants ($n = 100$) filled out the SQLS-R4, Mini Mental Status Examination (MMSE), and Brief Psychiatric Rating Scale (BPRS) under the supervision of one experienced occupational therapist. Using confirmatory factor analysis, we first determined that a 29-item model was more satisfactory than the original 33-item model based on the findings of better fit indices for the 29-item model. We then found that a three-correlated-factor structure was best for the SQLS-R4 after four models (namely, two-correlated-factor, three-correlated-factor, seven-correlated-factor, and second-order models) had been compared. In addition, the three constructs (psychosocial, physical, and vitality) were moderately to highly correlated with the constructs of the World Health Organization Quality of Life- (WHOQOL-) BREF ($r = -0.38$ to -0.69), except for one low correlation between the vitality construct of the SQLS-R4 and the psychological construct of the WHOQOL-BREF ($r = -0.26$). We tentatively conclude that the SQLS-R4 with a three-correlated-factor structure is a valid and reliable instrument for examining the quality of life of people with schizophrenia.

1. Introduction

Quality of life (QoL) measures have become more important for therapeutic interventions and clinical decisions [1, 2], especially for patients with chronic illness [3]. When people with schizophrenia confront their chronic disabling illness, it is important for healthcare professionals to understand their QoL. QoL, a subjective perception of an individual's health position within their cultural context and value system [4], can be used as one of the long-term goals of medical interventions [3].

Two kinds of QoL measures can be applied to people with schizophrenia: generic QoL measures and schizophrenia-specific QoL measures [5]. Although the schizophrenia-specific QoL measures cannot compare QoLs between different populations with disabilities (e.g., people with stroke and people with spinal cord injury), they focus on the core symptoms that people with schizophrenia encounter [5]. Therefore, the schizophrenia-specific QoL measures are particularly useful for understanding how the symptoms affect the QoL of people with schizophrenia.

Several schizophrenia-specific QoL measures have been developed, and the Schizophrenia Quality of Life Scale Revision 4 (SQLS-R4) has been suggested to be one of the most useful ones [5–7]. In addition to its items specifically designed for people with schizophrenia [5, 8], its other strengths include (1) practical and short content to fill out (10–15 minutes to complete); (2) improved psychometric properties after several revisions [6, 9]; (3) solid factor structure and internal reliability [7–12]; and (4) availability of cross-cultural comparisons by providing rigorously translated versions in 52 languages through standardized procedures: forward translation, reconciliation, and back translation [9].

However, as a newly developed QoL measure [8, 11], the construct of SQLS-R4 still needs to be confirmed. Although the SQLS-R4 has good psychometric properties [6, 10, 13], to the best of our knowledge, only one UK study [7] has used confirmatory factor analysis (CFA) to examine the construct of SQLS-R4. The advantage of using CFA is being able to compare several proposed models and to clarify the construct of the tested instruments [14]. Therefore, the CFA is suitable for understanding the constructs of measurements that are under development, such as the SQLS-R4. Although the SQLS-R4 was suggested to be two-dimensional [6, 7, 12, 13], Martin and Allan [7] indicated that some CFA fit indices are not acceptable (root mean square error of approximation [RMSEA] = 0.11 and weighted root mean square residual [WRMR] = 0.94). In addition, one Singaporean study [11] mentions that the cultural difference between Asia and the West may influence the psychometric properties of the SQLS-R4. Thus, the construct of the SQLS-R4 may differ in Asian and Western cultures. Therefore, for better application and interpretation of the SQLS-R4, we suggest that additional studies on the SQLS-R4 construct in Asian populations are needed.

The former version of the SQLS-R4, SQLS, is a 30-item self-reported measure compromising three domains (psychosocial, motivation and energy, and symptoms and side effects) [8]. Several revisions were carried out for the SQLS to improve its psychometric properties, and finally the SQLS-R4 with two factors was developed with different language versions [7, 9], including Taiwanese version [6, 13]. However, when Kuo et al. [6] examined the psychometric properties of the Taiwan version of SQLS-R4, they found that four items had weak corrected item-total correlation with their domains. Therefore, Kuo et al. [13] further removed the four items and used the retained items to do the exploratory factor analysis. They found that the Taiwan version of SQLS-R4 contained seven factors and proposed three dimensions (psychosocial, physical condition, and validity) to include the seven factors. Kuo et al. [13] proposed the physical condition as one of the dimensions because physical domain is a key component for QoL. Hence, current literature suggests different factor structures for the SQLS-R4 according to its item numbers (29 or 33 items) and underlying factors (2, 3, and 7 factors/dimensions).

Five CFA models of the SQLS-R4 construct are proposed in our study. In addition to the two-factor model, we propose three more models based on the findings and suggestions of one Taiwanese study [13]: a three-factor model (psychosocial, physical, and vitality), a seven-factor model (relationships with others, loneliness, depressed thinking, worry, exhaustion status, somatic concern, and vitality), and a second-order model with seven first-order factors (relationships with others, loneliness, depressed thinking, worry, exhaustion status, somatic concern, and vitality) embedded in three second-order factors (psychosocial, physical, and vitality). Moreover, four items have been found to be weak for the SQLS-R4 Taiwan version [13], and, thus, a comparison between a 33-item model and a 29-item model was conducted.

We investigated the SQLS-R4 construct for the population of Taiwan and suggest appropriate items to improve the SQLS-R4's psychometric properties. Specifically, we first compared 33-item, 29-item, three-factor, seven-factor, and second-order models. We then tested the determined underlying constructs for their concurrent validity with one generic QoL measure (World Health Organization Quality of Life [WHOQOL]-BREF).

2. Methods

The study was approved by the Institutional Review Board of National Cheng Kung University Hospital, and all the participants filled out and signed informed consents before beginning this study.

2.1. Participants and Procedure. Convenience sampling was used to recruit the participants from a psychiatric hospital in southern Taiwan. Like some other mental institutions in Taiwan, this psychiatric hospital was mainly designed to take long-term care of patients with chronic mental illness. Although symptoms remained relatively stable, most of the patients in this hospital were unable to totally live independently in community due to severity of symptoms, insufficient family support, or other issues. All the participants in our study were diagnosed with schizophrenia based on the DSM IV-TR [15] definition, and all were more than 18 years old (age range: 27 to 66). In addition, they all met the inclusion criteria of an illness duration > 2 years, no medication adjustment within the previous two months, a score ≥ 24 on the Mini Mental Status Examination (MMSE), and a score < 24 on the Brief Psychiatric Rating Scale (BPRS). Participants were excluded if they met the following exclusion criteria: (1) impaired cognitive ability to complete the questionnaires as assessed by one occupational therapist with more than 10 years of clinical experience using clinical observation and (2) with comorbid diagnoses of anxiety, depression, bipolar disorder, organic mental disorder, dementia, intellectual disability, and learning disability. All participants were asked to complete several questionnaires mentioned below. Finally, the data of 100 participants, a minimum criterion for performing CFA [16, 17], were used in the study.

2.2. Instruments

2.2.1. The Schizophrenia Quality of Life Scale Revision 4 (SQLS-R4). The SQLS was initially developed to resolve the lack of QoL measures for people with schizophrenia [8]. The original version of the SQLS contains 30 items distributed between three factors: psychosocial (15 items), motivation and vitality (7 items), and symptoms and side effects (8 items). It has a satisfactory internal consistency (α = 0.80–0.93) [8]. After several revisions that improved its psychometric properties, the latest version of the SQLS (SQLS-R4) contains 33 items distributed between two factors: psychosocial (20 items) and vitality (13 items) [9]. The SQLS-R4 is self-rated, and all but four items are coded on a 5-point scale in relation to their frequency of occurrence during the previous week: 0 = never and 4 = always. The exceptional 4 items are coded the opposite way: 0 = always and 4 = never. A higher SQLS-R4 score represents a worse QoL.

2.2.2. The WHO Questionnaire on the Quality of Life, Short Form (WHOQOL-BREF). We used the WHOQOL-BREF Taiwan version, which has 28 items (two items are domestic items, and other items are international items). Four domains (physical health, psychological health, social relations, and environment) are included in the WHOQOL-BREF. The psychometric properties of the WHOQOL-BREF Taiwan version have been tested (e.g., the internal consistency [Cronbach's α = 0.70–0.91], the test-retest reliability [r = 0.76–0.80], and the construct validity [CFI = 0.89]) and were found to be satisfactory [18]. In addition, a recent study found that the construct of the WHOQOL-BREF Taiwan version fit well with the schizophrenia population and is suitable for using to measure the QoL of people with schizophrenia [19]. A higher WHOQOL-BREF score represents a better QoL.

2.2.3. Mini Mental State Examination (MMSE). The MMSE contains 11 items and has a total score of 30. It is commonly used to screen the function of cognition; a score ≥ 24 suggests an intact cognition function. The test-retest reliability (r = 0.89–0.98) and interrater reliability (r = 0.83) have been examined for the Chinese version of the MMSE [20].

2.2.4. Brief Psychiatric Rating Scale (BPRS). The BPRS contains 16 items; it is designed to measure the severity of psychiatric symptoms. A lower BPRS score indicates a better psychological condition, and the internal consistency of the Chinese version of BPRS is good (Cronbach's α = 0.80) [21].

2.3. Data Analysis. The construct of the SQLS-R4 was examined using CFA models with maximum-likelihood estimations. Five CFA models were tested: Models 1 (33 items; Figure 1) and 2 (29 items; Figure 2) were two-correlated-factor models (psychosocial and vitality). Models 3 and 4 were three-correlated-factor (psychosocial, physical, and vitality; Figure 3) and seven-correlated factor (relationships with others, loneliness, depressed thinking, worry, exhaustion status, somatic concern, and vitality; Figure 4) models, respectively. Unlike Models 1 to 4, all first-order models, Model 5 (Figure 5) was a second-order model with three dimensions correlated in the second-order (psychosocial, physical, and vitality), and seven first-order factors embedded in the second-order factors (psychosocial: relationships with others, loneliness, depressed thinking, and worry; physical: exhaustion status and somatic concern; and vitality: vitality). The underlying factors of the proposed models were correlated based on the suggestions of Martin and Allan [7].

To examine the data-model fit for the five models, we used the χ^2 test and four additional indices: the comparative fit index (CFI), Tucker-Lewis index (TLI), root mean square error of approximation (RMSEA), and standardized root mean square residual (SRMR). The values of the CFI and TLI were > 0.9 [22], and those of the RMSEA and SRMR were < 0.08, which suggests that the data-model fit is acceptable [23, 24]. Moreover, to compare the five models, Akaike's information criterion (AIC) and expected cross-validation index (ECVI) were consulted; smaller values indicate a better fit [24].

After the construct of the SQLS-R4 had been determined, concurrent validity using Pearson correlation was done to strengthen the validity performance of the SQLS-R4. The correlation between each domain of the WHOQOL-BREF and each factor of the SQLS-R4 was tested, and an absolute correlation coefficient > 0.3 suggests a fair correlation [25].

The CFAs were done using Lisrel 8.8 (Scientific Software International, Lincolnwood, IL, USA), and Pearson correlation was done using SPSS 16.0 (SPSS Inc., Chicago, IL, USA).

Table 1: Participants' characteristics.

Variable	n or mean ± SD
Gender	
Male	66
Female	34
Education level	
Junior high school or below	44
Senior high school or above	56
Previously or currently employed?	
Yes	39
No	61
Marital status	
Single	76
Married	10
Other	14
Age (year)	49.2 ± 7.8
Age at onset of schizophrenia (year)	22.6 ± 5.8
Duration of schizophrenia (year)	26.6 ± 8.1
Duration of institutionalization for schizophrenia (year)	17.4 ± 8.7

3. Results

The age, age at onset of schizophrenia, duration of schizophrenia, and duration of institutionalization for schizophrenia of the participants are presented in Table 1. Two-thirds of the participants were male, sixty-one percent of them had never been employed, and more than three-quarters of them were single (Table 1).

For the model comparisons, we first determined that the 29-item SQLS-R4 (Model 2: AIC = 685.519; ECVI = 6.924) was a better data-model fit than was the 33-item SQLS-R4 (Model 1: AIC = 994.108; ECVI = 10.041) (Table 2). Thus, the remainder of the models examined (3, 4, and 5) had 29 items. All of Model 3's fit indices were acceptable (CFI = 0.967, TLI = 0.964, RMSEA = 0.068, SRMR = 0.072, AIC = 666.993, and ECVI = 6.737) and outperformed the other models (CFI = 0.928 to 0.963, TLI = 0.918 to 0.960, RMSEA = 0.072 to 0.107, SRMR = 0.073 to 0.132, AIC = 685.519 to 914.583, and ECVI = 6.924 to 9.238). Based on the results, the SQLS-R4 fit the first-order three-dimensional construct the best. In addition, the standardized factor loadings of Model 3 were all significant (Table 3).

The correlation between the SQLS-R4 and the WHOQOL-BREF was then examined. All the factors underlying the SQLS-R4 were significantly and fairly correlated with the dimensions in the WHOQOL-BREF (all Ps < 0.01 and absolute r > 0.3) except for the correlation between vitality and psychological (r = −0.26, P < 0.01) (Table 4).

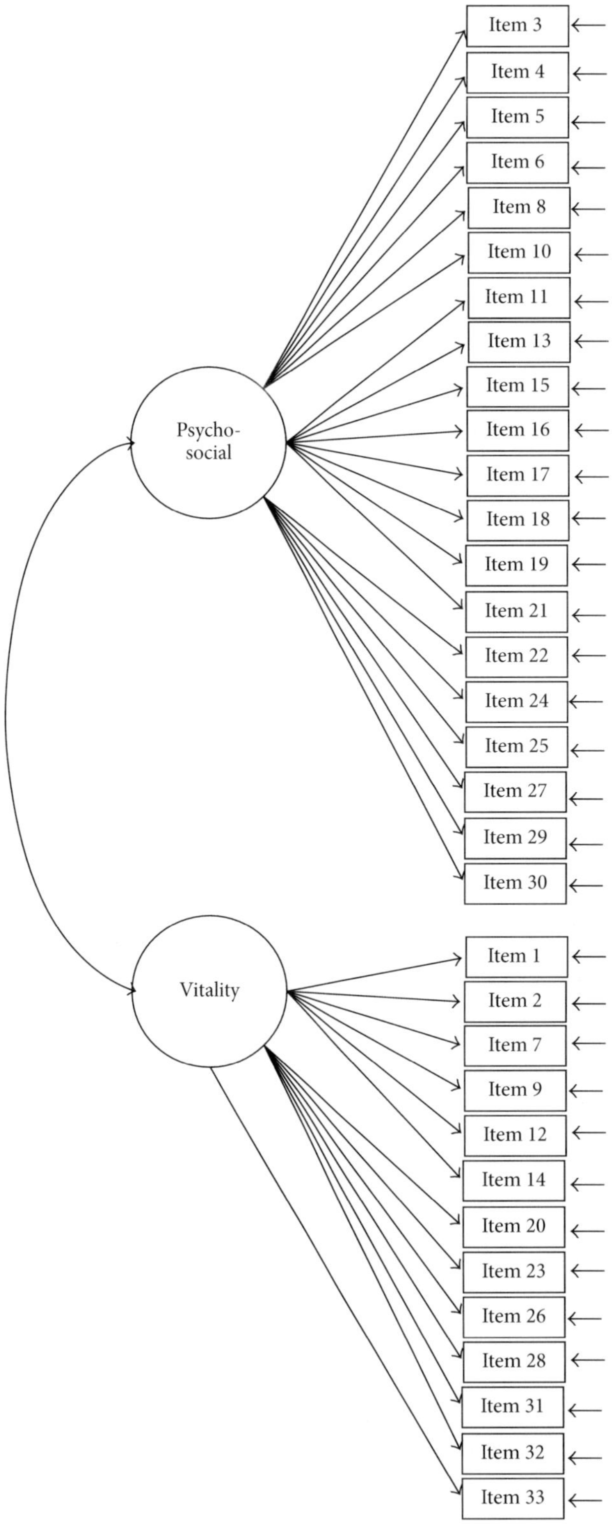

FIGURE 1: Model 1: the two-correlated-factor model with 33 items. Item descriptions are in Table 3.

4. Discussion

In this study, we examined the construct of a newly developed, schizophrenia-specific self-reported QoL measure (SQLS-R4) for people with schizophrenia in Taiwan. To the best of our knowledge, this is the first study that compares several possible factor structures of the SQLS-R4 using CFA and that confirms the construct of the SQLS-R4 for the Asian population. The proposed three-factor model (psychosocial, physical, and vitality) fit best with our data. Moreover, this

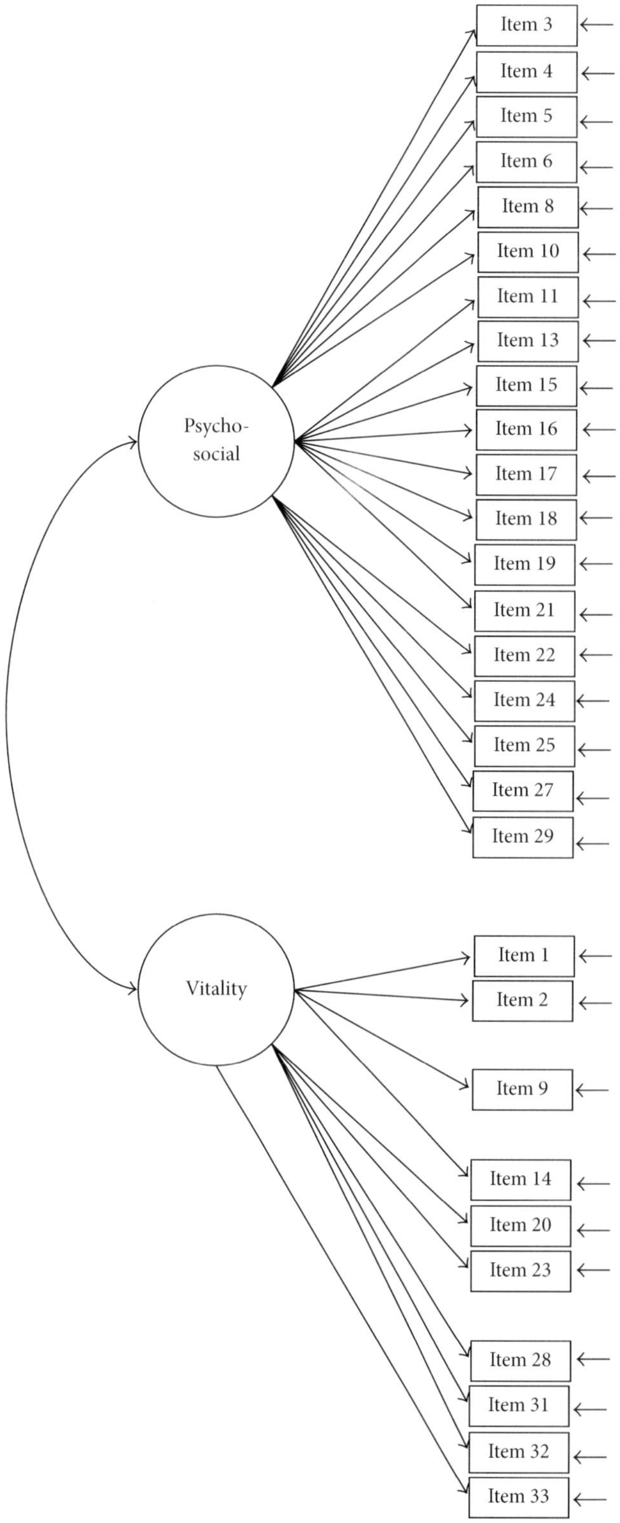

FIGURE 2: Model 2: the two-correlated-factor model with 29 items. Item descriptions are in Table 3.

proposed model was supported by the correlation between its 3 factors on the SQLS-R4 and the factors of the WHOQOL-BREF.

Based on our belief that the underlying concepts should all be correlated because of their relevance to QoL, we did not examine the uncorrelated-factor models. Similar findings were concluded by Martin and Allan [7], who proposed three-factor structures (namely, a one-factor structure, a two-correlated-factor model, and a two-uncorrelated-factor model) and found that the two-correlated factor model

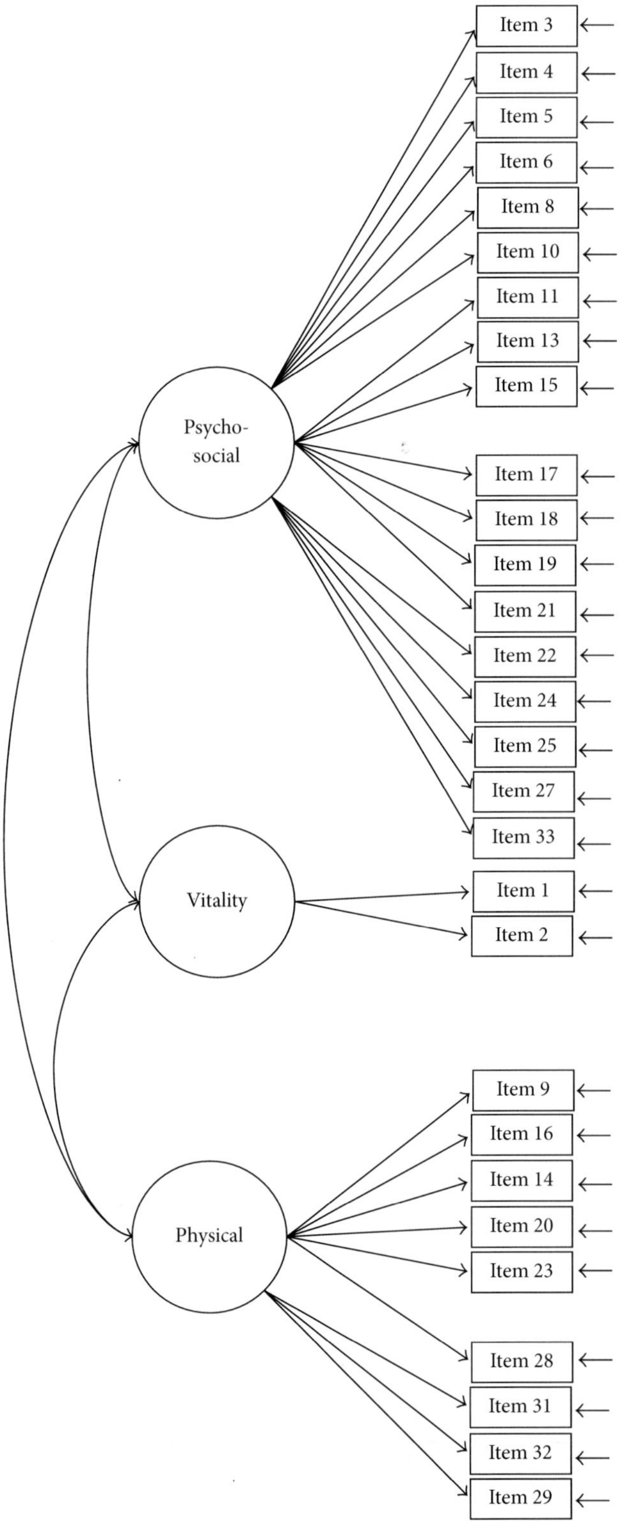

FIGURE 3: Model 3: the three-correlated-factor model with 29 items. Item descriptions are in Table 3.

had the best data-model fit. However, they also reported that the two-correlated-factor model was not good enough. Therefore, in our study, three more factor structures were compared, and we found that the three-correlated-factor model (psychosocial, physical, and vitality) was the best construct for the SQLS-R4. In addition, our results also suggested that four items on the SQLS-R4 (i.e., Item 7 [able to carry out daily activities]; Item 12 [feel I can cope]; Item 26 [feel happy]; and Item 30 [concerned about social life]) can be omitted. Items 26 and 30 are new to the SQLS-R4

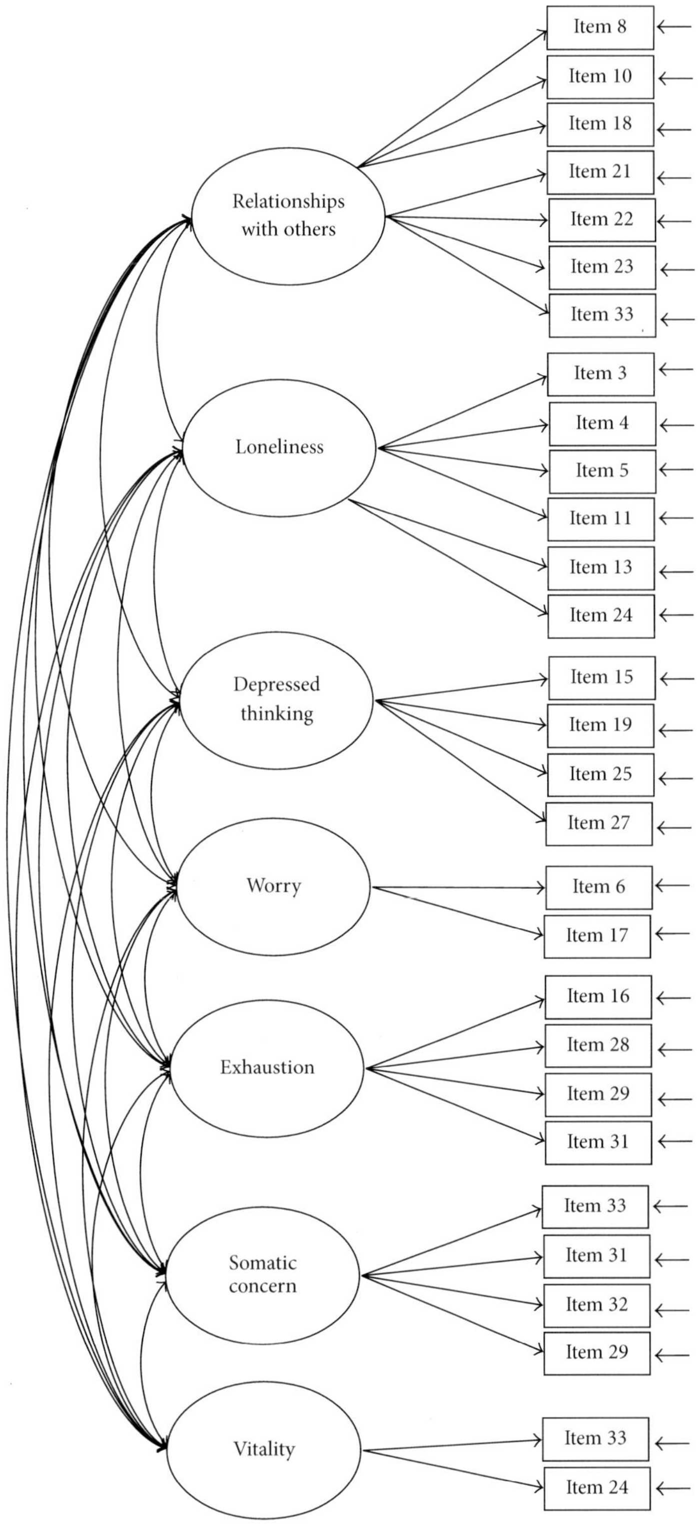

FIGURE 4: Model 4: the seven-correlated-factor model with 29 items. Item descriptions are in Table 3.

and have relatively low factor loadings (<0.3) in the vitality construct and psychosocial construct, in previous studies [6, 13]. The wordings of these two new items may still be under development, which might contribute to their unstable psychometric properties [24]. Another possible reason is that the participants in our study were institutionalized and may have had limited social lives as well as happy feelings. Thus, further studies may test these two items for people with schizophrenia who live in communities to verify our hypothesis. Items 7 and 12 were found to have higher

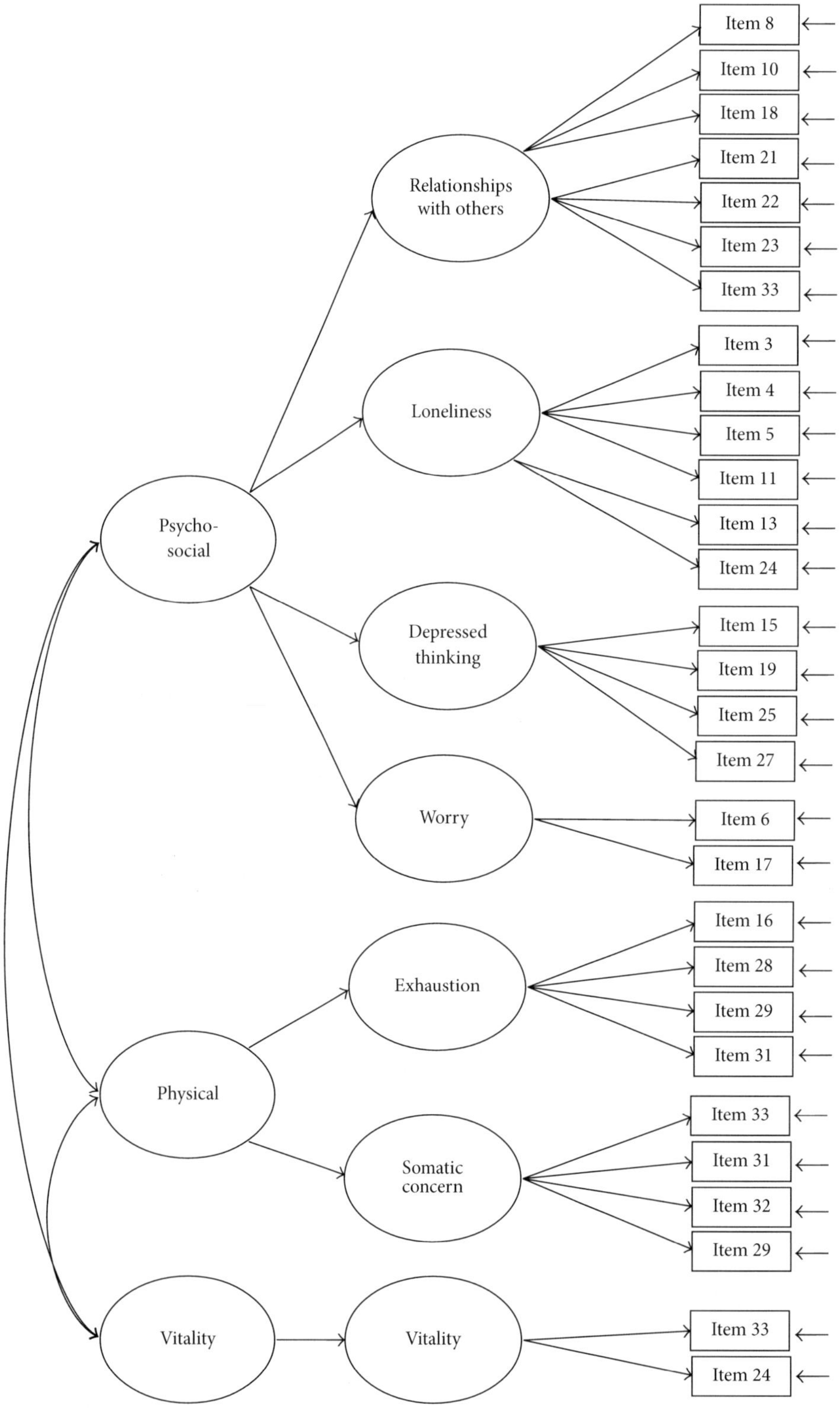

FIGURE 5: Model 5: the second-order model with 29 items. Item descriptions are in Table 3.

correlations with the total score of the motivation and energy domain in the SQLS for the UK version ($r = 0.67$ and 0.68) [8] and for English-speaking Asians ($r = 0.51$ and 0.42) [11] than for the Japanese version ($r = 0.39$ and 0.34) [10] and for Chinese-speaking Asians ($r = 0.21$ and 0.32) [11]. Therefore, the two items may be perceived differently from the vitality construct in Asian and Western cultures [6, 12].

The factor structure of the SQLS/SQLS-R4 has been revised several times [9], and its psychometric properties have been tested (e.g., Wilkinson et al. [8]; Kaneda et

TABLE 2: Model comparisons.

	Model number				
	1	2	3	4	5
χ^2 (*df*)	860.108 (494)	567.519 (376)	544.993 (374)	756.583 (356)	675.982 (368)
CFI	0.934	0.963	0.967	0.928	0.945
TLI	0.929	0.960	0.964	0.918	0.939
RMSEA	0.087	0.072	0.068	0.107	0.092
SRMR	0.090	0.073	0.072	0.132	0.074
AIC	994.108	685.519	666.993	914.583	809.982
ECVI	10.041	6.924	6.737	9.238	8.182

Model 1: two correlated factors (psychosocial and vitality) with 33 items.
Model 2: two correlated factors (psychosocial and vitality) with 29 items.
Model 3: three correlated factors (psychosocial, physical, and vitality) with 29 items.
Model 4: seven correlated factors (relationships with others, loneliness, exhaustion, depressed thinking, somatic concern, vitality, and worry) with 29 items.
Model 5: seven correlated factors (relationships with others, loneliness, exhaustion, depressed thinking, somatic concern, vitality, and worry) underlying three correlated dimensions (psychosocial, physical, and vitality) with 29 items.
CFI = comparative fit index; TLI = Tucker-Lewis index; RMSEA = root mean square error of approximation; SRMR = standardized root mean square residual; AIC = Akaike's information criterion; ECVI = expected cross-validation index.

TABLE 3: Standardized factor loadings on SQLS-R4 with three underlying constructs.

Item number	Item description	Standardized factor loadings		
		Psychosocial	Physical	Vitality
1	Lack energy	—	—	0.816
2	Couldn't be bothered	—	—	0.769
3	Worry about future	0.475	—	—
4	Lonely	0.574	—	—
5	Hopeless	0.654	—	—
6	Panicky	0.632	—	—
7	Able to carry out daily activities[a]	—	—	—
8	Took things people said the wrong way	0.552	—	—
9	Hard to concentrate	—	0.606	—
10	Difficult to mix with people	0.536	—	—
11	Down	0.753	—	—
12	Feel I can cope[a]	—	—	—
13	Mixed up and unsure	0.662	—	—
14	Slept well	—	0.261	—
15	Have mood swings	0.769	—	—
16	Concerned wouldn't get better	—	0.554	—
17	Worry	0.569	—	—
18	People avoid me	0.684	—	—
19	Upset about past	0.537	—	—
20	Poor memory	—	0.644	—
21	Cut off from world	0.543	—	—
22	Uncomfortable with people	0.740	—	—
23	Can't think clearly	0.512	—	—
24	Upsetting thoughts	0.766	—	—
25	Suicidal thoughts	0.562	—	—
26	Feel happy[a]	—	—	—
27	Depressed	0.740	—	—
28	Drowsy	—	0.654	—
29	Restless	—	0.577	—
30	Concerned about social life[a]	—	—	—
31	Tired	—	0.647	—
32	Physically weak	—	0.637	—
33	Wasn't leading normal life	0.604	—	—

All *Ps* < 0.01
[a]Items not in the three-correlated-factor model.

Table 4: Correlations between the SQLS-R4 and the WHOQOL-BREF.

	SQLS-R4		
	Psychosocial	Physical	Vitality
WHOQOL-BREF			
Physical	−0.50	−0.64	−0.39
Psychological	−0.41	−0.53	−0.26
Social	−0.38	−0.48	−0.38
Environment	−0.59	−0.69	−0.52

All $Ps < 0.01$.

al. [10]; and Kuo et al. [13]). Three methods have been used: concurrent validity [6, 10–12, 26], exploratory factor analysis [8, 13], and CFA [7]. Except for the CFA, concurrent validity and exploratory factor analysis indirectly tested the construct of the SQLS-R4. Concurrent validity is used to examine the relationship between several measures [27] (e.g., the relationship between the SQLS-R4 and the WHOQOL-BREF). Because the constructs of other measures (e.g., the WHOQOL-BREF) are not the same as that of the SQLS-R4, the SQLS-R4 construct cannot be precisely examined using concurrent validity. Exploratory factor analysis is used to explore the possible underlying factors of one measure [28], such as the SQLS-R4; it was suitable for identifying a set of latent constructs underlying the measured items on the SQLS-R4 without an a priori hypothesis factor structure. In other words, exploratory factor analysis explores rather than examines the construct of SQLS-R4. Therefore, we suggest that it would be more appropriate to compare our results with those of Martin and Allan [7], who also used CFA to examine the factor structure of the SQLS-R4.

The main difference between the best-fit structure of the SQLS-R4 in this study and the former structure of the SQLS-R4 is one construct (physical) added to our suggested structure. Although the structure of the SQLS-R4 is designed without a physical construct [8, 9], the definition of QoL includes the concept of physical performance [1, 4, 29]. Therefore, the construct of physical should also be emphasized for the SQLS-R4, as Kuo et al. [13]. have recommended. The physical construct is defined as an individual's ability to perform daily activities (e.g., self-care; rest) and is related to one's physical condition [29]. Thus, some items on the SQLS-R4 (e.g., physically weak; slept well; restless) are suitable for the physical construct, and they were verified in a report on health-related quality of life measures [29]. Because no published studies have examined the three-correlated-factor model of the SQLS-R4 for any Western population, we suggest that our three-correlated-factor model should be tested using Western populations to further understand the physical construct.

In addition to the CFA-based confirmation of the factor structure of the SQLS-R4, our concurrent validity test also supported the SQLS-R4 construct. Significantly moderate-to-high correlations were found between the SQLS-R4 constructs and the WHOQOL-BREF constructs, except for a low correlation between the vitality construct of the SQLS-R4 and the psychological construct of the WHOQOL-BREF ($r = -0.26$). Consistent with our findings, Chou et al. [30]. also found a nonsignificant correlation between the vitality construct of the SQLS-R4 and the psychological construct of the S-QoL. The content of vitality construct items (namely, "lack energy" and "couldn't be bothered") seems to describe more about physical condition and social interaction than about mental function, which may contribute to the low correlation.

This study has several limitations. There were only 100 participants in this study, the minimum required for a reliable CFA [16, 17]. However, because the replication of a factor structure is recommended for CFA [16], our findings for the SQLS-R4 construct can be seen as a preliminary outcome for the Asian population. Future studies may conduct other CFAs based on our findings to strengthen the construct of the SQLS-R4. Second, all the participants were inpatients from one psychiatric hospital; thus, our findings may not be generalizable to people with schizophrenia and living in the community. Third, we recruited only participants with intact cognitive ability (MMSE $\geq$ 24 and BPRS $<$ 24); therefore, the SQLS-R4 construct we suggested in this study cannot be generalized to those with impaired cognitive ability.

In conclusion, our results suggested a three-correlated-factor construct of SQLS-R4 for people with schizophrenia in Taiwan. In addition, the reliability and validity were good for the SQLS-R4. However, because our participants were all institutionalized, additional studies that examine the SQLS-R4 construct on outpatients with schizophrenia are needed. Moreover, comparing the SQLS-R4 construct for Asian and Western populations is also suggested.

Competing Interests

The authors declare that they have no competing interests.

References

[1] D. Basu, "Quality-of-life issues in mental health care: past, present, and future," *German Journal of Psychiatry*, vol. 7, no. 3, pp. 35–43, 2004.

[2] C.-Y. Lin, W.-M. Luh, C.-P. Cheng, A.-L. Yang, C.-T. Su, and H.-I. Ma, "Measurement equivalence across child self-reports and parent-proxy reports in the Chinese version of the pediatric quality of life inventory version 4.0," *Child Psychiatry and Human Development*, vol. 44, no. 5, pp. 583–590, 2013.

[3] A. O. Adelufosi, A. Ogunwale, O. Abayomi, and J. T. Mosanya, "Socio-demographic and clinical correlates of subjective quality of life among Nigerian outpatients with schizophrenia," *Psychiatry Research*, vol. 209, no. 3, pp. 320–325, 2013.

[4] The WHOQOL Group, "Study protocol for the World Health Organization project to develop a quality of life assessment instrument (WHOQOL)," *Quality of Life Research*, vol. 2, no. 2, pp. 153–159, 1993.

[5] J. Bobes, P. García-Portilla, P. A. Sáiz, T. Bascarán, and M. Bousoño, "Quality of life measures in schizophrenia," *European Psychiatry*, vol. 20, supplement 3, pp. S313–S317, 2005.

[6] P.-J. Kuo, M.-J. Chen-Sea, R.-B. Lu et al., "Validation of the Chinese version of the Schizophrenia Quality of Life Scale Revision 4 (SQLS-R4) in Taiwanese patients with schizophrenia," *Quality of Life Research*, vol. 16, no. 9, pp. 1533–1538, 2007.

[7] C. R. Martin and R. Allan, "Factor structure of the Schizophrenia Quality of Life Scale Revision 4 (SQLS-R4)," *Psychology, Health & Medicine*, vol. 12, no. 2, pp. 126–134, 2007.

[8] G. Wilkinson, B. Hesdon, D. Wild et al., "Self-report quality of life measure for people with schizophrenia: the SQLS," *British Journal of Psychiatry*, vol. 177, pp. 42–46, 2000.

[9] Oxford Outcomes Ltd, *The Revised Schizophrenia Quality of Life Questionnaire (SQLS-R4): User Manual for the SQLS-R4*, Oxford Outcomes, Cassington, UK, 2004.

[10] Y. Kaneda, A. Imakura, A. Fujii, and T. Ohmori, "Schizophrenia Quality of Life Scale: validation of the Japanese version," *Psychiatry Research*, vol. 113, no. 1-2, pp. 107–113, 2002.

[11] N. Luo, B.-K. Seng, F. Xie, S.-C. Li, and J. Thumboo, "Psychometric evaluation of the Schizophrenia Quality of Life Scale (SQLS) in English- and Chinese-speaking Asians in Singapore," *Quality of Life Research*, vol. 17, no. 1, pp. 115–122, 2008.

[12] N. A. Taha, M. I. Ibrahim, A. F. Rahman, A. A. Shafie, and A. H. Rahman, "Validation of the schizophrenia quality of life scale revision 4 among chronic schizophrenia patients in Malaysia," *Value in Health Regional Issues*, vol. 1, no. 1, pp. 82–86, 2012.

[13] P.-J. Kuo, H.-I. Ma, C.-C. Kuo, W.-C. Huang, and M.-S. Chung, "Factor analysis of the Schizophrenia Quality Of Life Scale Revision 4 (SQLS-R4) Chinese version and related factors," *International Journal of Psychiatry in Clinical Practice*, vol. 13, no. 4, pp. 278–284, 2009.

[14] K. A. Bollen, "Confirmatory factor analysis," in *Structure Equations with Latent Variables*, K. A. Bollen, Ed., pp. 226–315, John Wiley & Sons, New York, NY, USA, 1989.

[15] American Psychological Association, *Diagnostic and Statistical Manual of Mental Disorders*, vol. 1, American Psychiatric Association, Arlington, Va, USA, 4th edition, 2000.

[16] P. Kline, *A Psychometric Primer*, Free Association Books, London, UK, 1993.

[17] J. C. Loehlin, *Latent Variable Models: An Introduction to Factor, Path, and Structural Analysis*, Lawrence Erlbaum Associates, Mahwah, NJ, USA, 1998.

[18] G. Yao, C.-W. Chung, C.-F. Yu, and J.-D. Wang, "Development and verification of validity and reliability of the WHOQOL-BREF Taiwan version," *Journal of the Formosan Medical Association*, vol. 101, no. 5, pp. 342–351, 2002.

[19] Y.-C. Kao, Y.-P. Liu, M.-K. Chou, and T.-H. Cheng, "Subjective quality of life in patients with chronic schizophrenia: relationships between psychosocial and clinical characteristics," *Comprehensive Psychiatry*, vol. 52, no. 2, pp. 171–180, 2011.

[20] N.-W. Guo, H.-C. Liu, P.-F. Wong et al., "Chinese version and norms of the Mini-Mental State Examination," *Journal of Chinese Rehabilitative Medicine*, vol. 16, pp. 52–59, 1989 (Chinese).

[21] T.-J. Chang, H.-G. Hwu, and F.-W. Wei, "The inter-rater reliability of brief psychiatric rating scale (BPRS)," *Chinese Society Neurology and Psychiatry Bulletin*, vol. 12, pp. 29–36, 1986 (Chinese).

[22] M. A. Garcia-Barrera, R. W. Kamphaus, and D. Bandalos, "Theoretical and statistical derivation of a screener for the behavioral assessment of executive functions in children," *Psychological Assessment*, vol. 23, no. 1, pp. 64–79, 2011.

[23] L.-T. Hu and P. M. Bentler, "Cutoff criteria for fit indexes in covariance structure analysis: conventional criteria versus new alternatives," *Structural Equation Modeling*, vol. 6, no. 1, pp. 1–55, 1999.

[24] C.-Y. Lin, W.-M. Luh, C.-P. Cheng, A.-L. Yang, and H.-I. Ma, "Evaluating the wording effect and psychometric properties of the kid-kindl: using the multitrait-multimethod approach," *European Journal of Psychological Assessment*, vol. 30, no. 2, pp. 100–109, 2014.

[25] Y. H. Chan, "Biostatistics 104: correlational analysis," *Singapore Medical Journal*, vol. 44, no. 12, pp. 614–619, 2003.

[26] J. H. Kim, S. J. Yim, and S. K. Min, "The Korean version of the 4th Revision of Schizophrenia Quality of Life Scale: validation study and relationship with PANSS," *Journal of Korean Neuropsychiatry Association*, vol. 45, p. 401, 2006.

[27] L. G. Portney and M. P. Watkins, "Validity of measurements," in *Foundations of Clinical Research: Application to Practice*, L. G. Portney and M. P. Watkins, Eds., pp. 79–110, Prentice Hall Health, Upper Saddle River, NJ, USA, 2nd edition, 2000.

[28] B. G. Tabachnick and L. S. Fidell, "Principal components and factor analysis," in *Using Multivariate Statistics*, B. G. Tabachnick and L. S. Fidell, Eds., pp. 607–675, Pearson International, Boston, Mass, USA, 5th edition, 2007.

[29] M. J. Naughton and S. A. Shumaker, "The case for domains of function in quality of life assessment," *Quality of Life Research*, vol. 12, no. 1, pp. 73–80, 2003.

[30] C.-Y. Chou, M.-C. Ma, T.-T. Yang, and M.-J. Chen-Sea, "Psychometric validation of the S-QoL Chinese (Taiwan) version for patients with schizophrenia," *Quality of Life Research*, vol. 20, no. 5, pp. 763–767, 2011.

10

Pinnipeds and PTSD: An Analysis of a Human-Animal Interaction Case Study Program for a Veteran

Rachel A. Wortman, Theresa Vallone, Michele Karnes, Christine Walawander, Dion Daly, and Bonnie Fox-Garrity

Department of Occupational Therapy, D'Youville College, 320 Porter Avenue, Buffalo, NY 14201, USA

Correspondence should be addressed to Rachel A. Wortman; wortmanrachel@gmail.com

Academic Editor: Lynette Mackenzie

The objective of this study was to examine the impact of a pinniped (grey and harbor seals) facilitated human-animal interaction pilot program on the self-reported PTSD-like symptoms of a veteran. This study analyzed preexisting, deidentified data that represented the participant's scores on the Post-Traumatic Stress Disorder Checklist (PCL-5). The PCL-5 was completed as part of a pilot program operated in partnership between the Veteran and Military Affiliated Research Center (VMARC) and a local aquarium. Scores on the PCL-5 were collected prior to (T1), midway (T2), and immediately after (T3) completion of the *Project Seal to Heal* program. Changes in the scores of each item were reported for the participant, for aggregated items that represented different clusters of PTSD symptoms, and for overall scores. Results revealed decreased scores in 11 of the 20 PTSD symptom-related items, improvement in the sum scores for each criteria symptom cluster, and a 15-point decrease in the overall PCL-5 score, indicating clinical significance. These results serve as a call to motivate future research investigating pinniped interactions with veterans who have PTSD in order to determine therapeutic clinical application and outcomes.

1. Introduction

In 2013, the World Health Organization (WHO) published their Mental Health Action Plan for 2013–2020. In this report, WHO claims that there is "no health without mental health" (p. 6). Globally, it is estimated that one-fourth of families will be directly affected with at least one member of that family identifying as having a mental or behavior disorder. These effects are not only experienced by the individual and his or her loved ones, but by society overall [1, 2]. The United States' National Institute of Mental Health (NIMH) has projected that by 2030; global spending directly related to mental health will equal $6.0 trillion, in comparison to the 2010 global spending cost of $2.5 trillion. Moreover, poor mental health may perpetuate, or be perpetuated by, maladaptive behavior [3, 4]. These mutually influential healthcare concerns often occur in conjunction with other disorders and/or impairments, making them two of the largest contributors of global economic burden [3, 5].

One such mental health ailment that often alters behavior is posttraumatic stress disorder, or PTSD, which is currently defined as a stress disorder brought on by exposure to a traumatic event. As such, PTSD falls into the mental and behavioral health spectrum [6]. According to the WHO, approximately 3.6% of the world population is afflicted with PTSD. An estimated 7.0–8.0% of the US population contribute to that percentage [6–10]. Though there are many populations exposed to traumatic situations, the prevalence of PTSD within the United States military veteran population has not only increased public awareness of the disorder but has also reached astonishing levels.

The US Department of Veterans Affairs (USDVA) and the National Center for PTSD estimates that 11–20% of military personnel involved in Operations Iraqi Freedom (OIF) and Enduring Freedom (OEF) have been diagnosed with PTSD. This estimate does not include veterans who were involved in WWII, the Vietnam War, or the Gulf War [8]. Due to the overtaxing of specific mental capacities, veterans with PTSD have also been recognized to be more likely than those with other mental health diagnoses to demonstrate high-risk drug use and adverse clinical outcomes, such as injuries and overdoses [11]. Comorbidities such as depression, anxiety, and difficulty sleeping often accompany PTSD and can affect nearly every activity and interaction with which individuals engage. Despite growing trends of PTSD diagnosis within military populations, effective treatments to combat the disorder within this sector of the population have not followed suit [12].

Currently, the majority of veterans diagnosed with PTSD are treated with serotonin reuptake inhibitor antidepressants (SSRIs). However, SSRIs have been found to contribute little more than a placebo in the alleviation of mild to moderate symptoms [12, 13]. In fact, in 2007 it was reported that sertraline, an SSRI, provided no additional benefits when compared to a placebo, specifically when used by veterans who had PTSD [14]. Yet, seven years later in 2012, 89% of the US veterans who had a diagnosis of PTSD were treated with SSRIs. Simultaneously less than 20% of veterans who were diagnosed with PTSD also reported receiving adequate treatment, no matter the treatment type [15]. A diagnosis of PTSD often comes with the recommendation for psychotherapy, but in 2016, it was reported that only one-third of the troops who had identified as having PTSD went on to receive the minimum number of therapeutic sessions suggested after receiving their diagnosis. This was either due to personal choice or because there was a current shortage of healthcare professionals available to address the growing demand and backlog for the treatment of PTSD for veterans [16, 17]. The implication is that many veterans with PTSD either are not receiving treatment or are paying for a treatment that is ineffective.

This information notwithstanding, Global War on Terror (GWOT) veterans are making more claims for injury and/or illness than any veteran population of previous wars, and peak cost spent on veteran medical care specific to disability does not occur until decades after a military member has been discharged. For post-9/11 veterans discharged in 2013, it has been estimated that costs linked to medical treatment will exceed $1.0 trillion by 2053. Due to these unprecedented increases in veterans seeking assistance, it has been postulated that as of 2016, veteran healthcare cost approximations established by the US Department of Defense (DOD) are low [16]. Without exploration into new avenues of PTSD treatment alternatives, a perpetuation of massive economic, social, and environmental burdens will continue to cultivate [12, 16].

Global appreciation of the gravity and impact of mental health on economics and human well-being continues to expand. Analogously, a rise in new approaches to address these ailments has been steadily investigated. As human well-being is multifaceted, with many instrumental and contingent components, contrived inquiry into the establishment and maintenance of this well-being is beset with a multitude of complex challenges [18]. The investigation into methods of creatively addressing burdens linked to PTSD presents a unique opportunity for healthcare professionals.

Currently, there is an intercontinental proliferation of organizations compelling healthcare professional consciousness in the direction of new and innovative approaches for human health and well-being, simultaneously uniting global human constitution and obligations to conserve a salubrious planet with advantageous economic applications. Ecology, biodiversity, and environmental sustainability have all been recognized as essential underpinnings to public and environmental health. Changes in environments, including changes in organisms comprising those environments, can potentially directly and indirectly impact human health [19]. Few healthcare professions have the capacity to fully incorporate the necessity of a true holistic approach to human well-being, accounting for the complex and dynamic relationships between environments, behaviors, and overall health. However, occupational therapy stands as an aberration against this inclination.

In truth, occupational therapists stand at the precipice of utilizing their unique expertise to not only aid individuals but also, in turn, affect positive influences in global economics, ecological sustainability, and community well-being. This conviction has been expressed in the World Federation of Occupational Therapy's (WFOT) position statement on environmental sustainability. The WFOT takes the position that occupational therapists should not only attend to individual needs but also simultaneously promote well-being and environmental health [20]. Occupational therapists have the expertise and responsibility to recognize humans as both influencers of their environment and beings whom are influenced by their environment [18, 21].

It is vital that occupational therapists are cognizant of ecology and biodiversity, or the diversity of life, while fulfilling their core role addressing occupations and occupational performance. This is due to the fact that human occupations are transformed in response to the availability and condition of environmental resources. Efforts within the profession should be directed toward environmental sustainability while paralleling collaborative efforts directed toward optimal occupational performance of clients and communities. These efforts should also meet growing healthcare concerns within specific populations. Occupational therapists specialize in engaging a single component from an environment as the tool to facilitate a change in unhealthy or maladaptive human behavior. Biodiversity may serve as both the tool and the objective for augmented health. However, addressing all of the issues that accompany global shifts in ecology and biodiversity, while simultaneously addressing immediate healthcare demands, such as the increased burden of mental illnesses, can be daunting.

The Model of Human Occupations (MOHO) and the biophilia hypothesis serves as guiding conceptual frameworks for both mental health and as a tool for environmentally conscious healthcare practices, endorsing the dynamic interplay between organisms and their environment. MOHO is an occupational therapy-specific framework that encompasses the idea that occupational engagement is an open and dynamic system of interaction and change. Not only is the person seen as an input mechanism, and the occupation as the output result, but MOHO considers the environmental influence on the motivation, patterns, and performance of the individual [22]. Much as MOHO claims that humans have a need to engage in activities within their environments, biophilia attests that nature contains components that support life and that humans have a want and need to interact with natural organisms, as they are a part of the "self," meaning a part of the person [23–28]. Under the scope of these theories, emerging therapeutic practices have sprouted, including animal-assisted therapy (AAT) [27, 29].

Health benefits associated with AAT have started to be explored and have proven promising, with the bulk of AAT research focusing on domesticated, companion animals [30]. Inquiries into the efficacy of nonhuman animals in therapeutic interventions beyond the scope of companionship have begun to emerge, but are relatively limited. Central to these investigations is the realization that all humans are continuously influenced by, and dependent upon, nonhuman animals. Purportedly, nonhuman animals influence every day occupations, as they are, according to Huggett [31], a part of the "entirety of life" and, as such, are also a part of life support systems. This is an inherent virtue of AAT, the application of a component of life in a therapeutic capacity, in order to better that life, engaging biodiversity as the means and the end.

However, increased research of human-animal interactions (HAIs) is obligatory for therapeutic understanding of the potential success of AAT. There is also a need for new medicinal techniques, utilizing information garnered from the HAI research that concomitantly benefits the human client, while acknowledging the importance of an explicit nonhuman participant. To truly recruit a component of "life" as a therapeutic instrument in AAT, nonhuman animals that influence environmental health are required. Conceivably, many of these animals are wild and considered vulnerable in their relationship with humans, or made so indiscreetly through the impact of human behavior on their environment. Investigating HAIs, beyond companion animals, and with vulnerable nonhuman populations may prove to be beneficial [31].

According to the Millennium Ecosystem Assessment (MEA) [32], vulnerability is defined as "exposure to contingencies and stress, and the difficulty in coping with them" (p. 605). There are research articles and opinion publications addressing the potential employment of certain nonhuman animals in AAT which may fall under the scope of vulnerable, specifically aquatic animals [31, 33]. Aquatic animals are of special consideration for AAT application, as their health and well-being is often influenced by human activity and, in turn, ultimately an influencer on global human health [34].

The employment of oceanic mammals in therapeutic interactions has potential, as these nonhuman animals are under great ecological shifts amidst limited public awareness about such. In general, aquatic animals, when discussed in AAT research, are almost exclusively limited to bottlenose dolphins, a practice referred to as dolphin-assisted therapy (DAT) [35, 36]. Though DAT may be tangential to AAT in an aquatic environment, the engagement of pinnipeds (seals, sea lions, fur seals, and walrus) in a similar capacity has until now gone unexamined.

Pinnipeds play an important role in global biodiversity and environmental health [37–39]. When compared to dolphins, seals and sea lions are much more commonly rescued and kept in captivity when injured. These rescues, as well as human raise pinnipeds, may be considered a vulnerable population in need of care and are abundantly more accessible to the general public than dolphins [40–42]. Demeanor, accessibility, and other distinct characteristics among pinnipeds make them apt candidates for employment in AAT. Pinniped engagement in AAT, a possible alternative to DAT, has yet to be investigated, in any capacity, for therapeutic benefit in human populations [43–45].

Currently, there is a lack of research addressing the impact of interactions between veterans with PTSD-like symptoms and rescued or otherwise nonrelease seals. By utilizing the MOHO and the biophilia hypothesis in combination, this research sought to evaluate a veteran-pinniped HAI program at a local aquarium in order to identify (1) the impact of the pinniped HAI program for veterans identifying as having PTSD-like symptoms and (2) the implications for future occupational therapy research specific to pinniped HAIs.

2. Methods

Upon approval by the D'Youville College's Internal Review Board (IRB), the researcher requested use of a deidentified data set from the Veteran and Military Affiliated Research Center (VMARC) at a small private, liberal arts college in Buffalo, NY. The deidentified data was drawn from preexisting information gathered by the VMARC pertaining to a pinniped facilitated HAI program entitled *Project Seal to Heal*. This program was conducted by the VMARC in partnership with the Aquarium of Niagara Falls and included aquarium staff, a representative from the VMARC with knowledge and experience in PTSD mediation, and four seals, including one rescued grey seal, one rescued Pacific harbor seal, one rescued Atlantic harbor seal, and one harbor seal who was raised under human care.

Project Seal to Heal participants were introduced to only one of the four seals per session, with each session incorporating a different seal. Each session was in total one hour in duration, which encompassed the total time spent at the Aquarium. Participants were allotted direct and indirect interactions with the seals. Indirect interactions were educationally based, ranging in scope from broad to narrow topics. Broad topics included education regarding ocean ecology, pinniped taxonomy, pinniped distribution and habitat, pinniped anatomy and physiology, and conservation themes such as human/pinniped interface and implications. Narrow topics included education in husbandry tasks, which involves the actions required in order to care for wild animals in captivity, such as preparing meals for the seals and seal enrichment activities. Direct interactions were provided when participants shared space with and/or were in physical contact with the seals. Each participant was afforded a minimum of ten minutes of direct interaction with the seal, per session during which information was provided regarding the seal's personal history, preferences, and dislikes.

Table 1: Program seal to heal PCL-5 scores for T1, T2, and T3 ($n = 1$).

Participant number	PCL question number	PCL (T1)	PCL (T2)	(T1–T2)	PCL (T3)	(T2–T3)	(T1–T3)
3	1	1	2	−1	2	0	−1
	2	2	3	−1	1	2	1
	3	4	1	3	1	0	3
	4	4	3	1	2	1	2
	5	3	2	1	2	0	1
	6	4	2	2	1	1	3
	7	3	1	2	1	0	2
	8	4	4	0	3	1	1
	9	3	2	1	2	0	1
	10	2	3	−1	2	1	0
	11	3	3	0	2	1	1
	12	2	1	1	3	−2	−1
	13	4	2	2	4	−2	0
	14	1	1	0	1	0	0
	15	3	2	1	3	−1	0
	16	3	2	1	2	0	1
	17	4	4	0	3	1	1
	18	2	2	0	2	0	0
	19	4	4	0	4	0	0
	20	3	4	−1	3	1	0
	Sum	**59**	**48**	**11**	**44**	**4**	**15**

Key to PCL answers: 0 = not at all, 1 = a little bit, 2 = moderately, 3 = quite a bit, 4 = extremely; key to test and week identification: T1 = week 1, T2 = week 2, T3 = week 4.

Participants were involved in training the seal of that session, which included feeding, touching, and observing the seal's behavior.

Additionally, participants completed a self-reported questionnaire regarding their subjective rating of PTSD symptoms. These questionnaires were collected by and stored with the VMARC for program evaluation. No demographic or personal information beyond the PCL-5 scores were recorded on the deidentified data form, in order to maintain anonymity for the researcher. The specific questionnaire utilized during the program was the PTSD Checklist (PCL-5) (the appendix).

2.1. PCL-5. The PTSD checklist (PCL) is currently one of the most widely utilized self-report measurement tools for PTSD. The most contemporary version of the PCL-5 is used as a resource for a variety of purposes in unison with the fifth edition of the Diagnostic and Statistical Manual of Mental Disorders (DSM-5), including monitoring changes in symptoms related to PTSD during a range of treatment techniques and research [8, 46, 47]. As a self-report instrument, the PCL-5 contains 20 items measured on a Likert scale ranging from zero to four. The lowest score any one individual can receive is a zero, which would indicate no PTSD symptoms at all. The highest overall score that an individual can receive is an eighty, denoting severe and impactful symptoms of PTSD [46, 48]. The scoring to the items is organized parallel to the cluster criteria of PTSD symptoms. Questions one to five are related to PTSD diagnostic criterion B, questions six and seven are linked to criterion C, questions eight to fourteen align with criterion D, and questions fifteen to twenty are associated with criterion E. The PCL-5 has been established as a sound instrument for the measurement of PTSD symptoms, with an internal consistency of $\alpha = 0.94$, a test-retest reliability of $r = 0.82$, a convergent validity of $r = 0.74$ to 0.85, and a discriminant validity of $r = 0.31$ to 0.60 [46, 49]. When used for estimating changes in symptoms due to an intervention, a reduction of five points or more reflects a reliable statistical change, where a reduction of ten points or more is an indication of clinical significance [48, 50, 51].

2.2. Treatment of Data. Participants in *Project Seal to Heal* completed the PCL-5 at T1, T2, and T3 equating to three sets of scores. These were supplied to the researcher via an encrypted, electronic spreadsheet by the VMARC (Table 1). Prior to the transfer of this information, the VMARC changed the names of the program participants to a number code in order to ensure anonymity for this research. Demographic information was also not provided on the spreadsheet.

A range of numerical responses one to four corresponded to the Likert scale for the PCL-5. Zero corresponded to an answer of "not at all," one corresponded to an answer of "a little bit," two corresponded to "moderate," three correlated to "quite a bit," while an answer of four corresponded to "extremely." The raw data provided consisted of participant responses to the 20 questions on the PCL-5 for each time period in which data was collected. The data existed in a column that was designated by a "T" identifier corresponding to each data collection point, meaning "T1" represented the pretest data collected in week one, "T2" represented the midpoint data, and "T3" represented the posttest data. Pertinent data gained from the study was reported utilizing tables and graphs for easy comprehension of alterations in reported PTSD-like symptoms before, during, and after interactions with rescued seals.

From this information, the researcher calculated the difference in reported scores for each week the questionnaires were administered (Table 1). To do this, the researcher subtracted T2 from T1 in order to obtain the difference in reported scores from pretest to midpoint test. The researcher also subtracted T3 from T2 and from T1 in order to obtain the difference in reported scores for midpoint test to posttest, as well as from pretest to posttest. Any calculated differences greater than zero indicated that the participant had responded positively to the HAI for the specific question and the symptom corresponding to that question. Calculated differences less than zero indicated a negative response to the HAI, and a score of zero indicated no noticeable change to in the reported symptom. The calculated differences in scores could range from a 4.0 to a −4.0 (Table 1).

The calculated differences between T1, T2, and T3 were transferred to Table 2 by the researcher in order to tally an aggregate mean for each item on the PCL-5. From these means, the researcher determined if the symptom correlating to each of these PCL-5 items was influenced positively (a decrease in the aggregated symptom score), negatively (an increase in the aggregated symptom score), or not at all (a reported aggregated mean of zero in the symptom score).

Table 3 shows the sum of scores that were calculated corresponding to the PCL-5 questions, that, when clustered, corresponded to PTSD diagnostic criteria for symptomatology. These questions were clustered as such: questions one to five were added for the sum related to criteria B (intrusion symptoms), questions six and seven were added for the sum related to criteria C (symptoms correlating to persistent reexperiencing of the stressful event), questions eight to fourteen were added for the sum related to criteria D (symptoms correlating to negative alterations in mood and cognition), and questions fifteen to twenty were added for the sum related to criteria E (symptoms correlating to alterations in arousal and reactivity).

The accumulative items for each cluster of questions were calculated for T1, T2, and T3. The overall difference between T1 and T3 were calculated, in order to determine changes in the PCL-5 question clusters for PTSD criteria scores reported prior to participation in the program when compared to scores reported after completion of the program.

Additionally, the overall PCL-5 scores were examined for each week the participant completed the PCL-5. The highest overall score any one participant could receive was an 80, indicating the highest severity of symptoms, and the lowest a score a zero, which would indicate no reported symptoms at all.

3. Results

At the onset of *Project Seal to Heal*, four veterans were screened by the VMARC for participation in the six-week program. The VMARC supplied the researcher with the results from one veteran (identified as participant number three) who completed the four weeks of *Project Seal to Heal*. Due to adverse weather conditions, the program itself was limited to four weeks, and three of the participants were unable to attend all four sessions.

3.1. Individual PLC-5 Item Scores. Table 1 summarizes the scores supplied by the VMARC for each week that the PCL-5 was administered, as well as the difference between each item of the PCL-5 from T1, T2, and T3. It was noted that the program participant reported gave the highest score of 4.0 at T1 in six of the twenty questions, indicating that he/she was "extremely" impacted by the PTSD symptoms correlating to that specific PCL-5 question. The participant also at T1 gave the second highest score of a three for seven of the PCL-5 questions, indicating that the participant was impacted "quite a bit" from the symptom correlating to the question.

A "moderate" rating for symptoms was given in four of the questions. The participant did not give a zero for any question, but did answer with a one for the remaining two questions, indicating the symptom impacted his/her life "a little bit."

From these scores, the difference between each PCL-5 item score was calculated. These calculated scores were listed in the appropriate columns, labeled T1–T2, T2–T3, and T1–T3 as seen in Table 2, which illustrates the aggregated mean differences per item on the PCL-5. The mean illustrates the greatest areas of change in symptoms with consideration of the differences between data points weeks. Overall, there were two PCL-5 items found to slightly ($\bar{x} = 0.667$) negatively impact the PTSD symptoms, meaning an increase in the reported score. These occurred in repeated, disturbing, and unwanted memories of the event and loss of interest in enjoyable activities. These symptoms were originally rated as having a little to a moderate impact on symptoms, respectfully. Seven PCL-5 items indicated no mean change in the symptom ($\bar{x} = 0$). These included self-blaming for the stressful event, feeling distant or cut off from others, having difficulty experiencing feelings, irritable behavior, feeling irritable or easily startled, having difficulty concentrating, and having trouble falling asleep.

Nine of the PCL-5 mean item scores decreased, indicating an improvement in the symptom. This decreases ranged from $\bar{x} = 0.667$ to $\bar{x} = 2$, with the largest differential change ($\bar{x} = 2$) reported in symptoms related to suddenly feeling or acting as if the stressful event were occurring again, feeling very upset after experiencing a reminder of the stressful event, avoiding memories, thought, or feelings related to the stressful experience.

3.2. Criteria Symptom Clusters and Overall PCL-5. Table 3 illustrates sums of and alterations in the reported scores correlating to each cluster of symptom composing the PTSD

Table 2: PCL-5 aggregated mean ($\bar{x}$) item scores for the PCL-5 ($n = 1$).

PCL-5 question	T1–T2	T2–T3	T1–T3	Aggregate $\bar{x}$ [(T1–T2–T3)/3]	↑ $\bar{x}$ score	↓ $\bar{x}$ score	No change in $\bar{x}$ score
1	−1	0	−1	−0.667	X		
2	−1	2	1	0.667		X	
3	3	0	3	2		X	
4	1	1	2	2		X	
5	1	0	1	0.667		X	
6	2	1	3	2		X	
7	2	0	2	0.667		X	
8	0	1	1	0.667		X	
9	1	0	1	0.667		X	
10	1	1	0	0			X
11	0	1	1	0.667		X	
12	1	−2	−1	−0.667	X		
13	2	−2	0	0			X
14	0	0	0	0			X
15	1	−1	0	0			X
16	1	0	1	0.667		X	
17	0	1	1	0.667		X	
18	0	0	0	0			X
19	0	0	0	0			X
20	−1	1	0	0			X

Table key: T1 = week 1 (pretest), T2 = week 2 (midpoint), T3 = week 4 (posttest), $\bar{x}$ = mean, ↑ = increase, ↓ = decrease, X = indicated changed.

TABLE 3: Impact on PCL-5 accumulative sum (Σ) scores for PTSD criteria clusters and overall PCL-5 score ($n = 1$).

PTSD criteria	PCL-5 questions clusters for PTSD criteria	T1 Σ score	T2 Σ score	T3 Σ score	Overall difference from T1–T3 (week 1 to week 4)
B: Intrusion	1 to 5	14	11	8	−6
C: Persistent	6 and 7	7	3	2	−5
D: Negative alterations in cognition and mood	8 to 14	19	16	17	−2
E: Alterations in arousal and reactivity	15 to 20	19	18	17	−2
Total score	**1 to 20**	**59**	**48**	**44**	**−15**

Table key: T1 = week 1 (pretest), T2 = week 2 (midpoint), T3 = week 4 (posttest), Σ = sum (of cluster questions per PTSD criteria).

criteria recorded for T1, T2, and T3, as well as the overall difference from T1 to T3. From T1 to T3, results indicate that all criteria clusters reduced in the reported score, with the most significant reductions in score occurring in criteria B, intrusion (reduction of six points), and criteria C, persistent avoidance (reduction of five points). A reduction of two points was reported for criteria D (negative alterations in cognition and mood) and criteria E (alterations in arousal and reactivity). Though the total criteria scores all reduced, a deviation occurred in the reported symptoms of criteria D, in which the T3 score increased in comparison to the T2 score. However, criteria D at T3 remained lower than the T1 score. Further, Tables 1 and 2 show the overall score of the PCL-5 reduced from T1 to T2 by eleven points and from T2 to T3 by four points. This accounts for a reduction of fifteen points for the overall PCL-5 score.

4. Discussion

Previous research focusing on the engagement of nature or natural elements in order to address a variety of ailments have shown physiological, psychosocial, emotional, and mental benefits for the individuals who participated in those studies [12, 26, 52–57]. Specific to HAI, previous studies have found benefits in decreased symptoms of depression and anxiety, increased self-esteem, positive alterations in behavior, decreased feelings of isolation, increased feelings of empathy, increase in positive outlook, decrease in irritability, and an overall increase in perceived quality of life [6, 30, 58–63]. The results of this study support these previous findings with regard to the potential merit of HAIs for the veterans who have PTSD.

Results indicate that overall, participation in *Project Seal to Heal* was clinically significant in the reduction of PTSD-like symptoms for the veteran participant who completed the program. Comparisons of PCL-5 items for each cluster indicated the greatest positive impact from program participation for criteria B and C (intrusion and persistence). The specific symptoms most significantly and positively impacted included those of suddenly feeling or acting as if the stressful experience were occurring again; feeling very upset when reminded of the stressful event; avoiding memories, thoughts, or feelings related to the stressful experience; and avoiding external reminders of the stressful experience.

Though the majority of PCL-5 items indicated a decrease in the correlating symptoms, seven of the items indicated no change in the mean scores. This indicates that participation in the program possibly had no effect on those specific symptoms. These symptoms included blaming the self for the stressful event, feeling distant or cut off from others, having trouble experiencing positive feelings, experiencing irritable behavior and/or angry outbursts, feeling jumpy or easily startled, having difficulty concentrating, and having trouble falling or staying asleep.

The symptom related to PCL-5 item nineteen (difficulty concentrating) was of the most interest, as this item was reported as a four, or extremely disruptive in everyday life, for T1, T2, and T3. Additionally, item thirteen (feeling distant or cut off from other people) was initially reported as a four at T1, dipping to a two at T2, and then rising again to a four at T3. These items were the only two without an overall change of four when comparing T1 to T3. Although the items decreased only to return to the previously reported level, the implication is that participation in *Project Seal to Heal* may have no impact on that symptom when the symptom is initially reported at the highest level of severity.

There were also reported negative impacts on symptoms including those of repeated, disturbing, and unwanted memories of the stressful event and loss of interest in enjoyable activities (items one and twelve). However, the overall positive impact indicated on the PCL-5 suggests not only that *Project Seal to Heal* was clinically significant in the reduction of symptoms for the veteran participant but also that pinniped (seal) facilitated human-animal interaction programs merit further investigation by and within the therapeutic community.

5. Limitations

For this study, there were several limitations. The single participant sample size, lack of a control group, and no randomization make it impossible to generalize the results of the study. Another limitation is that only participants who are interested in seals were likely to partake in *Project Seal to Heal.* This may lead to potential bias in reported symptom alterations as individuals who have a positive outlook on animals may already have a predisposition to receive or experience a change in their ailment. Additionally, a limitation lies in the fact that the participant only had interactions with captive grey and harbor seals; thus, the results cannot be generalized to all pinnipeds. Beyond that, this study is limited by the cultural beliefs of the geological location, inland northern East Coast United States, and the language of that community when specifically addressing and interacting with marine environments and pinnipeds.

6. Conclusion

The results found in this study indicate that participation in the *Project Seal to Heal* program was clinically significant for the reduction of PTSD-like symptoms for the veteran who completed the program. The PTSD symptoms corresponding to the diagnostic criteria that were most notably impacted were those related to intrusion and persistence in reliving the stressful event. However, participation in the program had a negative noted effect on two symptoms and no noticeable impact on six symptoms. The results of the study cannot be generalized due to small sample size, no control group, limited pinniped species inclusion, and no randomization. The findings do support continued research in pinniped facilitated HAI in order to address the growing burden of PTSD within the veteran community. The findings are of interest to occupational therapists as engagement of this particular animal in a therapeutic intervention may be advantageous in addressing global healthcare needs in mental health, as well as attending to the WFOT's call for practitioners to address immediate healthcare demands while simultaneously confronting environmental health.

Table 4

In the past month, how much were, you bothered by	Not at all	A little bit	Moderately	Quite a bit	Extremely
(1) Repeated, disturbing, and unwanted memories of the stressful experience?	0	1	2	3	4
(2) Repeated, disturbing dreams of the stressful experience?	0	1	2	3	4
(3) Suddenly feeling or acting as if the stressful experience were actually happening again (as if you were actually back there reliving it)?	0	1	2	3	4
(4) Feeling very upset when something reminded you of the stressful experience?	0	1	2	3	4
(5) Having strong physical reactions when something reminded you of the stressful experience (e.g., heart pounding, trouble breathing, and sweating)?	0	1	2	3	4
(6) Avoiding memories, thoughts, or feelings related to stressful experience?	0	1	2	3	4
(7) Avoiding external reminders of the stressful experience (e.g., people, places, conversations, activities, objects, or situations)?	0	1	2	3	4
(8) Trouble remembering important parts of the stressful experience?	0	1	2	3	4
(9) Having strong negative beliefs about yourself, other people, or the world (e.g., having thoughts such as: I am bad, there is something seriously wrong with me, no one can be trusted, the world is completely dangerous)?	0	1	2	3	4
(10) Blaming yourself or someone else for the stressful experience or what happened after it?	0	1	2	3	4
(11) Having strong negative feelings such as fear, horror, anger, guilt, or shame?	0	1	2	3	4
(12) Loss of interest in activities that you used to enjoy?	0	1	2	3	4
(13) Feeling distant or cut off from other people?	0	1	2	3	4
(14) Trouble experiencing positive feelings (e.g., being unable to feel happiness or have loving feelings for people close to you)?	0	1	2	3	4
(15) Irritable behavior, angry outbursts, or acting aggressively?	0	1	2	3	4
(16) Taking too many risks or doing things that could cause you harm?	0	1	2	3	4
(17) Being "superalert" or watchful or on guard?	0	1	2	3	4
(18) Feeling jumpy or easily startled?	0	1	2	3	4
(19) Having difficulty concentrating?	0	1	2	3	4
(20) Trouble falling or staying asleep?	0	1	2	3	4

Source: US Department of Veteran Affairs (VA), National Center for PTSD, (2014). *PTSD checklist for DSM-5 (PCL-5)*. Retrieved from http://www.ptsd.va.gov/professional/assessment/adult-sr/ptsd-checklist.asp.

Appendix

The PTSD Checklist for DSM-5 (PCL-5) Self-Reported Questionnaire (Items One to Twenty)

Instructions: Table 4 shows a list of problems that people sometimes have in response to a very stressful experience. Please read each problem carefully and then circle the numbers to the right to indicate how much you have been bothered by that problem *in the past month*.

Acknowledgments

This research/manuscript makes reference to and was conducted in correlation with the thesis entitled *Pinnipeds and PTSD: An Analysis of a Human-Animal Interaction Program for Veterans*. This research was supported by the Aquarium of Niagara Falls and the Veteran and Military Affiliated Research Center at D'Youville College. A large thank you goes to the Department of Occupational Therapy staff at D'Youville who provided guidance, expertise, and insight that improved the manuscript.

References

[1] World Health Organization (WHO), *Comprehensive Mental Health Action Plan 2013–2020*, WHO, Geneva, Switzerland, 2013, http://apps.who.int/iris/bitstream/10665/89966/1/9789241506021_eng.pdf.

[2] World Health Organization (WHO), *The World Health Report 2001: Mental Health: New Understanding, New Hope*, WHO, Geneva, Switzerland, 2001, http://www.who.int/whr/2001/en/whr01_en/whr01-en.pdf?ua=1.

[3] T. Insel, *Post by Former NIMH director Thomas Insel: The Global Cost of Mental Illness*, National Institute of Mental Health (NIMH), 2011, http://www.nimg.nih.gov/about/director/2011/the-global-cost-of-mental-illness.shtml.

[4] Z. Wilson, "Out of the shadows-making mental health a global development priority: editorial," *Mental Health Matters*, vol. 3, no. 3, pp. 1–4, 2016.

[5] American Hospital Association (AHA), *Bringing Behavioral Health into the Care Continuum: Opportunities to Improve Quality, Cost and Outcomes*, AHA, Washington, DC, 2012.

[6] M. E. O'Haire, N. A. Guérin, and A. C. Kirkham, "Animal-assisted intervention for trauma: a systematic literature review," *Frontiers in Psychology*, vol. 6, 2015.

[7] J. L. Gradus, *Epidemiology of PTSD. U.S*, Department of Veterans Affairs (VA), 2016, http://www.ptsd.va.gov/professional/PTSD-overview/epidemiological-facts-ptsd.asp.

[8] U.S. Department of Veteran Affairs (VA), National Center for PTSD, *Understanding PTSD and PTSD treatment*, U.S. Department of Veteran Affairs, National Center for PTSD, 2016, http://www.ptsd.va.gov/public/understanding_ptsd/booklet.pdf.

[9] PTSD United, *PTSD Statistics*, PTSD United, 2013, http://ptsdunited.org/ptsd-statistics-2/.

[10] World Health Organization, "WHO releases guidance on mental health care after trauma," *Saudi Medical Journal*, vol. 34, no. 9, p. 975, 2013.

[11] K. H. Seal, Y. Shi, G. Cohen et al., "Association of mental health disorders with prescription opioids and high-risk opioid use in US veterans of Iraq and Afghanistan," *JAMA*, vol. 307, no. 9, pp. 940–947, 2012.

[12] W. J. Nichols, *Blue Mind: The Surprising Science that Shows How Being near, in, on, or under Water Can Make you Happier, Healthier, More Connected, and Better at What You Do*, Back Bay Books, New York, NY, 2014.

[13] I. Kirsch, B. J. Deacon, T. B. Huedo-Medina, A. Scoboria, T. J. Moore, and B. T. Johnson, "Initial severity and antidepressant benefits: a meta-analysis of data submitted to the Food and Drug Administration," *PLoS Medicine*, vol. 5, no. 2, article e45, 2008.

[14] M. J. Friedman, C. R. Marmar, D. G. Baker, C. R. Sikes, and G. M. Farfel, "Randomized, double-blind comparison of sertraline and placebo for posttraumatic stress disorder in a department of veterans affairs setting," *The Journal of Clinical Psychiatry*, vol. 68, no. 05, pp. 711–720, 2007.

[15] W. Alexander, "Pharmacotherapy for post-traumatic stress disorder in combat veterans: focus on antidepressants and atypical antipsychotic agents," *Pharmacy and Therapeutics*, vol. 37, no. 1, pp. 32–38, 2012.

[16] N. C. Crawford, *Costs of War: US Budgetary Costs of Wars Through 2016: $4.79 Trillion and Counting*, Watson Institute Internarial & Public Affairs and Brown University, 2016, http://watson.brown.edu/costsofwar/files/cow/imce/papers/2016/Costs%20of%20War%20through%202016%20FINAL%20final%20v2.pdf.

[17] K. A. Hepner, E. M. Sloss, C. P. Roth et al., "Quality of care for PTSD and depression in the military health system: phase I report," *Rand Health quarterly*, vol. 6, no. 1, p. 14, 2016.

[18] M. Aoyama, M. J. Hudson, and K. C. Hoover, "Occupation mediates ecosystem services with human well-being," *Journal of Occupational Science*, vol. 19, no. 3, pp. 213–225, 2012.

[19] R. R. N. Alves and I. M. L. Rosa, "Biodiversity, traditional medicine and public health: where do they meet?," *Journal of Ethnobiology and Ethnomedicine*, vol. 3, no. 1, p. 14, 2007.

[20] World Federation of Occupational Therapists (WFOT), *Environmental Sustainability, Sustainable Practice within Occupational Therapy [Position Statement]*, World Federation of Occupational Therapists, Taiwan, 2012.

[21] M. J. Hudson and M. Aoyama, "Occupational therapy and the current ecological crisis," *British Journal of Occupational Therapy*, vol. 71, no. 12, pp. 545–548, 2008.

[22] G. Kielhofner, *A Model of Human Occupation: Theory and Application (4th)*, Lippincott Williams & Wilkins, Philadelphia, PA, 2008.

[23] H. Frumkin and R. Louv, *The Powerful Link between Conserving Land and Preserving Health*, Land Trust Alliance, Washington, D.C., 2007.

[24] E. Gullone, "The biophilia hypothesis and life in the 21st century: increasing mental health or increasing pathology?," *Journal of Happiness Studies*, vol. 1, no. 3, pp. 293–322, 2000.

[25] N. Hensley, "Cultivating biophilia: utilizing direct experience to promote environmental sustainability," *Journal of Sustainability Education*, vol. 9, 2015.

[26] T. Kamidin, A. Muda, S. Roslan, and M. M. Konting, "Ecopsychology elements in environmental education as to strengthen attitudes towards the environment," *Journal of ASIAN Behavioural Studies*, vol. 1, no. 1, pp. 17–27, 2016.

[27] A. Pryor, M. Townsend, C. Maller, and K. Field, "Health and well-being naturally: 'contact with nature' in health promotion for targeted individuals, communities and populations," *Health Promotion Journal of Australia*, vol. 17, no. 2, pp. 114–123, 2006.

[28] E. O. Wilson, *Biophilia. Massachusetts, United States*, Harvard University Press, 1984.

[29] N. Satiansukpong, M. Pongsaksri, S. Sung-U et al., "Thai elephant-assisted therapy program: the feasibility in assisting an individual with autism," *World Federation of Occupational Therapists Bulletin*, vol. 58, no. 1, pp. 17–26, 2008.

[30] J. Nimer and B. Lundahl, "Animal-assisted therapy: a meta-analysis," *Anthrozoös*, vol. 20, no. 3, pp. 225–238, 2007.

[31] R. J. Huggett, *Global Ecology. Ecology: Encyclopedia of Life Support Systems (EOLSS)*, vol. 1, Eolss Publishers Co. Ltd., Oxford, United Kingdom, 2009.

[32] Millennium Ecosystem Assessment (MEA), *Ecosystems and Human Well-Being*, vol. 200, Island Press, Washington, DC, 2005.

[33] B. L. Fiksdal, D. Houlihan, and A. C. Barnes, "Dolphin-assisted therapy: claims versus evidence," *Autism Research and Treatment*, vol. 2012, Article ID 839792, 7 pages, 2012.

[34] C. J. Dawe, "Implications of aquatic animal health for human health," *Environmental Health Perspectives*, vol. 86, pp. 245–255, 1990.

[35] Intergovernmental Panel on Climate Change (IPCC), "Climate change 2014: Synthesis Report," in *Contribution of Working Groups I, II and III to the Fifth Assessment Report of the Intergovernmental Panel on Climate Change*, Core Writing Team, R. K. Pachauri, and L. A. Meyer, Eds., IPCC, Geneva, Switzerland, 2014.

[36] D. P. Tittensor, C. Mora, W. Jetz et al., "Global patterns and predictors of marine biodiversity across taxa," *Nature*, vol. 466, no. 7310, pp. 1098–1101, 2010.

[37] Northeast Fisheries Science Center (NEFSC), *Protected Species: Seals*, National Oceanic and Atmospheric Administration, Northeast Fisheries Science Center, 2016, http://nefsc.noaa.gov/ecosys/ecosystem-ecology/pinnipeds.html.

[38] M. Riedman, *The Pinnipeds: Seals, Sea Lions, and Walruses (No. 12)*, University of California Press, Oxford, England, 1990.

[39] A. W. Trites, "The role of pinnipeds in the ecosystem," in *Pinniped Populations, Eastern North Pacific: Status, Trends and Issues*, G. Stone, J. Goebel, and S. Webster, Eds., vol. 2110, pp. 31–39, A symposium of the 127th Annual Meeting of the American Fisheries Society, 1997.

[40] K. M. Kovacs, A. Aguilar, D. Aurioles et al., "Global threats to pinnipeds," *Marine Mammal Science*, vol. 28, no. 2, pp. 414–436, 2012.

[41] M. Penel and F. Delbour, "Are California sea lions (*Zalophus californianus*) sensitive to the attentional state of their caretakers?," *Animal Behavior and Cognition*, vol. 1, no. 4, pp. 434–445, 2014.

[42] D. J. St. Aubin, J. R. Geraci, and V. J. Lounsbury, *Rescue, Rehabilitation, and Release of Marine Mammals: an Analysis of Current Views and Practices*, U.S. of Commerce, National Oceanic and Atmospheric Administration, National Marine Fisheries Service, Office of Protected Resources, 1996, http://www.nmfs.noaa.gov/pr/pdfs/health/rescue.pdf.

[43] K. Cale, *Phoca vitulina (On-line)*, Animal Diversity Web, 2012, http://apnimaldiversity.org/accounts/Phoca_vitulina/.

[44] T. Götz and V. M. Janik, "Repeated elicitation of the acoustic startle reflex leads to sensitisation in subsequent avoidance behaviour and induces fear conditioning," *BMC Neuroscience*, vol. 12, no. 1, p. 30, 2011.

[45] V. Servais, "Some comments on context embodiment in zootherapy: the case of the Autidolfijn project," *Anthrozoös*, vol. 12, no. 1, pp. 5–15, 1999.

[46] C. A. Blevins, F. W. Weathers, M. T. Davis, T. K. Witte, and J. L. Domino, "The posttraumatic stress disorder checklist for *DSM-5* (PCL-5): development and initial psychometric evaluation," *Journal of Traumatic Stress*, vol. 28, no. 6, pp. 489–498, 2015.

[47] S. M. Keen, C. J. Kutter, B. L. Niles, and K. E. Krinsley, "Psychometric properties of PTSD checklist in sample of male veterans," *The Journal of Rehabilitation Research and Development*, vol. 45, no. 3, pp. 465–474, 2008.

[48] F. W. Weathers, B. T. Litz, T. M. Keane, P. A. Palmieri, B. P. Marx, and P. P. Schnurr, *The PTSD Checklist for DSM-5 (PCL-5)*, U.S. Department of Veterans Affairs, 2013, http://www.ptsd.va.gov/professional/assessment/adult-sr/ptsd-checklist.asp.

[49] T. L. Biehn, *Examining the Underlying Dimensions of Posttraumatic Stress Disorder and Major Depressive Disorder Using the Proposed DSM-5 Diagnostic Criteria*, Doctoral dissertation, University of Toledo, 2014.

[50] U.S. Department of Veteran Affairs (VA), National Center for PTSD, *Using the PTSD Checklist for DSM-IV (PCL)*, U.S. Department of Veteran Affairs (VA), National Center for PTSD, 2014, http://www.vsias.org/wp-content/uploads/2015/07/DP-063015_Using-the-PCL.pdf.

[51] U.S. Department of Veteran Affairs (VA), National Center for PTSD, *PTSD Checklist for DSM-5 (PCL-5)*, U.S. Department of Veteran Affairs (VA), National Center for PTSD, 2014, http://www.ptsd.va.gov/professional/assessment/adult-sr/ptsd-checklist.asp.

[52] K. Frances, "Outdoor recreation as an occupation to improve quality of life for people with enduring mental health problems," *British Journal of Occupational Therapy*, vol. 69, no. 4, pp. 182–186, 2006.

[53] A. Pedretti-Burls, "Ecotherapy: a therapeutic and educative model," *Journal of Mediterranean Ecology*, vol. 8, pp. 19–25, 2007.

[54] J. Vining, "The connection to other animals and caring for nature," *Human Ecology Review*, vol. 10, no. 20, pp. 87–99, 2003.

[55] J. Lloret, "Human health benefits supplied by Mediterranean marine biodiversity," *Marine Pollution Bulletin*, vol. 60, no. 10, pp. 1640–1646, 2010.

[56] J. Barton and J. Pretty, "What is the best dose of nature and green exercise for improving mental health? A multi-study analysis," *Environmental Science & Technology*, vol. 44, no. 10, pp. 3947–3955, 2010.

[57] D. Cracknell, M. P. White, S. Pahl, W. J. Nichols, and M. H. Depledge, "Marine biota and psychological well-being: a preliminary examination of dose–response effects in an aquarium setting," *Environment and Behavior*, vol. 48, no. 10, pp. 1242–1269, 2016.

[58] A. Beetz, K. Uvnäs-Moberg, H. Julius, and K. Kotrschal, "Psychosocial and psychophysiological effects of human-animal interactions: the possible role of oxytocin," *Frontiers in Psychology*, vol. 3, p. 234, 2012.

[59] G. Hosey and V. Melfi, "Human-animal interactions, relationships and bonds: a review and analysis of the literature," *International Journal of Comparative Psychology*, vol. 27, no. 1, pp. 117–142, 2014.

[60] B. P. Velde, J. Cipriani, and G. Fisher, "Resident and therapist views of animal-assisted therapy: implications for occupational therapy practice," *Australian Occupational Therapy Journal*, vol. 52, no. 1, pp. 43–50, 2005.

[61] K. A. Kruger and J. A. Serpell, "Animal-assisted interventions in mental health: definitions and theoretical foundations," in *Fine, A. H. Handbook on Animal-Assisted Therapy*, pp. 21–38, Elsevier, London, UK, 3rd edition, 2010.

[62] H. Kamioka, S. Okada, K. Tsutani et al., "Effectiveness of animal-assisted therapy: a systematic review of randomized controlled trials," *Complementary Therapies in Medicine*, vol. 22, no. 2, pp. 371–390, 2014.

[63] M. Samfira and I. Petroman, "Therapeutic value of the human being-animal relationship," *Scientific Papers Animal Science and Biotechnologies*, vol. 44, no. 2, pp. 512–515, 2011.

11

A Cognitive Occupation-Based Programme for People with Multiple Sclerosis: A Study to Test Feasibility and Clinical Outcomes

Sean Reilly and Sinéad M. Hynes

Discipline of Occupational Therapy, National University of Ireland Galway, Galway, Ireland

Correspondence should be addressed to Sinéad M. Hynes; sinead.hynes@nuigalway.ie

Academic Editor: Jodie A. Copley

Cognitive impairments are common in MS and affect personal, social, and occupational functioning. There is a developing body of evidence highlighting the role of cognitive rehabilitation, but there is still no evidence for a validated holistic approach. The aim of this study was to assess the effectiveness of Cognitive Occupation-Based Programme for People with Multiple Sclerosis (COB-MS) for improving daily life and cognitive impairment. This study used an experimental pretest/posttest design with eight-week follow-up. Participants were recruited from MS networks using convenience sampling. The primary outcome measure was the GAS. Secondary outcomes included the OSA-DLS, CVLT-II, BVMT-R, SDMT, TMT, BRIEF-A, and EMQ-R. Twelve participants were recruited, aged 39–73 years (mean: 55.08; SD: 9.61). There were statistically significant improvements in the GAS ($p < .002$), CVLT-II: total free recall ($p < .000$), short delay free recall ($p < .018$), long delay free recall ($p < .008$), BVMT-R total recall ($p < .000$), TMT part B ($p < .044$), and EMQ-R ($p < .006$). Except for the BRIEF-A, clinically significant improvements were observed in secondary outcome measures at posttest and follow-up. Limitations include selection bias and subtle practice effects in cognitive measures. Results suggest that a larger scale study is justified considering improvements seen in daily life and cognitive measures.

1. Background

Multiple Sclerosis (MS) is a demyelinating disease of the central nervous system, characterised by the development of lesions in the brain and spinal cord [1]. According to Amato et al. [2], the prevalence of cognitive difficulties in MS ranges from 43% to 70%. The most commonly affected cognitive domains in people with MS are memory, attention, processing speed, and executive functions [3]. Cognitive difficulties affect the daily lives of people with MS in several ways. Cognitive impairment resulting from MS has been found to be associated with impaired social functioning [4], reduced employability [5], and decreased quality of life [6].

Cognitive rehabilitation (CR) is an intervention that aims to improve cognitive impairment through using compensatory and restorative approaches [7]. There are many unique factors to be considered when developing interventions for people with MS such as the disease's fluctuating nature, associated fatigue, and the emotional well-being of the person [8]. To date, most studies examining CR in MS have mainly involved computer-based interventions [9–12], although others have investigated non-computer-based (face to face) interventions that use educational methods [13, 14]. Research has found that computer-based interventions, specifically targeting the domain of attention (e.g., [9, 10]), are effective at improving outcomes on cognitive measures for people with MS. Computer-based interventions that target several cognitive domains [15] also found significant improvements in objective and subjective cognitive outcome measures. In contrast, many computerised interventions that specifically target memory did not lead to improvements (e.g., [16, 17]). It is apparent that non-computer-based interventions are more beneficial for improving memory [18] and several cognitive domains [19, 20] than computerised interventions. Group interventions and frequent professional contact appear to be important components in the effectiveness of CR for people with MS.

Despite the findings from individual studies being generally positive, the pooled results of a meta-analysis in a Cochrane review [21] suggest that the effectiveness of cognitive rehabilitation for people with MS is far from being conclusive. In two recent reviews [22, 23], the authors found low-level evidence that CR reduces cognitive difficulties in MS. Both reviews concluded that CR in MS is in its relative infancy. There is a clear need for more randomised control trials of sound methodological quality before conclusions can be drawn on the possibility of improving function through CR. In addition, both reviews recommended that future studies should examine interventions that aim to increase occupational participation and use outcomes that measure impact on daily life—cognitive interventions adopting a specific approach may not necessarily generalise to functional domains. Findings and recommendations provided the rationale for the current study.

From the current evidence and recommendations provided in the literature, there was a clear need for a holistic cognitive intervention targeting several domains using a functional approach that is measured by and focuses on occupational participation. A Cognitive Occupation-Based Programme for People with Multiple Sclerosis (COB-MS) was developed in response to this noted clinical treatment gap, and it focuses on facilitating people with MS to engage more effectively in everyday occupations that they find difficult as a result of their cognition [24].

Thus, the purpose of this current study was to establish clinical outcomes of COB-MS in relation to daily life and cognition. This study will contribute towards COB-MS' proof of principle and add to the paucity of research in the field of MS and CR.

Specifically, the following research questions were addressed:

(i) Will people who receive COB-MS have improved daily life scores?

(ii) Will people who receive COB-MS see improvements in their cognition?

We were interested if any gains seen were also maintained at follow-up of 8 weeks.

2. Method

2.1. Recruitment. Information regarding the study was available to participants through MS networks such as the monthly MS Ireland newsletter, biannual MS Ireland eZine, and research section of MS Ireland website and Facebook page. Recruitment posters were also hung, with permission, in the outpatient department of University Hospital Galway. Study details and the second author's contact information were available on all recruitment material.

2.2. Participants. Participants were self-selected by contacting the second author via phone or email if they were interested in taking part. To be part of the convenience sample, participants had to meet the following inclusion criteria: (i) be aged 18 years of age or older, (ii) be fluent in written and spoken English, (iii) have a diagnosis of MS, (iv) have mild cognitive difficulties as shown by a score of >22 on the MSNQ, (v) be clinically stable, (vi) can provide informed consent, (vii) do not have neurologic history other than MS, including evidence of current dementia, (viii) do not have history of major depressive disorder, schizophrenia, or bipolar disorder I or II, (ix) do not have history of diagnosed substance use or dependence disorder, and (x) live in the community. Exclusion criteria were the following: (i) cognitive impairment that would affect reliable participation or capacity to give informed consent and (ii) being incarcerated or institutionalised.

Eligibility was determined by the second author during the initial contact. If deemed ineligible, the participant was thanked for their time and the reasons were explained. For eligible participants who were satisfied with the study requirements, verbal consent was sought and their availability was noted to allow for scheduling of COB-MS sessions. Once individual and group sessions were confirmed by the second author, the first author then contacted the participants via phone to schedule the baseline assessment. The first author posted an information sheet to participants for the study. The first author also went through the information sheet with participants at the beginning of the baseline assessment and answered any questions the participants had before signing the written consent form.

2.3. COB-MS Programme. The COB-MS programme consists of eight sessions: two being individual and six being group-based. The focus of the COB-MS is on managing the demands of employment and daily life by using compensatory strategies and routines and learning new techniques that can be integrated into daily occupations and contexts in order to make it meaningful to the participant. The programme was facilitated by the second author. The programme consisted of eight sessions over 9 weeks, beginning one week after baseline assessments and finishing one week before posttest assessments. The COB-MS programme takes a three-pronged approach to cognitive rehabilitation using education, remediation, and adaption to help people meet their goals while managing their cognitive challenges. The programme is informed by the Person-Environment-Occupational Performance model [25].

Table 1 summarises the content of each of the 60-minute sessions.

2.4. Outcome Measures. Participants completed a total of eight assessments. The Goal Attainment Scaling (GAS) [26] was the primary outcome measure of this current study and allowed participants to set meaningful goals related to daily life, which could be measured in a systematic way. Given the emphasis placed on goal-setting in COB-MS and the importance of personal goals as a source of motivation for participants, goal achievement reflected the practical benefit of COB-MS.

Table 1

Session	Brief content
Session 1 (individual)	*Focus on you* (i) Initial meeting with the OT: briefing on what will be involved in COB-MS (ii) Goal setting with the person on occupations that they wish to target
Session 2 (group)	*You and your cognition* (i) Education about the brain and cognition (ii) Discussion on how MS can impact cognitive function (iii) Discussion on the impact of cognitive difficulties on day-to-day occupations
Session 3 (group)	*You, the centerpiece* (i) How the cognitive difficulties affect you? (ii) What changes can be made by you? (iii) Discussion and application of strategies
Session 4 (group)	*You, the person* (i) Further concepts on what changes can be made by you (ii) Internal strategies to practice and apply (iii) Discussion around sleep and sleep diaries
Session 5 (group)	*Your environment* (i) How does the environment impact cognition? (ii) What can we change that might help? (iii) Application of external memory strategies (iv) Managing distraction and the impact of other factors
Session 6 (group)	*Focus on doing* (i) How are our occupations and daily life affected? (ii) What can we do to help integrate strategies into daily life? (iii) Examples of how to adapt or remediate occupations
Session 7 (group)	*Seeking new challenges* (i) Seek new challenges with strategies that support success (ii) Set goals for yourself (iii) Stay motivated, maintain progress and on-going adaptation (iv) Group conclusion and debrief
Session 8 (individual)	*Testing the application* (i) Review goals and strategies used (ii) Plan for future (iii) Discussion around useful groups and services (iv) Debrief and summary

Secondary outcomes included measures of occupational competence [Occupational Self-Assessment-Daily Living Scales (OSA-DLS) [27]], verbal memory [California Verbal Learning Test-II (CVLT-II) [28]], visual memory [Brief Visuospatial Memory Test-Revised (BVMT-R) [29]], processing speed [Symbol Digit Modality Test (SDMT) [30]], divided attention [Trail Making Test (TMT) [31]], perceived executive functioning [Behaviour Rating Inventory of Executive Function-Adult Version (BRIEF-A) [32]], and self-reported memory difficulties [Everyday Memory Questionnaire-Revised (EMQ-R) [33]].

Data was collected by the researcher at three time points: one week before the first COB-MS session (baseline), one week after the final COB-MS session (posttest), and eight weeks after the final COB-MS session (follow-up). Except for the GAS, all assessments were administered at three time points, with alternate forms used where possible.

2.5. Statistical Analysis. SPSS Version 23 was utilised to analyse the data. Descriptive statistics were used to describe the characteristics of the sample regarding gender, age, education, work status, MS type, disease duration, and MSNQ score. To answer the research questions, inferential statistics were utilised. The Friedman test measured changes in mean daily life and cognitive scores over three time points, whereas the Wilcoxon signed-rank test measured changes over two time points.

3. Results

In total, 1 male and 11 female participants received COB-MS. The types of MS varied between participants and included relapsing remitting ($n = 5$) or primary progressive ($n = 3$) types. Four participants were unsure of their MS type. Participants' work status also varied and included long term disability ($n = 5$), staying at home parent ($n = 3$), or being retired ($n = 4$).

A full data set was obtained, as the twelve participants completed outcome measures at each of the three time points. Descriptive statistics were expressed as a mean, standard

Table 2: Demographic data of the sample.

	Mean	SD	Minimum	Maximum
Age (years)	55.08	9.61	39	73
Duration (years)	14.25	7.61	3	31
Education (years)	16.42	2.31	13	20
MSNQ	26.58	2.27	23	30

Table 3: Wilcoxon signed-rank test results for the GAS.

	Time 1			Time 3			z-value	p value
	Mean	SD	Median	Mean	SD	Median		
GAS	37.02	0.88	37.5	56.23	10.60	52.7	−3.061	.002*

* p value is statistically significant at $p < .05$.

Table 4: Friedman test results for the OSA-DLS.

	Time 1			Time 2			Time 3			p value
	Mean	SD	Median	Mean	SD	Median	Mean	SD	Median	
Competence	30.58	7.50	31.00	31.67	6.77	33.00	31.33	7.55	34.00	.822
Importance	31.42	6.54	31.00	31.92	8.59	35.00	31.67	8.19	31.00	1.000

deviation (SD), minimum, and maximum. Table 2 illustrates the demographic data of the sample in relation to age, disease duration, education, and MSNQ score.

3.1. Daily Life. After receiving COB-MS, participants' goal achievement improvement in scores on the GAS (Table 3) was statistically significant ($z = -3.061$; $p = .02$). This shows that the meaningful goals set in relation to daily life were achieved by follow-up. Table 4 shows that occupational competence scores on the OSA-DLS were clinically significant as posttest and follow-up scores were greater than baseline.

3.2. Cognition. Findings from cognitive outcome measures are shown in Table 5. Statistically significant improvements were observed in verbal memory on the CVLT-II: in total free recall ($p = .000$), short delay free recall ($p = .018$), and long delay free recall ($p = .008$). In visual memory, a statistically significant difference was obtained on the BVMT-R in total recall ($p = .000$). In part B of the TMT, improvements in divided attention were statistically significant ($p = .044$). Although results for part A of the TMT and the SDMT were not statistically significant, results show that processing speed improved across the three time points. Participants reported significantly fewer memory difficulties in daily life on the EMQ-R ($p = .006$). In contrast to the trend of results, perceived executive functioning scores on the BRIEF-A at follow-up did not improve when compared to baseline.

3.3. Post Hoc Tests. After establishing that there were statistically significant differences somewhere among the three time points in Friedman test results for the CVLT-II, BVMT-R, TMT, and EMQ-R, post hoc tests were used to identify changes between individual time points (Table 6). Wilcoxon signed-rank tests were used to compare Time 1 with Time 2, Time 2 with Time 3, and Time 1 with Time 3.

To control for Type 1 errors, a Bonferroni adjustment was applied to the alpha values. This involved dividing the original alpha level of .05 by the total number of tests used (.05/3 = .01666). Thus, the adjusted alpha level for determining statistical significance was .0167.

4. Discussion

Results suggest that people who receive COB-MS have significantly higher mean daily life scores at posttest and eight-week follow-up. The GAS, which was the primary outcome measure of the study, showed a statistically significant increase in goal achievement with a large effect size. This adds to the findings of Mantynen et al. who observed similar changes in the GAS and showed that personal goals for their computer-based and non-computer-based interventions were well achieved [34]. However, it is important to note that the goals set by participants in this study related to leisure, self-care, and productivity occupations in their daily lives and not just the intervention as seen in Mantynen et al.'s work [34]. Therefore, the improvements observed in the GAS in this study reflect the practical benefit of COB-MS and acknowledge the real-world implications of COB-MS in daily life.

Although there was no statistically significant increase in the OSA-DLS, scores at posttest and follow-up were greater than baseline and are indicative of clinical significance. With regard to the trend of competence scores in the OSA-DLS, it appears that people who receive COB-MS feel that they improve their ability to sustain a pattern of occupational behaviour, which is both satisfying and productive. Therefore, the perceived ability to perform activities of daily living (ADLs) and instrumental activities of daily living (IADLs) increased after receiving COB-MS. Similarly, the importance placed on daily life occupations was also greater at posttest and follow-up. Unfortunately, no comparisons with other

Table 5: Friedman test results for cognitive outcome measures.

	Time 1			Time 2			Time 3			p value
	Mean	SD	Median	Mean	SD	Median	Mean	SD	Median	
CVLT-II										
Total free recall	45.92	6.83	45.00	58.00	7.10	56.00	54.50	9.85	52.00	.000*
Short delay free recall	9.00	2.09	9.00	12.17	2.41	13.00	11.25	3.22	13.00	.018*
Long delay free recall	9.67	2.81	10.00	12.33	2.06	13.00	11.58	2.84	12.00	.008*
BVMT-R										
Total recall	45.67	9.87	44.00	51.33	12.61	52.00	57.33	10.22	60.00	.000*
Delayed recall	48.83	12.77	49.00	52.42	14.87	56.00	57.58	8.22	61.00	.103
SDMT	38.42	8.08	38.00	39.83	10.20	37.00	41.75	9.28	37.00	.127
TMT										
Part A	35.92	12.07	31.00	34.33	11.51	33.00	33.75	15.39	33.00	.368
Part B	95.92	47.96	79.00	69.17	31.57	56.00	67.33	27.58	62.00	.044*
BRIEF-A										
Behavioural regulation index	58.83	9.71	58.00	57.58	8.55	60.00	59.33	7.98	61.00	.376
Metacognition index	61.58	11.31	61.00	61.08	7.83	63.00	63.00	7.94	63.00	.862
Global executive composite	61.17	10.05	63.00	60.25	8.01	62.00	61.25	8.21	61.00	.320
EMQ-R	19.83	10.85	18.00	15.67	12.46	14.00	16.00	11.07	14.00	.006*

* p value is statistically significant at $p < .05$.

Table 6: Wilcoxon signed-rank test results for post hoc tests.

	Time 1	Time 2	Time 3
CVLT-II: total free recall	.002*	.181	.003*
CVLT-II: short delay free recall	.008*	.058	.052
CVLT-II: long delay free recall	.012*	.311	.044
BVMT-R: total recall	.028	.012*	.022
TMT: part B	.077	.610	.016*
EMQ-R	.040	.563	.022

* p value is statistically significant at $p < .0167$.

studies can be made as the OSA-DLS was not used as an outcome measure in previously reviewed literature. However, there is an abundance of literature pertaining to the Model of Human Occupation which illustrates the meaning of the OSA-DLS results [35]. It has been stated by Lee et al. that a person's motivation for occupation, often referred to as volition, is influenced by personal causation, values, and interests [36]. Volition is also recognised as a fundamental factor in the achievement of goals. Thus, this is in line with findings in the current study as higher competence scores (personal causation) and importance scores (values and interests) appear to have contributed towards people achieving their daily life goals after receiving COB-MS.

With regard to cognition, results suggest that people who receive COB-MS have statistically significant improvements in verbal memory scores at posttest and follow-up, as shown on the CVLT-II. This finding is similar to verbal memory improvements seen in computer-based interventions [11, 37], non-computer-based interventions [38, 39], and studies that investigated computer-based and non-computer-based interventions [40, 41]. While one may think that an intervention that specifically trained memory would result in better verbal memory outcomes than a nonspecific intervention, this is not the case. For example, two computer-based interventions specifically targeting memory failed to find statistically significant improvements in verbal memory [12, 17], whereas the nonspecific intervention in this current study did. This observation supports the argument that interventions for people with MS are more effective in the presence of a healthcare professional [20].

Findings from this current study also suggest that people who receive COB-MS improve statistically in visual memory, as shown in the BVMT-R. These findings are reminiscent of those by computer-based interventions [15, 40] and interventions using a combination of computer-based and non-computer-based training [37, 41, 42]. Once again, there is evidence supporting the argument by Jonsson et al., as interventions that involved frequent input from a healthcare professional appear to be more effective for improving visual memory [39]. It appears that regular contact with a professional is required as people may not comply with the intervention if they are not monitored weekly [14]. In addition, qualitative research suggests that people enjoy the social element of group interventions [13], which is absent in individual and computer-based interventions. In COB-MS, each session involves discussion around cognitive difficulties, whereby the facilitator explains various strategies and techniques that can be applied to improve occupational performance in daily life. A group-based design is a feasible and cost-efficient method to deliver interventions in a healthcare setting, making the COB-MS meaningful to frontline health professionals. The format of the COB-MS, importantly, allows for individualisation through the two individual sessions coupled with goal setting.

Although results pertaining to processing speed and working memory on the SDMT did not improve statistically, they were nonetheless clinically significant. From the literature reviewed which utilised the SDMT as an outcome measure, no study identified a statistically significant improvement [9, 10, 14, 16, 38]. However, it is interesting to note that people who received COB-MS improved in the SDMT at each time point (follow-up > posttest > baseline). Considering that there are minimal practice effects in the SDMT [43], it would appear that the 8-week gap between posttest and follow-up allowed people to integrate and generalise strategies learned in COB-MS into their daily lives. This finding validates the purpose of a follow-up assessment in the current study.

There was also a clinically significant improvement for processing speed in part A of the TMT. Similar to the SDMT, participants performed better at each time point. It must be noted that, at one-month intervals, part A is susceptible to practice effects after the first trial [44]. However, according to the same research by Craddick and Stern [44], there were no practice effects for part B in the current study as it was only utilised at three time points. Thus, it was positive to discover statistically significant improvements for divided attention in part B after receiving COB-MS. While clinical improvements in the TMT were frequently observed in the literature [10, 34, 41], few studies identified statistically significant changes. Although Amato et al. identified statistically significant improvements in both parts of the TMT, their computer-based intervention specifically targeted attention, which means that the results were unsurprising [9].

Results suggest that people who receive COB-MS perceive fewer difficulties with memory in daily life. Although a statistically significant improvement was observed after the Friedman test, the improvement was not statistically significant when using a Bonferroni adjustment. This is similar to Carr et al. who also identified a clinically but not statistically significant improvement [13]. It is possible that the small sample size in both studies may have led to the lack of a statistically significant difference. Furthermore, the use of a Bonferroni adjustment to reduce the chance of Type 1 error made the significance level more conservative. However, it is correct practice to use a Bonferroni adjustment when making multiple comparisons.

Although participants perceived fewer difficulties with executive functioning at posttest, scores at follow-up show that there was a greater frequency of difficulties reported in comparison with baseline. However, similar to the OSA-DLS, it is difficult to draw comparisons as the BRIEF-A was not used as an outcome measure in previously reviewed literature. While some studies have identified statistically significant improvements in objective executive functioning [41, 42], it has been argued by Sullivan et al. that subjective cognitive functioning often correlates poorly with the objective equivalent [45]. It may have been that, given the period of reflection that comes with follow-up assessment, participants became more aware of the metacognitive domains (e.g., planning and monitoring) and their difficulties in these areas. The subjective scores they provided may not necessarily reflect objective measurement but an increased insight and awareness of difficulties.

The results from this study suggest that people who receive COB-MS improve significantly (statistically or clinically), in all daily life outcome measures and most cognitive outcome measures, at posttest and follow-up. These findings are encouraging given the fact that this was a pilot study with a small number of participants. Considering that a nonspecific intervention was used in this study, it is not surprising that there were only two statistically significant improvements in cognitive outcome measures. As MS is a degenerative disease, cognitive difficulties are likely to worsen [1]. Therefore, it could be argued that a nonspecific intervention that addresses daily life, by targeting difficulties with cognition, will produce longer lasting benefits for people with MS rather than attempting to improve a specific cognitive domain. Thus, the validity of COB-MS is supported by statistically significant improvements in the primary outcome measure, the GAS, and clinically significant improvements in the OSA-DLS. However, there are some factors that limit the generalisability of findings.

Firstly, there is a high risk of self-selecting bias in this study. Therefore, the participants may have been highly motivated to learn and apply strategies from COB-MS in their daily lives. However, treatment contamination is incredibly difficult to control when recruiting community-dwelling participants. Although the prevalence of MS is reported to be three times more common in females [46], there was only one male participant and this limits generalisability to males. The lack of disease course data on the entire sample as well as the substantial variation in disease duration is also noted as a limitation. Another significant limitation that relates to participant selection is the use of the MSNQ. This measurement device was used as a self-report screening tool for cognitive impairment as part of the inclusion criteria, whereby participants required a score of at least 22 or more. However, the observation of ceiling effects in the results suggests that this cut-off score may have been too low, and previous studies have shown weak correlations between subjective and objective cognitive impairments [47, 48]. Nonetheless, it was decided to include people who had self-reported cognitive impairment (as shown in the MSNQ) without objective evidence because (i) this was a pilot study, which aimed to ensure that COB-MS was feasible in the largest possible sample of people with MS, (ii) some people may have experienced cognitive difficulties in daily life but would not be classified as impaired on an objective measure, and (iii) it was felt that the people would be more motivated to learn if they felt they had cognitive difficulties.

Secondly, despite using alternative assessment forms (CVLT-II and BVMT-R) and research stating minimal practice effects (SDMT and TMT part B), subtle practice effects cannot be completely ruled out in cognitive outcome measures. There are two types of practice effects: "test-specific," which refers to people knowing the assessment format, and "item-specific," which refers to people learning the actual content of the assessment (e.g., word lists or geometric figures [49, 50]). Although item-specific practice effects were mitigated by using alternative forms, test-specific practice effects were unavoidable. For example, at baseline assessments, participants were unaware that there was a delayed recall in the CVLT-II. However, at posttest and follow-up, it is likely that participants knew that they would have to recall the words and may have been internally listing them. In addition, the use of nonparametric tests to analyse outcomes is a limitation. The Friedman test and Wilcoxon signed-rank test are less sensitive than the equivalent parametric techniques, one-way repeated-measures ANOVA and paired-samples t-test, respectively. Thus, it is possible that statistically significant differences may have been missed [51].

5. Conclusion

Future research should use outcome measures related to daily life. It was highlighted in the literature review that it is unclear whether improvements in cognitive outcome measures are indicative of improvements in daily life [52]. The use of daily life assessments would also facilitate comparisons between studies, an issue that was observed in the current study. In addition, subjective cognitive assessments should continue to be used. Although Sullivan et al. argue that subjective and objective cognitive assessments correlate poorly with each other [45], findings from this current study suggest that they trend in the same direction. It appears that different concepts are being measured, with objective tools measuring how a person performs in a structured test, whereas subjective devices measure how a person feels they perform in daily life. Furthermore, outcome assessors should be blinded, and a follow-up period of approximately 6–12 months should be used to determine if improvements are maintained over the long term.

Occupational therapists and people with MS reported that COB-MS may be more beneficial for people who are newly diagnosed [24]. Thus, future studies of COB-MS could consider comparing its effectiveness for people who are newly diagnosed versus people who have been diagnosed for some time. Considering that Chiaravalloti et al. [18] found that people with moderate cognitive impairment benefitted more than those with mild cognitive impairment, it may be worth comparing the effectiveness of COB-MS for a group of moderately versus mildly impaired participants. These recommendations could also be integrated into occupational therapy practice, whereby COB-MS is provided to people with MS who are newly diagnosed and/or have similar levels of cognitive impairment. Previous studies found that older participants were more adherent in completing CR at home than younger participants [15, 41]. Therefore, future COB-MS studies should monitor completion of homework activities to determine adherence to the programme. In addition, the paucity of qualitative research indicates that participants of future COB-MS studies should be interviewed to determine benefits of the programme that cannot be detected in quantitative measures, as shown in Carr et al. [13].

The primary implication for occupational therapy practice is that this study provides an occupation-based intervention that is specific to the cognitive difficulties faced by people with MS. COB-MS is a step-by-step evidence-based intervention that can be facilitated by occupational therapists and enable people to identify, understand, and implement strategies to simultaneously manage cognitive impairment and improve function in daily life.

To conclude, this pilot study established the clinical outcomes of COB-MS in relation to daily life and cognition. This study provides foundational evidence to support COB-MS as the most suitable intervention for people with MS who experience cognitive difficulties in daily life and adds to the paucity of research in the field of MS and CR.

Disclosure

A poster presentation of these finding was presented at European Committee for Treatment and Research in Multiple Sclerosis 2017.

Acknowledgments

This research was supported by funding from the National University of Ireland Galway Millennium Fund 2016/2017.

References

[1] B. K. Tsang and R. McDonnell, "Multiple sclerosis: diagnosis, management and prognosis," *Australian family physician*, vol. 40, no. 12, pp. 948–959, 2011.

[2] M. P. Amato, V. Zipoli, and E. Portaccio, "Multiple sclerosis-related cognitive changes: a review of cross-sectional and longitudinal studies," *Journal of the Neurological Sciences*, vol. 245, no. 1-2, pp. 41–46, 2006.

[3] D. W. Langdon, "Cognition in multiple sclerosis," *Current Opinion in Neurology*, vol. 24, no. 3, pp. 244–249, 2011.

[4] M. Filippi, G. Riccitelli, F. Mattioli et al., "Multiple sclerosis: effects of cognitive rehabilitation on structural and functional MR imaging measures—an explorative study," *Radiology*, vol. 262, no. 3, pp. 932–940, 2012.

[5] N. D. Chiaravalloti and J. DeLuca, "Cognitive impairment in multiple sclerosis," *The Lancet Neurology*, vol. 7, no. 12, pp. 1139–1151, 2008.

[6] A. Brenk, K. Laun, and C. G. Haase, "Short-term cognitive training improves mental efficiency and mood in patients with multiple sclerosis," *European Neurology*, vol. 60, no. 6, pp. 304–309, 2008.

[7] S. H. Pierson and N. Griffith, "Treatment of cognitive impairment in multiple sclerosis," *Behavioural Neurology*, vol. 17, no. 1, pp. 53–67, 2006.

[8] T. A. M. Siepman, A. C. J. W. Janssens, I. De Koning, C. H. Polman, J. B. Boringa, and R. Q. Hintzen, "The role of disability and depression in cognitive functioning within 2 years after multiple sclerosis diagnosis," *Journal of Neurology*, vol. 255, no. 6, pp. 910–916, 2008.

[9] M. P. Amato, B. Goretti, R. G. Viterbo et al., "Computer-assisted rehabilitation of attention in patients with multiple sclerosis: Results of a randomized, double-blind trial," *Multiple Sclerosis Journal*, vol. 20, no. 1, pp. 91–98, 2014.

[10] A. Cerasa, M. C. Gioia, P. Valentino et al., "Computer-assisted cognitive rehabilitation of attention deficits for multiple sclerosis: a randomized trial with fMRI correlates," *Neurorehabilitation and Neural Repair*, vol. 27, no. 4, pp. 284–295, 2013.

[11] M. Lanz, J. Kraus, H. Hahn, B. Schwarze, G. Schwendemann, and H. Hildebrandt, "Cognitive training in MS: effects and relation to brain atrophy," *Aktuelle Neurologie*, vol. 32, no. S 4, 2005.

[12] L. Mendozzi, L. Pugnetti, A. Motta et al., "Computer-assisted memory retraining of patients with multiple sclerosis," *Italian Journal of Neurological Sciences*, vol. 19, no. 6, pp. S431–S438, 1998.

[13] S. E. Carr, R. Das Nair, A. F. Schwartz, and N. B. Lincoln, "Group memory rehabilitation for people with multiple sclerosis: A feasibility randomized controlled trial," *Clinical Rehabilitation*, vol. 28, no. 6, pp. 552–561, 2014.

[14] N. B. Lincoln, A. Dent, J. Harding et al., "Evaluation of cognitive assessment and cognitive intervention for people with multiple sclerosis," *Journal of Neurology, Neurosurgery & Psychiatry*, vol. 72, no. 1, pp. 93–98, 2002.

[15] E. Shatil, A. Metzer, O. Horvitz, and A. Miller, "Home-based personalized cognitive training in MS patients: A study of adherence and cognitive performance," *NeuroRehabilitation*, vol. 26, no. 2, pp. 143–153, 2010.

[16] L. M. Hancock, J. M. Bruce, A. S. Bruce, and S. G. Lynch, "Processing speed and working memory training in multiple sclerosis: A double-blind randomized controlled pilot study," *Journal of Clinical and Experimental Neuropsychology*, vol. 37, no. 2, pp. 113–127, 2015.

[17] A. Solari, A. Motta, L. Mendozzi et al., "Computer-aided retraining of memory and attention in people with multiple sclerosis: a randomized, double-blind controlled trial," *Journal of the Neurological Sciences*, vol. 222, no. 1-2, pp. 99–104, 2004.

[18] N. D. Chiaravalloti, J. DeLuca, N. B. Moore, and J. H. Ricker, "Treating learning impairments improves memory performance in multiple sclerosis: A randomized clinical trial," *Multiple Sclerosis Journal*, vol. 11, no. 1, pp. 58–68, 2005.

[19] F. Fink, E. Rischkau, M. Butt, J. Klein, P. Eling, and H. Hildebrandt, "Efficacy of an executive function intervention programme in MS: A placebo-controlled and pseudo-randomized trial," *Multiple Sclerosis Journal*, vol. 16, no. 9, pp. 1148–1151, 2010.

[20] E. Shevil and M. Finlayson, "Pilot study of a cognitive intervention program for persons with multiple sclerosis," *Health Education Research*, vol. 25, no. 1, pp. 41–53, 2010.

[21] E. M. Rosti-Otajärvi and P. I. Hämäläinen, "Neuropsychological rehabilitation for multiple sclerosis.," *Cochrane Database of Systematic Reviews*, vol. 2, p. CD009131, 2014.

[22] R. das Nair, K. J. Martin, and N. B. Lincoln, "Memory rehabilitation for people with multiple sclerosis," *The Cochrane Library*, 2016.

[23] A. R. O'Brien, N. Chiaravalloti, Y. Goverover, and J. DeLuca, "Evidenced-Based Cognitive Rehabilitation for Persons With Multiple Sclerosis: A Review of the Literature," *Archives of Physical Medicine and Rehabilitation*, vol. 89, no. 4, pp. 761–769, 2008.

[24] S. M. Hynes and S. J. Forwell, "A Cognitive Occupation-Based Programme for People with Multiple Sclerosis (COB-MS): the development of a new occupational therapy intervention," in Press.

[25] C. Christiansen, C. M. Baum, and J. Bass, "The Person-Environment-Occupational-Performance Model," in *Foundations for Practice in Occupational Therapy*, S. E. A. Duncan, Ed., pp. 93–104, Elsevier, London, UK, 5th edition, 2011.

[26] T. J. Kiresuk and R. E. Sherman, "Goal attainment scaling: A general method for evaluating comprehensive community mental health programs," *Community Mental Health Journal*, vol. 4, no. 6, pp. 443–453, 1968.

[27] P. Scott, *Occupational Self Assessment - Daily Living Scales*, Model of Human Occupation, Clearinghouse, 2016.

[28] J. Baños, "California Verbal Learning Test-Second Edition D. Delis, J. Kramer, E. Kaplan, B. Ober. San Antonio, TX. The Psychological Corporation, 2000," *Archives of Clinical Neuropsychology*, vol. 17, no. 5, pp. 509–512.

[29] R. H. Benedict, *Brief visuospatial memory test–revised: professional manual*, PAR, 1997.

[30] A. Smith, *Symbol digit modality test (SDMT): manual (revised)*, Psychological Services, Los Angeles, Cakif, USA, 1982.

[31] R. M. Reitan and D. Wolfson, "The Trail Making Test as an initial screening procedure for neuropsychological impairment in older children," *Archives of Clinical Neuropsychology*, vol. 19, no. 2, pp. 281–288, 2004.

[32] R. M. Roth, P. K. Isquith, and G. A. Gioia, *Behavior Rating Inventory of Executive Function - Adult Version, Professional Manual*, Psychological Assessment Resources, 2005.

[33] J. Royle and N. B. Lincoln, "The Everyday Memory Questionnaire - Revised: Development of a 13-item scale," *Disability and Rehabilitation*, vol. 30, no. 2, pp. 114–121, 2008.

[34] A. Mantynen, E. Rosti-Otajärvi, K. Koivisto, A. Lilja, H. Huhtala, and P. Hämäläinen, "Neuropsychological rehabilitation does not improve cognitive performance but reduces perceived cognitive deficits in patients with multiple sclerosis: A randomised, controlled, multi-centre trial," *Multiple Sclerosis Journal*, vol. 20, no. 1, pp. 99–107, 2014.

[35] G. Kielhofner, *A model of human occupation: Theory and application*, Williams and Wilkins, Baltimore, MD, USA, 4th edition, 2008.

[36] S. W. Lee, R. Taylor, G. Kielhofner, and G. Fisher, "Theory use in practice: a national survey of therapists who use the model of human occupation," *The American Journal of Occupational Therapy*, vol. 62, no. 1, pp. 106–117, 2008.

[37] H. Brissart, M. Leroy, E. Morele, C. Baumann, E. Spitz, and M. Debouverie, "Cognitive rehabilitation in Multiple sclerosis," *Neurocase*, vol. 19, no. 6, pp. 553–565, 2013.

[38] A. K. Stuifbergen, H. Becker, F. Perez, J. Morison, V. Kullberg, and A. Todd, "A randomized controlled trial of a cognitive rehabilitation intervention for persons with multiple sclerosis," *Clinical Rehabilitation*, vol. 26, no. 10, pp. 882–893, 2012.

[39] A. Jonsson, E. M. Korfitzen, A. Heltberg, M. H. Ravnborg, and E. Byskov-Ottosen, "Effects of neuropsychological treatment in patients with multiple sclerosis," *Acta Neurologica Scandinavica*, vol. 88, no. 6, pp. 394–400, 1993.

[40] A. Vogt, L. Kappos, P. Calabrese et al., "Working memory training in patients with multiple sclerosis - Comparison of two different training schedules," *Restorative Neurology and Neuroscience*, vol. 27, no. 3, pp. 225–235, 2009.

[41] J. Gich, J. Freixanet, R. García et al., "A randomized, controlled, single-blind, 6-month pilot study to evaluate the efficacy of MS-Line!: A cognitive rehabilitation programme for patients with multiple sclerosis," *Multiple Sclerosis Journal*, vol. 21, no. 10, pp. 1332–1343, 2015.

[42] N. Tesar, K. Bandion, and U. Baumhackl, "Efficacy of a neuropsychological training programme for patients with multiple sclerosis - A randomised controlled trial," *Wiener Klinische Wochenschrift*, vol. 117, no. 21-22, pp. 747–754, 2005.

[43] R. H. B. Benedict, J. A. Duquin, S. Jurgensen et al., "Repeated assessment of neuropsychological deficits in multiple sclerosis using the symbol digit modalities test and the MS neuropsychological screening questionnaire," *Multiple Sclerosis Journal*, vol. 14, no. 7, pp. 940–946, 2008.

[44] R. A. Craddick and M. R. Stern, "Practice effects on the trail making test," *Perceptual and Motor Skills*, vol. 17, no. 3, pp. 651–653, 1963.

[45] M. J. L. Sullivan, K. Edgley, and E. Dehoux, "A survey of multiple sclerosis. Part 1: Perceived cognitive problems and compensatory strategy use," *Canadian Journal of Rehabilitation*, vol. 4, no. 2, pp. 99–105, 1990.

[46] A. D. Sadovnick, "European Charcot Foundation Lecture: The natural history of multiple sclerosis and gender," *Journal of the Neurological Sciences*, vol. 286, no. 1-2, pp. 1–5, 2009.

[47] J. M. Bruce, A. S. Bruce, L. Hancock, and S. Lynch, "Self-reported memory problems in multiple sclerosis: influence of psychiatric status and normative dissociative experiences," *Archives of Clinical Neuropsychology*, vol. 25, no. 1, pp. 39–48, 2010.

[48] S. W. Kinsinger, E. Lattie, and D. C. Mohr, "Relationship between depression, fatigue, subjective cognitive impairment, and objective neuropsychological functioning in patients with multiple sclerosis," *Neuropsychology*, vol. 24, no. 5, pp. 573–580, 2010.

[49] R. H. B. Benedict and D. J. Zgaljardic, "Practice effects during repeated administrations of memory tests with and without alternate forms," *Journal of Clinical and Experimental Neuropsychology*, vol. 20, no. 3, pp. 339–352, 1998.

[50] D. J. Zgaljardic and R. H. B. Benedict, "Evaluation of practice effects in language and spatial processing test performance," *Applied Neuropsychology*, vol. 8, no. 4, pp. 218–223, 2001.

[51] J. Pallant, *SPSS survival manual: A step by step guide to data analysis using IBM SPSS*, McGraw-Hill Education, Berkshire, UK, 5th edition, 2013.

[52] B. A. Wilson, "Neuropsychological rehabilitation," *Annual Review of Clinical Psychology*, vol. 4, pp. 141–162, 2008.

12

Evidence-Based Practice in Primary Care Occupational Therapy: A Cross-Sectional Survey in Sweden

Ann-Charlotte Lindström[1] and Susanne Bernhardsson[2,3]

[1]*Närhälsan Rehabilitation Sörhaga, Alingsås, Sweden*
[2]*Närhälsan Research and Development Primary Health Care, Region Västra Götaland, Gothenburg, Sweden*
[3]*Institute of Neuroscience and Physiology, Department of Health and Rehabilitation, Unit of Physiotherapy, University of Gothenburg, The Sahlgrenska Academy, Gothenburg, Sweden*

Correspondence should be addressed to Susanne Bernhardsson; susanne.bernhardsson@vgregion.se

Academic Editor: Jodie A. Copley

Introduction. Understanding of attitudes, knowledge, and behaviour related to evidence-based practice (EBP) and guidelines in Swedish occupational therapy is limited. The study aims were to investigate attitudes, knowledge, and behaviour related to evidence-based practice and guidelines of Swedish occupational therapists in primary care. *Methods.* A web-based survey of 94 Swedish primary care occupational therapists (response rate 53.7%). Data were analysed using logistic regressions. *Results.* Attitudes towards EBP and guidelines were highly positive (97%–98%). About half of the respondents reported confidence in finding and using evidence. Almost two-thirds reported being aware of guidelines and 47% knowing where to find guidelines. Four-fifths stated that they had easy access to guidelines and 75% that they used guidelines frequently. Men were more likely to feel confident to find research (OR 8.58, 95% CI 1.03 to 71.66; $p = 0.047$) and have easy access to guidelines (OR 9.10, 95% CI 1.94 to 42.83; $p = 0.005$). Occupational therapists older than 50 years were more likely to integrate patient preferences with guideline use (OR 6.44, 95% CI 1.14 to 36.57; $p = 0.035$). Few reported reading scientific articles, and many expressed uncertainty in finding research. The main barrier for using guidelines was reported to be lack of time. *Conclusion.* Although attitudes among primary care occupational therapists towards EBP are positive and a large proportion report using guidelines, many state that they want to learn more and improve their evidence-based practice skills. The findings suggest that education measures need to be taken to address the identified shortcomings.

1. Introduction

Evidence-based practice (EBP) means the integration of best available evidence from clinical research with clinical expertise and patients' preferences [1]. In recent years, EBP has become an expectation of most healthcare professionals and a vehicle to advance the profession and ensure that occupational therapists deliver quality services to their patients [2, 3]. Applying EBP ensures that clinicians use effective interventions to achieve desired outcomes and contributes to best quality care [4].

However, despite the spread of EBP during recent decades, research findings are not routinely used in occupational therapy practice [5–8]. To do so requires that clinicians have the necessary knowledge and skills to access, appraise, and apply research evidence in their clinical decision making, as well as sufficient time [9]. Applying EBP in occupational therapy is particularly challenging since research evidence for most interventions is limited [10]. Occupational therapy research has traditionally been more interpretive in approach, frequently involving case-based action with qualitative outcomes rather than effectiveness studies of interventions, and the profession has been slow to adopt research-informed practice [11]. Many factors affect whether occupational therapy practice is based on research evidence: individual factors such as attitude, preferences, educational level, context, knowledge, and skills, as well as organisational factors such as attitudes of managers and colleagues. Factors relating to both the individual and the organisation, e.g., support and time available to search for research evidence, are particularly important [10].

Knowledge and skills related to EBP vary among different countries, and various barriers for applying EBP have been identified [3–5, 9, 12]. A systematic review showed that attitudes toward EBP among occupational therapists in different countries vary [5]. While several of the included studies reported positive attitudes to various extents, some reported negative attitudes, particularly related to the perceived difficulty of understanding and applying EBP in clinical practice. In Sweden, hospital-employed occupational therapists have been shown to hold positive attitudes toward EBP, but lack of time is a key obstacle to integrating the research component of EBP into practice [13]. No study on EBP has been performed in a Swedish primary care occupational therapy context.

The use of clinical practice guidelines is a widely used strategy to implement EBP, and high quality guidelines provide evidence-based recommendations to support the clinician in choosing effective interventions. Over time, these types of guidelines have shifted from opinion-based to research-informed [14], thus constituting an excellent point of departure for integrating research findings with the other EBP components. An increasing number of guidelines are being produced that include recommendations for occupational therapy, for example, by the American Association of Occupational Therapists [15], the British Royal College of Occupational Therapists [16], and the Swedish National Association of Occupational Therapists [17]. However, implementation, uptake, and use of guidelines tend to vary based on different factors related to the guideline itself, the user/clinician, the patient, and the practice context [18].

There is a lack of knowledge about attitudes, access, knowledge, determinants, and use of EBP and clinical practice guidelines in primary care occupational therapy in Sweden, and whether any associations exist with demographic characteristics. Knowledge about these factors is important so that current trends in occupational therapy practice can be identified [12]. This knowledge also provides a basis for developing effective implementation strategies for clinical practice guidelines in order to increase the extent to which occupational therapy practice is evidence-based. Primary care occupational therapists in Sweden treat a wide variety of conditions and practice autonomously, without need for a doctor's referral, and applying EBP and using guidelines in everyday patient work are important so that patients are treated with effective methods and receive equal care. Therefore, the aim of this study was to investigate attitudes, knowledge, and behaviour related to EBP and guidelines among Swedish occupational therapists in primary care.

2. Methods

2.1. Participants and Setting. Eligible participants in this survey were occupational therapists employed in primary care by the Region Västra Götaland and currently practicing occupational therapy ($n = 193$). This is Sweden's second largest county council, providing healthcare services to nearly 1.7 million inhabitants in western Sweden. Individuals on parental leave and long-term sick leave ($n = 16$) and those involved in development of regional clinical practice guidelines ($n = 2$) were excluded. Data were collected during November–December 2016.

2.2. Data Collection. Eligible participants were invited to respond to the web-based survey, using the survey software esMaker® (Entergate AB, Halmstad, Sweden). Three reminder notices were sent via e-mail during a two-month period. A statement in the survey informed the respondents that their response was assumed as informed consent. The survey was filled out anonymously, and responses could not be traced back to the respondents. According to Swedish law, ethical approval for this type of research was not required.

Questions for the survey were drawn from a validated EBP questionnaire, originally developed by Jette et al. [19] to examine EBP and guideline variables among American physiotherapists. The questionnaire had been previously translated, adapted, and validated for a Swedish primary care context [20] and used to survey Swedish physiotherapists [21]. It was for the present study minimally modified for use with occupational therapists in the same context. The questionnaire comprised eight items on participant characteristics and 23 items reflecting various aspects of EBP and guidelines in the following domains: attitudes, knowledge, behaviour, and prerequisites and barriers related to EBP resources and guidelines. Most items were rated on 5-point Likert type scales ranging from "strongly disagree" to "strongly agree," with a "neutral" category in the middle. The item on frequency of use of guidelines ranged from "very infrequently" to "very frequently." The items on awareness that guidelines exist and knowing how and where to find them were answered with "yes," "to some extent," or "no."

2.3. Data Analysis. Frequencies and distributions were analyzed with descriptive statistics. Bivariate logistic regression analyses were performed to explore associations with demographic variables. Associations between attitudinal, knowledge, and behavioural variables and frequent guideline use were also explored. Variables identified as significant in univariate analyses were tested for correlation against a criteria of Spearman's rho < 0.7 to qualify for inclusion in a multivariable model. They were entered in a multivariable model, using the stepwise forward conditional method. Interaction effects were tested at the 1% level.

Before analysis, response categories for the dependent variable "use of guidelines" were dichotomised into "frequent use" versus "infrequent use" (including "sometimes") and for independent variables into "agree" versus "disagree." Responses for the items with 3-point scales were dichotomised into "yes" versus "no/to some extent." The significance level was set to 0.05. Missing data were handled with listwise deletion. Statistical analyses were performed using IBM SPSS version 22.0.

3. Results

3.1. Respondents. Of the 175 occupational therapists invited to participate, 94 responded: response rate 53.7%. Participant characteristics are shown in Table 1. Internal missing values ranged from 0 to 5 (0% to 5.3%).

3.2. Attitudes, Knowledge, and Behaviour Related to EBP. Response frequencies for all variables are presented in Table 2. Most respondents agreed that EBP is necessary to practice (97%) and helps in decision making (92%). Approximately half of the respondents disagreed that EBP creates unreasonable demands (51%). Most (97%) agreed to wanting to improve their skills to apply EBP in their practice. Fifty-two percent agreed to feeling confident in their ability to find relevant research for their clinical questions, and 56% reported feeling confident about treating patients according to current best evidence.

Fifty percent stated that they agreed that the use of research was encouraged at their workplace, whereas 32% disagreed. Forty-six percent agreed that they knew how to access databases through the electronic library, whereas 45% disagreed.

Eighty-two percent of the respondents reported reading fewer than two articles and the rest of the respondents (19%) read 2–5 articles in an average month. Ninety percent reported performing fewer than two, 9% 2–5, and 1% 6–10 database searches per month on average.

Table 1: Participant characteristics ($n = 94$).

Characteristic	n	%
Sex		
Women	85	90.4
Men	9	9.6
Age (years)		
20–29	7	7.4
30–39	29	30.9
40–49	22	23.4
50–59	24	25.5
>60	12	12.8
Education level/degree		
Lower level degree	16	17.0
Bachelor's degree	74	78.7
Master's degree	4	4.3
PhD student or PhD	0	0.0
Certified specialist	8	8.6
Years of experience in primary care occupational therapy		
<3	31	33.0
3–5	11	11.7
6–10	13	13.8
11–15	12	12.8
16–20	11	11.7
>20	16	17.0

3.3. Attitudes, Knowledge, and Behaviour Related to Guidelines. All of the respondents agreed that it is important to use guidelines. Sixty-five percent stated that they were aware of guidelines relevant to their work and 32% that they were partially aware. Nearly half of the respondents (47%) knew where to find guidelines on the Internet, and 44% knew this to some extent. Eighty-one percent agreed to having easy access to relevant guidelines at their workplace. Seventy-five percent reported knowing how to integrate patient preferences with guidelines.

All of the respondents agreed that guidelines are important for the patient to get the best treatment possible. Ninety-five percent agreed that guidelines facilitate their work, and 99% agreed that guidelines are important so that patients receive equal treatment. Seventy-five percent of the respondents reported using guidelines frequently or very frequently, 21% sometimes, and 3% infrequently or never.

Therapists who perceived that they had easy access to guidelines, as well as those who felt confident in their ability to treat patients according to evidence, were more likely to use guidelines frequently (Table 3). Other variables that were associated with frequent guideline use in univariate analyses did not remain significant in the final multiple regression model. No significant interaction effects between those variables and demographic variables were found.

Reported barriers for using guidelines are shown in Figure 1. The most important barrier was lack of time, cited by 72% of the respondents. This was followed by a perceived paucity of guidelines relevant for primary care occupational therapy, that it takes too much time to read guidelines, and that guidelines are too general and unspecific. The category "too much recipe" represents the perception that many patients do not fit a specific guideline, e.g., due to comorbidity or other complex situations.

3.4. Associations with Demographic Variables. Few demographic characteristics were associated with EBP and guideline variables. Men were more likely than women to report self-efficacy in finding research (OR 8.58, 95% CI 1.03 to 71.66; $p = 0.047$) and having easy access to guidelines (OR 9.10, 95% CI 1.94 to 42.83; $p = 0.005$). Occupational therapists older than 50 years were more likely to report knowing how to integrate patient preferences with guideline use than younger therapists (OR 6.44, 95% CI 1.14 to 36.57; $p = 0.035$). No significant association was found between EBP variables and therapist experience.

4. Discussion

The study provides new knowledge on EBP and guideline use among primary care occupational therapists. Key findings of this study are that attitudes toward EBP and guidelines were highly positive and that a large majority of the respondents were aware of relevant guidelines and knew where to find them. Four-fifths reported having easy access to guidelines, and three quarters claimed to use guidelines frequently. The largest barrier for using guidelines was lack of time. Two factors were found to predict frequent guideline use: feeling able to treat patients according to evidence and having easy access to guidelines.

TABLE 2: Distribution of questionnaire responses.

Variable	n	Response frequencies*				
Attitudes to EBP		*Strongly disagree*	*Disagree*	*Neutral*	*Agree*	*Strongly agree*
EBP is necessary to practice	94	0 (0.0%)	0 (0.0%)	3 (3.2%)	45 (47.9%)	46 (48.9%)
EBP creates unreasonable demands	94	12 (12.8%)	36 (38.3%)	19 (20.2%)	26 (27.7%)	1 (1.1%)
EBP helps decision making	94	0 (0.0%)	0 (0.0%)	8 (8.5%)	53 (56.4%)	33 (35.1%)
Want to learn/improve skills	92	0 (0.0%)	0 (0.0%)	3 (3.3%)	34 (37.0%)	55 (59.8%)
Strong evidence is lacking for most treatments	90	6 (6.7%)	27 (30.0%)	12 (5.2%)	38 (42.2%)	7 (7.8%)
Self-efficacy to find research	94	8 (8.5%)	25 (26.6%)	12 (12.8%)	39 (41.5%)	10 (10.6%)
Self-efficacy to treat patients according to evidence	93	2 (2.2%)	18 (19.4%)	21 (22.6%)	48 (51.6%)	4 (4.3%)
Knowledge about EBP		*Strongly disagree*	*Disagree*	*Neutral*	*Agree*	*Strongly agree*
Know how to access databases	92	25 (27.2%)	16 (17.4%)	9 (9.8%)	31 (33.7%)	11 (12.0%)
Behaviour related to EBP		*≤1/month*	*2–5/month*	*6–10/month*	*11–15/month*	*16+/month*
Read articles, no. of articles per month	92	75 (81.5%)	17 (18.5%)	0 (0.0%)	0 (0.0%)	0 (0.0%)
Search databases, no. of searches per month	93	84 (90.3%)	9 (8.6%)	1 (1.1%)	0 (0.0%)	0 (0.0%)
Prerequisites for EBP		*Strongly disagree*	*Disagree*	*Neutral*	*Agree*	*Strongly agree*
EBP encouraged at workplace	94	10 (10.6%)	20 (21.3%)	17 (18.1%)	35 (37.2%)	12 (12.9%)
Attitudes to guidelines		*Strongly disagree*	*Disagree*	*Neutral*	*Agree*	*Strongly agree*
Important that guidelines exist	93	0 (0.0%)	2 (2.2%)	0 (0%)	12 (12.9%)	79 (84.9%)
Important to use guidelines	91	0 (0.0%)	0 (0%)	0 (0%)	26 (28.6%)	65 (71.4%)
Guidelines are important to facilitate practice	94	0 (0.0%)	1 (1.1%)	3 (3.2%)	41 (43.6%)	49 (52.1%)
Knowledge about guidelines		*Strongly disagree*	*Disagree*	*Neutral*	*Agree*	*Strongly agree*
Know how to integrate pat. pref. w/ guidelines	92	0 (0.0%)	0 (0.0%)	23 (25.0%)	59 (64.1%)	10 (10.9%)
		No	*To some extent*	*Yes*		
Aware that guidelines exist	93	3 (3.2%)	30 (32.3%)	60 (64.5%)		
Know where to find guidelines	93	8 (8.6%)	41 (44.1%)	44 (47.3%)		
Prerequisites for use of guidelines		*Strongly disagree*	*Disagree*	*Neutral*	*Agree*	*Strongly agree*
Have easy access to guidelines	92	3 (3.3%)	5 (5.4%)	10 (10.9%)	54 (58.7%)	20 (21.7%)
Behaviour related to guidelines		*Very infrequently or never*	*Infrequently*	*Sometimes*	*Frequently*	*Very frequently or always*
Use guidelines	93	2 (2.2%)	1 (1.1%)	20 (21.5%)	51 (54.8%)	19 (20.4%)

*Data are numbers (percentages).

TABLE 3: Significant associations in univariate analyses and in the final multiple logistic regression model. Dependent variable: frequent use of guidelines.

Independent variable	Level	n	Univariate associations Odds ratio (95% CI)	p	B (SE)	Multiple associations Odds ratio (95% CI)	p
Strong evidence is lacking for most interventions	Disagree	89	3.43 (1.05–11.25)	0.042			
	Agree		Reference				
Self-efficacy to treat patients according to evidence	Agree	92	3.30 (1.23–8.87)	0.018	1.93 (0.71)	6.91 (1.73–27.60)	0.006
	Disagree		Reference			Reference	
Know where to find guidelines	Yes	92	6.57 (1.43–30.25)	0.016			
	No		Reference				
Easy access to guidelines	Agree	91	11.27 (3.50–36.36)	<0.001	2.92 (0.73)	18.57 (4.40–78.26)	<0.001
	Disagree		Reference			Reference	
Know how to integrate patient preferences with guidelines	Agree	91	4.28 (1.53–11.97)	0.006			
	Disagree		Reference				

[b]Nagelkerke $R^2 = 0.42$, overall correctly predicted = 75.3%, B = unstandardised regression coefficient, SE = standard error, CI = confidence interval.

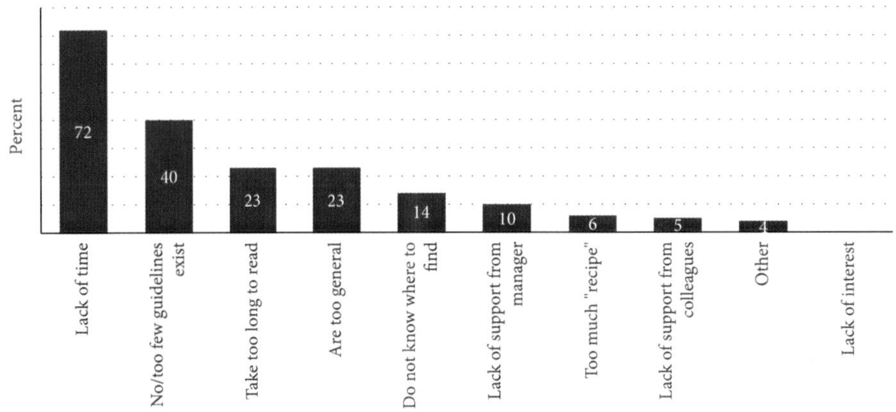

FIGURE 1: Reported barriers for using guidelines.

Although the vast majority of the occupational therapists had very positive attitudes to both EBP and guidelines, EBP-related behaviour did not reflect these attitudes. Only a small proportion said that they searched the literature and read scientific articles. These findings may be related to EBP not being taught consistently at undergraduate occupational therapy programs. The reported high awareness of guidelines, knowledge of where to find them, and easy access to them were likely related to a guideline project that had been ongoing within the county council over the past few years. That project involved the development of several practice guidelines that were published on a dedicated website, in order to make the guidelines easily accessible. Awareness and access are important prerequisites of guideline use, which in fact also was quite high; three quarters of the respondents reporting using guidelines frequently, with another fifth using guidelines sometimes.

The finding that men were more likely than women to report self-efficacy to find research and having easy access to guidelines needs to be interpreted with caution, because gender distribution of the sample was quite skewed, less than one-tenth were men. In addition, the confidence intervals for the odds ratios were quite wide. The finding that older occupational therapists were more likely to know how to integrate patient preferences with guideline use may be understandable, in that younger therapists did not have as much experience with different kinds of patients and therefore may not be skilled in incorporating their preferences into therapy.

Only two variables, self-efficacy to treat patients according to evidence and having easy access to guidelines, remained significantly associated with frequent use of guidelines in the final regression model. While easy access to guidelines is an obvious prerequisite of using them, feeling confident in one's ability to treat patients according to evidence is an interesting finding and less easily explainable. The opposite would have been more logical—feeling confident to treat according to evidence would reduce the need for guidelines. However, the link may be more easily understood when considering that those who are keen on and able to treat according to evidence are probably also more likely to want to rely on guidelines that include evidence-based recommendations.

The findings of positive attitudes toward EBP but limited perceived knowledge and skills are supported by research from other countries. McCluskey [9] reported that half of the occupational therapists in an Australian survey rated their level of EBP knowledge and skills as low. Lyons et al. [4] reported positive attitudes towards research among Australian paediatric occupational therapists, but poor confidence in research knowledge and in how to implement research findings into practice. In South Africa, Buchanan [22] showed positive perceptions toward EBP among occupational therapists but poor confidence in EBP skills, attributed primarily to limited knowledge and skills.

In our study, most respondents estimated their EBP knowledge from moderate to high; yet nearly all expressed a desire to learn more about EBP. Similar findings were shown in the study by Lyons et al. [4], where the respondents held positive attitudes toward research and wanted to access new information to guide practice.

Our study suggests a gap between positive attitudes towards EBP and sufficient knowledge to apply EBP by searching for and reading scientific literature. This gap was also identified by Upton et al. [5], who found that occupational therapists across several countries generally hold positive attitudes toward EBP but that these attitudes do not necessarily translate into practice. Salls et al. [8] showed that although a large majority of American occupational therapists considered EBP important to their practice, use of research findings to inform practice remained limited.

Our study, like most studies on EBP in occupational therapy, was conducted among practicing clinicians. In students, it is likely that search and appraisal skills are taught already in undergraduate training and that both attitudes and behaviours related to EBP therefore are more positive than those of practicing therapists. Stronge and Cahill [3] found that students in Ireland had a clear understanding of EBP and were willing to practice EBP in their future and that many accessed evidence on a weekly basis. However, Crabtree et al. [23] showed that although a master-level EBP training program improved basic EBP skills and knowledge among Canadian students, those skills were not retained after eight weeks of fieldwork. To support both students and recent graduates entering clinical practice, those findings, as well as the findings of our study, underscore the importance of continued training of clinicians in EBP skills.

Occupational therapists are expected to base their practice on the best available evidence [24, 25]. In our study, half of the respondents disagreed that applying EBP in daily practice is an unreasonable requirement, representing a positive attitude to EBP. However, nearly one-third considered it an unreasonable requirement. The reason for this negative attitude is not known, but a plausible explanation is a perceived lack of time, which was identified as a major barrier to EBP.

The multiple barriers identified for using EBP and guidelines are consistent with previous research. Lack of time was by far the most important barrier, and a quarter of the respondents also stated that it took too much time to read guidelines. Upton et al. [5] identified lack of time, availability and accessibility to research, and limited research skills as main barriers for applying EBP among occupational therapists. Lyons et al. [4] reported lack of time to read research and to implement new ideas as the greatest barriers for applying EBP in clinical practice among Australian occupational therapists. Lack of skills to understand statistics and to evaluate research quality was also among the top perceived barriers. Among South African occupational therapists, reported barriers include lack of time, knowledge, and convenient access to evidence [22]. In US occupational therapists, lack of time, high continuing education costs, weak research analysis skills, and placing higher value on clinical experience than on research have been reported as import barriers [26]. In Sweden, Heiwe et al. [13] identified lack of time, statistical knowledge, and research and appraisal skills as important barriers for EBP among hospital-based occupational therapists. Similar barriers have also consistently been reported in other healthcare professions, for example, physiotherapists [21, 27, 28], physicians [29, 30], and nurses [31].

The finding that some therapists felt that guideline use was too "recipe-like" may be indicative of the complexity of clinical reasoning and decision making and why therapists may not be using research evidence as the predominant method of achieving EBP. Planning individual therapy requires integration of research evidence with a range of different information sources such as the patient and their circumstances and experiences and the setting, in order to be both evidence-based and client-centred. Clinical reasoning, involving the thinking process of planning, conducting, and reflecting on clinical practice [32], is an essential part of making decisions about occupational therapy service delivery. It often draws on factual knowledge, tacit and practical know-how, and gut response to clients and their situations in an attempt to synthesize these different modes through metacognition [33]. Clinical reasoning is a skill that evolves with experience and has been suggested to differ between novice and experienced occupational therapists [34]. Even though our study failed to show any differences related to age or experience, it is likely that older and more experienced therapists rely more on their experience and less on research evidence than do their younger colleagues. Integrating the three EBP components is not self-evident. The research evidence component is conceptually different from the other two components; it denotes published, collective evidence, whereas clinical expertise and patient preferences mostly relate to the individual level [35]. Viewed in this light, the level of guideline use showed in this study forms a solid basis for integration with the other components. Treatment decisions should be made jointly with the patient, and their preferences and values should be elicited as part of this dialogue so that treatment can be adequately individualised and person-centred. This is particularly important in occupational therapy where several treatment options may be appropriate and research evidence for some treatments remains limited [36]. Communication and a good patient-therapist dialogue then become even more important and lay the ground for collaborative rehabilitation [37].

The history and tradition of occupational therapy is another barrier that may impede EBP. Occupational therapy is a profession that tends to rely on professional craft and personal knowledge which may reduce the importance attached to EBP [38]. Welch and Dawson [38] found that research knowledge was not included in British occupational therapists' construct of a good practitioner and that they lacked confidence in EBP. However, they also showed that practice-embedded collaborative learning was a way to develop this confidence and facilitate the therapists' use of research knowledge in their clinical reasoning. Furthermore, as suggested by Miller and Willis [11], the occupational therapy profession has produced less research in comparison to other health professionals such as physicians, nurses, and physiotherapists, which may constitute a significant barrier for occupational therapists to adopt and apply EBP. The low volume of research produced likely contributes to the low evidence grade for many occupational therapy interventions, the paucity of clinical practice guidelines, and to the fairly high proportion of respondents in our survey who did not feel confident in finding and using evidence to treat their patients.

In our study, nearly half of the respondents reported that guidelines were lacking for their specific patient population. Many also perceived that existing guidelines were too general in their recommendations. These are barriers related to guideline development that can and should be addressed by policy makers and guideline development teams, who could make further efforts to ensure that more relevant guidelines are developed and that they are specific in scope and recommendations.

4.1. Strengths and Limitations. Study limitations include a relatively low response rate and the lack of nonresponse analysis. With the exception of gender, we had no data on characteristics or outcome variables for those who did not respond to the survey. Men were overrepresented among respondents (10%) vs. nonrespondents (3%). Perhaps, those who responded to the survey were more positive toward EBP than those who did not respond. A further limitation is that, as in all questionnaire-based surveys, data were self-reported. Only publically employed occupational therapists were surveyed; attitudes and behaviour among private practitioners may differ.

A strength of the study is the use of a validated and reliable EBP questionnaire [20], which has previously been used among physiotherapists in Sweden [21]. Advantages of this questionnaire is that it targets practicing clinicians rather than students and that it, in addition to EBP variables, includes items on guidelines. Its forerunner, an EBP questionnaire developed by Jette et al. [19], has been used in a multitude of studies, particularly in physiotherapy [13, 39–42].

The study participants are likely to be similar in characteristics, attitudes, and behaviours to the national population of occupational therapists in primary care in Sweden; the findings can therefore probably be generalised to the rest of Sweden and possibly other countries with similar healthcare systems and practices. Still, the relatively low sample size calls for caution on an overly broad generalisation of the findings.

4.2. Implications for Practice and Research. The study findings have several implications for both clinicians and researchers in primary care occupational therapy. The prerequisites for applying EBP to a greater extent create high demands for the coming years, on both practicing therapists, their managers, as well as students and recent graduates who are entering the job market. Because today's occupational therapy, students learn EBP skills in their undergraduate training, efforts on improving EBP skills, and behaviour should focus on continued professional development efforts among practicing occupational therapists in primary care. Such practitioner training should be comprehensive, contextually relevant, and collaborative to help practitioners implement and integrate EBP into clinical practice and is more likely to change practice patterns if conducted in workplace settings [43]. The importance of integrating different sources of evidence into clinical reasoning should be emphasised.

The insight provided by this study into the reported attitudes towards knowledge of and barriers for EBP and guidelines can facilitate the development of strategies for increasing the use of EBP among occupational therapists. The identified barriers related to EBP could be addressed in several ways. The barriers related to the use of guidelines would be particularly relevant to address in guideline development work: making the guidelines brief, specific, and with clear links to the underpinning evidence.

The major barrier of perceived time constraints, which could be both a personal and a contextual or organisational barrier, needs to be addressed. This barrier is not likely to be reduced without organisational or managerial support, for instance, by provision of protected work time for searching and appraising literature and other EBP activities. One such activity that may be both effective and cost-effective, in that it requires minimal resources, could be the organisation of journal clubs. This is a form of EBP teaching that allows participants to keep up-to-date with current, clinically relevant, research evidence as well as to improve their research appraisal skills. Journal clubs have been shown to be acceptable to occupational therapists and other allied health professionals and to be likely to be used with enthusiasm to achieve EBP [44].

4.3. Future Research. To minimise bias from self-reported data, there is a need to develop objective measures for assessing implementation of EBP. For a deeper understanding of EBP behaviours, as well as barriers and facilitators for applying EBP, a qualitative approach using individual interviews or focus groups is suggested. Furthermore, research is needed to address the remaining knowledge gaps with regard to occupational therapy interventions. Many of the interventions that occupational therapists use have yet to be underpinned by substantial research evidence, due to the limited number of studies performed as well as problems with research design.

5. Conclusions

This study provides new knowledge about attitudes, knowledge, behaviour, prerequisites, and barriers to EBP and guidelines among Swedish primary care occupational therapists that are likely to be transferable to other countries with similar healthcare systems. In spite of very positive attitudes and a fairly high use of clinical guidelines, the large proportion of occupational therapists who wanted to learn more about EBP, the small proportion who searched for and read scientific articles, and the fairly poor self-efficacy in finding research and in treating patients according to research evidence sends a signal to managers and decision makers that measures need to be taken to address these shortcomings. The study findings highlight the importance of continual professional development and training in EBP skills, with focus on search and appraisal of literature as well as on integrating different sources of evidence into clinical reasoning. In addition, more research is needed to address knowledge gaps that remain with regard to occupational therapy interventions.

Acknowledgments

This work was partially supported by the Research and Development Centre of Gothenburg and Södra Bohuslän. The authors wish to thank all the occupational therapists in primary care in the region of Västra Götaland for participating in the study and for taking the time to answer the questionnaire.

References

[1] D. L. Sackett, W. M. C. Rosenberg, J. A. M. Gray, R. B. Haynes, and W. S. Richardson, "Evidence based medicine: what it is and what it isn't," *BMJ*, vol. 312, no. 7023, pp. 71-72, 1996.

[2] P. A. Crist, "Adapting research instruction to support the scholarship of practice: practice-scholar partnerships,"

Occupational Therapy In Health Care, vol. 24, no. 1, pp. 39–55, 2010.

[3] M. Stronge and M. Cahill, "Self-reported knowledge, attitudes and behaviour towards evidence-based practice of occupational therapy students in Ireland," *Occupational Therapy International*, vol. 19, no. 1, pp. 7–16, 2012.

[4] C. Lyons, T. Brown, M. H. Tseng, J. Casey, and R. McDonald, "Evidence-based practice and research utilisation: perceived research knowledge, attitudes, practices and barriers among Australian paediatric occupational therapists," *Australian Occupational Therapy Journal*, vol. 58, no. 3, pp. 178–186, 2011.

[5] D. Upton, D. Stephens, B. Williams, and L. Scurlock-Evans, "Occupational therapists' attitudes, knowledge, and implementation of evidence-based practice: a systematic review of published research," *British Journal of Occupational Therapy*, vol. 77, no. 1, pp. 24–38, 2014.

[6] K. A. V. Cameron, S. Ballantyne, A. Kulbitsky, M. Margolis-Gal, T. Daugherty, and F. Ludwig, "Utilization of evidence-based practice by registered occupational therapists," *Occupational Therapy International*, vol. 12, no. 3, pp. 123–136, 2005.

[7] D. B. Philibert, P. Snyder, D. Judd, and M. M. Windsor, "Practitioners' reading patterns, attitudes, and use of research reported in occupational therapy journals," *American Journal of Occupational Therapy*, vol. 57, no. 4, pp. 450–458, 2003.

[8] J. Salls, C. Dolhi, L. Silverman, and M. Hansen, "The use of evidence-based practice by occupational therapists," *Occupational Therapy In Health Care*, vol. 23, no. 2, pp. 134–145, 2009.

[9] A. McCluskey, "Occupational therapists report a low level of knowledge, skill and involvement in evidence-based practice," *Australian Occupational Therapy Journal*, vol. 50, no. 1, pp. 3–12, 2003.

[10] A. Thomas and M. Law, "Research utilization and evidence-based practice in occupational therapy: a scoping study," *American Journal of Occupational Therapy*, vol. 67, no. 4, pp. e55–e65, 2013.

[11] E. Miller and M. Willis, "The Cochrane Collaboration and occupational therapy: an emerging partnership," *British Journal of Occupational Therapy*, vol. 63, no. 6, pp. 288–290, 2000.

[12] S. Mulligan, B. P. White, and S. Arthanat, "An examination of occupation-based, client-centered, evidence-based occupational therapy practices in New Hampshire," *OTJR: Occupation, Participation and Health*, vol. 34, no. 2, pp. 106–116, 2014.

[13] S. Heiwe, K. N. Kajermo, R. Tyni-Lenne et al., "Evidence-based practice: attitudes, knowledge and behaviour among allied health care professionals," *International Journal for Quality in Health Care*, vol. 23, no. 2, pp. 198–209, 2011.

[14] T. Kredo, S. Bernhardsson, S. Machingaidze et al., "Guide to clinical practice guidelines: the current state of play," *International Journal for Quality in Health Care*, vol. 28, no. 1, pp. 122–128, 2016.

[15] The American Association of Occupational Therapists, "Practice guidelines," Bethesda, MD, USA, August 2018, https://www.aota.org/Practice/Researchers/practice-guidelines.aspx.

[16] Royal College of Occupational Therapists, "RCOT practice guidelines," London, UK, August 2018, https://www.rcot.co.uk/practice-resources/rcot-practice-guidelines.

[17] Arbetsterapeuterna, "Riktlinjer," The National Association of Occupational Therapists, Stockholm, Sweden, August 2018, https://www.arbetsterapeuterna.se/Min-profession/riktlinjer/.

[18] M. Stergiou-Kita, "Implementing clinical practice guidelines in occupational therapy practice: recommendations from the research evidence," *Australian Occupational Therapy Journal*, vol. 57, no. 2, pp. 76–87, 2010.

[19] D. U. Jette, K. Bacon, C. Batty et al., "Evidence-based practice: beliefs, attitudes, knowledge, and behaviors of physical therapists," *Physical Therapy*, vol. 83, no. 9, pp. 786–805, 2003.

[20] S. Bernhardsson and M. E. H. Larsson, "Measuring evidence-based practice in physical therapy: translation, adaptation, further development, validation, and reliability test of a questionnaire," *Physical Therapy*, vol. 93, no. 6, pp. 819–832, 2013.

[21] S. Bernhardsson, K. Johansson, P. Nilsen, B. Oberg, and M. E. H. Larsson, "Determinants of guideline use in primary care physical therapy: a cross-sectional survey of attitudes, knowledge, and behavior," *Physical Therapy*, vol. 94, no. 3, pp. 343–354, 2014.

[22] H. Buchanan, *Evidence-Based Practice in Occupational Therapy in South Africa and the Western Cape, [Ph.D. thesis]*, University of Cape Town, Cape Town, South Africa, 2011.

[23] J. L. Crabtree, M. Justiss, and S. Swinehart, "Occupational therapy master-level students' evidence-based practice knowledge and skills before and after fieldwork," *Occupational Therapy In Health Care*, vol. 26, no. 2-3, pp. 138–149, 2012.

[24] *Code of Ethics for Occupational Therapists*, Swedish Association of Occupational Therapists, Nacka, Sweden, 2012, https://www.arbetsterapeuterna.se/Global/Forlag/Etisk%20kod/CodeofEthics2012_final2016.pdf.

[25] W. Coster, "International conference on evidence-based practice: a collaborative effort of the American Occupational Therapy Association, the American Occupational Therapy Foundation, and the Agency for Healthcare Research and Quality," *American Journal of Occupational Therapy*, vol. 59, no. 3, pp. 356–358, 2005.

[26] A. MacEwan Dysart and G. S. Tomlin, "Factors related to evidence-based practice among U.S. occupational therapy clinicians," *American Journal of Occupational Therapy*, vol. 56, no. 3, pp. 275–284, 2002.

[27] L. Scurlock-Evans, P. Upton, and D. Upton, "Evidence-based practice in physiotherapy: a systematic review of barriers, enablers and interventions," *Physiotherapy*, vol. 100, no. 3, pp. 208–219, 2014.

[28] T. M. da Silva, L. da Cunha Menezes Costa, A. N. Garcia, and L. O. P. Costa, "What do physical therapists think about evidence-based practice? A systematic review," *Manual Therapy*, vol. 20, no. 3, pp. 388–401, 2015.

[29] H. Sadeghi-Bazargani, J. S. Tabrizi, and S. Azami-Aghdash, "Barriers to evidence-based medicine: a systematic review," *Journal of Evaluation in Clinical Practice*, vol. 20, no. 6, pp. 793–802, 2014.

[30] S. Zwolsman, E. te Pas, L. Hooft, M. W. D. Waard, and N. van Dijk, "Barriers to GPs' use of evidence-based medicine: a systematic review," *British Journal of General Practice*, vol. 62, no. 600, pp. e511–e521, 2012.

[31] F. Sadoughi, T. Azadi, and T. Azadi, "Barriers to using electronic evidence based literature in nursing practice: a systematised review," *Health Information & Libraries Journal*, vol. 34, no. 3, pp. 187–199, 2017.

[32] J. C. Rogers, "Teaching clinical reasoning for practice in geriatrics," *Physical & Occupational Therapy In Geriatrics*, vol. 1, no. 3, pp. 29–37, 1982.

[33] C. Unsworth and A. Baker, "A systematic review of professional reasoning literature in occupational therapy," *British Journal of Occupational Therapy*, vol. 79, no. 1, pp. 5–16, 2016.

[34] D. Gibson, B. Velde, T. Hoff, D. Kvashay, P. L. Manross, and V. Moreau, "Clinical reasoning of a novice versus an experienced occupational therapist: a qualitative study," *Occupational Therapy In Health Care*, vol. 12, no. 4, pp. 15–31, 2000.

[35] J. Rycroft-Malone, K. Seers, A. Titchen, G. Harvey, A. Kitson, and B. McCormack, "What counts as evidence in evidence-based practice?," *Journal of Advanced Nursing*, vol. 47, no. 1, pp. 81–90, 2004.

[36] M. P. Dijkers, S. L. Murphy, and J. Krellman, "Evidence-based practice for rehabilitation professionals: concepts and controversies," *Archives of Physical Medicine and Rehabilitation*, vol. 93, no. 8, pp. S164–S176, 2012.

[37] S. Bernhardsson, K. S. Samsson, K. Johansson, B. Öberg, and M. E. H. Larsson, "A preference for dialogue: exploring the influence of patient preferences on clinical decision making and treatment in primary care physiotherapy," *European Journal of Physiotherapy*, 2018.

[38] A. Welch and P. Dawson, "Closing the gap: collaborative learning as a strategy to embed evidence within occupational therapy practice," *Journal of Evaluation in Clinical Practice*, vol. 12, no. 2, pp. 227–238, 2006.

[39] N. M. Salbach, S. B. Jaglal, N. Korner-Bitensky, S. Rappolt, and D. Davis, "Practitioner and organizational barriers to evidence-based practice of physical therapists for people with stroke," *Physical Therapy*, vol. 87, no. 10, pp. 1284–1303, 2007.

[40] R. Iles and M. Davidson, "Evidence based practice: a survey of physiotherapists' current practice," *Physiotherapy Research International*, vol. 11, no. 2, pp. 93–103, 2006.

[41] R. Ramirez-Velez, M. C. Bagur-Calafat, J. E. Correa-Bautista, and M. Girabent-Farres, "Barriers against incorporating evidence-based practice in physical therapy in Colombia: current state and factors associated," *BMC Medical Education*, vol. 15, no. 1, p. 220, 2015.

[42] T. M. Silva, L. C. M. Costa, and L. O. P. Costa, "Evidence-based practice: a survey regarding behavior, knowledge, skills, resources, opinions and perceived barriers of Brazilian physical therapists from São Paulo state," *Brazilian Journal of Physical Therapy*, vol. 19, no. 4, pp. 294–303, 2015.

[43] C. T. Myers and J. Lotz, "Practitioner training for use of evidence-based practice in occupational therapy," *Occupational Therapy In Health Care*, vol. 31, no. 3, pp. 214–237, 2017.

[44] L. M. Lizarondo, K. Grimmer-Somers, and S. Kumar, "Exploring the perspectives of allied health practitioners toward the use of journal clubs as a medium for promoting evidence-based practice: a qualitative study," *BMC Medical Education*, vol. 11, no. 1, p. 66, 2011.

13

Identification of Sensory Processing and Integration Symptom Clusters: A Preliminary Study

Lucy Jane Miller,[1] Sarah A. Schoen,[1] Shelley Mulligan,[2] and Jillian Sullivan[3]

[1] *STAR Institute, 5420 S. Quebec Street, Suite 105, Greenwood Village, CO 80111, USA*
[2] *Department of Occupational Therapy, 4 Library Way, University of New Hampshire, Durham, NH 03824, USA*
[3] *Northeastern University, 312E Robinson Hall, 360 Huntington Ave., Boston, MA 02115, USA*

Correspondence should be addressed to Sarah A. Schoen; sarah.schoen@spdstar.org

Academic Editor: Claudia Hilton

Rationale. This study explored subtypes of sensory processing disorder (SPD) by examining the clinical presentations of cluster groups that emerged from scores of children with SPD on the Sensory Processing 3-Dimension (SP-3D) Inventory. *Method.* A nonexperimental design was used involving data extraction from the records of 252 children with SPD. Exploratory cluster analyses were conducted with scores from the SP-3D Inventory which measures sensory overresponsivity (SOR), sensory underresponsivity (SUR), sensory craving (SC), postural disorder, dyspraxia, and sensory discrimination. Scores related to adaptive behavior, social-emotional functioning, and attention among children with different sensory modulation patterns were then examined and compared. *Results.* Three distinct cluster groups emerged from the data: High SOR only, High SUR with SOR, and High SC with SOR. All groups showed low performance within multiple domains of adaptive behavior. Atypical behaviors associated with social-emotional functioning and attention varied among the groups. *Implications.* The SP-3D Inventory shows promise as a tool for assisting in identifying patterns of sensory dysfunction and for guiding intervention. Better characterization can guide intervention precision and facilitate homogenous samples for research.

1. Introduction

Current estimates indicate that 5% to 16.5% of the general population [1, 2] have symptoms associated with sensory processing challenges and these estimates are higher for clinical populations such as autism spectrum disorder (ASD) [3] and attention deficit hyperactivity disorder (ADHD) [4]. Sensory processing is part of normal development and reflects one's ability to interpret and respond to daily sensory experiences [5]. The integration of sensory information contributes to successful functioning in daily life reflected in our ability to self-regulate, interact socially [2], and develop adaptive behavioral skills/abilities [6]. Thus, sensory processing is only considered a problem when it interferes with functioning in daily life. In fact, the autism literature has been recently characterized as a form of atypical sensory processing that enhances daily life called enhanced perception linked to superior sensory acuity [7]. However, some subtypes of sensory processing have been associated with impairments in activities of daily living [6] and with other kinds of behavioral problems [8]. An increase in recognition of sensory processing challenges [7] supports the need to articulate patterns of dysfunction and associated functional deficits across clinical populations. Clinically meaningful descriptions will facilitate increased understanding of the clinical presentation, which can provide more specificity for guiding intervention and greater homogeneity of samples for research.

Interest in understanding and defining the patterns of sensory processing dysfunction has been prevalent since Ayres first developed the Southern California Sensory Integration Tests [9], followed by the Sensory Integration and Praxis Tests [SIPT] [10]. With the publication of the sensory profile [11], responsivity patterns characteristic of individuals with sensory modulation challenges were included. Davies and Tucker [12] summarized the evidence from 1986 to 2006, and they found that the literature was limited by the specific assessment tools used because no single study included a comprehensive assessment of sensory function and sensory-based motor performance. Thus, it is difficult to arrive at a consensus regarding factors or cluster groups across studies due to the varied constructs evaluated by different assessment tools, as well as due to heterogeneity and comorbidities in the samples studied [13].

Sensory processing dysfunction includes a heterogeneous set of symptoms that affects the manner in which individuals use sensory information for emotion regulation, motor performance, social interaction, and daily life functioning at home, at school, and in the community [14–16]. Some research to date has described the neurodevelopmental, behavioral, and functional characteristics and correlates of children who present with sensory processing challenges. For example, a systematic review by Koenig and Rudney [17] found that children with sensory overresponsive (SOR) patterns and sensory-related motor dysfunction have more difficulty with social participation and performance of activities of daily living than children with sensory underresponsivity (SUR). Reynolds and Lane [18] also found SOR to be associated with poor performance of activities of daily living. Elbasan et al. [19] associated disruption in performance in activities of daily living with visual and tactile discrimination problems, postural problems, and dyspraxia.

SOR in the tactile and auditory domains has been given the most attention in the literature. SOR has been associated with anxiety in children and adolescents previously classified as Asperger's syndrome (e.g., high functioning autism) [20] as well as with problems acquiring a number of adaptive behavior and functional skills [18, 21, 22]. SOR has also been associated with children who have attention deficit disorders [17, 22–24]. Although we are beginning to understand the clinical presentations of each sensory processing pattern in various clinical conditions, there is a need for further clarification of relations among patterns and differential association with occupational performance in children without comorbid diagnoses [12].

This study fills the gap in research elucidated by Davies and Tucker [25] by using a comprehensive assessment of sensory processing functions including sensory modulation, sensory discrimination, and sensory-based motor abilities, called the Sensory Processing 3-Dimension Inventory [26], previously called the Sensory Processing Scale [27]. We use a more homogeneous sample, since samples with different diagnoses and comorbidities may present differently, and our investigation of patterns includes constructs related to functioning in everyday life. Thus, the present study expands upon previous studies by examining characteristics within sensory modulation dysfunction related to adaptive behavior, social-emotional functioning, and inattention/overactivity; the study by Mailloux and colleagues [28] examined patterns of dyspraxia and sensory discrimination and the study by Mailloux and colleagues [28, 29] only examined sensory modulation. Knowledge of the patterns of dysfunction and associated functional impairments provides greater homogeneity of samples in research studies which allows for comparisons of results across studies [12]. Clinicians also need this information to increase treatment specificity and communication among parents, teachers, and other professionals.

Cluster analysis was used to determine whether a sample of children with known sensory processing challenges could be organized into clinically meaningful groups based on similarities and differences. Cluster analyses are exploratory, multivariate data reduction strategies that are commonly used to discover groupings of individuals across a variety of clinical conditions that tend to be heterogeneous in nature [30]. Cluster analysis facilitates the identification of patterns within groups and is useful in evaluating diagnostic taxonomies [31, 32]. Information regarding patterns of dysfunction is helpful so that interventions can be tailored to meet specific sensory processing and associated functional challenges of each group identified. Researchers can also use information from cluster analyses to form more homogeneous samples in treatment effectiveness studies and when investigating the underlying neurological mechanisms of a disorder. The following research questions were addressed: (a) what distinct and clinical meaningful cluster groups emerge based on scores from the SP-3D Inventory? and (b) what are the characteristics of children within each of the cluster groupings with respect to dimensions adaptive behavior, social-emotional functioning, and inattention/overactivity?

2. Method

2.1. Procedures and Participants. The study was conducted at Sensory Therapies And Research (STAR) Institute for Sensory Processing Disorder in Greenwood Village, CO, and involved retrospective data extraction from the charts of clients with SPD seen from 2007 to 2013. The data collected were from caregiver report measures used in routine clinical care. Chart review and data entry of deidentified information were completed by research assistants, supervised by a senior researcher following procedures approved by the Rocky Mountain University of Health Professions Institutional Review Board.

The sample consisted of data from 252 children ages 4 to 14 years ($M = 6.9$ years, SD = 2.05) who did not meet criteria for an autism spectrum disorder, a neurologic or orthopedic syndrome, or a mental health diagnosis based on parent report of medical history from a community pediatrician. Males made up 180 of the 252 participants (71.4%) and 80% of the sample were Caucasian. Socioeconomic status was based on parent education, with 61% of parents reporting that they had a high school education and 39% a college education or above. All participants completed a 2-hour, comprehensive performance-based occupational therapy evaluation including a standardized assessment of motor functioning, norm-referenced parent-rating scales of sensory, adaptive, and problem behaviors, and clinical observations of sensory processing, postural control, and motor performance. Only those children who had complete data on the Sensory Processing Three-Dimension Inventory were included. This sample was representative of a clinical sample of children with SPD referred to the STAR Institute for sensory and behavioral challenges that significantly interfered with daily functioning at home, at school, and/or in the community.

2.2. Instrumentation

Sensory Processing Three-Dimension Inventory. The Sensory Processing Three-Dimension (SP-3D) Inventory [33, 34] utilizes parent report to measure all subtypes of SPD based on the nosology [13], with six subscales: sensory overresponsivity (SOR), sensory underresponsivity (SUR), sensory craving (SC), postural disorder (PD), dyspraxia (DYS), and sensory discrimination disorder (SDD). For the three modulation subscales (SOR, SUR, and SC) and one sensory discrimination subscale, items address behaviors believed to be associated with the processing of the input from the visual, tactile, vestibular, proprioception, auditory, gustatory, and olfactory sensory domains. Scoring utilizes a binary system which requires the informant to indicate whether any of the behavioral descriptions/items apply to their child (applicable = 1; not applicable = 0). The SP-3D Inventory takes approximately 20 minutes to complete and consists of 182 items. Total scores reflect the sum of items endorsed by the parent on each subscale or SPD subtype, and higher scores suggest greater impairment. Scores for this study were transformed into percentages of total items endorsed to account for the variability in total number of items on each subscale, which were as follows: SOR-47 items; SUR-21 items, SC-28 items, SDD-26 items; posture disorder-23 items; and dyspraxia-37 items. Previous research demonstrates acceptable internal consistency reliability (α = .63–.75) and discriminative validity (Cohen's d = .56–1.53 [33, 35]. Principal axis factor analysis also confirmed the internal structure of the modulation subscales [33]. For this sample, internal consistency reliability for the subscales ranged from $\alpha = .80$ to $\alpha = .92$).

Adaptive Behavior Assessment Scale-II. The Adaptive Behavior Assessment Scale (ABAS-II) [36] is a norm-referenced, caregiver rating scale for individuals from birth to 21 years. The ABAS-II provides a comprehensive assessment of a child's adaptive behavior including functioning in ten related adaptive skill areas: communication, community use, functional academics, school/home living, health and safety, leisure, self-care, self-direction, social, and work. Three composite scores, conceptual, social, and practical, make up the General Adaptive Composite (GAC). Higher scores reflect *better* adaptive functioning. Internal consistency reliability for the GAC and all adaptive skill areas was found to be high for all age groups (α = .79–.99). Data in the test manual supports the tool's reliability and validity.

Behavior Assessment System for Children-2. The Behavior Assessment System for Children-2 (BASC-2) [26] is a norm-referenced measure of emotional and behavioral disorders for children 4 to 18 years. The parent-rating measure assesses a child's problem behaviors in the community and at home, including hyperactivity, aggression, conduct problems, anxiety, depression, somatization, attention problems, learning problems, atypicality, and withdrawal. The four composite scores are externalizing problems, internalizing problems, adaptive skills, and behavioral symptoms index. Higher scores indicate *greater* impairment. For this study, the adaptive subscale was not used because the content is similar to the ABAS-II, and the conduct disorder subscale score was not reported because the age range was limited to children 6 years and older. Reliability and validity data are reported to be strong including internal consistency reliability of the scales with Cronbach α values ranging from .88 to .94 [26].

The Swanson, Nolan, and Pelham Parent-Rating Scale. The Swanson, Nolan, and Pelham Parent-Rating Scale (SNAP-IV) [27] is an 18-item, parent report used to characterize ADHD features. It has two subscales characterizing each of the ADHD subtypes; 9 items represent the hyperactive/impulsive subtype, and 9 items represent the inattentive subtype. A 4-point Likert scale is used to rate behaviors from 0, not at all, to 3, very much. Internal consistency reliability for the parent report form is high $\alpha = .94$ [30] with Cronbach α values for the inattentive and hyperactive/impulsive subscales .90 and .79, respectively [30]. Studies of predictive validity, sensitivity, and specificity support the tool as an acceptable measure of behaviors associated with ADHD [30].

2.3. Data Analysis. A Ward's agglomerative hierarchical cluster analysis was first conducted using the items from all subscales of the SP-3D Inventory to identify potential cluster solutions based on squared Euclidean values in a distance matrix [37]. Next, a K-means clustering algorithm based on the results from the hierarchical analysis (as described by [38]) was conducted to derive the final clusters. No meaningful cluster groupings emerged using all six of the SP3D Inventory subscales. Cluster analysis is considered an exploratory and somewhat subjective technique which evaluates children's scores on all variables by how close or distant they are from other children [39]. A lack of meaningful cluster groups may have occurred because of the inherent heterogeneity of children with SPD, that is, children having many different combinations of the various subtypes. To explore the data further with less variability, cluster analysis was repeated using only the scales representing sensory modulation behaviors. When there appears to be no interpretable solution, the literature suggests carefully considering the variables that are included in the analysis [39, 40]. Since sensory modulation has a strong theoretical foundation and is a common sensory processing symptomatology, cluster analysis was rerun using the three modulation subscales. A 3-cluster solution which grouped children based on the scoring of items on the SOR, SUR, and SC subscales best fit the data (based on effect size attributed to each cluster variable). Subsequent analyses then examined the specific characteristics of each cluster group, and differences in their scores from the ABAS-II, BASC-2, and SNAP-IV as well as from the other three SP3D Inventory subscales (e.g., posture, dyspraxia, and sensory discrimination).

One-way ANOVAs were performed to assess cluster group differences. Games-Howell post hoc tests were used when the Brown-Forsythe test for robustness of the median was significant. Due to the exploratory nature of this investigation, and to minimize the potential for Type II errors, an alpha level of $p < 0.05$ was used to determine statistical

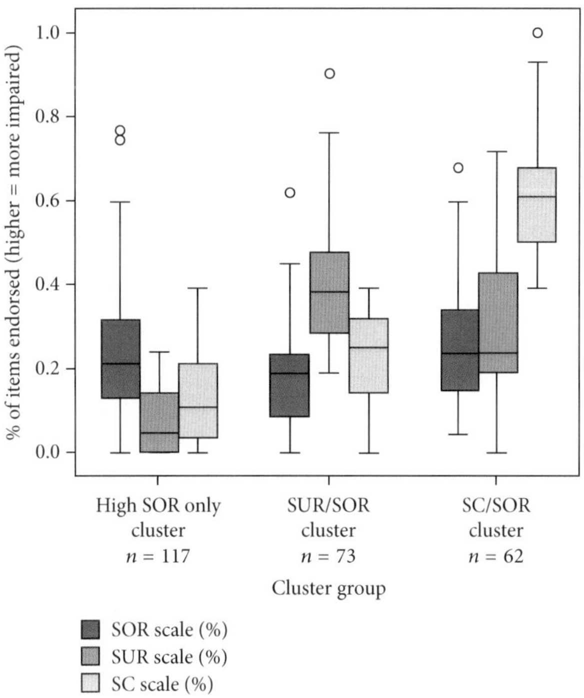

FIGURE 1: Cluster groupings.

differences despite multiple comparisons, as suggested by [41].

3. Results

The distance matrix from the hierarchical cluster analysis provided support for a three-cluster solution: (a) High SOR only cluster ($n = 117$); (b) High SUR plus SOR cluster ($n = 73$); and (c) High SC plus SOR cluster ($n = 62$) (see Figure 1).

In terms of demographics, the High SOR only group was 70.9% male with a mean age of 7.28 (SD = 2.23). The High SUR plus SOR (SUR/SOR) cluster group was 64.4% male with a mean age of 6.78 (SD = 1.92), and the High SC plus SOR (SC/SOR) cluster group was 80.6% male with a mean age of 6.37 (SD = 1.67). A one-way ANOVA confirmed cluster group differences for age, $F(2, 249) = 4.37$, $p = 0.014$, with the High SOR only cluster group being significantly older than the SC cluster group ($p = 0.004$) but not significantly different from the SUR cluster group ($p = 0.099$). Chi-square analysis showed no significant differences in gender distribution among the groups, $\chi^2(2) = 4.37$, $p = 0.11$.

The three-cluster solution in the K-means analysis produced groups that significantly differed in their SP-3D Inventory SOR subscale score, $F(2, 249) = 3.45$, $p = 0.033$; $\eta^2 = .011$, SUR subscale score, $F(2, 249) = 142.89$, $p < 0.001$, $\eta^2 = .376$, and SC subscale score $F(2, 249) = 326.93$, $p < 0.001$, $\eta^2 = .724$. Games-Howell post hoc tests showed that the High SC/SOR cluster group had more SOR behaviors than was found in the High SUR/SOR cluster group ($p = 0.028$) although the High SOR only cluster group did not significantly differ from the other cluster groups on their SOR subscale scores ($p > 0.05$). Thus, all cluster groups had some behaviors related to overresponsivity. Sensory craving behaviors were much more prevalent in the High SC/SOR cluster group and sensory underresponsivity subscale behaviors were more prevalent in the High SUR/SOR cluster group ($p < 0.01$). Table 1 summarizes the findings for the SP-3D Inventory by cluster group.

Using one-way ANOVAs, significant group differences among the three-cluster groups were found on the SP-3D Inventory postural subscale, $F(2, 249) = 7.33$, $p < 0.01$; praxis subscale, $F(2, 249) = 23.96$, $p < 0.001$; and sensory discrimination subscale, $F(2, 249) = 28.21$, $p < 0.001$. Post hoc tests revealed that, in comparison with the High SOR only cluster group, the High SC/SOR and High SUR/SC groups showed significantly higher (more impairment) scores on the postural, praxis, and sensory discrimination disorder subscales ($p < 0.01$ for all). The High SUR/SOR and High SC/SOR cluster groups did not significantly differ from each other on the total scores for the postural, praxis, or discrimination subscales.

Data from the SP3D Inventory was available from a previous study [26] for a nonrepresentative typically developing sample of children ($n = 140$) for comparison to the clinical sample. All subscale scores for the High SUR/SOR and High SC/SOR cluster groups are more than two standard deviations above the typical mean. Subscale scores for the High SOR only group were most elevated for sensory overresponsivity. See Table 1.

An exploratory analysis was conducted of frequency of item endorsement across the three-cluster groups to discover trends within the data. Significant or near significant differences were identified for several items. The High SUR/SOR cluster group had more problems with dressing and undressing ($p = 0.019$) such as placing arm or leg correctly in clothing ($p = 0.044$), completing fasteners ($p = 0.066$), and tending to look disheveled ($p = 0.012$). They also tended to prefer sedentary activities ($p < 0.001$) and had difficulty climbing on or over objects ($p = 0.010$) and licking an ice cream cone ($p = 0.067$). The High SC/SOR cluster group tended to crave tactile stimuli (examining toys by touching and feeling; $p = 0.082$) and had more problems grading force needed for a task ($p = 0.079$), maintaining or copying rhythmical movements ($p = 0.149$), and differentiating printed figures that appear similar ($p = 0.011$).

The Adaptive Behavior Assessment System-II (ABAS-II) scores were available for 170 (67% of the sample) children, and they are summarized in Table 2. A one-way ANOVA showed no group differences on the General Adaptive Composite (GAC) nor any of the other composite scores ($p > 0.1$ for all). However, the mean GAC score was more than one standard deviation below the mean suggesting below-average functioning in adaptive behavior for all cluster groups. Scores on the conceptual composite (i.e., self-direction, functional academics, and communication) and the social composite (i.e., social skills and leisure activities) were at or below one standard deviation for the High SUR/SOR and High SC/SOR cluster groups and within normal limits for the High SOR only cluster group. The communication subscale of the ABAS-II showed significant differences $F(2, 167) = 3.41$,

Table 1: Mean scores from SP3D Inventory group.

Variable	SOR only group Mean (SD)	SUR/SOR group Mean (SD)	SC/SOR group Mean (SD)	Typical group Mean (SD)
SP3D Inventory	*n* = 117	*n* = 73	*n* = 62	*n* = 140
SOR scale	10.6 (6.9)	8.89 (6.48)	11.95 (7.07)	2.25 (2.43)
SUR scale	1.73 (1.61)	8.42 (3.08)	6.35 (3.94)	0.96 (2.13)
SC scale	3.53 (3.18)	6.33 (3.05)	17.03 (4.13)	0.58 (1.14)
Posture scale	4.09 (4.29)	6.22 (5.05)	6.6 (5.35)	0.64 (1.91)
Praxis scale	7.49 (6.26)	14.23 (8)	12.15 (6.41)	1.57 (3.36)
Discrimination scale	1.87 (2.16)	4.1 (3.25)	4.74 (2.91)	0.48 (1.65)

Table 2: Mean scores from the ABAS II by cluster group.

Variable	SOR only group Mean (SD)	SUR/SOR group Mean (SD)	SC/SOR group Mean (SD)
ABAS II	*n* = 72	*n* = 49	*n* = 49
General Adaptive Composite	82.1 (16.2)	79.0 (17.1)	77.8 (12.6)
Conceptual composite	87.2 (15.4)	83.7 (15.9)	83.1 (12.7)
Communication	8.8 (3.2)	7.4 (3.3)	7.6 (3.3)
Functional academic	8.5 (3.3)	8.3 (3.5)	8.3 (2.6)
Self-direction	6.3 (3.6)	6.3 (3.1)	5.7 (2.5)
Social composite	88.3 (16.6)	82.9 (18.1)	84.7 (14.1)
Leisure	8.6 (3.0)	7.6 (3.3)	7.9 (2.8)
Social	7.1 (3.3)	6.6 (3.5)	6.9 (3.0)
Practical composite	79.6 (16.9)	75.9 (17.5)	75.9 (12.1)
Community use	7.6 (3.5)	7.1 (3.3)	6.9 (3.1)
Home living	6.4 (3.5)	5.9 (3.2)	5.8 (2.5)
Health and safety	8.3 (3.5)	6.6 (3.6)	6.9 (2.9)
Self-care	5.1 (2.7)	5.1 (2.9)	4.8 (2.0)

Note. Atypical on ABAS-II composite scores is ≤85. Atypical on ABAS-II subscales is ≤7.

$p = 0.035$; among the groups with the High SUR/SOR cluster group scoring lower than the High SOR only group ($p = 0.05$). On the health and safety subscale, the High SUR/SOR group ($p = 0.034$) and High SC/SOR group ($p = 0.06$) had lower scores than the High SOR only group. Subscale mean scores for each of the three-cluster groups on self-direction, home living, and self-care were more than one standard deviation below the mean, while functional academics, communication, and leisure mean scores fell within the typical range for all three-cluster groups.

The Behavior Assessment System for Children-2 (BASC-2) scores were available for 188 of the subjects (74.6% of the total sample) and are presented in Table 3. For composite scores, one-way ANOVAs confirmed cluster group differences for externalizing behavior: $F(2, 185) = 19.74$, $p < 0.001$; internalizing behavior: $F(2, 185) = 5.22$, $p = 0.006$; and for the behavioral symptoms index: $F(2, 185) = 15.63$, $p < 0.001$. For externalizing, post hoc tests revealed that the High SC/SOR cluster group had more symptoms than the High SOR only and High SUR/SOR groups ($p < 0.001$; <0.002, resp.). For internalizing and externalizing composites, High SC/SOR cluster was the only cluster whose mean score fell in the clinically significant range, and this group had greater symptoms than both the High SUR/SOR group ($p = 0.008$) and the High SOR only group ($p = 0.041$). For the behavioral index composite, the High SUR/SOR and High SC/SOR cluster group's means fell in the clinically significant range. Both the High SUR/SOR cluster ($p = 0.003$) and the High SC/SOR cluster ($p < 0.001$) groups had greater symptoms than the High SOR only cluster group.

At the subscale level, Games-Howell post hoc tests revealed that hyperactivity showed the biggest difference between groups, with the High SC/SOR cluster showing the most symptoms compared to the High SUR/SOR cluster ($p < 0.001$) and the High SOR only group ($p < 0.001$). The High SOR only and High SUR/SOR groups differed but only marginally ($p = 0.06$). On the aggression subscale, only the High SC/SOR cluster group was in the clinically significantly range, while both the High SUR/SOR and High SC/SOR cluster groups had hyperactivity scores falling in the clinically significant range. The BASC-2 anxiety subscale showed that the High SC/SOR cluster group had the most symptoms, reaching statistical significance when compared to the High SUR cluster group ($p = 0.006$). The High SUR/SOR and High SOR only cluster groups did not differ on this subscale ($p = 0.32$). On the depression subscale, the High SC/SOR

Table 3: Mean scores from BASC-2 by cluster group.

Variable	SOR only group Mean (SD)	SUR/SOR group Mean (SD)	SC/SOR group Mean (SD)
BASC-2	*n* = 78	*n* = 57	*n* = 53
Externalizing composite	54.1 (10.5)	58.9 (11.4)	66.4 (11.5)
Hyperactivity	56.9 (11.3)	61.4 (11.2)	72.7 (12.0)
Aggression	52.6 (10.1)	56.7 (12.4)	61.2 (21.1)
Conduct problems	49.3 (13.1)	55.0 (11.9)	53.0 (9.3)
Internalizing composite	57.0 (11.9)	55.3 (11.6)	62.4 (12.8)
Anxiety	56.8 (13.0)	52.6 (11.5)	60.4 (14.2)
Depression	57.4 (11.9)	58.2 (11.4)	64.8 (13.4)
Somatization	51.9 (13.0)	52.7 (12.2)	53.8 (12.2)
Behavioral index composite	58.1 (10.2)	64.2 (10.4)	68.7 (12.2)
Atypicality	55.5 (11.1)	65.7 (14.3)	65.4 (16.0)
Withdrawal	58.1 (13.9)	60.2 (15.3)	56.5 (15.1)
Attention	56.0 (10.9)	62.4 (7.5)	64.6 (8.6)

Note. Atypical on BASC-2 is ≥60.

group again showed the most symptoms, with significant differences between the High SC/SOR group and the SUR ($p = 0.018$) and SOR ($p = 0.004$) groups. On the behavior atypicality and attention subscales, the High SOR only group had scores falling in the typical range, which was significantly different than the High SUR/SOR and High SC/SOR groups ($p < 0.001$ for both). The High SC/SOR and High SUR/SOR cluster groups did not significantly differ from each other on these scales. Withdrawal was in the clinically significant range for the High SUR/SOR cluster group only, and none of the groups had atypical conduct problems or somatization symptoms.

The SNAP-IV scores were available for 78 (31%) children in the sample with the results showing cluster group differences on the SNAP-IV total score, $F(2, 76) = 24.49$, $p < 0.001$. The High SC/SOR group had more symptoms on the SNAP-IV than the High SOR only ($p < 0.001$) and the High SUR/SOR ($p = 0.009$) groups, and the High SUR/SOR cluster had more symptoms than the High SOR only group ($p = 0.002$). In examining specific ADHD behaviors, post hoc tests indicated that the High SC/SOR cluster group had more hyperactivity symptoms than either the High SUR/SOR cluster group ($p < 0.001$) or the High SOR only cluster group ($p < 0.001$), but the High SC/SOR cluster group was not significantly different from the High SUR/SOR group on inattention ($p = 0.942$). The High SOR only group had fewer hyperactivity and inattention symptoms than the High SUR/SOR group ($p = 0.044$; $p = 0.008$, resp.) and fewer than the High SC/SOR group ($p < 0.001$; $p = 0.003$, resp.). Only fifty-five percent of this sample qualified for an ADHD diagnosis.

4. Discussion

Clusters that emerged from the analysis partially support the sensory modulation patterns, described by Miller et al. [13]. Although all three groups had symptoms of sensory overresponsivity, SUR and SC seemed to suggest distinct groups with the third group differentiated by elevated SOR symptoms only and fewer other sensory and motor symptoms, while distinct groups representing postural disorder, dyspraxia, and sensory discrimination disorder did not emerge from the analyses. Other methodology that has been used to examine sensory processing constructs was conducted by Su and Parham [42] using the Sensory Processing Measure [43], a similar measure of sensory processing challenges. In this study, Su and Parham used confirmatory factor analysis to test whether sensory questionnaire items represent distinct sensory processing constructs using a sample of 454 children from 2 to 10 years of age. They found that items associated with individual sensory systems, tactile, vestibular-proprioceptive, visual, and auditory systems, formed distinct factors rather than patterns of sensory processing such as sensory over- or underresponsivity and sensory discrimination.

Previous research has suggested that postural disorder and dyspraxia may be a single construct [44] and perhaps there is too much overlap in the SP-3D Inventory items from these two subscales to form distinct cluster groupings. Moreover, underlying sensory discrimination problems such as tactile discrimination has commonly been associated with motor planning deficits (called somatopraxis; see [28, 45]) which may be an explanation for the lack of sensory-based motor clusters emerging from this SP-3D Inventory data.

Upon examination of the characteristics of each of the sensory modulation cluster groups that did emerge, some differences were found related to postural, praxis, and sensory discrimination functions, adaptive behavior, and social-emotional and attention/hyperactivity behaviors. The High SOR only group had elevated overresponsivity scores but fewer symptoms related to postural disorder, dyspraxia, and sensory discrimination and all scores falling within normal limits on the BASC-2. The High SOR only group did have atypical scores on scales measuring performance in activities of daily living and self-direction. The High SUR/SOR group had many atypical adaptive behavior scores, with the lowest social composite score, similar delays in daily living skills and self-direction, and additional delays in health and safety and community use. Dyspraxia and postural symptoms were common in this group especially with a preference for sedentary activities and poor participation in dressing, undressing, and climbing. Inattention and withdrawal also scored high in this group. The High SC/SOR group had the greatest number of adaptive behaviors and behavioral symptoms and was differentiated from the other groups by clinically significant externalizing and internalizing behaviors, specifically hyperactivity, aggression, depression, and anxiety. The High SC/SOR cluster showed problems related to grading force, performing rhythmical movements, and visual discrimination. In adaptive behavior, the High SC/SOR group showed symptoms within all three composite scores measuring social, conceptual, and practical daily living skill domains.

A previous study of sensory modulation dysfunction phenotypes by James et al. [29] supported two of the cluster groups, SC and SUR, that were found in our study. Similarly, defining characteristics of the SC cluster included aggression, inattention, and many externalizing behaviors. Additionally, SOR was present in both clusters identified by James et al. [29] as it was in this study. Our results also support the coexistence of sensory modulation symptoms with motor problems, building on findings in previous studies [28, 29]. Clinically, it is not surprising that the SUR and SC cluster groups had associated motor difficulties as children who crave sensory input tend to engage in a great deal of nonproductive, nonpurposeful movement.

The finding that children fitting the High SC/SOR cluster also often have praxis problems may dispel the notion that sensory craving is just a compensatory behavioral strategy that is employed to counteract sensory over- or underresponsivity. Other evidence supporting our results [18, 46] suggests that SC comprises its own symptom cluster which can be associated with sensory based motor challenges and externalizing behaviors. For the High SUR/SOR cluster, we suggest that the lack of awareness to body sensations coupled with a reduced or slowed reactivity to external environmental sensory demands affects their motor skill acquisition and motor planning.

The High SUR/SOR and High SC/SOR cluster groups had more symptoms in social-emotional and fewer adaptive behavior abilities than the High SOR only cluster group, although all three-cluster groups had challenges in adaptive behavior. Individuals in the High SC/SOR cluster group tended to be more aggressive, hyperactive, anxious, and depressed than individuals in the other two cluster groups. We found more attention problems in the High SUR/SOR and High SC/SOR cluster groups unlike a previous study that found an association between inattention and only sensory overresponsivity [28, 29].

Of interest is that children in the High SC/SOR cluster were slightly younger than the other two cluster groups. One possibility is that individuals with SC tend to be more disruptive and thus may be identified at an earlier age. Children with SUR are usually quiet and passive and may not be identified until daily life requirements (functions) at school or at home become intolerable. Another possibility is that sensory craving or externalizing behavior tends to decline as children with age, similar to the decline in hyperactivity that tends to occur in children with ADHD as they get older [47].

Sensory processing challenges are increasingly recognized as a component of other disorders such as ADHD [24, 48] and ASD [49, 50]. Studies aiming to describe phenotypic characteristics may assist in differentiating clinical conditions. Research describing sensory patterns in ASD suggest cluster groups based on sensory domain involvement such as tactile, auditory, and movement sensitivity [32]. Other studies suggest patterns based on severity of symptoms as well as reflecting the cooccurrence of hyperresponsiveness (e.g., SOR) and hyporesponsiveness (e.g., SUR) responsivity possibly similar to the SUR/SOR cluster group identified in this study [51, 52]. Furthermore, behavioral manifestations of sensory symptoms in ASD have been shown to be more severe than those in individuals without a comorbid diagnosis [53].

This study suggests that ADHD and children with sensory processing challenges have some characteristics in common but also may differ. Research examining ADHD symptoms within individuals with sensory processing challenges shows an overlap with behaviors such as hyperactivity, inattention, and motor incoordination cooccurring with sensory issues [54]. In this study, many children who did not meet criteria for an ADHD diagnosis fell within each of the clusters. Similarly, Ben-Sasson et al. [55] identified a group of children with elevated ADHD symptoms *only* as well as a group with elevated SOR symptoms *only*, thus supporting the independence and uniqueness of each disorder.

Delineation of patterns of sensory processing dysfunction will help to facilitate outcomes research because in order to compare the effectiveness of intervention approaches, homogenous samples are necessary [12]. The clusters identified in this study represent different symptom presentations which likely require differing intervention strategies, so a greater understanding of the distinguishing characteristics of children within each pattern will help guide intervention. Finally, clarifying various patterns of dysfunction sets the stage for the study of the neuroanatomical and neurophysiological underpinnings of these cluster groups [56].

Limitations within the study design must be considered in the interpretation of findings. First, data were collected retrospectively from just one private clinic in Colorado and therefore may not be representative of all clinical samples of children with sensory processing challenges. The BASC-2, ABAS-II, and SNAP-IV were available only for a subset of the participants resulting in smaller samples of children with data from these questionnaires. These findings should be replicated in other clinic settings and with different samples. The age range in this study was broad, so that if developmental changes exist within sensory symptom presentation, an examination of scores by age may yield different outcomes. Finally, the SP-3D Inventory is a new tool, and extensive study of its reliability and validity is needed to support its use as a comprehensive parent report measure of sensory processing. Future studies should focus on delineation of sensory domain characteristics of overresponsivity within the cluster groups to determine if this helps to further define the cluster groupings. Additionally, correlational studies are suggested to help determine if having both SUR and SOR or both SC and SOR put children at greater risk for behavioral and adaptive behavior problems compared to SUR or SC alone.

5. Conclusions and Implications for Occupational Therapy Practice

This study provides information to the categorization of patterns of children with sensory processing challenges who do not meet criteria for other clinical diagnoses. This work assists in enhancing the clarity of communication used to describe children with sensory processing challenges both within and outside the occupational therapy profession. The results supported three distinct groups all with symptoms of sensory overresponsivity (e.g., High SOR only, High SUR/SOR cluster, and High SC/SOR cluster), and within these patterns, differing symptoms related to motor challenges and sensory discrimination challenges were found. All three-cluster groups had some challenges in occupational performance with individuals in the High SUR/SOR and High SC/SOR clusters displaying more challenges than children in the High SOR only group. This study builds on previous work by further elucidating patterns of sensory processing dysfunction and associated functional and behavioral symptoms that characterize each group. A greater understanding of the strengths and challenges inherent within each pattern is useful for guiding the delivery of appropriate occupational therapy interventions and for selecting homogenous participants for research.

Acknowledgments

The authors thank the children and families who participated in the study. They also wish to thank their research assistants Andrea Valdez, Shannon Hampton, and Aryanna Wiggins for their tireless effort on this manuscript. Primary funding for this work was provided by the Wallace Research Foundation. Additional support was provided by the National Institutes of Health Grant R21 HD41614-01 to Lucy Jane Miller and by the National Institutes of Health Grant T32MH15442 to the University of Colorado Denver in support of Sarah A. Schoen.

References

[1] A. Ben-Sasson, L. Hen, R. Fluss, S. A. Cermak, B. Engel-Yeger, and E. Gal, "A meta-analysis of sensory modulation symptoms in individuals with autism spectrum disorders," *Journal of Autism and Developmental Disorders*, vol. 39, no. 1, pp. 1–11, 2009.

[2] R. R. Ahn, L. J. Miller, S. Milberger, and D. N. McIntosh, "Prevalence of parents' perceptions of sensory processing disorders among kindergarten children," *American Journal of Occupational Therapy*, vol. 58, no. 3, pp. 287–293, 2004.

[3] S. D. Tomchek and W. Dunn, "Sensory processing in children with and without autism: a comparative study using the short sensory profile," *The American Journal of Occupational Therapy*, vol. 61, no. 2, pp. 190–200, 2007.

[4] S. J. Lane, S. Reynolds, and L. Thacker, "Sensory over-responsivity and ADHD: Differentiating using electrodermal responses, cortisol, and anxiety," *Frontiers in Integrative Neuroscience*, vol. 4, no. 8, 2010.

[5] L. J. Miller, *Sensational kids: Hope and help for children with sensory processing disorder*, Penguin Group (USA) Inc., New York, NY, USA, 2014.

[6] T. Bar-Shalita, J.-J. Vatine, and S. Parush, "Sensory modulation disorder: A risk factor for participation in daily life activities," *Developmental Medicine & Child Neurology*, vol. 50, no. 12, pp. 932–937, 2008.

[7] L. Mottron, M. Dawson, I. Soulières, B. Hubert, and J. Burack, "Enhanced perceptual functioning in autism: an update, and eight principles of autistic perception," *Journal of Autism and Developmental Disorders*, vol. 36, no. 1, pp. 27–43, 2006.

[8] S. G. Hofmann and S. Bitran, "Sensory-processing sensitivity in social anxiety disorder: Relationship to harm avoidance and diagnostic subtypes," *Journal of Anxiety Disorders*, vol. 21, no. 7, pp. 944–954, 2007.

[9] A. J. Ayres, *Southern California Sensory Integration Tests manual*, Western Psychological Services, Las Angeles, CA, USA, 1972.

[10] A. J. Ayres, *Sensory Integration and Praxis Tests (SIPT)*, Western Psychological services, California, calif, USA, 1989.

[11] W. Dunn, *The Sensory Profile*, Psychological Corporation, San Antonio , TX, USA, 1999.

[12] P. L. Davies and R. Tucker, "Evidence review to investigate the support for subtypes of children with difficulty processing and integrating sensory information," *American Journal of Occupational Therapy*, vol. 64, pp. 391–402, 2010.

[13] L. J. Miller, M. E. Anzalone, S. J. Lane, S. A. Cermak, and E. T. Osten, "Concept evolution in sensory integration: A proposed nosology for diagnosis," *American Journal of Occupational Therapy*, vol. 61, no. 2, pp. 135–142, 2007.

[14] A. Ben-Sasson, T. W. Soto, F. Martínez-Pedraza, and A. S. Carter, "Early sensory over-responsivity in toddlers with autism spectrum disorders as a predictor of family impairment and parenting stress," *Journal of Child Psychology and Psychiatry and Allied Disciplines*, vol. 54, no. 8, pp. 846–853, 2013.

[15] A. S. Carter, A. Ben-Sasson, and M. J. Briggs-Gowan, "Sensory over-responsivity, psychopathology, and family impairment in school-aged children," *Journal of the American Academy of Child and Adolescent Psychiatry*, vol. 50, no. 12, pp. 1210–1219, 2011.

[16] L. Gourley, C. Wind, E. M. Henninger, and S. Chinitz, "Sensory Processing Difficulties, Behavioral Problems, and Parental Stress in a Clinical Population of Young Children," *Journal of Child and Family Studies*, vol. 22, no. 7, pp. 912–921, 2013.

[17] K. P. Koenig and S. G. Rudney, "Performance challenges for children and adolescents with difficulty processing and integrating sensory information: A systematic review," *American Journal of Occupational Therapy*, vol. 64, no. 3, pp. 430–442, 2010.

[18] S. Reynolds and S. J. Lane, "Diagnostic validity of sensory over-responsivity: A review of the literature and case reports," *Journal of Autism and Developmental Disorders*, vol. 38, no. 3, pp. 516–529, 2008.

[19] B. Elbasan, H. Kayihan, and I. Duzgun, "Sensory integration and activities of daily living in children with developmental coordination disorder," *Italian Journal of Pediatrics*, vol. 38, no. 1, article no. 14, 2012.

[20] B. Pfeiffer, M. Kinnealey, C. Reed, and G. Herzberg, "Sensory modulation and affective disorders in children and adolescents with Asperger's disorder," *American Journal of Occupational Therapy*, vol. 59, no. 3, pp. 335–345, 2005.

[21] S. J. Rogers, S. Hepburn, and E. Wehner, "Parent Reports of Sensory Symptoms in Toddlers with Autism and Those with Other Developmental Disorders," *Journal of Autism and Developmental Disorders*, vol. 33, no. 6, pp. 631–642, 2003.

[22] S. Reynolds and S. J. Lane, "Sensory overresponsivity and anxiety in children with ADHD," *American Journal of Occupational Therapy*, vol. 63, no. 4, pp. 433–440, 2009.

[23] R. Iwanaga, H. Ozawa, C. Kawasaki, and R. Tsuchida, "Characteristics of the sensory-motor, verbal and cognitive abilities of preschool boys with attention deficit/hyperactivity disorder combined type," *Psychiatry and Clinical Neurosciences*, vol. 60, no. 1, pp. 37–45, 2006.

[24] A. Ghanizadeh, "Sensory processing problems in children with ADHD, a systematic review," *Psychiatry Investigation*, vol. 8, no. 2, pp. 89–94, 2011.

[25] P. L. Davies and R. Tucker, "Evidence review to investigate the support for subtypes of children with difficulty processing and integrating sensory information," *American Journal of Occupational Therapy*, vol. 64, no. 3, pp. 391–402, 2010.

[26] C. R. Reynolds and R. W. Kamphaus, *Behavior Assessment System for Children-2*, AGS Publishing, Circle Pines, MN, USA, 2003.

[27] J. M. Swanson, SNAP-IV Scale, 1995, Irvine, CA: University of California Development Center.

[28] Z. Mailloux, S. Mulligan, S. S. Roley et al., "Verification and clarification of patterns of sensory integrative dysfunction," *American Journal of Occupational Therapy*, vol. 65, no. 2, pp. 143–151, 2011.

[29] K. James, L. J. Miller, R. Schaaf, D. M. Nielsen, and S. A. Schoen, "Phenotypes within sensory modulation dysfunction," *Comprehensive Psychiatry*, vol. 52, no. 6, pp. 715–724, 2011.

[30] R. Bussing, M. Fernandez, M. Harwood et al., "Parent and teacher SNAP-IV ratings of attention deficit hyperactivity disorder symptoms: psychometric properties and normative ratings from a school district sample," *Assessment*, vol. 15, no. 3, pp. 317–328, 2008.

[31] A. S. Carter, M. J. Briggs-Gowan, and N. O. Davis, "Assessment of young children's social-emotional development and psychopathology: recent advances and recommendations for practice," *Journal of Child Psychology and Psychiatry and Allied Disciplines*, vol. 45, no. 1, pp. 109–134, 2004.

[32] A. E. Lane, R. L. Young, A. E. Z. Baker, and M. T. Angley, "Sensory processing subtypes in autism: association with adaptive behavior," *Journal of Autism and Developmental Disorders*, vol. 40, no. 1, pp. 112–122, 2010.

[33] S. A. Schoen, L. J. Miller, and J. Sullivan, "The development and psychometric properties of the Sensory Processing Scale Inventory: A report measure of sensory modulation," *Journal of Intellectual and Developmental Disability*, pp. 1–10, 2016.

[34] S. A. Schoen, L. J. Miller, and J. Sullivan, "The development and psychometric properties of the Sensory Processing Scale Inventory: A report measure of sensory modulation," *Journal of Intellectual and Developmental Disability*, vol. 42, no. 1, pp. 12–21, 2017.

[35] S. A. Schoen, L. J. Miller, and K. E. Green, "Pilot study of the sensory over-responsivity scales: Assessment and inventory," *American Journal of Occupational Therapy*, vol. 62, no. 4, pp. 393–406, 2008.

[36] P. L. Harrison and T. Oakland, *Adaptive Behavior Assessment System-II*, Psychological Corporation, San Antonio , TX, USA, 2003.

[37] P. A. J. Gore, "Handbook of applied multivariate statistics and mathematical modeling," in *Handbook of applied multivariate and mathematical modeling*, H. E. A. Tinsley and and S. D. Brown, Eds., pp. 298–318, Academic Press, Cambridge, MA, USA, 2000.

[38] J. Mandara, "The typological approach in child and family psychology: A review of theory, methods, and research," *Clinical Child and Family Psychology Review*, vol. 6, no. 2, pp. 129–146, 2003.

[39] M. Norusis, "IBM SPSS* statistics 19," in *Advanced Statistical Procedures Companion*, pp. 375–404, Addison Wesley, Boston, Mass, USA, 2011.

[40] O. Yim and K. T. Ramdeen, "Hierarchical Cluster Analysis: Comparison of Three Linkage Measures and Application to Psychological Data," *The Quantitative Methods for Psychology*, vol. 11, no. 1, pp. 8–21, 2015.

[41] R. Bender and S. Lange, "Adjusting for multiple testing—when and how?" *Journal of Clinical Epidemiology*, vol. 54, no. 4, pp. 343–349, 2001.

[42] C.-T. Su and L. D. Parham, "Validity of sensory systems as distinct constructs," *American Journal of Occupational Therapy*, vol. 68, no. 5, pp. 546–554, 2014.

[43] L. D. Parham and C. Ecker, *Sensory Processing Measure (SPM): Manual*, Western Psychological Services, Los Angeles, CA, USA, 2007.

[44] J. Lai, A. G. Fisher, L. C. Magalhães, and A. C. Bundy, "Construct Validity of the Sensory Integration and Praxis Tests," *The Occupational Therapy Journal of Research*, vol. 16, no. 2, pp. 75–97, 2016.

[45] A. van Jaarsveld, "Patterns of sensory integration dysfunction in children from South Africa," *South African Journal of Occupational Therapy*, p. 44, 2014.

[46] M. Liss, C. Saulnier, D. Fein, and M. Kinsbourne, "Sensory and attention abnormalities in autistic spectrum disorders," *Autism*, vol. 10, no. 2, pp. 155–172, 2006.

[47] S. V. Faraone, J. Biederman, and E. Mick, "The age-dependent decline of attention deficit hyperactivity disorder: a meta-analysis of follow-up studies," *Psychological Medicine*, vol. 36, no. 2, pp. 159–165, 2006.

[48] B. Pfeiffer, B. P. Daly, E. G. Nicholls, and D. F. Gullo, "Assessing sensory processing problems in children with and without attention deficit hyperactivity disorder," *Physical & Occupational Therapy in Pediatrics*, vol. 35, no. 1, pp. 1–12, 2015.

[49] A. Ben-Sasson, S. A. Cermak, G. I. Orsmond et al., "Extreme sensory modulation behaviors in toddlers with autism spectrum disorders," *The American Journal of Occupational Therapy*, vol. 61, no. 5, pp. 584–592, 2007.

[50] A. E. Z. Baker, A. Lane, M. T. Angley, and R. L. Young, "The relationship between sensory processing patterns and behavioural responsiveness in autistic disorder: A pilot study," *Journal of Autism and Developmental Disorders*, vol. 38, no. 5, pp. 867–875, 2008.

[51] K. Ausderau, J. Sideris, M. Furlong, L. M. Little, J. Bulluck, and G. T. Baranek, "National survey of sensory features in

children with ASD: Factor structure of the sensory experience questionnaire (3.0)," *Journal of Autism and Developmental Disorders*, vol. 44, no. 4, pp. 915–925, 2014.

[52] K. K. Ausderau, M. Furlong, J. Sideris et al., "Sensory subtypes in children with autism spectrum disorder: Latent profile transition analysis using a national survey of sensory features," *Journal of Child Psychology and Psychiatry and Allied Disciplines*, vol. 55, no. 8, pp. 935–944, 2014.

[53] S. A. Schoen, L. J. Miller, B. A. Brett-Green, and D. M. Nielsen, "Physiological and behavioral differences in sensory processing: A comparison of children with Autism Spectrum Disorder and Sensory Modulation Disorder," *Frontiers in Integrative Neuroscience*, vol. 3, article no. 29, 2009.

[54] A. Yochman, O. Alon-Beery, A. Sribman, and S. Parush, "Differential diagnosis of sensory modulation disorder (SMD) and attention deficit hyperactivity disorder (ADHD): Participation, sensation, and attention," *Frontiers in Human Neuroscience*, vol. 7, 2013.

[55] A. Ben-Sasson, T. W. Soto, A. E. Heberle, A. S. Carter, and M. J. Briggs-Gowan, "Early and Concurrent Features of ADHD and Sensory Over-Responsivity Symptom Clusters," *Journal of Attention Disorders*, vol. 21, no. 10, pp. 835–845, 2014.

[56] L. F. Koziol, D. E. Budding, and D. Chidekel, "Sensory integration, sensory processing, and sensory modulation disorders: Putative functional neuroanatomic underpinnings," *The Cerebellum*, vol. 10, no. 4, pp. 770–792, 2011.

14

Exploring Cultural Competence amongst OT Students

Pragashnie Govender, December M. Mpanza, Tarryn Carey, Kwenzile Jiyane, Bicolé Andrews, and Sam Mashele

Discipline of Occupational Therapy, School of Health Sciences, University of KwaZulu-Natal, Westville Campus, Westville, South Africa

Correspondence should be addressed to Pragashnie Govender; naidoopg@ukzn.ac.za

Academic Editor: Kathleen M. Matuska

Occupational therapy relies primarily on communication between the therapist and client for effective intervention. Adequate communication may be influenced by language and cultural differences between the therapist and client. Cultural competence in relation to language and culture is thus a vital part in practice. Limited research exists on cultural competence in occupational therapy students. This study thus aimed to explore the cultural competence of final year students and their perceptions of their own cultural competence, with respect to language and culture in their practice as students. An explorative qualitative study design was utilised with a nonprobability purposeful sample of 21 final year undergraduate students at a tertiary institute in South Africa. Three focus groups were conducted, comprising between 6 and 8 students in each group. Thematic analysis using inductive reasoning was undertaken in order to analyse the students' experiences and understanding of cultural competence. Findings of the study suggest that cultural competence, in relation to language and culture, influences the occupational therapy intervention process. It was shown to both positively and negatively influence intervention through supporting or hindering rapport building, client centeredness, and effective intervention.

1. Introduction

The concept of cultural competence, which in this study relates to the understanding of the influence of different languages and cultures, forms an essential component in the practice of any health care profession. Clear communication is necessary, between the clinician and client, for exchange of vital information for effective intervention [1]. Occupational therapy is one such profession which relies primarily on the interchange of communication between the therapist and client. Clients are viewed as unique beings, where their difficulties are as a result of a combination of factors and where the management of the client may rely on an understanding of the client's culture and family, including continued communication and/or support with the client and family [2]. Communication difficulties resulting from language and cultural differences between the therapist and client can thus have a significant impact on cultural competence and the occupational therapy intervention process. This is of concern in the South African context, given the country's multicultural population and eleven official languages. According to Penn [3], more than 80% of interactions between physicians and patients in South Africa take place across linguistic and cultural differences and therefore directly influence the patient-therapist relationship and quality of care. It is thus imperative that health practitioners and occupational therapists in general bridge these gaps in language and cultural differences in practice to gain a sense of cultural competence. To the authors' knowledge there has been only one other study conducted on cultural competence amongst student occupational therapists within South Africa [4] and one other study on cultural competence on professional South African occupational therapists [5]; thus limited evidence exists on how therapists in South Africa view language and culture as influencing practice and how students perceive and negotiate cultural competence in practice.

2. Literature Review

Occupational therapy is a diverse profession which relies on a functional relationship with the client whilst examining the

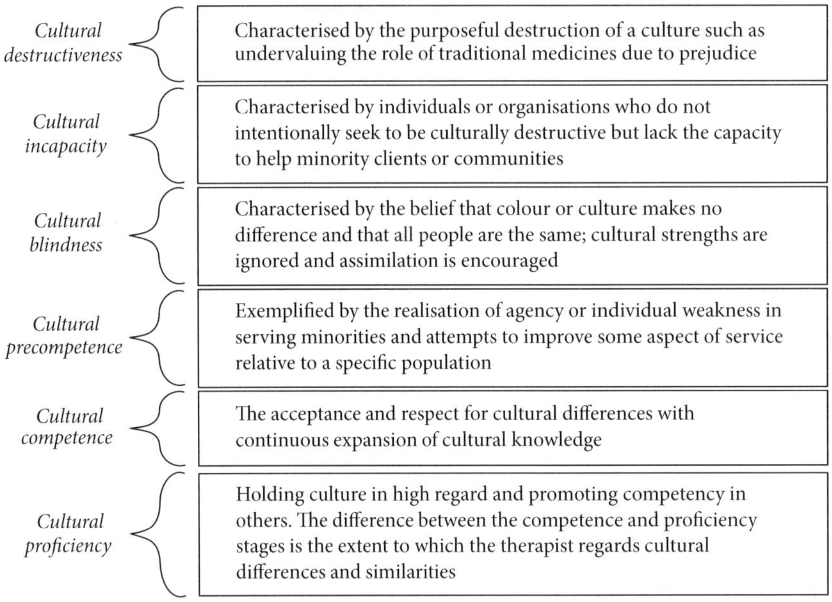

FIGURE 1: Cultural competence continuum [12, 13].

physiological, psychological, and environmental components that are unique to that person [1]. Intervention is thus more effective when the therapist can communicate with the patient about treatment [1]. Effective communication results when all participants in the communication process understand the content of what is being communicated [6]. A therapist speaking a different language to their client would thus have difficulty in fully grasping the client's cultural context without fully understanding the client's language first. Language is also a primary purveyor of culture. A study conducted by Levin [7] found that there was a link between language and culture. If language becomes a barrier between the practitioner and client, then the difference in their cultures could become a barrier as well. In situations such as these, cultural sensitivity needs to be applied. Moore [8] emphasised that to be culturally sensitive, one needs to be willing to consider the cultural background of the client and have at least the basic knowledge of the client's culture or beliefs within the society they practice. The Occupational Therapy Association of South Africa (OTASA) Code of Ethics and Professional Conduct [9] indicates that "occupational therapy services shall not allow prejudice or discrimination towards a patient/client based on race, culture, language, age, sexual orientation, disability, socioeconomic status." Ulrey and Amason [10] suggest that health care providers may not be aware of the client's cultural values, beliefs, and attitudes and learn as they experience it within the field of practice to become culturally competent.

Cultural competence is defined as "the process by which individuals and systems respond respectfully and effectively to people of all cultures, languages, classes, races and ethnic backgrounds in a way that recognizes, affirms, and values the worth of the individual and protects and preserves the dignity of each." [11]. It is thus imperative for students to be sufficiently exposed to different cultures and languages to build cultural competence which can be a lifelong learning process. Cultural competence, according to Cross [12], is described in six stages through which an individual develops along a continuum from cultural destructiveness to cultural proficiency. The stages are further defined as per Wittman and Velde's [13] definition of each stage (Figure 1).

Therapists in any of the first three stages, that is, destructiveness, incapacity, or blindness, may be considered to be culturally incompetent [13]. Evidence indicates that lack of cultural competence in the therapist can impact on therapeutic outcomes, treatment implementation, compliance, and follow-up [14]. Cheung et al. [15] conducted a study assessing perceptions of cultural competence amongst 51 occupational therapy students in England, in which they found a majority of students having reported limited awareness of and exposure to other cultures and insufficient training in cultural competence.

Cultural competence requires the health care practitioner to understand his/her own cultural values before understanding other cultures, their communication, behaviour, and the impact of their culture on the individual's health care beliefs. Language and cultural barriers are a common concern in clinical practice both in South Africa and internationally. With communication difficulties between the patient and the health care provider, there is often the use of interpreters either trained or untrained which could result in treatment being effective or ineffective.

A study conducted in the western United States explored the perspectives of 495 primary care physicians and their use of various methods to bridge language and cultural barriers between themselves and their clients [16]. In this study, authors found that in a place of cultural and ethnic diversity where physicians had access to the services of trained interpreters, a significantly higher quality of patient-physician communication and care occurred. Health care providers are exposed to diverse cultures and experience challenges to providing culturally and linguistically appropriate care to result in cultural competence. Occupational therapy as a profession thus needs to focus on providing culturally and linguistically appropriate care in order to provide holistic and culturally competent intervention.

3. Material and Methods

An explorative qualitative study design was utilised to explore occupational therapy undergraduate students' perceptions of cultural competence in relation to language and culture and the influence on their practice in the province of KwaZulu-Natal in South Africa. Nonprobability purposive sampling was used to select the study population of 24 final year undergraduate occupational therapy students from the school of health sciences at a tertiary institution in the province. From this sample, 21 participants agreed to participation in the study. The target population was comprised of a diverse group of students that speak different home languages and who hail from variable cultural backgrounds. Occupational therapy final year students were selected as they would have had at least three years of exposure to various service learning sites as part of their occupational therapy undergraduate training at the time. These service learning sites that the undergraduate students are exposed to during training are multicultural settings comprising hospitals, clinics, community sites, rehabilitation facilities, geriatric homes, and schools, serving a culturally and linguistically diverse population.

Three focus groups comprising a maximum of eight students were conducted spanning approximately one hour. Participants were divided into engineered heterogeneous focus groups to ensure cultural diversity. Questions posed to the groups included the following:

(i) The experience of students working with clients of a similar and divergent language and culture compared to their own.

(ii) The student's opinions on the influence they believed language and culture have on occupational therapy practice/intervention.

(iii) The opinion of students on the positive and negative aspects that language and culture have on their OT practice and how they dealt with this in practice.

(iv) Student's understanding of the term cultural competence.

(v) Student's opinions of their preparedness to deal with clients of varied cultures and language backgrounds.

(vi) Student's learnings of language and cultural influences in their practice and how they have negotiated this in OT practice.

Students responded to these questions and shared their fieldwork experiences of the past three years. Furthermore, probes were used to elicit deep reflection of their personal experiences rather than actual observations during fieldwork.

Audio voice recordings of each focus group, with participant consent, occurred and data were transcribed verbatim by authors. Transcriptions of the focus groups were proof-read by all authors prior to being analysed, to ensure investigator triangulation of results. Qualitative data collected from the focus groups were then thematically analysed using inductive reasoning. The process of thematic analysis involved the use of four levels of coding, including initial codes, creation of subcategories, categories, and themes. Trustworthiness was achieved through examination and comparison of data collected to existing bodies of knowledge on the topic (credibility). Transferability was achieved through the authors' documentation and justification of the methodological approach and the critical processes and procedures that helped them to construct and create meaning associated with the study. Dependability was achieved through regular peer briefings which ensure analytical triangulation. These strategies allowed for validation and congruency of research findings by all team members. To ensure confirmability steps were taken by the authors to ensure that the study findings are representative of the experiences of the participants' rather than being influenced by the researchers [17]. Four of the authors were final year occupational therapy students at the time of the study. Therefore, steps were taken to reduce bias; these included bracketing through reflexive journaling prior to and during data collection and triangulation during the data analysis process.

Ethical clearance was obtained from the University of KwaZulu-Natal Research Ethics Committee (Ethical Approval number SHSEC 007/16). Additionally, consent to access students in this study was obtained via gatekeeper permission from the registrar of the institution. Prior to consent from participants, an information document stating participant's rights, ethics, aims, and procedures of the study was forwarded to the participants. Those that volunteered to participate signed informed consent and were assured of confidentiality and no physical or emotional risk to them and that that they could withdraw from the study at any time.

4. Findings

Demographic Profile of OT Students. Of the 21 students that participated in the study, 19 (90%) were female and two (10%) were male. The median age of the participants was 20 years. In terms of home language, 11 (52%) participants were English-speaking, eight (38%) spoke isiZulu, one (5%) spoke SiSwati, and one (5%) was Sepedi-speaking. Of the participants, 10 (48%) spoke English as a second language, 4 (19%) spoke Afrikaans as a second language, one (5%) spoke Hindi as a second language, and six (28%) identified themselves as having no second language. Identified cultures and language of participants are highlighted in Figures 2 and 3, respectively.

Seven themes emerged, of which many were common to the content of the reflexive journals of student authors. These included "culture as an influence on intervention," "culture and language on client centeredness," and "is it lost in translation." Refer to an overview of themes presented in Figure 4 and described in detail below.

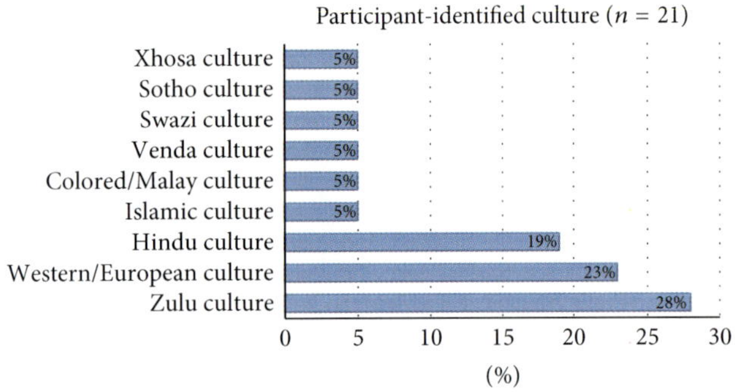

Figure 2: Participants identified culture ($n = 21$).

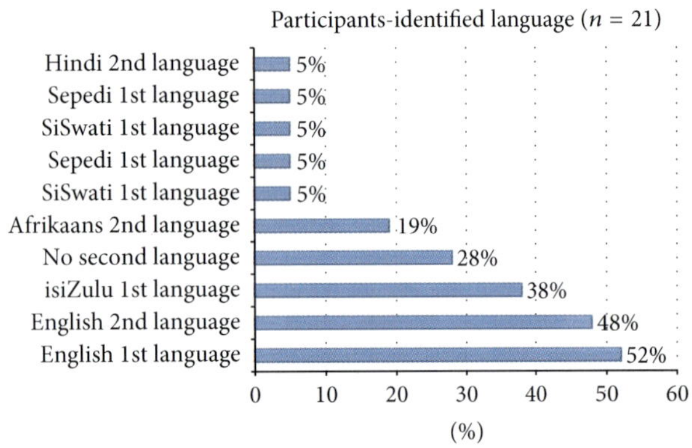

Figure 3: Participants identified language ($n = 21$).

Theme 1 (culture as an influence on intervention). Participants described culture as *"a mixture of beliefs,"* one's traditions, values, and interests. *It is "how we explain things, how we make sense of the world and everything...around us"* (Thami). This description was similar to the views expressed in the reflexive journal of four student authors which were documented prior to commencing data collection. As students, participants indicated that they had been exposed to diverse cultures both in the lectures and during service learning which had broadened their cultural knowledge and understanding: *"When I got a Zulu patient, I got to learn more about my culture, about how they...do their practices instead of how I do at home"* (Maggie). Sadie expressed that *"Even though they are the same colour as me does not mean they are the same culture."* Ashrena added that *"It gives you the opportunity to go back and learn about them and that's just increasing your knowledge into different cultures."*

Culture was further identified by participants to influence intervention both positively and negatively. *"There is some sort of emotional attachment...with people of the same culture"* (Thami) and *"They sort of take advantage of the fact that they are similar"* (Ashrena). Four student authors shared the same view; they identified culture to have a strong influence in the OT intervention.

Participants indicated that they acknowledge that culture itself is evolving. It is *"very dynamic, it changes and it differs"* (Fatima) from individual to individual and as they have grown and evolved, so has their perceptions of culture: *"...culture is changing as it goes...changing all the time"* (Sadie).

Theme 2 (the language debate). Participants understood language as the way in which they communicate and understand; it is the words and gestures used to get a message across. As Thami indicated *"...that one has a problem...I was like my goodness, the kid barely speaks...and then somebody one day was just like, oh ya, she's not from here."*

Participants, furthermore, found themselves frustrated by the linguistic barriers experienced. *"It's frustrating, not just frustrating for you, it is also frustrating for the person because they want to understand what you telling them...So it's a mutual frustration"* (Fatima).

Contrastingly, language for some participants had a positive impact on intervention; it assisted in building rapport with clients and had even resulted in participants learning a new language in order to connect to their clients. *"...It almost brought us together that all of us were talking different languages because we were all like trying to find a base that we could work from"* (Ashley). Sadie added *"working with a different language is it forces you to try and learn that language."*

Theme 3 (culture and language on client centeredness). Some participants viewed cultural and linguistic understanding within the South African context as aiding client-therapist rapport and understanding of their client's context within practice for more client directed therapy: *"Activities that we choose at the end of the day some of them have to be client centred and the only way you gonna know what your patient likes or doesn't like is if you actually communicate with them. So to make your therapy more client directed rather than therapist directed"* (Zandile).

However, majority of participants including the student authors viewed language and culture as detrimental to client centeredness when disregarded in intervention: *"I'm not familiar with games others (cultures) do. So that affects my plan of my treatment and it tends not to be client-centred but more of therapist-centred"* (Prince). Participant's further expressed that clients found comfort in familiarity which positively influenced client centeredness: *"The patient sort of gelled more with someone of the same culture as themselves... a familiarity thing"* (Thami). On the other hand, differences between the client's need and the therapists goals would result in the therapist's disregard of client centeredness: *"Because they (the client) are in need of something from you as a therapist and so they just accept whatever you may come with"* (Prince). The client's cultural and health beliefs were also perceived by participants as affecting client centeredness as one student reflects on an interaction with a client: *"...that man from Ubhumbulu sent a lightning bolt and I had a stroke so I need to go to Inyanga (*Inyanga *is a traditional healer using cultural practices to speak to ancestors) to cure"* (Thami). The participant was thus concerned that this cultural practice will affect interventions and acceptance of the therapeutic management offered.

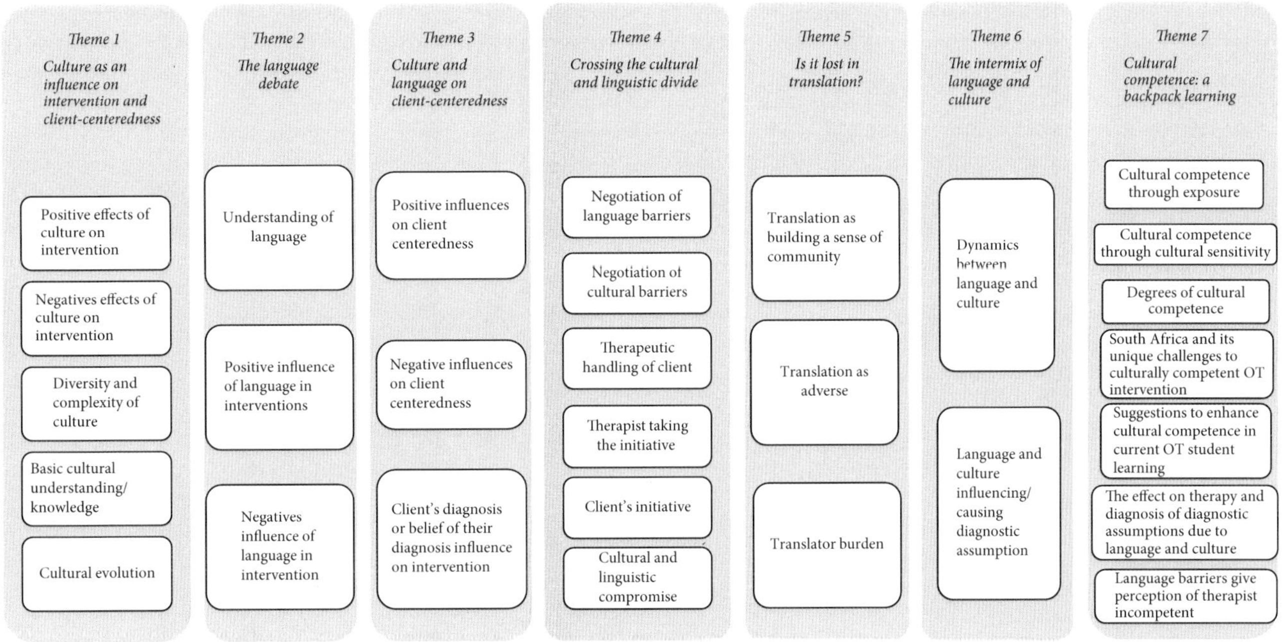

FIGURE 4: Themes and subthemes.

Theme 4 (crossing the cultural and linguistic divide). Participants made use of various strategies to negotiate language and cultural barriers which included translators, demonstration, effective handling of the client, learning written phrases, using digital applications for translation, researching language and culture, engaging with colleagues, and increasing intervention time to compensate for language barriers. Participants expressed the following:

> *A lot of it is done through body language um obviously if you get a translator that is amazing, on community I got another one of the students to write down the different instructions for me. (Ashley)*

> *I've learned (about) culture from my classmates. (Ashley)*

> *I'll go use the internet as a resource, books and other people of that culture so I just research about that. (Sadie)*

A small percentage of participants stated that research alone was not enough to bridge the cultural and linguistic gap: As Sipho indicated, *"Like do some research on it...you always get told that and then you go to Google and find a book and there's never any information about it and how it impacts therapy."*

Majority of participants, however, viewed themselves as personally responsible for taking the initiative to learn the culture and language and meet the client halfway:

> *It's up to me if I want to go deep or I want to be superficial. (Sthabile)*

> *You bring yourself down to their level, there's no 'my language' 'my culture' all of that, that's the thing, I don't think it's up to the client, I don't think it's up to the OT, I think it's up to both of you to try get there cause if one of you is not willing then it's not gonna work. (Ashley)*

Theme 5 (is it lost in translation?). Participants and two student authors highlighted the influence of translators in therapy in their attempt to be culturally competent. Translators were mostly seen to have a negative impact when attempting to build a therapeutic rapport with clients as well as resulting in therapists' exclusion which negatively influences therapeutic use of self in therapy.

> *You losing the intervention you doing coz they (the translator) then end up almost taking over. (Sipho)*

> *...the caregiver just always looks towards the translator and they actually never build that connection with you... (Shanon)*

> *Sometimes as a therapist you happen to go out of the loop which a therapist should never be. (Fatima)*

The burden placed on the translator, as viewed by the participants, was a further negative to translation:

> *...they say the long things...I'm not gonna remember everything, so I take the short cut and end up not giving the full message. (Maggie)*

> *It is difficult especially when they have their own client to treat, and they are taking the time out of all the stuff that they need to do. (Sipho)*

Theme 6 (the intermix of language and culture). Throughout the focus group discussions, participants revealed that they view language and culture as synonymous with each other or as having a dynamic influence on each other: *"There is definitely a link between language and culture even though they are 2 separate things"* (Sadie).

Participants found that they could bridge the cultural gap with language: *"To communicate with patients in their language it helps you understand their context and once you understand their context you're able to go deeper into their culture"* (Thando).

Theme 7 (cultural competence: a backpack of learning). Opinions of students varied on what it meant to be culturally competent, with majority of participants perceiving themselves as culturally incompetent, but with a willingness to engage in lifelong learning and growing towards the ideal of cultural competence: *"I don't know if you can ever be fully culturally competent but I feel like you can aspire towards cultural competence by using cultural sensitivity...it is something you should always work towards"* (Ashley). Penny indicated *"I don't even think that I am competence (competent) in all areas in my own culture."*

However, participants still displayed cultural awareness, growth, and sensitivity due to exposure to and learning of different languages and cultures: *"I am definitely cultural sensitive...I don't just barge in with who I am and what I bring"* (Sadie). Ashrena added *"As you grow with the degree and learn about more culture and you become more emotionally attached to other cultures as well."*

Majority of students felt that they had been provided with appropriate information and exposure to cultures and language during their training but some students including student authors still viewed this as insufficient: *"We get into the OT course and then we experience all these cultural forms and diversity, but it's not deep enough, we don't know deep enough"* (Sthabile). Phindile felt that this process is complex, *"...for the course teaching us about being competent, it's not that simple or easy."*

Cultural competence in occupational therapy practice specific to the South African context was found to challenge students: *"I also think with the tests we have....they are like not adapted for everyone...they don't incorporate everyone there is in South Africa"* (Prince). Sarah added *"It has been tough working with such a diverse population."*

5. Discussion

The findings of this study indicate that the student cohort who formed the study sample have been exposed to varied cultures through their undergraduate training. Cultural differences were found to negatively affect intervention, where, in some cases, clients refused intervention due to the cultural difference thus causing frustration for both the participants and their clients. These findings are aligned to other findings from a study by Mabuza et al. [18] on community placement areas of South African Universities, in which he demonstrated that, in some instances due to cultural or religious norms, treatment was often refused. Additionally, a study conducted by Levin [19] identified that cultural misinterpretation occurred, so did negative attitudes between the therapist and client, in some therapist-client encounters. However, culture was viewed by participants as having positive implications on intervention where it had improved rapport, intervention, and therapist's cultural knowledge, through exposure to various cultures. Consequently, this was influenced most often by the therapist's initiative in the interventions and in establishing rapport with clients that they encountered.

Language is considered to provide the means by which humans communicate, and communication plays a pivotal role in the health profession in developing trust and cooperation between the practitioner and client [20]. This is in keeping with findings of this study which highlighted that when trying to speak the client's language, participants noted positive changes in the client-therapist rapport building. It forced participants to learn a language to improve their intervention. Language was still, however, the greatest concern of the participants as this barrier negatively impacts intervention and their ability to be culturally competent. Participants found therapeutic opportunities were missed and the intervention provided was superficial or even incorrect. The findings are consistent with those of Ong et al. [21] and Schlemmer and Mash [22] who found that patient care and clinical outcomes suffered due to the language barrier. It is noteworthy to the authors to note the lack of distinction between language and culture in the study where students viewed both of these concepts as one entity or as one influencing the other. This corresponds with the literature that highlights that language is a primary purveyor of culture and the connection between language and culture is extensively rooted [20].

Occupational therapists view clients holistically, taking into account their linguistic and cultural context in order to create a client centred intervention. Majority of participants showed that when communicating effectively they were able to provide client centred intervention which was similarly found in a study conducted on occupational therapy students in the University of Free State in South Africa [4]. It is of a concern that some participants struggling with linguistic and cultural understanding were unable to provide the client centred therapy they felt their clients deserved. Furthermore, failure to consider a client's identified problems was noted by a few participants resulting in inaccurate history taking and misinterpretation of diagnosis which has also been well documented in the literature [23, 24]. This disregard for client centeredness, in most of the cases reported, would result in the acceptance of the student's cultural incompetence by the client due to client desperation and need for their help. It is thus important that practitioners find a way to cross the linguistic and cultural divide to meet the needs of the people with whom they work [7]. Whilst therapists try to bridge the cultural divide, they may consider that clients often "warm up" to therapists of similar culture which positively influences client centeredness as noted in this study. This could be essential where rapport is difficult to build. Furthermore, in bridging the gap between language and culture, cultural brokering which serves as a mediator is said to be valuable [25]. Responses from participants revealed the use of this technique as well as various other measures to bridge the gap of a cultural or linguistic divide, which included use of translators, use of research, and use of body language. Using translation was found to be useful in intervention for some, however, majority reported that it resulted in dilution of the information and therapist exclusion from the intervention process. Other studies [11, 26] also found that the use of translators affected rapport and accuracy of data being translated making it superficial, thus, impeding on assessment and intervention outcomes. The most notable finding was in the ability of students to take the initiative to learn the language of their clients for improved therapeutic outcomes. This is similar to a study by Tjale and De Villiers [27] that highlighted that self-empowerment in terms of culture and language was a factor that enables the health practitioner to provide effective intervention, as this encourages client's willingness to participate and influences positive rapport with clients.

Overall this cohort of students showed cultural sensitivity and understood cultures as diverse, forever evolving, complex, and specific to each individual. This alone showed a high level of precultural competence according to Cross [12] cultural competence model. Students however viewed themselves as generally culturally incompetent. Cheung et al. [15] study found that the majority of students reported having limited exposure to other cultures and insufficient training in cultural competence.

Two similar studies [4, 5], from a South African perceptive, also showed that students felt they did not have enough exposure to cultural issues in both university-based education and fieldwork. Students in these studies did not feel sufficiently equipped with respect to cultural competence as a result of the occupational therapy curricula at their institutions. These findings are in contrast to the findings of this study as participants suggested they had felt prepared through exposure and training at this particular institution. Wohl [28] suggested that health practitioners may not fully know all their client's cultural customs and attitudes; they become equipped through experience as they become exposed. These findings [28] support the participant's responses that cultural competence may not be fully obtained but enhanced through exposure to various cultures and that it is a continuous learning journey of collecting knowledge as they experience it, carrying this knowledge into all their practice, as expressed by one participant *"it's like a little backpack you carry with you everywhere"*.

6. Conclusion

In this study, the authors aimed to explore the perspectives of final year occupational therapy students on the issue of cultural competence. Whilst occupational therapy students are exposed to diverse languages and cultures in various fieldwork placements within their undergraduate training, students still viewed themselves as being culturally incompetent. Instead, students displayed cultural sensitivity, due to the belief that culture and its many subcultures are too diverse and evolving to ever reach an ideal state of cultural competence. Cultural incompetence related to language barriers and misunderstanding of the client's culture have been viewed as negatively influencing the intervention process specifically in rapport building, accurate assessments, and client centred activity choices. The negative influence of cultural incompetence could be exacerbated when attending to difficult clients. However, clients of similar culture to their therapists often build rapport easily; therefore, situations where therapists of similar culture act as mediators can be considered a step closer to client centeredness intervention. The authors found that participants use the term language and culture interchangeably indicating a strong perceived link between language and culture as influencing their ability to achieve cultural competence and client centred intervention. Participants thus viewed it as essential to take responsibility or initiative to deal with linguistic and cultural barriers to achieve cultural sensitivity and strive towards cultural competence. Negotiation of barriers was found to include body language, use of translators, research on the Internet, and learning from others. Participants were thus found to show cultural awareness and cultural sensitivity on a precultural competence level in this study. As a way forward further studies can address how cultural competence is enacted in daily practice of occupational therapists; there may also be the need for adaptations to existing OT curricula on cultural competence in more formal ways to ensure a more comprehensive understanding of the concept by exploring terms such as cultural awareness, cultural sensitivity, and cultural knowledge. Finally, we encourage the occupational therapy community to engage in critical debate on whether a state of cultural competence may ever be possible within occupational therapy practice and how this may contribute to the professions identity.

7. Limitations of the Study

The study was limited to one cohort of students in a particular context and the authors did not assess or observe actual behaviours of the students within the framework of cultural competence. Thus, participants may have recalled and expressed their experiences differently to their actual behaviour or attitudes.

References

[1] B. Richardson and B. Smith, "Communication in occupational therapy during diagnosis & treatment using the case study of an injured violinist," http://mathcs.ups.edu/~bryans/Current/Journal_Spring_2009/BRichardson_2009.pdf, 2009.

[2] J. M. Lum, A. P. Williams, S. Rappolt, M. D. Landry, R. Deber, and M. Verrier, "Meeting the challenge of diversity: results

from the 2003 survey of occupational therapists in Ontario," *Occupational Therapy Now*, vol. 6, no. 4, pp. 13–17, 2004.
[3] C. Penn, "Factors affecting he success of mediated medical interviews in South Africa," *Current Allergy & Clinical Immunology*, vol. 20, no. 2, pp. 66–71, 2007.
[4] E. J. van Rensburg, T. van der Merwe, and M. Nel, "Cultural competence among occupational therapy students at the University of the Free State, South Africa," *Acta Academica*, vol. 44, no. 3, pp. 119–155, 2012.
[5] A. E. Leendertz, *Cultural competency: perceptions of South African trained occupational therapists [Ph.D. thesis]*, 2013.
[6] S. M. Lee, *A Review of Language and Other Communication Barriers in Health Care*, US Department of Health and Human Services, Portland, Ore, USA, 2003.
[7] M. E. Levin, "Language as a barrier to care for Xhosa-speaking patients at a South African paediatric teaching hospital," *South African Medical Journal*, vol. 96, no. 10, pp. 1076–1079, 2006.
[8] S. E. Moore, "Cultural sensitivity treatment and research issues with black adolescent drug users," *Child & Adolescent Social Work Journal*, vol. 9, no. 3, pp. 249–260, 1992.
[9] Occupational Therapy Association of South Africa, *Code of Ethics and Professional Conduct*, OTASA, Cape Town, South Africa, 2005, http://coteceurope.eu/COTEC%20Docs/Publications/Reference_list.pdf.
[10] K. L. Ulrey and P. Amason, "Intercultural communication between patients and health care providers: An exploration of intercultural communication effectiveness, cultural sensitivity, stress, and anxiety," *Health Communication*, vol. 13, no. 4, pp. 449–463, 2001.
[11] R. Murden, A. Norman, J. Ross, E. Sturdivant, M. Kedia, and S. Shah, "Occupational therapy students' perceptions of their cultural awareness and competency," *Occupational Therapy International*, vol. 15, no. 3, pp. 191–203, 2008.
[12] T. L. Cross, "Towards a culturally competent system of care: a monograph on effective services for minority children who are severely emotionally disturbed," https://eric.ed.gov/?id=ED330171, 1989.
[13] P. Wittman and B. P. Velde, "Attaining cultural competence, critical thinking, and intellectual development: A challenge for occupational therapists," *American Journal of Occupational Therapy*, vol. 56, no. 4, pp. 454–456, 2002.
[14] J. P. Muñoz, "Culturally responsive caring in occupational therapy," *Occupational Therapy International*, vol. 14, no. 4, pp. 256–280, 2007.
[15] Y. Cheung, S. Shah, and S. Muncer, "An exploratory investigation of undergraduate students' perceptions of cultural awareness," *The British Journal of Occupational Therapy*, vol. 65, no. 12, pp. 543–550, 2002.
[16] J. Hornberger, H. Itakura, and S. R. Wilson, "Bridging language and cultural barriers between physicians and patients," *Public Health Reports*, vol. 112, no. 5, pp. 410–417, 1997.
[17] A. K. Shenton, "Strategies for ensuring trustworthiness in qualitative research projects," *Education for Information*, vol. 22, no. 2, pp. 63–75, 2004.
[18] L. H. Mabuza, P. Diab, S. Reid et al., "Communities' views, attitudes and recommendations on community-based education of undergraduate health sciences students in South Africa: a qualitative study," *African Journal of Primary Health Care and Family Medicine*, vol. 5, no. 1, article 456, 2013.
[19] M. E. Levin, "Impact of language and culture on the quality of medical communication and care," *Current Allergy and Clinical Immunology*, vol. 20, no. 2, article 54, 2007.
[20] A. Bischoff, P. A. Bovier, R. Isah, G. Françoise, E. Ariel, and L. Louis, "Language barriers between nurses and asylum seekers: their impact on symptom reporting and referral," *Social Science and Medicine*, vol. 57, no. 3, pp. 503–512, 2003.
[21] L. M. Ong, J. C. De Haes, A. M. Hoos, and F. B. Lammes, "Doctor-patient communication: a review of the literature," *Social Science & Medicine*, vol. 40, no. 7, pp. 903–918, 1995.
[22] A. Schlemmer and B. Mash, "The effects of a language barrier in a South African district hospital," *South African Medical Journal*, vol. 96, no. 10, pp. 1084–1087, 2006.
[23] C. Watson, "Why warriors lie down and die: towards an understanding of why the Aboriginal people of Arnhem Land face the greatest crisis in health and education since European contact: R. Trudgen," *Australian Journal of Rural Health*, vol. 9, no. 3, pp. 141-142, 2001.
[24] G. Flores, "Culture and the patient-physician relationship: achieving cultural competency in health care," *Journal of Pediatrics*, vol. 136, no. 1, pp. 14–23, 2000.
[25] K. Singleton and E. Krause, "Understanding cultural and linguistic barriers to health literacy," *The Online Journal of Issues in Nursing*, vol. 14, no. 3, 2009.
[26] O. Carrasquillo, E. J. Orav, T. A. Brennan, and H. R. Burstin, "Impact of language barriers on patient satisfaction in an emergency department," *Journal of General Internal Medicine*, vol. 14, no. 2, pp. 82–87, 1999.
[27] A. Tjale and L. De Villiers, *Cultural Issues in Health and Health Care: A Resource Book for Southern Africa*, Juta and Company, 2004.
[28] J. Wohl, "Integration of cultural awareness into psychotherapy," *American Journal of Psychotherapy*, vol. 43, no. 3, pp. 343–355, 1989.

15

A Systematic Review of Translation and Cross-Cultural Adaptation of Instruments for the Selection of Assistive Technologies

Bárbara Iansã de Lima Barroso,[1] **Cláudia Regina Cabral Galvão**,[1] **Luiz Bueno da Silva**,[2] **and Selma Lancman**[3]

[1]*Graduate Student of the Graduate Program in Rehabilitation Sciences, Faculty of Medicine FMUSP, University of São Paulo, São Paulo, SP, Brazil*
[2]*Professor of the Postgraduate Program in Production Engineering, Federal University of Paraíba UFPB, João Pessoa, PB, Brazil*
[3]*Professor of the Postgraduate Program in Rehabilitation Sciences. Faculty of Medicine FMUSP, University of São Paulo, São Paulo, SP, Brazil*

Correspondence should be addressed to Bárbara Iansã de Lima Barroso; barbarabarroso@yahoo.com.br

Academic Editor: Lynette Mackenzie

This article presents a systematic review, for which research was carried out in the following electronic databases: Web of Science, Scopus, PubMed, and ERIC, in which several articles were found ($n = 560$). The results were analyzed based on the information obtained in the titles and abstracts, and the remaining studies were read in full for the analysis. The aim of this article was to identify the different questionnaires used for selecting items of assistive technology, describe and evaluate the translation and transcultural adaptation procedures, characterize the thematic domains of each resource, evaluate the cultural adaptation process adopted, and describe the psychometric properties. Data extraction and evaluation of the methodological quality of the eligible studies were performed in accordance with the COSMIN verification list with a checklist of 4 points. The publication of systematic review studies and others that synthesize research results is fundamental to provide support for change in the behavior of professionals in the field of health, and not only to access the available literature but also to incorporate this information into daily clinical practice. The results of this review could provide subsidies that would enable the planning, execution, identification, and choice of specific instruments for a determined study within the context of assistive technology, with a view to helping researchers and health professionals in clinical and investigatory practices.

1. Introduction

According to the World Health Organization (WHO, 2008) [1], approximately 10% of the world population has some type of deficiency, and, of this total, only 3% of them require rehabilitation and receive some aid in underdeveloped countries. In Brazil, disability affects 23.9% of the population (IBGE, 2010) [2].

In 2001, the WHO approved the classification system—International Classification of Functioning, Disability and Health (ICF)—which is a tool for understanding human functionality and incapacity, recommended for identifying structural and environmental conditions and personal characteristics that interfere with functionality [3]. This has changed the approach based on diseases and prioritizes focus on functionality and autonomy [4].

Considering the functions of the human body, autonomy mainly involves each individual's capacity to care for themselves: performing tasks enabling them to adapt to situations and take responsibility for their own acts, thereby improving their mobility, communication, and autonomy; reinforcing their social participation, professional productivity, and sense of control of their own lives [3].

Measurement instruments were used to obtain standardized data that enabled comparison of results between different populations [5], and they are an economic and effective way to acquire reliable and valid measurement results [6]. These instruments transform subjective measurements into quantifiable objective data that can be analyzed, enabling verification of the impacts on health intervention processes, and comparisons would therefore require fewer financial resources.

Researchers conducting exploratory researches have to decide whether to use previously developed instruments or to construct one specifically suited to their studies. As the process of creating a new instrument is complex, and provided that there are validated instruments for assessing the same phenomenon, the process of translation and adaptation to the desired culture is recommended [7].

Cook and Polgar [8] defined assistive technology as the science that deals with the application of any item, part, equipment, service, or product system of high or low technology that is commercially acquired, modified, or custom-made, and which is used for increasing, maintaining, promoting, or developing the functional capacity of disabled people.

Compared with other North American and European countries, Brazil has few instruments to help researchers and professionals in the field of rehabilitation with the process of prescribing, indicating, and selecting assistive technology items. Evaluation and rehabilitation processes have limitations, since achieving their real objectives is known to depend on the adequate selection and use of suitable instruments. To use the evaluation instruments available in the literature in assistive technology and in other areas of health, they must be suited to the purpose by following the guidelines for cultural adaptation, translation, and test measurement properties [4, 9–11]. However, to use in a new different country, culture, and/or language, cultural adaptation requires a methodology making it possible to achieve: equivalence [10], solving cultural and idiomatic differences, and a process for standardization and validation of the measurement properties [4, 12, 13].

Cultural adaptation must result in a reliable valid instrument, similar to the original, capable of being used as a reference in clinical research and replicated in different cultures; i.e., a tool that can be used to compare results obtained in different countries [5]. The influential cultural, psychosocial, financial, physiological, and biomechanical factors of distinct cultures must be sufficiently understood to help rehabilitation professionals make decisions during therapeutic processes [9, 11].

In this article, we proposed to conduct a systematic review to identify different questionnaires used for selecting assistive technology items, describe and evaluate translation and transcultural adaptation procedures and evaluate the process adopted, characterize the thematic domains of each instrument and describe the psychometric properties found in the studies [11, 12]. This review may result in subsidies for planning, identifying, and choosing specific instruments for a determined study, within the context of assistive technology, and be helpful to researchers and health professionals in their clinical and investigatory practices.

2. Materials and Methods

This bibliographic research was defined as a systematic review. To conduct this research, the authors adopted the Preferred Reporting Items for Systematic Reviews and Meta-Analyses (PRISMA) criteria. According to Liberati et al. [14], PRISMA assists systematic review writing and is essential for precisely and reliably summarizing proofs of the efficacy and safety of health interventions.

The literature search was performed during two periods between 19th July, 2016 and 31st August, 2017 (the date it was updated), and there was a manual addition of them between 6th and 12th of July, 2018, updating the files of this review.

According to the PRISMA-P committee guidelines [15], this research was registered with the International Prospective Register of Systematic Reviews (PROSPERO) on 19th July, 2016 and updated on 31st August, 2017. Registration number CRD42016043065.

Although the PRISMA recommendations were primarily developed for textual presentation of systematic reviews of interventions, studies of prognosis [16] and clinical diagnosis [17], transcultural adaptations [18], measurement properties [19], and others [11, 20] have used them extensively.

2.1. Search Strategy. The following electronic databases were sequentially searched for articles, without any language restriction: Web of Science, Scopus, PubMed/MEDLINE, and the Educational Resources Information Center (ERIC), with terms used based on Medical Subject Headings (MeSH) descriptors. The literary bibliography was searched using the following descriptors: "Assistive technology" AND "Cross-cultural adaptation" OR "Assistive technology device" AND "Translation" OR "Validation" AND "Successful Rehabilitation" OR "Assistive technology selection". Variations in the descriptors served to find a broader range of significant results for this research.

2.2. Inclusion and Exclusion Criteria. The inclusion criteria adopted were as follows: articles must be indexed in the selected data bases, be available in the free form of the text, written in any language, they must not have data filters, be without restrictions relative to the manuscript's place of origin, and without exclusion criteria due to language in the translation and cultural adaptation process.

Due to the inclusion and exclusion criteria employed in our systematic review, a small number of articles [21–25] were not included in our overall sample ($n = 560$). Therefore, the findings of these articles were not included in our final analysis. Given our large article sample, we do not anticipate that this omission caused any substantial change in our results. Yet, to mitigate this issue, we intend to include these articles in a future review to measure their specific impact.

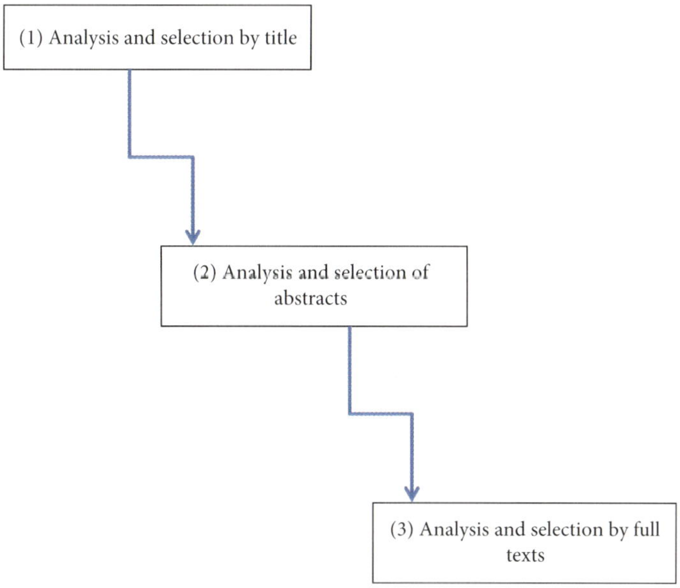

FIGURE 1: The selection process hierarchically included the following strategies.

2.3. Eligibility Criteria—Selection of Studies. The studies considered and fulfilled the following criteria: (1) quantitative cross-sectional researches and (2) studies investigating the translation and cross-cultural adaptation process of instruments for selecting assistive technology for disabled people.

2.4. Data Extraction and Quality Evaluation. Two researchers screened paper titles and abstracts and applied the eligibility criteria. The papers that did not meet the eligibility criteria were excluded. The selection process hierarchically included the following strategies: (1) analysis and selection by title, (2) analysis and selection of abstracts, and (3) analysis and selection by full texts (Figure 1).

One reviewer extracted the data independently at the time of the search and again after the data analysis. Subsequently, a second researcher independently analyzed and reviewed the data. Consequently, no third reviewer or final arbitration was required. One researcher conducted data extraction of all eligible studies, which were summarized in table depicting their descriptive characteristics.

Data was extracted with the purpose of finding out how the translation, cross-cultural adaptation procedures, and all measurement properties of each study included were performed. Moreover, Consensus-based Standards for selecting health Measurement Instruments (COSMIN) [4] were used to classify the translation, cross-cultural adaptation procedures, and psychometric measurement properties, respectively. The evidence of validity was analyzed according to the following criteria [4, 5, 10, 13, 14, 17, 20]: for internal consistency, Cronbach's alpha >0.70 (ideal) [4, 5, 20, 26], and also in accordance with the COSMIN guidelines [4, 12].

2.5. Consensus-Based Standards for Selecting Health Measurement Instruments (COSMIN). In the literature, the taxonomy of measurement properties presented a great variety; however, in this study, the authors used the definitions proposed by COSMIN to evaluate the psychometric properties of instruments. The authors chose to describe the test performed, results and criteria for evaluating the psychometric properties of instruments developed, adapted, and validated [4, 5, 13, 27].

A 4-point classification scale was used to mark and classify the methodological quality of each measurement property: (A) internal consistency, (B) reliability, (C) measurement error, (D) content validity, (E) structural validity, (F) hypothesis tests, (G) cross-cultural validity, (H) criterion validity, and (I) responsiveness. Each box was finally classified by the lowest score attributed to any of the items [4, 13, 28]. Apart from the above-mentioned boxes, another field had to be completed for each measurement property, with the aim of identifying the population's clinical-epidemiological profile, analyzing mean age, distribution by gender, disease characteristics, country of origin, and language [4, 28–30].

3. Results

In the initial research, 560 potentially eligible studies were identified in the systematic review (Figure 2). Of these, 319 were excluded because they were duplicates; 241 remained, of which 210 were discarded after reading the title and abstract, leaving 22 studies. Of these, two were excluded because they were not available in full. Thus, the 20 remaining studies were read in full, after which 15 were discarded because they did not fit in with the eligibility criteria. Finally, only five researches were included in the qualitative synthesis because they fulfilled the inclusion criteria.

The five studies of translation and cross-cultural adaptation evaluated after reading the full texts were the following: Quebec User Evaluation of Satisfaction with Assistive Technology (QUEST 2.0), translated and adapted from English into Brazilian Portuguese [31]; Psychosocial Impact of Assistive Devices Scale (PIADS), from English into Canadian

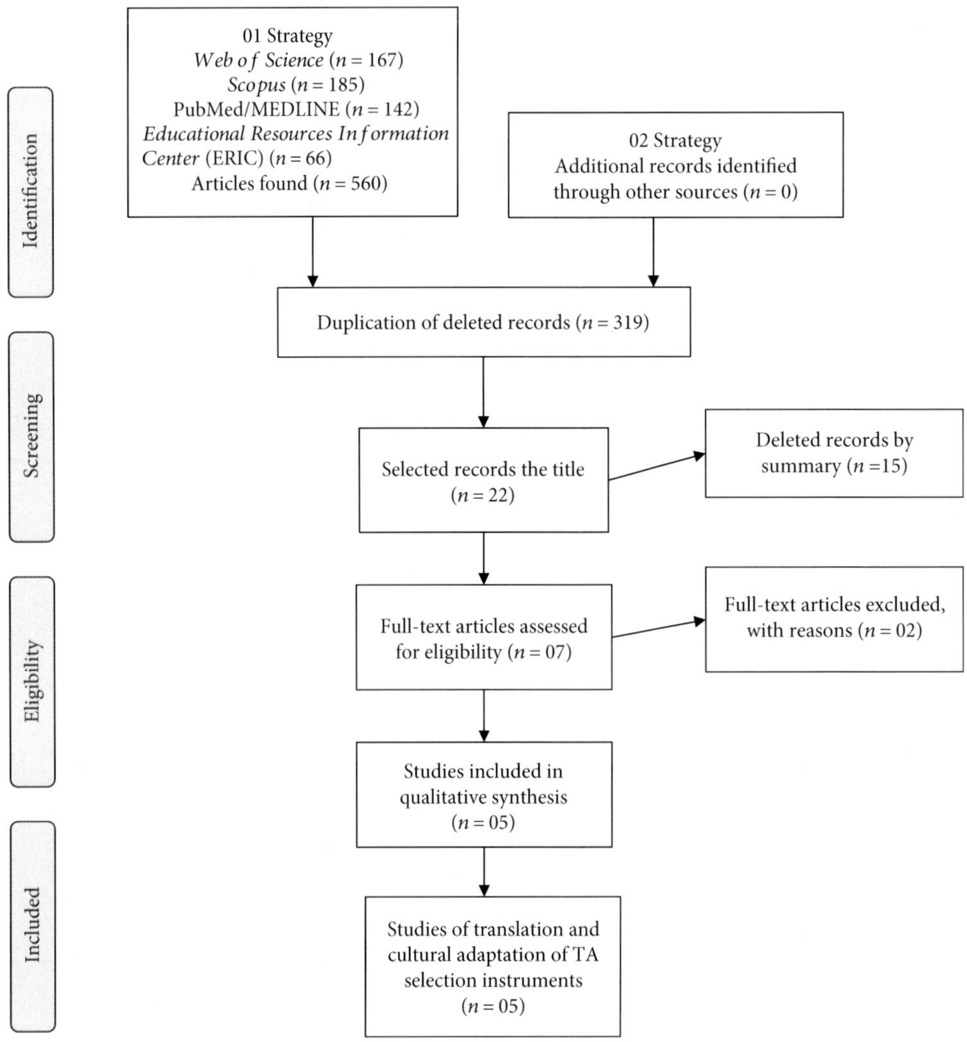

FIGURE 2: PRISMA 2009 Flow Diagram—selection process for the studies included in the analysis.

French [32]; Quebec User Evaluation of Satisfaction with Assistive Technology 1.0 (QUEST1.0), from English into Danish [33]; Family Impact of Assistive Technology Scale, from English into Turkish [34]; and Quebec User Evaluation of Satisfaction with Assistive Technology (QUEST 2.0), from English into Chinese (Mandarin) and adapted to Taiwanese [35], as demonstrated in Table 1.

In Table 2, the translations and transcultural adaptations evaluated were presented according to the guidelines proposed by Mokkink et al.—COSMIN committee [4, 12].

3.1. Internal Consistency. The five instruments [31–35] were tested for internal consistency; however, only three [32, 34, 35] were classified as "excellent", because they fulfilled the COSMIN requisites. The translation and validation of the Quebec User Evaluation of Satisfaction with Assistive Technology (QUEST 2.0) [31], translated from English into Portuguese, was classified as "good", because it had partially completed the checklist of the guidelines. The methodological quality of the Quebec User Evaluation of Satisfaction with Assistive Technology (QUEST 1.0) [33] was "fair" in all the subclassification of (Box A).

The intraclass correlation coefficient (ICC) and Cronbach's alpha (α) were used to evaluate the reliability and internal consistency in the majority of the studies selected in this review [31, 32, 34, 35], and ρ for Cronbach's alpha ($\alpha = 0.70$) was adopted as the minimum acceptable value [32].

One research [35] also used Cronbach's alpha relative to the ICC values; four studies performed the test [31, 32, 34, 35], and the value ≥ 0.70 was appropriately obtained [35]. The ICC demonstrated an error of measurement and agreement, as the relationship between the true and the observed variance. There was no consensus regarding the value the ICC indicated as an acceptable degree of reliability; however, the majority of the authors agreed that to appropriate values, at least (≥ 0.70) was required [11, 26, 30].

The study "Translation and validation of the Quebec User Evaluation of Satisfaction with Assistive Technology" (QUEST 2.0) [31], translated from English into Brazilian Portuguese, and the "Translation, cross-cultural adaptation, and content validation of the QUEST 1.0" [33] did not present the reproducibility/reliability tests of the instruments.

Table 1: Translation and cross-cultural adaptations [4, 6, 10, 12].

Authors/year	Assistive technology tools	Language	Sample	Translation	Synthesis	Back translation	Expert committee review	Pretesting
de Carvalho et al. [31]/2014.	Quebec User Evaluation of Satisfaction with Assistive Technology (QUEST 2.0)	From English to Brazilian Portuguese	121	+	+	+	+	+
Demers et al. [32]/2002.	Psychosocial Impact of Assistive Devices Scale (PIADS)	From English to French Canadian	304	+	+	+	+	+
Brandt [33]/2005.	Quebec User Evaluation of Satisfaction with Assistive Technology (QUEST 1.0)	North American English to Danish	10	+	+	+	+	+
Bek et al. [34]/2012.	Family Impact of Assistive Technology Scale (FIATS)	North American English into Turkish	55	+	+	+	+	+
Mao et al. [35]/2010.	Quebec User Evaluation of Satisfaction with Assistive Technology (QUEST 2.0)	From English to Chinese (Mandarin)	105	+	+	+	+	+

+ = positive rating; − = negative rating; 0 = no information available; ? = unclear.

In order to know more about the ICC of QUEST 2.0 [31], the authors of this review sent e-mails to the main authors, asking about the application of the ICC and/or Kappa to measure the internal consistency and/or other forms for evaluating the point at which individuals could be distinguished from one another in spite of measurement errors. The author sent her dissertation data, informing that she used test (a) to evaluate the internal consistency of the instrument, which indicated the level of the instrument, or of the questions of which it was composed, and that it was sensitive in capturing the change in values after removing each item [36]. For this systematic review, this data was not tabulated because, according to [4], it was not available in the article analyzed [31].

3.2. Reliability. The reliability of all the instruments was tested. The Quebec User Evaluation of Satisfaction with Assistive Technology (QUEST 1.0) [33] was classified as "poor" because it used a sample below the number ($n = 10$) indicated and did not apply the statistical methods indicated.

The test-retest ICC reliability of the Turkish version of the Family Impact of Assistive Technology Scale (FIATS) [34], translated and validated from North American English into Turkish ($n = 55$), obtained the validity and reliability score of 0.931 (95% 0.881–0.960), with an excellent estimate. The Psychosocial Impact of Assistive Devices Scale (PIADS) [32] instrument, translated and validated from North American English into Canadian French ($n = 304$), achieved good stability in the ICC (0.77–0.90) and internal consistency (0.75–0.94) tests. For the Quebec User Evaluation of Satisfaction with Assistive Technology (QUEST 2.0) [31] instrument, translated and validated from North American English into Brazilian Portuguese ($n = 121$), the test-retest stability, which was performed two months later, was analyzed by the Spearman correlation test, demonstrating a high correlation ($\rho > 0.6$) for the majority of the items. These three instruments [31, 32, 34] were classified as "good".

The Quebec User Evaluation of Satisfaction with Assistive Technology (QUEST 2.0) [35], translated from North American English into Chinese (mandarin) ($n = 105$), although it specifically achieved an ICC of (0.90, 0.97, 0.95), positive total scores of the device, services and T-QUEST, and good test-retest stability were classified as "good".

Further, to the Taiwanese QUEST 2.0 [35], the exploratory factorial analysis revealed that the T-QUEST had a two-factor structure for the service device and construction of user satisfaction, which constituted 53.42% of the variance explained.

3.3. Measurement Error. Measurement error was verified in all the instruments, and only three were considered "excellent"—PIADS [32], FIATS [34], and QUEST 2.0—translated from North American English into Chinese (mandarin) [35].

Further, to the Quebec User Evaluation of Satisfaction with Assistive Technology (QUEST 2.0) [31], despite the appropriate sample number ($n = 121$) indicated by the guidelines (≥100) [4, 12], the statistical quality was classified as "fair". Whereas, the Quebec User Evaluation of Satisfaction with Assistive Technology (QUEST 1.0) [33] was classified as "poor", due to the sample ($n = 10$) and lack of statistical tests.

3.4. Content Validity. The content validity was analyzed in the five articles; however, there was a difference related to the COSMIN checklist score. The manuscript [33] was classified as "fair", due to small methodological failures in the study presentation. The researches [31, 32] were classified as "good", and the studies [34, 35] as "excellent"; therefore, they achieved positive points in the entire checklist.

3.5. Structural Validity. After verification, the article [33] was classified as "poor", because it presented no statistical resources. The research [31] was classified as "good" and the studies [32, 34, 35] as "excellent". These results represented

TABLE 2: Evaluation of the methodological quality of the included studies through the COSMIN checklist with 4-point rating scale: consensus-based standard for the selection of health measurement instruments [4, 12].

Instruments	Authors/year/language	Internal consistency (A)	Reliability (B)	Measurement error (C)	Content validity (D)	Structural validity (E)	Cross-cultural validity (G)	Criterion validity (H)	Responsiveness (I)
Quebec User Evaluation of Satisfaction with Assistive Technology (QUEST 2.0)	de Carvalho et al. [31]/2014. From English to Brazilian Portuguese	Good	Good	Fair	Good	Good	Excellent	Good	Good
Psychosocial Impact of Assistive Devices Scale (PIADS)	Demers et al. [32]/2002. From English to French Canadian	Excellent	Good	Excellent	Good	Excellent	Excellent	Excellent	Excellent
Quebec User Evaluation of Satisfaction with Assistive Technology (QUEST 1.0)	Brandt [33]/2005. North American English to Danish	Fair	Poor	Poor	Fair	Poor	Good	Poor	Poor
Family Impact of Assistive Technology Scale (FIATS)	Bek et al. [34]/2012. North American English into Turkish	Excellent	Good	Excellent	Excellent	Excellent	Excellent	Excellent	Excellent
Quebec User Evaluation of Satisfaction with Assistive Technology (QUEST 2.0)	Mao et al. [35]/2010. From English to Chinese (Mandarin)	Excellent	Good	Excellent	Excellent	Excellent	Excellent	Excellent	Excellent

The following property was not used in the study: box F. Hypotheses testing.

excellent structural validity for all the questions tested in these instruments.

3.6. Cross-Cultural Validity. The field for transcultural validity received the highest positive value among the items analyzed. Four instruments were adapted to their respective cultures: Brazilian [31], Canadian [32], Turkish [34], and Chinese [35], according to the method recommended [4, 12] and were classified as "excellent".

The Quebec User Evaluation of Satisfaction with Assistive Technology (QUEST 1.0) [33] transcultural adaptation was classified as "good", although its sample size was inadequate (<50).

3.7. Criterion Validity. The Quebec User Evaluation of Satisfaction with Assistive Technology (QUEST 1.0) [33] was classified as "poor", due to the sample's size (<50), lack of statistical analyses, and other measures of interpretability, with the clinically important minimum difference.

The ceiling and floor effects, reflecting interpretability of the questions, were verified in the Quebec User Evaluation of Satisfaction with Assistive Technology (QUEST 2.0) instrument [31], which was classified as "good". The reliability or internal consistency of the instrument items was tested by Cronbach's alpha coefficient for each factor, for each item removed, and for total score. The Spearman correlation was used to analyze precision during the test-retest procedure, showing a relationship between the first and second applications of the instrument, thus corroborating Nunnally's psychometric theory [31, 37], which recommends a minimum of ten individuals for each existent item in a scale. In this research, the sample consisted of ($n = 121$).

The Psychosocial Impact of Assistive Devices Scale (PIADS) [32], Family Impact of Assistive Technology Scale (FIATS) [34], and Chinese Quebec User Evaluation of Satisfaction with Assistive Technology (QUEST 2.0) [35] instruments were classified as "excellent". Their hypotheses and statistical methods were formulated and tested.

3.8. Responsiveness. In this item, the article [33] was classified as "poor", the research [31] as "good", and the studies [32, 34, 35] as "excellent".

4. Discussion

The World Health Organization (WHO) recommends the translation and cross-cultural adaptation of the existent instruments available for selection, into different languages and cultures, thereby favoring communication between different researchers and the comparison of data obtained at an international level [38].

Standardized assessments are the tools that facilitate the process of prescribing and monitoring the use of assistive technology resources in occupational therapy and other professions. They favor the understanding of the demands of the subjects and allow professionals to identify which important areas will be considered in an evaluation process, and the degree of satisfaction and functional improvement after a certain period of use of the AT device [39].

The use of a standardized evaluation allows the foundation of new research and the development of products, as well as the verification of its impact in the formulation of public policies and the identification of the sustainability of rehabilitation programs in assistive technology. The results produced, when valid and reliable, favor the credibility of the professional area for the generation of the measured results and their influences [39–42].

The systematic review of the properties of measurement is a process in which the content and properties of measurements by the measurement instruments are critically and comparatively evaluated in detail. The systematic reviews of these properties are useful tools for selecting a measurement instrument for a certain purpose [26].

Five different studies [31–35] were found, of which three concerned the same instrument of assistive technology selection: the Quebec User Evaluation of Satisfaction with Assistive Technology (QUEST)—one, in version 1.0, and two, in version 2.0. In all of the five articles, some of their measurement properties were tested. However, the use of an instrument in a new country or a new culture—albeit within the same country—requires a method that guarantees equivalence between the original versions. Therefore, the instrument content must undergo cross-cultural adaptation and validation to guarantee maximum faithfulness [4, 6, 10, 12, 13, 33].

The COSMIN initiative was created in 2005, which was inspired by the lack of clarity in the literature about terminologies and definitions of measurement properties. A large number of instruments for the measurement of results—many of them similar—are used for measuring the same mechanisms developed with focus on the same population of patients, with criteria that are not always coherent with the culture and the need for the local population to be researched and/or attended [4, 12].

The COSMIN checklist may be used to evaluate the methodological quality of studies regarding the properties of measurement of health status or to compare their properties in various measurement instruments during a systematic review. The methodological quality of the high- and low-quality studies selected must be analyzed and possible bias indicated [4, 43].

As far as the stages of translation and cross-cultural adaptation proposed by [4, 12] are concerned (these are presented in Table 2), all the measurement properties were checked. For Coster and Mancini [7]and Guillemin et al. [10], the maximum equivalence between the original instrument and its translated and adapted version must guide the entire process to prevent (frequently subtle) forms of interpretation, causing distortion in both the process of using the instrument and in the values obtained [37].

Generally speaking, the most used test was the intraclass correlation coefficient (ICC), which is calculated based on a ratio of variance. Four studies used the test [31, 32, 34, 35], and the value ≥ 0.70 was obtained in an appropriate manner. They were classified as "good" [4, 12, 15]. No instrument completely tested all the properties of the measure of reliability, and none were able to achieve the classification "excellent" (Table 2).

The criteria most tested, based on the COSMIN classification, were those of internal consistency, content validity, and cross-cultural validity. Internal consistency is the interrelationship between the components of the questionnaires, content validity includes face validity, and cross-cultural validity is the capacity of an instrument to obtain similar results with different individuals and evaluators. This may be evaluated by the reliability and agreement of the construct [4, 12].

All the instruments performed the pretest [31–33, 35] or pilot-test (as it was denominated in the study [34]). The majority of the studies adequately described the sample [31–33, 35], and only one [34] was not in agreement with COSMIN [4, 12, 13].

To generalize the results of the transcultural adaptation process, the COSMIN checklist recommends that the participants involved in the pretest should be clinically and epidemiologically described in terms of age, sex, characteristics of the disease/deficiency, and source of participant recruitment (hospital, clinic, rehabilitation center, university, therapeutic community, etc.).

The authors also observed that in some instruments [31–34] the retro-translation was done by two different person, who were natives of the original language of the instrument to be translated. The instrument [35] did not mention the quantity of translators and related that the process was performed by a committee [4, 12, 43, 44].

It is recommended that the translation procedure should be done by two different person in an independent manner. Comparison between two different translations assures the precision of the original version, with a more appropriate process, and maintenance of the semantic equivalence. It is important for the translators or the team not to communicate with one another about the work during the translations that will be compared afterwards [12, 13, 44].

Although the searches were conducted in the most used databases, using all the 27 items of the checklist included in the report of the systematic review and meta-analysis [12, 13, 18], some studies may not have been included in this systematic review.

5. Conclusion

This systematic review presented assistive technology instruments that have undergone the process of translation and cross-cultural adaptation. The publication of systematic reviews that synthesize the results of research is fundamental for bringing about a change in practices and behaviors among health care professionals. As such, the present review may provide subsidies for planning, identifying, and choosing specific instruments for a determined objective, within the context of the assistive technology field, while also being helpful for researchers and health professionals in their clinical and investigatory practices. This transformation requires that these professionals not only consult the available literature but also incorporate the information and knowledge provided by it into their daily clinical practice.

QUEST may be considered as the instrument that is most translated and adapted to other cultures and appropriate for use, when compared with other questionnaires tested for the same purpose. This happens because QUEST's properties of measurement were properly tested and most stages of cultural adaptation were performed.

It is important to emphasize, though, that due to the inclusion and exclusion criteria employed in our systematic review, a small number of articles (five) about PIADS were not included in our overall sample ($n = 560$). As such, it is possible that, because of this involuntary omission, some relevant findings may have not been included in the analysis performed in our review. Consequently, a future study will have to measure the impact of these missing papers. Yet, given our large article sample and our adopted strategy for decreasing the number of the studies in favor of assuring the quality of the results, we do not anticipate a priori that this omission may have caused any substantial change in our results and conclusions.

Finally, we want to mention that our study may have limitations related to a few types of assistive technology instruments, because our research was limited to questionnaires involving a limited set. Therefore, we suggest that further reviews should be conducted and that a meta-analysis should be included, which will present evidence and characteristics of different assistive technology instruments.

Acknowledgments

This project is linked to the Announcement of Assistive Technology in Brazil and Studies on Deficiency (PGPTA) No. 59/2014, Program of Support to Postgraduate and Scientific and Technological Research in Assistive Technology in Brazil (PGPTA/CAPES). Special thanks to the Foundation for Research Support of the State of São Paulo (FAPESP) for the financing of this article through the project Financing: Building the Intersectoriality in the Field of Worker's Health: Prospects of Professionals in the Service Network of the City of São Paulo No. 2014/25985-2. The authors would like to thank Dr. Miguel Nicolelis' review of the manuscript.

References

[1] Organização Mundial de Saúde (OMS) and Organização Panamericana de Saúde (OPAS), *CIF Classificação Internacional de Funcionalidade, Incapacidade e Saúde*, Universidade de São Paulo, Edusp, São Paulo, Brazil, 2008.

[2] IBGE, Instituto Brasileiro de Geografia e Estatística, "Censo 2010- resultados-resumo," 2012, https://downloads.ibge.gov.br/.

[3] J. A. Ruaro, M. B. Ruaro, D. E. Souza, A. R. Fréz, and R. O. Guerra, "An overview and profile of the ICF's use in Brazil: a decade of history," *Brazilian Journal of Physical Therapy*, vol. 16, no. 6, pp. 454–462, 2012.

[4] L. B. Mokkink, C. B. Terwee, D. L. Patrick et al., "The COSMIN checklist for assessing the methodological quality of studies on measurement properties of health status

measurement instruments: an international Delphi study," *Quality of Life Research*, vol. 19, no. 4, pp. 539–549, 2010.

[5] L. Gjersing, J. R. M. Caplehorn, and T. Clausen, "Cross-cultural adaptation of research instruments: language, setting, time and statistical considerations," *BMC Medical Research Methodology*, vol. 10, no. 1, p. 13, 2010.

[6] D. E. Beaton, C. Bombardier, F. Guillemin, and M. B. Ferraz, "Guidelines for the process of cross-cultural adaptation of self-report measures," *Spine*, vol. 25, no. 24, pp. 3186–3191, 2000.

[7] W. J. Coster and M. C. Mancini, "Recomendações para a tradução e adaptação transcultural de instrumentos para a pesquisa e a prática em terapia ocupacional," *Revista de Terapia Ocupacional da Universidade de São Paulo*, vol. 26, no. 1, pp. 50–57, 2015.

[8] A. M. Cook and J. M. Polgar, *Assistive Technologies: Principles and Practice*, Mosby, St. Louis, MO, USA, 4th edition, 2015.

[9] R. O. Pinto, M. P. Pattussi, L. do Prado Fontoura et al., "Validation of an instrument to evaluate health promotion at schools," *Revista de Saúde Pública*, vol. 50, 2016.

[10] F. Guillemin, C. Bombardier, and D. Beaton, "Cross-cultural adaptation of health-related quality of life measures: literature review and proposed guidelines," *Journal of Clinical Epidemiology*, vol. 46, no. 12, pp. 1417–1432, 1993.

[11] R. F. Sampaio and M. C. Mancini, "Systematic review studies: a guide for careful synthesis of the scientific evidence," *Brazilian Journal of Physical Therapy*, vol. 11, no. 1, pp. 83–89, 2007.

[12] L. B. Mokkink, C. A. C. Prinsen, L. M. Bouter, H. C. W. Vet, and C. B. Terwee, "The Consensus-based Standards for the selection of health Measurement Instruments (COSMIN) and how to select an outcome measurement instrument," *Brazilian Journal of Physical Therapy*, vol. 20, no. 2, pp. 105–113, 2016.

[13] C. B. Terwee, L. B. Mokkink, D. L. Knol, R. W. J. G. Ostelo, L. M. Bouter, and H. C. W. de Vet, "Rating the methodological quality in systematic reviews of studies on measurement properties: a scoring system for the COSMIN checklist," *Quality of Life Research*, vol. 21, no. 4, pp. 651–657, 2012.

[14] A. Liberati, D. G. Altman, J. Tetzlaff et al., "The PRISMA statement for reporting systematic reviews and meta-analyses of studies that evaluate health care interventions: explanation and elaboration," *Annals of Internal Medicine*, vol. 151, no. 4, pp. W65–W94, 2009.

[15] L. Shamseer, D. Moher, M. Clarke et al., "Preferred reporting items for systematic review and meta-analysis protocols (PRISMA-P) 2015: elaboration and explanation," *BMJ*, vol. 349, article g7647, 2015.

[16] L. H. M. Pengel, R. D. Herbert, C. G. Maher, and K. M. Refshauge, "Acute low back pain: systematic review of its prognosis," *BMJ*, vol. 327, no. 7410, pp. 323–320, 2003.

[17] M. J. Hancock, C. G. Maher, J. Latimer et al., "Systematic review of tests to identify the disc, SIJ or facet joint as the source of low back pain," *European Spine Journal*, vol. 16, no. 10, pp. 1539–1550, 2007.

[18] L. C. M. Costa, C. G. Maher, J. H. McAuley, and L. O. P. Costa, "Systematic review of cross-cultural adaptations of McGill Pain Questionnaire reveals a paucity of clinimetric testing," *Journal of Clinical Epidemiology*, vol. 62, no. 9, pp. 934–943, 2009.

[19] L. O. P. Costa, C. G. Maher, J. Latimer, and R. J. E. M. Smeets, "Reproducibility of rehabilitative ultrasound imaging for the measurement of abdominal muscle activity: a systematic review," *Physical Therapy*, vol. 89, no. 8, pp. 756–769, 2009.

[20] M. E. Reichenheim and C. L. Moraes, "Operationalizing the cross-cultural adaptation of epidemological measurement instruments," *Revista de Saúde Pública*, vol. 41, no. 4, pp. 665–673, 2007.

[21] R. Andrich, F. Pedroni, and G. Vanni, "Psychosocial impact of assistive devices: Italian localization of the PIADS instrument," in *Assistive Technology - Shaping the Future*, G. M. Craddock, L. P. McCormack, R. B. Reilly, and H. T. P. Knops, Eds., pp. 917–921, IOS Press, Amsterdam, Netherlands, 2003.

[22] A. C. Martins, "Adaptação cultural e linguística da versão Portuguesa do PIADS: escala do impacto psicossocial das tecnologias de apoio (P-PIADS)," *Integrar*, vol. 21-22, pp. 120–124, 2004.

[23] Y.-J. Hsieh and J. A. Lenker, "The psychosocial impact of assistive devices scale (PIADS): translation and psychometric evaluation of a Chinese (Taiwanese) version," *Disability and Rehabilitation: Assistive Technology*, vol. 1, no. 1-2, pp. 49–57, 2006.

[24] E. M. Orellano and J. W. Jutai, "Cross-cultural adaptation of the psychosocial impact of assistive device scale (PIADS) for Puerto Rican assistive technology users," *Assistive Technology*, vol. 25, no. 4, pp. 194–203, 2013.

[25] A. Zahid and B. Boyle, "Using impact measurement to establish confidence in emergent assistive technology services - first phase translation of the PIADS outcome measurement tool for implementation in an Arabic context," in *Assistive Technology: From Research to Practice*, vol. 33 of Assistive Technology Research Series, , pp. 1071–1077, IOS Press, 2013.

[26] J. Hair, R. E. Anderson, R. Tatham, and W. Black, *Análise Multivariada de Dados*, Porto Alegre, Brazil, Bookman, 2005.

[27] M. E. Cornélio, N. M. C. Alexandre, and T. M. São-João, "Instrumentos de medida en cardiología adaptados a la lengua portuguesa de Brasil: una revisión sistemática," *Revista da Escola de Enfermagem da USP*, vol. 48, no. 2, pp. 368–376, 2014.

[28] E. Lima, L. F. Teixeira-Salmela, L. Simões, A. C. C. Guerra, and A. Lemos, "Assessment of the measurement properties of the post stroke motor function instruments available in Brazil: a systematic review," *Brazilian Journal of Physical Therapy*, vol. 20, no. 2, pp. 114–125, 2016.

[29] C. Maher, "PRISMA: helping to deliver information that physical therapists need," *Physical Therapy*, vol. 89, no. 9, pp. 870–872, 2009.

[30] C. B. Terwee, S. D. M. Bot, M. R. de Boer et al., "Quality criteria were proposed for measurement properties of health status questionnaires," *Journal of Clinical Epidemiology*, vol. 60, no. 1, pp. 34–42, 2007.

[31] K. E. C. de Carvalho, M. B. Gois Júnior, and K. N. Sá, "Translation and validation of the *Quebec User Evaluation of Satisfaction with Assistive Technology* (QUEST 2.0) into Portuguese," *Revista Brasileira de Reumatologia*, vol. 54, no. 4, pp. 260–267, 2014.

[32] L. Demers, M. Monette, M. Descent, J. Jutai, and C. Wolfson, "The Psychosocial Impact of Assistive Devices Scale (PIADS): translation and preliminary psychometric evaluation of a Canadian–French version," *Quality of Life Research*, vol. 11, no. 6, pp. 583–592, 2002.

[33] Å. Brandt, "Translation, cross-cultural adaptation, and content validation of the QUEST," *Technology and Disability*, vol. 17, pp. 205–216, 2005.

[34] N. Bek, I. E. Simsek, S. Erel, Y. Yakut, and F. Uygur, "Turkish version of impact on family scale: a study of reliability and validity," *Health and Quality of Life Outcomes*, vol. 7, no. 1, p. 4, 2009.

[35] H. F. Mao, W. Y. Chen, G. Yao, S. L. Huang, C. C. Lin, and W. N. W. Huang, "Cross-cultural adaptation and validation of the Quebec User Evaluation of Satisfaction with Assistive Technology (QUEST 2.0): the development of the Taiwanese version," *Clinical Rehabilitation*, vol. 24, no. 5, pp. 412–421, 2010.

[36] C. KEC, *Tradução para a língua Portuguesa do Brasil e validação do Quebec User Evaluation of Satisfaction with Assistive Technology (Quest 2.0), [M.S. thesis]*, Escola Bahiana de Medicina e Saúde Pública, Programa de Pós-Graduação em Medicina e Saúde Humana, Salvador, Brazil, 2013, http://pos.bahiana.edu.br/upload/Disserta%C3%A7%C3%A3o%20de%20Mestrado%20-%20Karla%20Emmanuelle.pdf.

[37] L. Demers, R. Wessels, R. Weiss-Lambrou, B. Ska, and L. P. De Witte, "Key dimensions of client satisfaction with assistive technology: a cross-validation of a Canadian measure in the Netherlands," *Journal of Rehabilitation Medicine*, vol. 33, no. 4, pp. 187–191, 2001.

[38] The WHOQOL Group, "The World Health Organization Quality of Life assessment (WHOQOL): position paper from the World Health Organization," *Social Science & Medicine*, vol. 41, no. 10, pp. 1403–1409, 1995.

[39] A. M. Cook and J. M. Polgar, "Principles of assistive technology: introducing the human activity assistive technology model," in *Assistive Technologies: Principles and Practice*, pp. 1–15, Elsevier, 2015.

[40] C. M. Frattali, "Perspectives on functional assessment: its use for policy making," *Disability and Rehabilitation*, vol. 15, no. 1, pp. 1–9, 1993.

[41] M. R. Schmeler, *Development and testing of a clinical outcome measurement tool to assess wheeled mobility and seating intervention, [Ph.D. thesis]*, School of Health and Rehabilitation Sciences, University of Pittsburgh, Pittsburgh, PA, USA, 2005, http://d-scholarship.pitt.edu/9562/.

[42] M. R. Schmeler, M. B. Holm, and T. L. Mills, "Wheelchair functional outcomes measures & functioning everyday with a wheelchair tools," in *2006 Canadian Seating & Mobility Conference*, pp. 42–45, Toronto, ON, Canada, 2006.

[43] M. R. de Boer, A. C. Moll, H. C. W. de Vet, C. B. Terwee, H. J. M. Volker-Dieben, and G. H. M. B. van Rens, "Psychometric properties of vision-related quality of life questionnaires: a systematic review," *Ophthalmic and Physiological Optics*, vol. 24, no. 4, pp. 257–273, 2004.

[44] L. B. Mokkink, C. B. Terwee, D. L. Patrick et al., "The COSMIN study reached international consensus on taxonomy, terminology, and definitions of measurement properties for health-related patient-reported outcomes," *Journal of Clinical Epidemiology*, vol. 63, no. 7, pp. 737–745, 2010.

16

Translational Research for Occupational Therapy: Using SPRE in Hippotherapy for Children with Developmental Disabilities

Deborah Weissman-Miller, Rosalie J. Miller, and Mary P. Shotwell

School of Occupational Therapy, Brenau University, 500 Washington Street SE, Gainesville, GA 30501, USA

Correspondence should be addressed to Deborah Weissman-Miller; dweissman-miller@brenau.edu

Academic Editor: Jodie A. Copley

Translational research is redefined in this paper using a combination of methods in statistics and data science to enhance the understanding of outcomes and practice in occupational therapy. These new methods are applied, using larger data and smaller single-subject data, to a study in hippotherapy for children with developmental disabilities (DD). The Centers for Disease Control and Prevention estimates DD affects nearly 10 million children, aged 2–19, where diagnoses may be comorbid. Hippotherapy is defined here as a treatment strategy in occupational therapy using equine movement to achieve functional outcomes. Semiparametric ratio estimator (SPRE), a single-subject statistical and small data science model, is used to derive a "change point" indicating where the participant adapts to treatment, from which predictions are made. Data analyzed here is from an institutional review board approved pilot study using the Hippotherapy Evaluation and Assessment Tool measure, where outcomes are given separately for each of four measured domains and the total scores of each participant. Analysis with SPRE, using statistical methods to predict a "change point" and data science graphical interpretations of data, shows the translational comparisons between results from larger mean values and the very different results from smaller values for each HEAT domain in terms of relationships and statistical probabilities.

1. Introduction

Translational research is often defined as translating research done in the laboratory so it can be applied in clinical practice in medicine. Translational research also applies to the adoption of best practices in the community. For the entire history of occupational therapy (OT), there have not been sufficient statistics to "translate" OT and its perspective into a relevant scientific viewpoint [1]. Traditional statistical results from large datasets have not been able to show that engaging in meaningful occupation has statistically significantly improved a client's situation. However, translational research in occupational therapy may now be defined by new statistical and data science methodology available to analyze the data. Until recently, occupational therapy outcomes have been analyzed by means of larger data, such as t-tests and randomized controlled trials. These types of analyses are uniquely suited to public health and medicine but are not appropriate for the usual approach of occupational therapy treating one client, or a small group, at a time to determine the occupation meaningful to the client and design therapy accordingly. A goal in occupational therapy in this paper is to combine resources from treatment data with a new single-subject and small group design in statistics. This new single-subject design may also be used as small datasets in data science to promote enhancements in graphical analysis of prevention and therapies. In occupational therapy, translational research aims to "translate" findings in statistical and data science research results from larger group data into meaningful comparative results from smaller single-subject datasets that have been extracted from a portion of the group data and that influence clinical observation as part of occupational therapy practice. Translational research can implement "data to practice" outcomes to produce new treatment options for patients.

A fundamental model for this approach is the use of the new semiparametric ratio estimator (SPRE) as a single-subject statistical and small data science model to define, analyze, graph, and predict occupational therapy data to provide a pathway to meaningful treatment. SPRE, as the semiparametric ratio estimator discussed by Weissman-Miller et al. [2], in Weissman-Miller [3], and in Weissman-Miller [4], provides a statistical science model to determine the "change point" where the participant adapts to treatment. In the SPRE model, the change point is derived from a backwards stepwise ordinary least squares regression, which provides minimum bias. The change point is determined from the highest or lowest F statistic, according to Weissman-Miller et al. [2] as

$$F = t^2 = \frac{\text{MSReg}}{\hat{\sigma}^2}, \tag{1}$$

where F is the F-distribution, also known as Snedecor's F, which is a continuous probability distribution used here to determine the highest or lowest f statistic from the ordinary least squares regression, t^2 is Student's t-distribution that is a continuous probability distribution that arises when estimating the mean of a normally distributed population in situations where there is a small sample size, MSReg is the mean square due to regression, and $\hat{\sigma}^2$ is estimated population variance.

The result is associated with the relevant distributional p value [3] at the value of the time interval in the session number. From the change point, nonlinear estimates are given in the SPRE model using a new response function given from the cumulative distribution function of the Weibull distribution. These point estimates are given using a ratio of the Weibull distribution times the prior estimated outcome [3]. The new response function $G_k, \tau(t)$ is given as

$$\left(1 - e^{-(t/\tau)^k}\right), \tag{2}$$

when ε is the number 2.71828, the base of the natural logs, t is time, τ is the value of the change point, in this SPRE analysis (using the hereditary integral), and k determines the curvature of the distributional predictions.

Then the point estimation may be given as a ratio (R) of the Weibull distributions times the prior outcome.

The predictive equation from Weissman-Miller et al. [2] is then

$$\hat{\theta}_t = R \cdot \theta_{t_i}, \tag{3}$$

where $\hat{\theta}_t$ is outcomes beyond τ that are point estimates, R is ratio of Weibull distributions (varying by t = time), and θ_{t_i} is population parameter at the prior time.

Any OT data will fit the SPRE model if the sessions, a minimum of 13 to 14, are reasonably evenly spaced. The OT data must be taken from a measure that will yield results for the specified research question. Then, the raw data is entered into Excel and finally saved as a comma separated file (CSV). This type of file can be read directly by the SPRE program written in the R software language. The initial worksheet data is saved as an Excel worksheet. The final data for each participant is saved in a new worksheet as a CSV file. It can be seen in Figure 1 that the data headings for the SPRE R code are labeled FData and Session for the participant Partic.c, taken from an Excel file of this participant's data. These results will vary according to the input data, but the format for the SPRE R program is always the same, where the "FData" and "Session" are highlighted together and arranged in ascending or descending order following the order of the original raw data coded in Excel. Then, the session numbers are always arranged together with the original raw data that allows for accurate predictions of the change point [3].

Context for This Study. This study took place in the context of exploring the effectiveness of hippotherapy practice and a newly developed measure called the Hippotherapy Evaluation and Assessment Tool (HEAT). Hippotherapy is "therapy with the help of a horse" derived from the Greek word hippos, meaning "horse" [5]. Classic hippotherapy treatments, used in the rehabilitation of musculoskeletal, neuromuscular, and cardiopulmonary dysfunctions, use the movement of the horse and promote the patient's response to its dynamic movement [6]. The purported benefits of hippotherapy impact multiple body systems [7]. Literature identifies common tools used to measure multiple body system deficits ranging from static posture to dynamic motor behavior, sensory processing, and psychosocial/behavioral difficulties. Postural effects of hippotherapy are frequently evaluated using the *Pediatric Balance Scale* (PBS) [8] or the *Sitting Assessment Scale* (SAS) [9]. The *Gross Motor Function Measure* (MFM) [10] is often used to measure dynamic motor behavior. The *Sensory Profile* (SP) [11] and the *Sensory Processing Measure* (SPM) [12] assess sensory processing patterns. Psychosocial and behavioral domains are frequently evaluated with the *Pediatric Evaluation of Disability Inventory* (PEDI) [13]. The assessment used in the research described in this paper is the HEAT (*Hippotherapy Evaluation and Assessment Tool*) as given by Malone et al. [14].

Data Organization in SPRE for Statistical and Data Science. It should be noted that while any OT data can be input into Excel, the data is often statistically transformed depending upon the OT practice area for analysis in SPRE. For data in the HEAT measure [14], the raw data in Figure 1 was analyzed as

$$\text{HEATTOTAL/HEATStaticPosture}. \tag{4}$$

The data in Figure 1 are data for Partic.c, computing the ratio using (4) and arranging the data. These results will vary according to the input data, but the format for SPRE R program is always the same.

The important part of using SPRE as statistics and data science is that each participant is their own control, which means that the efficacy of data no longer depends on having a homogeneous participant pool. In this case, participants with varying comorbidities can be analyzed separately as single-subjects. Of course, total data can be taken and then analyzed for a small group. This approach, combining single-subject data, is much more effective for occupational therapy than pre-post analyses involving participants with comorbidities and very useful for translational research.

The usefulness of SPRE can also be seen in this paper where the participants have been diagnosed with comorbidities, because these participants can all be included in the

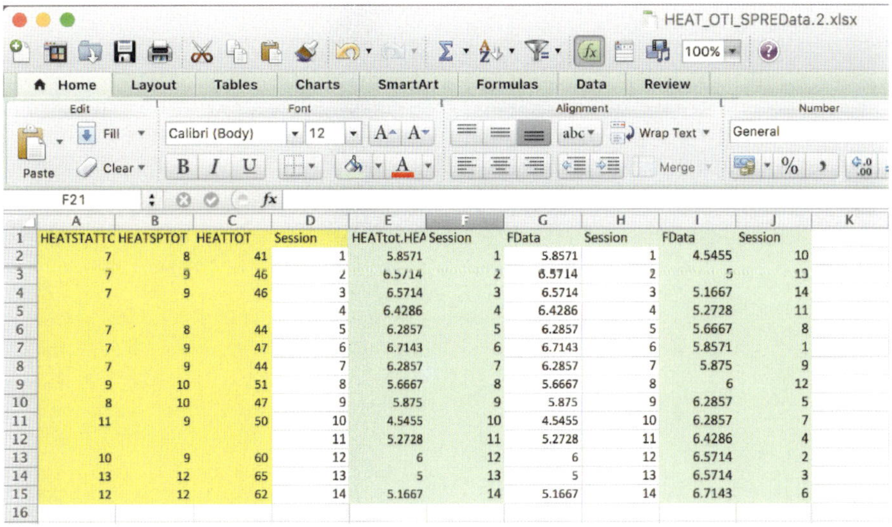

	A	B	C	D	E	F	G	H	I	J
1	HEATSTATTC	HEATSPTOT	HEATTOT	Session	HEATtot.HEA	Session	FData	Session	FData	Session
2	7	8	41	1	5.8571	1	5.8571	1	4.5455	10
3	7	9	46	2	6.5714	2	6.5714	2	5	13
4	7	9	46	3	6.5714	3	6.5714	3	5.1667	14
5				4	6.4286	4	6.4286	4	5.2728	11
6	7	8	44	5	6.2857	5	6.2857	5	5.6667	8
7	7	9	47	6	6.7143	6	6.7143	6	5.8571	1
8	7	9	44	7	6.2857	7	6.2857	7	5.875	9
9	9	10	51	8	5.6667	8	5.6667	8	6	12
10	8	10	47	9	5.875	9	5.875	9	6.2857	5
11	11	9	50	10	4.5455	10	4.5455	10	6.2857	7
12				11	5.2728	11	5.2728	11	6.4286	4
13	10	9	60	12	6	12	6	12	6.5714	2
14	13	12	65	13	5	13	5	13	6.5714	3
15	12	12	62	14	5.1667	14	5.1667	14	6.7143	6
16										

FIGURE 1: Excel (CSV) data for static posture of Partic.c for SPRE from raw data to arranged data.

same study, while they are analyzed separately. To facilitate the use of SPRE in a clinical setting, an "R" statistical program [15] has been written to compute data results collected from participants and prepared using Microsoft Excel [16]. This "R" program includes predictions and comparative graphical analytical tools that are a mainstay of data science. The question arises: what is the difference, in this context, between statistical and data science? An answer is that statistical science is fundamentally about a model. Data is trimmed and outliers are often discarded altogether to better fit the model. An example of this is the linear regression model, where missing data is not considered in the dataset and data outliers may be discarded as demonstrated in Weisberg [17]. In the small datasets used in occupational therapy, and particularly in single-subject design, there is a limit to the number of sessions that can be provided within time and duration of treatment constraints. Discarding sessions with missing data or with data that seems "outside the norm" provides too little data for analysis, according to Weissman-Miller and Holmes [18]. Furthermore, the whole of the data represents the participant's actual results. Discarding any of that data to fit a model may be considered in the same way as discarding some of the occupational therapists' descriptive notes on a participant because they do not fit the therapists' own assumptions. Using SPRE, missing data may be imputed using an approach described by Weissman-Miller and Holmes [18], where an error function for the data is derived. In doing this, the translational data and results are taken from the participant's actual complete data.

2. Materials and Methods

2.1. Design of the Study. This SPRE analysis is part of a research project which contributed to validity and reliability of a newly developed Hippotherapy Evaluation and Assessment Tool (HEAT). The HEAT is intended to provide a common tool for therapists to measure ongoing progress as well as outcomes in hippotherapy practice. In the original IRB approved protocol from which this analysis is taken, a non-experimental repeated measures study used data collected from 21 children receiving hippotherapy services in order to establish predictive validity of this new hippotherapy measure (HEAT). Research questions included the following: (1) Do scores on the HEAT show a statistically significant change over repeated measures? (2) Based on the F-statistic, can researchers predict the number of treatment sessions a client will need before they reach a "plateau" in progress? Once data was collected, it was analyzed using several techniques for all the data, such as a Kruskal-Wallis ANOVA (nonparametric ANOVA equivalent), the SPRE model using an ordinary least squares (OLS) linear regression, and a stepwise prediction method based on a ratio of a Weibull parametric cumulative distribution as given by Weissman-Miller et al. [2] and Weissman-Miller [3].

2.2. Summary of the Original Hippotherapy Evaluation and Assessment Tool (HEAT) Measure. The Hippotherapy Evaluation and Assessment Tool (HEAT) was developed by the third author of this paper (Shotwell) in response to the need for a comprehensive assessment to measure the outcomes of hippotherapy and used as part of graduate thesis research [19]. Using the literature in hippotherapy as a guide for what items should be on the HEAT, Shotwell, along with her graduate students [19], found that 45% of the literature discussed dynamic motor performance as an outcome of hippotherapy, 20% of the literature showed improvements in static posture, 20% of the articles represented changes in sensory processing, and the smallest percentage of outcomes (15%) was represented by psychosocial or behavioral changes. The final version of the HEAT is a 100-point measure containing four domains: (a) dynamic motor behavior; (b) static posture; (c) sensory processing; and (d) psychosocial/behavioral performance.

The overall purpose of the recent Malone et al. [14] research study was to further explore two forms of criterion-related validity of the HEAT in terms of (a) predictive validity within a repeated measures design and (b) further analysis of HEAT's concurrent validity in comparison to other "gold standard" measures. The repeated measures design portion provided an opportunity to apply the SPRE model to small group research.

2.3. Sampling and Recruitment. Malone et al. [14] used purposive sampling to recruit 21 children, male ($n = 8$) and female ($n = 13$), between the ages of 2 and 19 years who were engaged in hippotherapy services. According to Portney and Watkins [20], purposive sampling is a technique researchers use to select subjects on the basis of specific criteria. In this study, researchers wanted to test a variety of subjects with specifically different degrees of limitation. Purposive sampling was well suited to analysis using SPRE for a heterogeneous single-subject design. Children who had participated in hippotherapy were recruited from outpatient rehabilitation facilities and barns in the Southeastern US, to ensure familiarity with horses. Inclusion criteria required that participants speak English, unless a translator was available. No targeted gender, ethnicity, or diagnosis group was excluded. Attempts were made to recruit children with diagnoses typically seen in hippotherapy practice including autism; cerebral palsy; attention deficit hyperactivity disorder; Down syndrome; and other genetic disorders.

2.4. Data Collection and Analysis of the HEAT Sample Data. Data were collected over the course of 14 weeks during hippotherapy sessions using the HEAT. The Pediatric Evaluation of Disability Inventory (PEDI) was also administered during the first and last sessions in order to explore concurrent and predictive validity. Paired t-tests were performed to investigate HEAT's ability to show change over time. This quasi-experimental repeated measures study used data collected from 21 children receiving hippotherapy services. The quasi-experimental design was employed for this study because there was no random assignment or comparison group. To establish predictive validity of the HEAT, four research questions provided the framework for data collection from each participant. These questions included the following.

(1) Is there a difference in HEAT scores pre-post? (1a) Do scores on HEAT show statistically significant change over time? (1b) Does hippotherapy intervention show changes in functional behaviors as measured by the PEDI scores? (2) Is the HEAT a valid measure with respect to comparison with an "occupation-based measure" such as the PEDI? Once data was collected, statistical analysis consisted of (a) paired t-tests, (b) semiparametric ratio estimator (SPRE) model, and (c) exploratory correlations. Since children participating in hippotherapy are often unlike each other, a group design comparing them to each other would be flawed. It would be more appropriate that the client be their own control and their pretest scores compared to their posttest scores. Since the HEAT measure is intended for repeated measures, stability over time is explored as shown in Malone et al. [14].

Pre-post differences show that three of the four domains of the HEAT had statistically significant results except for static posture ($p = 0.071$). The paired t-test results in Table 1 give the statistical significance and an overall summary of the results of HEATTOTAL and each subdomain. The majority of the t-tests exploring differences in each domain in the HEAT were statistically significant. While this is useful information showing the sufficiency of the HEAT measure, this type of analysis does not provide a look into the "black box" of therapeutic result over time. From the overall result in Table 1, for 12 participants from this at risk dataset who completed sessions 1 and 14 for the pre-post sessions [14], we can determine what happened, but not why the results may have changed over time, or how the therapy may be improved. An advanced statistical technique, the semiparametric ratio estimator (SPRE) was conducted to further determine the HEAT's sensitivity and stability. Individual analyses by the SPRE model provided further comparison and insight between observational notes and numerical data on HEAT resulting in translational research of the data.

2.5. Design of the Study for Translational Research. Data obtained through the data collection process using the HEAT measure was entered in SPSS [21] to analyze 12 participants' pre-post results using paired t-tests. These results were statistically significant except for HEAT static posture ($p = 0.071$). Other statistical measures were used to analyze data for the total participant sample, $n = 21$. The next question addressed was what kind of change the participants' scores showed over time using the SPRE program written in R from Excel software. The R Development Core Team [15] computer software language provides a wide variety of statistical and graphical techniques that provide a basis for comparing individual results both numerically and graphically in statistics and data science. For the translational analysis in this paper, a subset of the sample ($n = 5$) was initially selected to investigate the potential for determining comparative results. The five participants were selected by the completeness of their datasets for use in SPRE analyses. In addition, the biostatistician was blinded to the identity of each participant, to reduce possible bias. The Excel data for each of these five participants was analyzed using the R program for SPRE. This program is used through R Studio [22]. To read the data, the Excel program must be saved as a "csv" or data file. Then, listing the dataset and sourcing the R program will read the dataset, for example,

```
Dataset <- read.csv("Falls.d.Final2_2014.csv")
source("test175.R")
```

The data name in the parentheses is your data. An illustration of this method in R Studio is given in Figure 1.

2.6. Analysis of a Subset of Selected Participants. Of the five randomly selected participants, four had had 14 sessions and one had had 13 sessions. Four participants were missing some data. The use of SPRE as a single-subject design model easily allows for the imputation of missing data. In this analysis, data was imputed using an approach given by Weissman-Miller and Holmes [18], so that "complete" datasets were

TABLE 1: Paired t-test results of the HEAT pretest/posttest results.

Items for T-tests	N	t	df	Sig.
HEAT total session 1 versus HEAT total session 14	12	−4.033	11	.002**
HEAT static posture session 1 versus HEAT static posture session 14	12	−2.000	11	.071
HEAT sensory processing session 1 versus HEAT sensory processing session 14	12	−2.568	11	.026**
HEAT psychosocial/behavioral session 1 versus HEAT psychosocial/behavioral session 14	12	−4.696	11	.001**

∗∗ is used by SPSS to signify statistical significance.

analyzed in SPRE to derive the "change point" for each of the 5 participants and the predictions of future efficacy of the treatment. In this study, the error estimates for missing data varied between 0.0005 and 0.0526 for the participants. The first consideration is to minimize the order of magnitude of the experimental data as much as possible before using LERP (linear interpolation) to fill in the necessary data between 2 existing raw data points. Therefore, the interpolation should be made almost at the last step of data preparation, where the order of magnitude of the ratio from (4) will be small. The most important part of this analysis is given by the error function. The error function for these data points is derived from Parnell [23] and computed from the second derivative of a cubic polynomial function derived from numerical analysis. The details and a complete analysis using data from fall prevention in elders are given in the paper by Weissman-Miller and Holmes [18]. The fundamental question is whether imputation of data, using a small local linearized segment of the original data points, distorts the data fit of the SPRE model. Since many, if not most, single-subject designs for small datasets have missing data, the basic idea in this analysis is to provide an error function, associated with each imputed data point, which can determine any potential for distortion. This assumption provides an answer in each case, not whether or not to impute data, but if the imputed data points have sufficiently small error functions. Then the SPRE model results can be considered sufficient, as in this analysis of the HEAT data for each participant.

The total data for each participant, across all domains, was run through the SPRE software program, producing numerical and graphic results. Then, each of the subdomains in the HEAT measure was analyzed for each participant. The results of these analyses for one of the HEAT domains were surprising and led to the interpretation of translational research in occupational therapy in this paper.

3. Results

A graphic representation of the SPRE model, using a single participant's data from one domain, shows the change point in Figure 2.

This is a regression problem in which the expected value of the dependent variable is assumed to have a different functional form in specific neighborhoods of the explanatory variable space. According to Weissman-Miller [3], in the SPRE model, the determination of the change point is a structural change that shows the dynamic nature of participants with comorbidities. The highest or lowest change point from which this participant's predictions are made is at session 5. The ability to calculate p values for the data points from the regression analysis and make predictions is a unique strength of the SPRE model.

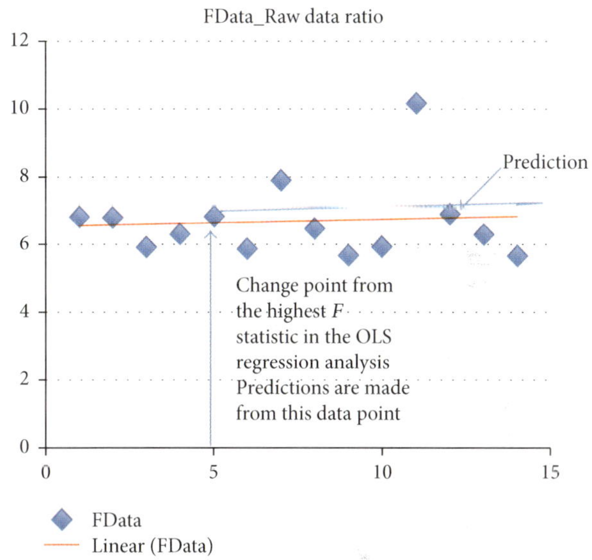

FIGURE 2: Partic.c_Sensory Processing plot of regression on data with change point and prediction.

3.1. Results of the HEATTOTAL Variable.

The HEATTOTAL variable is analyzed using SPRE. The outcomes for the total scores are positive for four individuals and have a normal distribution of the data, as shown by the scatter of the residuals, except for one participant. Because there is only one negative single-subject prediction among these five participants, the question is as follows: What is the total number of negative predictions among the 21 final participants' scores? In this study there were only three negative HEATTOTAL scores in the entire dataset. Therefore, the mean data from these three would have a very small or negligible impact on the statistical significance of all the HEAT data analyzed as a whole dataset.

TABLE 2: Analysis of the HEATTOTAL of individual participants.

Participant	Domain	Change point number	R^2	p value	Prediction direction	Residuals
Partic.a	Total	14	0.5875	0.00139	Positive	Normal distribution
Partic.b	Total	14	0.8275	0.00000644	Positive	Normal distribution
Partic.c	Total	1	0.2933	0.1656	Positive	Normal distribution
Partic.d	Total	13	0.7777	0.00000303	Positive	Normal distribution
Partic.e	Total	1	0.4153	0.4298	Negative	Normal distribution

TABLE 3: SPRE analysis of 5 participants for the static posture variable.

Participant	Domain	Change point number	R^2	p value	Prediction direction	Residuals
Partic.a	Static	14	0.524	*0.0034*	Positive	Normal distribution
Partic.b	Static	14	0.235	0.0788	Positive	Normal distribution
Partic.c	Static	13	0.454	0.212	Negative	~normal/outliers
Partic.d	Static	14	0.9996	*0.0125*	Positive	Normal distribution
Partic.e	Static	13 (of 13)	0.1282	0.2296	Negative	Normal distribution

In addition, when looking at one of five negative results, that is, still a relatively small impact when considering the mean data for all five participants, the paired t-test results give the statistical significance and an overall glance for the results of HEATTOTAL and each subdomain. While this is useful information as to the sufficiency of the HEAT measure, this type of analysis does not provide a look into the "black box" of therapeutic results. From overall results in Table 1 from Malone et al. [14], we can determine what happened, but not why the results may have changed over time, or how the therapy may be improved.

The results of HEATTOTAL for the random five participants are given in Table 2. Individual participants' data were analyzed using the SPRE as described by Weissman-Miller et al. [2] and by Weissman-Miller [3]. The participants have been described as Partic.a, and so on.

The value of being able to analyze the data using SPRE is that if the mean of all the data from all participants is analyzed and it is positive, there would also be a mean change point and p value. This type of analysis would validate the HEAT measure as a whole. However, SPRE can also be used on individual totals as well as each domain for each participant as shown in Table 2. The values for each participant are small for each domain, and the p values do reflect the statistical significance of the level of function for that individual. However each p value would not reflect the significance of the measure for all domains for all participants.

3.2. SPRE Analysis of Individual Participants in the Static Variable Domain. Individual participants' data were analyzed using SPRE. A summary of variable outcomes is given in Table 3.

It can be seen that there were two negative predictions among the five participants. Analyzing only the total data from one variable is quite different from taking the total of all of a participant's data. In this case, we can see that the participant named Partic.e is still negative, but the participant named Partic.c is also negative. When all of Partic.c's data was totaled, her prediction direction was positive, as can be seen in Table 2. The predicted difference for all the total data for one participant can be quite different when compared to the total of only one domain of data. In this way, translational research in occupational therapy begins to be implemented by "translating" comparative findings in statistical science research results into more meaningful occupational therapy practice and outcomes for each single participant. In this analysis, the analytical tool SPRE shows that Partic.c's static posture may be a problem that should be reviewed by the therapist.

3.3. SPRE Analysis of a Single Participant for All Domains. Partic.c's individual data were analyzed using SPRE. A summary of variable outcomes is given in Table 4.

An analysis was performed of each domain: static posture, dynamic motor behavior, sensory processing, and psychosocial/behavior for the participant (Partic.c). Her static posture prediction was negative, while the predictions for the remaining domains were positive. The comparative results show that the residuals of the data for the sensory processing domain are reasonably normal with outliers and the predictions are positive in this case. The outliers of the sensory processing domain may indicate that sensory processing is a problem for this participant. These relationships should be further investigated both graphically and statistically to determine the necessity for specific and targeted occupational therapy treatment.

3.4. SPRE Numerical and Graphic Results for the Partic.c. The SPRE analysis in Figure 3 is for Partic.c, for static posture. The plot in the upper right side of the figure, labeled "SPRE residuals," shows standardized residuals against theoretical quantiles of the data for this variable.

In Figure 4, the sensory processing data is analyzed in SPRE and plotted using the same format. The plots have a very similar shape although the outlying standardized residuals are different.

In Figure 5, the upper right hand plot plots the residuals against the fitted values for static posture.

TABLE 4: SPRE analysis of one participant for each variable.

Participant	Domain	Change point number	R^2	p value	Prediction direction	Residuals
Partic.c	Static	13	0.454	0.212	Negative	~normal/ladder
Partic.c	Dynamic	13	0.222	0.238	Positive	Normal
Partic.c	Sensory processing	5	0.328	0.065	Positive	Nonnormal/outliers
Partic.c	Psych/Soc	3	0.548	0.153	Positive	Normal

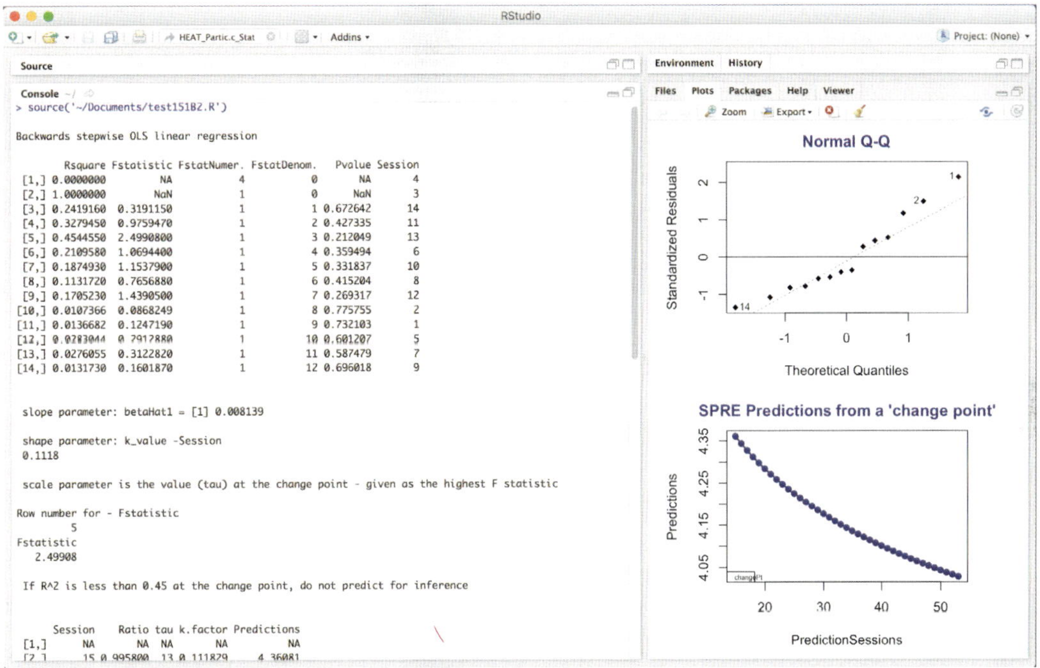

FIGURE 3: HEAT standardized residuals analysis for Partic.c _Static posture in SPRE.

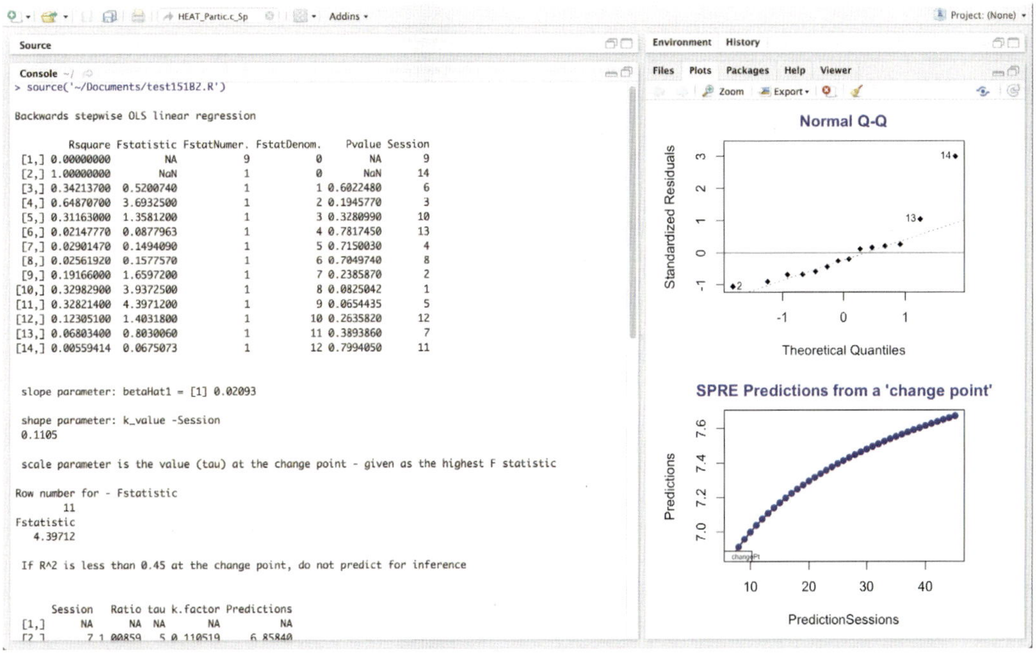

FIGURE 4: HEAT standardized residuals analysis for Partic.c _ sensory processing in SPRE.

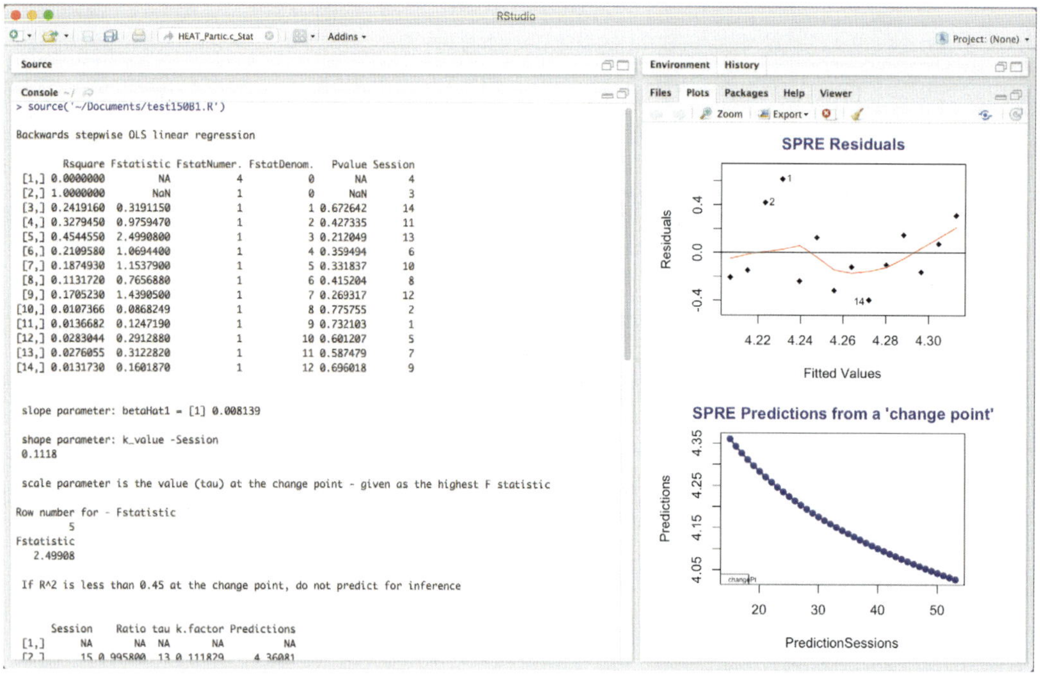

FIGURE 5: HEAT residuals analysis for Partic.c _ Static posture in SPRE.

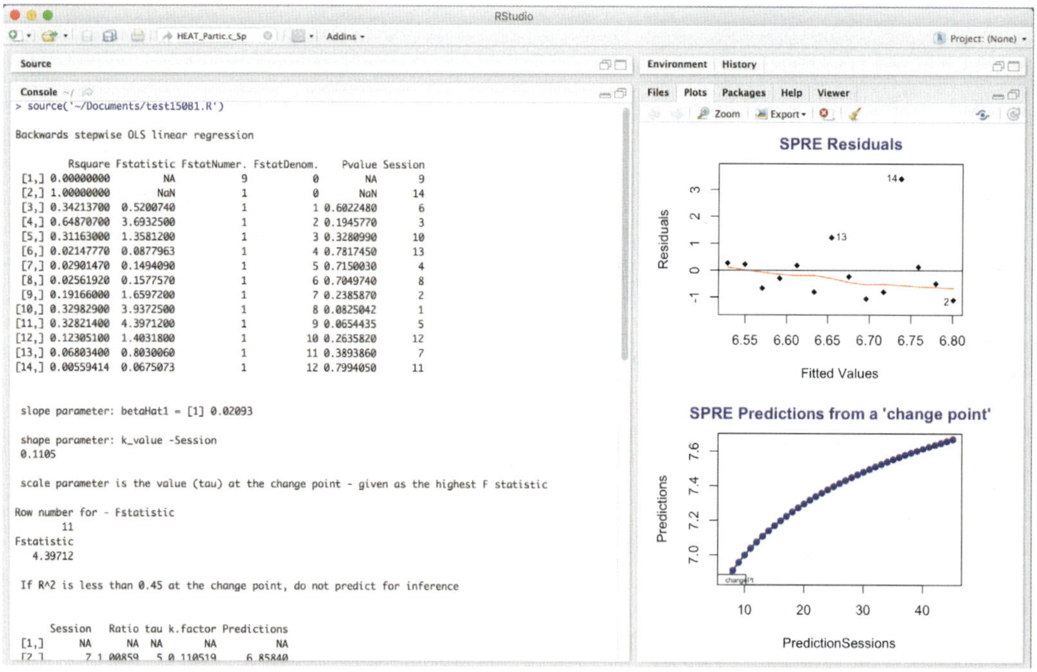

FIGURE 6: HEAT residuals analysis for Partic.c _ sensory processing in SPRE.

In Figure 6, the upper right hand plot plots the residuals against the fitted values for sensory processing.

These four plots show very different information. In Figures 3 and 4, the normal Q-Q plots have very similar shape. While Figure 3 shows a reasonably normal distribution with 2 potential outliers, Figure 4 also shows much of the data following the normal curve but with more defined outliers. Looking at these two plots from a data science perspective, the comparative resemblance of the shape indicates a possible relationship between the static posture and the sensory processing variables.

However, in investigating the data further, Figure 5 now indicates that these residuals from the regression analysis are from data in a normal distribution, with the same 2 potential outliers. However, the residuals in Figure 6 point to a real problem in the residuals of the data analysis results for this participant in this domain. This type of plot shows that the residuals from the data for this variable are not randomly scattered and therefore not from a normal distribution. Furthermore, the variance is not constant (when these residuals are shaped like a cone). This means that when one plots the individual error against the predicted value, the variance of the error predicted value should be constant. In fact, the SPRE residuals in Figure 6, which show nearly a straight line below 0.0, are so unlike the randomly scattered shape of the residuals in Figure 5 above and below 0.0, that it indicates a problem with the sensory processing for this participant. Additionally, the negative slope to the prediction for static posture in Figure 3 together with a normal distribution of the residuals of the data indicates a potential problem with static posture for this participant. Likewise, the extreme nonnormality of the residuals in sensory processing in Figure 6 indicates that sensory processing for Partic.c is a problem, even though the predictions are positive.

The findings from Figures 3–6 taken together indicate a problem in each of these two domains for this participant. This indicates a potential problematic therapeutic relationship between static posture and sensory processing in this case, based on comparative findings and anomalies from a statistical and data science approach to identifying a therapeutic problem for this participant.

4. Discussion

In this paper, translational research findings are applied from a combination of numerical methods in statistics and graphical methods in data science. This is particularly true when the use of the SPRE model has proceeded from the analysis of the total sum of the HEAT measure to the analysis of the individual variables for each participant. The result of this translational process from analyzing the larger mean to the specific and personal data has been to uncover a relation between two of the variables in that participant's responses and to determine potential therapeutic needs.

Following these discoveries in Partic.c's outcomes, a connection was considered between static posture and sensory processing, as both constructs take into account proprioception and vestibular function. According to Case-Smith [24], developing the vestibular-proprioceptive-visual connections provides the beginnings of postural control and continues to refine, resulting in further development of balance and fluidity in dynamic postural control. This study and others [see Snyder et al. [25] and Austin et al. [26]] indicate a correlation between posture and sensory processing domains on the HEAT, suggesting that the HEAT could be sensitive enough to identify challenges with sensory processing despite only 20 of the 100 points measuring this domain.

Referring to the occupational therapy case descriptive notes, it was seen that, toward the end of the intervention period, Partic.c's father and younger sibling began attending and watching the treatment session. These occupational therapy case notes were reviewed to provide a therapeutic context for the statistical changes in posture that were measured and for which there was a negative prediction in SPRE. During these last 3-4 sessions, her posture decreased when she looked toward her dad and little sister. Her scores on static posture declined (though the distribution of all HEAT 14 scores was normal with outliers). Her scores on HEAT sensory processing also decreased at session five of the 14 sessions.

Analyzing the outcomes for this participant using the SPRE results pointed to a relationship between static posture and sensory processing that was then confirmed by research literature. Furthermore, the negative predictive direction from the predictions in the SPRE analysis was explained by the occupational therapy descriptive notes during therapy. In this study, translational research "translates" comparative findings in statistical and data science research results into meaningful occupational therapy research, practice, and a better understanding of outcomes. In this sense, translational research may provide insights into implementing "data to practice" outcomes to produce new treatment options for patients.

Competing Interests

The authors declare that there is no conflict of interests regarding the publication of this paper.

References

[1] W. R. Dunton, "The need for and the value of research in occupational therapy," *Occupational Therapy and Rehabilitation*, vol. 13, no. 5, pp. 325–328, 1934.

[2] D. Weissman-Miller, M. P. Shotwell, and R. J. Miller, "New single-subject and small-n design in occupational therapy: application to weight loss in obesity," *American Journal of Occupational Therapy*, vol. 66, no. 4, pp. 455–462, 2012.

[3] D. Weissman-Miller, "Novel point estimation from a semiparametric ratio estimator (SPRE): long-term health outcomes from short-term linear data, with application to weight loss in obesity," *The International Journal of Biostatistics*, vol. 9, no. 2, pp. 175–184, 2013.

[4] D. Weissman-Miller, "On predicting survival in prostate cancer: using an extended maximum spacing method at the change point of the semiparametric ratio estimator (SPRE)," *International Journal of Statistics and Probability*, vol. 5, no. 2, 2016.

[5] American Hippotherapy Association (AHA), February 2015, http://www.americanhippotherapyassociation.org/.

[6] A. C. Granados and I. F. Agís, "Why children with special needs feel better with hippotherapy sessions: a conceptual review," *Journal of Alternative and Complementary Medicine*, vol. 17, no. 3, pp. 191–197, 2011.

[7] D. Debuse, C. Chandler, and C. Gibb, "An exploration of German and British physiotherapists' views on the effects of hippotherapy and their measurement," *Physiotherapy Theory and Practice*, vol. 21, no. 4, pp. 219–242, 2005.

[8] D. J. Silkwood-Sherer, C. B. Killian, T. M. Long, and K. S. Martin, "Hippotherapy—an intervention to habilitate balance deficits in children with movement disorders: a clinical trial," *Physical Therapy*, vol. 92, no. 5, pp. 707–717, 2012.

[9] D. Hamill, K. A. Washington, and O. R. White, "The effect of hippotherapy on postural control in sitting for children with

cerebral palsy," *Physical & Occupational Therapy in Pediatrics*, vol. 27, no. 4, pp. 23–42, 2007.

[10] D. B. Bertoti, "Effect of therapeutic horseback riding on posture in children with cerebral palsy," *Physical Therapy*, vol. 68, no. 10, pp. 1505–1512, 1988.

[11] M. B. Holm, J. M. Baird, Y. J. Kim et al., "Therapeutic horseback riding outcomes of parent-identified goals for children with autism spectrum disorder: an ABA′ multiple case design examining dosing and generalization to the home and community," *Journal of Autism and Developmental Disorders*, vol. 44, no. 4, pp. 937–947, 2014.

[12] M. M. Bass, C. A. Duchowny, and M. M. Llabre, "The effect of therapeutic horseback riding on social functioning in children with autism," *Journal of Autism and Developmental Disorders*, vol. 39, no. 9, pp. 1261–1267, 2009.

[13] E. S. Park, D.-W. Rha, J. S. Shin, S. Kim, and S. Jung, "Effects of hippotherapy on gross motor function and functional performance of children with cerebral palsy," *Yonsei Medical Journal*, vol. 55, no. 6, pp. 1736–1742, 2014.

[14] T. Malone, E. Maney, C. MacSpadden, E. Moss, B. O'Kelley, and E. Post, *Predictive validity of the Hippotherapy Evaluation and Assessment Tool (HEAT) [M.S. thesis]*, Brenau University, Gainesville, Ga, USA, 2016.

[15] R Development Core Team, *R: A Language and Environment for Statistical Computing*, R Foundation for Statistical Computing, Vienna, Austria, 2010, http://www.R-Project.org.

[16] Microsoft Excel, *Microsoft Corporation*, One Microsoft Way, Redmond, Wash, USA, 2016.

[17] S. Weisberg, *Applied Linear Regression*, Wiley-Interscience, Hoboken, NJ, USA, 2005.

[18] D. Weissman-Miller and W. Holmes, "Novel low-error interpolation method for a fall prevention program using the single-subject design statistical model SPRE," *International Journal of Current Research in Life Sciences*, vol. 4, pp. 429–435, 2015.

[19] H. Cox, T. Morgan, E. Smith, and R. Wiles, *Effects of hippotherapy on people with cerebral palsy from the users' perspective: a qualitative study [M.S. thesis]*, Brenau University, 2011.

[20] L. G. Portney and M. P. Watkins, "Validity of measurements," in *Foundations of Clinical Research: Applications to Practice*, L. G. Portney and M. P. Watkins, Eds., pp. 97–116, Pearson Education, Upper Saddle River, NJ, USA, 2009.

[21] IBM, *IBM SPSS Statistics for Windows, Version 22.0*, IBM, Armonk, NY, USA, 2013.

[22] R Studio v.0.96, 2014, http://www.rstudio.com.

[23] C. Parnell, "St. Andrews University, Numerical Analysis," March 2015, http://www-solar.mcs.st-andrews.ac.uk/~clare/Lectures/num-analysis/Numan_chap3.pdf.

[24] J. Case-Smith, "Development of childhood occupations," in *Occupational Therapy for Children*, J. Case-Smith and J. C. O'Brien, Eds., pp. 56–83, Elsevier, Maryland Heights, Mo, USA, 6th edition, 2010.

[25] J. Snyder, D. Smith, K. Mapp, and K. Wade, *Establishing concurrent validity of the hippotherapy assessment and evaluation tool [M.S. thesis]*, Brenau University, 2012.

[26] A. Austin, K. Bridges, D. Pledger, and L. Truitt, *Concurrent validity of the hippotherapy assessment and evaluation tool [M.S. thesis]*, Brenau University, 2013.

17

Principal Approaches to Understanding Occupation and Occupational Science Found in the Chilean Journal of Occupational Therapy (2001–2012)

Rodolfo Morrison,[1,2] Silvia Gómez,[1,2] Enrique Henny,[2,3] María Jesús Tapia,[1,2] and Laura Rueda[1,2]

[1] *Department of Occupational Therapy and Occupational Science, Faculty of Medicine, University of Chile, Santiago, Chile*
[2] *Chilean Society of Occupational Science, Santiago, Chile*
[3] *Tedes Center, Santiago, Chile*

Correspondence should be addressed to Rodolfo Morrison; morrison.rodolfo@gmail.com

Academic Editor: Claudia Hilton

Background. The progression of occupational science in Chile is documented in the main scientific publication of the field, the Chilean Journal of Occupational Therapy (RChTO). *Objective.* Identify approaches to understanding and applying occupation and occupational science as elucidated in the RChTO. *Methodology.* A systematic qualitative review of the journal (2001–2012) identified articles elucidating an approach to understanding and application operationally defined as references to specific authors, theories, models/paradigms, definitions, and other fields that support approaches to O/OS. *Results.* The study identified two main approaches. The first considers occupation/occupational science from a practical perspective or as a means to explain human behavior; the second considers occupation/occupational science as an object of study. Each approach is further divided into categories. *Conclusion.* This study provides a novel perspective on regional use of occupational science concepts. These findings contribute to our understanding of this science in context and to recognition of the cultural relevance of these scientific concepts.

1. Introduction

Rapid technological advances and the emergence of the information society have changed the landscape for the scientific community. It is more important than ever to elucidate the international perspectives and bodies of knowledge that form the foundation of any discipline. Given the abundance of information available, it is essential to provide clear guidelines for discourse and academic research.

Occupational therapy in Chile has been influenced by occupational science concepts that were developed in other regions but are applicable to the Chilean context. However, undergraduate occupational therapy programs tend to teach a limited number of theoretical frameworks [1]. Moreover, within our country, there has been little discussion of the various ways that occupational science and occupation can be understood and the local implications of these alternative perspectives [2–4].

The challenge for Chilean occupational therapists is to stimulate local discussion of these ideas and develop a theoretical framework that will support undergraduate and postgraduate occupational science/occupational therapy education. This content would provide students with a sound theoretical foundation, strengthen professional identity, and create effective connections between theory and practice [5–11].

Meeting this challenge requires recognizing the place of occupational science in professional education. Studies have shown that occupational therapists rarely use occupational therapy-specific theories to justify their practices, depending instead on concepts borrowed from other disciplines. This situation can be improved if occupational science concepts, foundations, and theories are taught explicitly [12] in occupational therapy education programs, along with their therapeutic applications to occupational behaviors.

As members of the Occupational Science Education Committee, we propose that it is essential to analyze the Chilean understanding of occupational science. Chilean perspectives are reflected in the Chilean Journal of Occupational Therapy (RChTO), which is our highest-impact scientific journal in the discipline [13]. This study explores the question: What approaches to understanding and applying occupational science/occupation are referenced in RChTO articles?

Theoretical Framework. As the objective of this study is to identify approaches to understanding and applying occupational science, we will define some relevant concepts.

Occupational science is the academic study of occupation [14]. It provides a theoretical and scientific foundation for occupational therapy practice, approaching occupation as an inherent human phenomenon. Because of its focus on human behavior, occupational science is considered a social science, like anthropology, psychology, or sociology [15].

One of the first approaches used in occupational science was to study the form, function, and meaning of occupation [14]. Form references to directly observable aspects of occupation. For example, occupational scientists may compare how different cultures or social groups perform a given occupation. Function refers to the contributions of an occupation to human development, health, or quality of life. Meaning refers to the subjective experience of participating in an occupation, which is constructed symbolically within a culture.

Understanding the evolution of occupational science/occupational therapy requires epistemological reflection. Contemporary analysis also involves social, economic, and political dimensions, as the discipline has broadened from an individual-centered perspective to consider the contribution of the community and context [16].

Occupational science/occupation is addressed in many ways in the literature. One way to sift through these perspectives is to investigate how concepts are applied, understood, and studied within the field, seeking to identify different approaches to understanding and application.

Several authors [17–19], reflecting on currents of thought, define approaches to understanding and application as ideologies, viewpoints, or theoretical concepts which explain phenomena that are shared, followed, and reproduced [18] within a discipline [19] through conferences, scientific journals, or other means. Authors sharing an approach may develop their own branches of the fundamental theory but use a common explanatory model [17]. Therefore, an approach is distinctive within a discipline [20], and there is general agreement on the basic conceptual elements and theoretical foundations [18].

Occupational therapy paradigms represent unified concepts set forth by authors seeking to define the nature and purpose of the discipline. These concepts are based on the principles articulated in publications such as those listed in the bibliography. Paradigms provide conceptualizations that organize theories and explain their applications [20].

Approaches to understanding and application represent a distinctive vision of the world. Different approaches may share instruments or theoretical categories. The procedures used in different approaches are based on their underlying world view [18]. Authors sometimes explicitly identify an approach as separate from another approach to understanding and application, alluding to the controversies over different approaches [19].

2. Methods

A systematic qualitative review [21] of the RChTO was performed. This method is based on grounded theory [22], which identifies the core concepts within systematically collected data on a topic. Such an approach does not require an a priori hypothesis but rather seeks to identify a new theory, in this case, approaches to the study of occupation. Other reviews have found this method effective for discovering patterns in the occupational science literature [23].

Inclusion criteria for articles were as follows: (a) keyword(s) and/or title referring to OS/O concepts; (b) published articles between 2001 and 2012; and (c) being available in full-text format.

Articles were analyzed using the operational definition of approach to understanding and application:

(i) *Authors refer explicitly* to a viewpoint on occupational science/occupation.

(ii) *Theories are explicitly identified*, such as epistemological assumptions in the context of a given paradigm; general theories on society or history; theories or assumptions on measurement, observation, data collection, or empirical evidence; theoretically based inferences; or construction of theoretical concepts [24].

(iii) *Conceptual models and paradigms are used.* For instance, theoretical or conceptual elements extracted from a general theory are cited; a model is used to understand an issue; or an explicit theoretical position from a specific approach is applied.

(iv) *Definitions of occupational science/occupation are provided.* A definition is an attempt to explain an idea or term by providing a precise and exhaustive reflection. Therefore, a definition is a cohesive description of the complex state of an object, circumstance, or idea that can be validated through examination.

(v) *Conceptualizations of occupational science/occupation are developed.* A conceptualization is an abstract, simplified perspective on our understanding of some aspect of the world. These abstract ideas stem from the experience and conscious understanding of the world [24, 25]. Conceptualizations may include new propositions and concepts or syntheses of existing ideas on occupational science/occupation.

The research team held several meetings to agree on our understanding and synthesis of the content and capture the issues highlighted by the authors. Finally, the articles were categorized according to similarities and differences.

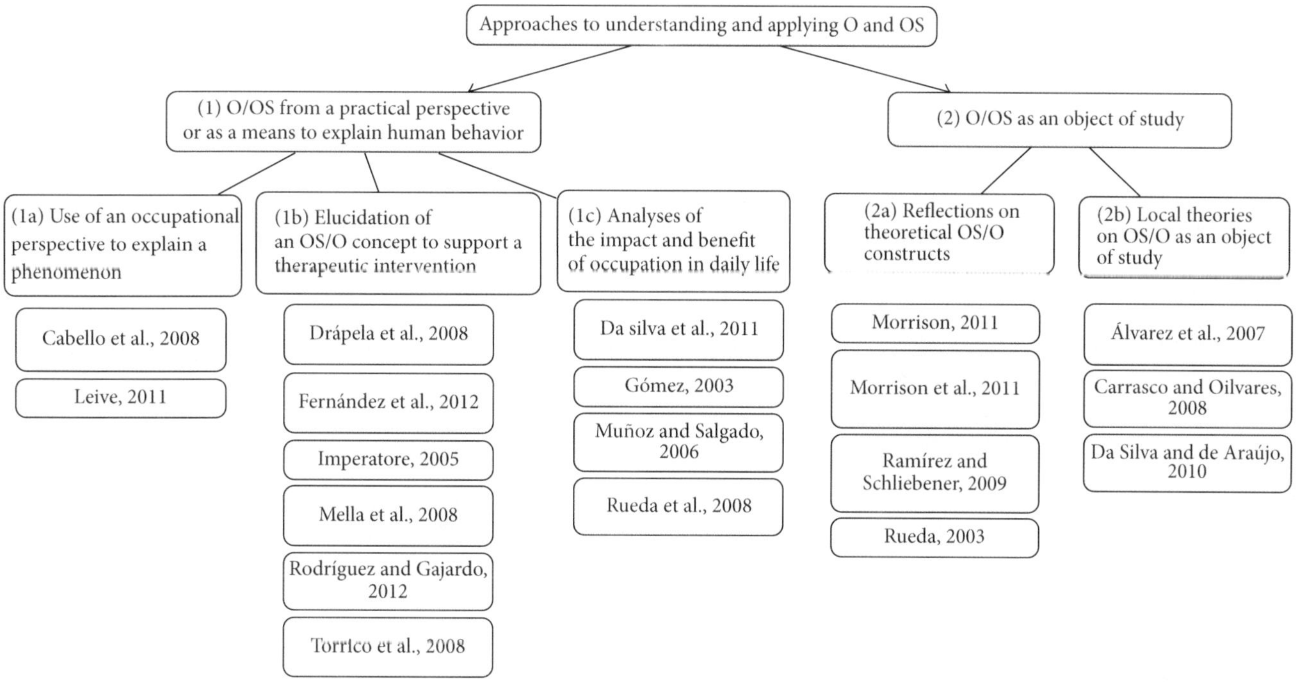

FIGURE 1: Approaches used by various authors, highlighting the two main approaches and the categories.

The research team systematically carried out specific tasks, including cross-reviewing notes, working in parallel and in dyads, outlining meeting minutes, summarizing findings, and critically reviewing these summaries.

The process can be summarized as follows:

(i) Article selection.

(ii) Identification and labeling of references to occupational science/occupation, including authors referenced, in each full-text article.

(iii) Summaries of findings regarding the approaches cited, including the key ideas and citations to support each point.

(iv) Triangulation of information gathered by the research team.

(v) Analysis and synthesis of articles in weekly meetings.

(vi) Categorization of articles.

(vii) Naming the approach to understanding and application for each group.

3. Analysis and Results

Of the 95 articles published in the journal between 2001 and 2012, 19 met the inclusion criteria. The analysis identified two main approaches. The first considers occupation/occupational science from a practical perspective or as a means to explain human behavior (12 articles); the second considers occupation/occupational science as an object of study (7 articles). Both approaches were then divided into categories, as shown in Figure 1 and described below.

(1) Occupation or Occupational Science Considered from a Practical Perspective or as a Means to Explain Human Behavior. These approaches represent first-order analyses, that is, studies performed by authors who instead of asking "what is occupation?" attempt to assign attributes to the concept and provide bibliographic references to support their analysis. These authors approach occupational science/occupation from a practical standpoint and as a way to explain human behavior.

This approach is divided into categories: (a) use of an occupational perspective to explain a phenomenon; (b) elucidation of an occupational science/occupation concept to support a therapeutic intervention; and (c) analyses of the impact and benefit of occupation in daily life.

(1a) Use of an Occupational Perspective to Explain a Particular Phenomenon. This category is based on a concrete situation, a specific conception of occupation, or a local reality. Occupation is used to explain a social behavior from the perspective of a previously defined theoretical construct. Authors that use this approach include Leive [26] and Cabello et al. [27].

In terms of conceptualizations and definitions of occupational science/occupation, Leive [26] focuses on the occupations of families. Occupations are evolving, flexible, orchestrated in parallel with other occupations, and purposeful. Therefore, behaviors that are involuntary, such as sleeping, are not occupations. However, going to sleep and waking up are occupations, as these acts possess a temporal-spatial structure, organization, and biological dimension.

To support this idea, Leive cites the following: Pierce's [28] concept of cooccupation, an occupation that requires synchrony within the occupational patterns of a cohabitating group; Zemke and Clark [14], emphasizing the crucial role of the environment in the construction of occupation, especially the family environment for children; Esdaile and Olson [29], noting that if occupational problems occur, the family dynamic is affected, including the orchestration of caregiver-child cooccupations and other familial roles; and Evans and Rodger [30], noting that the degree of synchronization between the caregiver and child impacts the construction of everyday occupations.

Occupations are performed as part of a routine that depends partly on others. An occupation has a name provided by society that reflects its meaning, is flexible in the face of daily requirements, is performed at a given time, and can be executed with mastery.

Occupations are made up of various tasks. Performing these tasks impacts growth and development. The conditions for existence underlying an occupation include the presence of cooccupations, such as a child going to sleep, which require a certain profile of person, such as a caregiver, to assist in performing them.

Leive asserts that it is necessary to develop certain behaviors before performing some occupations (e.g., going to sleep independently) and that synchrony between the caregiver and child constructs the child's occupation. Moreover, a suitable environment is required (such as the environment surrounding a child and caregiver). Finally, a routine is necessary to configure an occupation, which occurs through a progressive process.

For Cabello et al. [27], occupations are understood as part of everyday life and are performed habitually. Occupations are influenced by the occupations of others and modeled over time. As such, parents influence their children's occupations. The structure of an occupation impacts the family and children, driving behaviors. Occupational modeling consists of imitation (acting; doing) and imagination (preparing for action; thinking) and is influenced by interpersonal relationships. When there is disequilibrium, such as when a family member has a disability, occupations can become risk factors.

The authors cite concepts from Christiansen [31] to suggest that occupations impact social development and the emergence of habits and personal identity. Problems with participation in occupations are risk factors that affect the health of family members, especially children. The authors draw upon Nelson and Jepson-Thomas [32], noting that learning is an adaptive process that occurs through the performance of occupations.

Occupations and occupational knowledge impact a person's health. Occupations influence one's ability to adapt to society, develop habits, and identity and maintain relationships. Occupational modeling arises through interactions between people.

This perspective differs from those that follow because it does not (explicitly) take occupation as a therapeutic tool, but it allows accounting for different phenomena, a function that is also taken by authors in the following categories.

(1b) Elucidation of an Occupational or Occupational Science Concept to Support a Specific Therapeutic Intervention. This group of authors proposes that a theoretical construct of occupation can be used to explain a behavior and perform a therapeutic intervention in a particular population. Authors using this approach include Drápela et al. [33]; Fernández et al. [34]; Imperatore [35]; Mella et al. [36]; Rodríguez and Gajardo [37]; and Torrico et al. [38].

In terms of definitions and conceptualizations of occupational science/occupation, Drápela et al. [33], in their investigation of persons deprived of their liberty, where they identified the meanings associated with criminal activity, indicate that occupation is human performance in response to the vital needs of an individual that allows one to meet social demands, express oneself, and develop an identity. Occupations provide a path towards meaning in life and the development of personal, cultural, and social identity. Occupations consist of meaningful activities; their effects include a sense of efficacy, and they are essential for achieving personal objectives and forging a strong self-concept. These elements are therefore developed through occupation in an occupational therapy intervention. In this way, in occupational therapy intervention, through the occupation, the previous elements are identified.

Fernández et al. [34] suggest that, in order for an occupation to be meaningful, it should support identity construction, provide a sense of belonging, and promote empowerment. This research is focused on productive enterprises of people suffering from mental health problems and shows how therapeutic intervention favors these enterprises and contributes to social rehabilitation.

Imperatore [35] reflects on occupation as the object of occupational science study in the context of sensory integration disorders, especially the impact of such disorders on occupation selection. The author notes that occupation consists of form, function, and meaning, based on concepts [14]. The author presents factors that influence occupation selection, with an emphasis on the "occupational metamorphosis" concept [39], which explains relationships among biological factors such as sensory-seeking behaviors. Thus, occupation functions as a therapeutic tool that affects a person's biology as well as their occupational performance. For this reason, therapeutic intervention by means of the occupation is a central axis in the treatment of sensory integration disorders.

The author cites Zemke [40], reflecting on the organization of occupation in space and time and its relationship with sensory processing. Time is described as the perception of change, including perception of simultaneity, subjective present, sequencing, and duration.

Mella et al. [36], in their investigation of persons deprived of liberty, focus on other considerations regarding occupation. For these authors, occupation (a) is a right and a fundamental element of society in everyday life; (b) has individual meaning and value provided by one's culture and context; (c) includes everyday tasks (self-care, leisure, and contributions to social and economic development of one's community); and (d) represents an intervention space for occupational therapy, as it serves as a potential rehabilitation tool consisting of an organized set of specific tasks and activities.

In the process of therapeutic intervention, the occupation guarantees the right to social integration, allows for emergence of a social order, and supports individual and social wellbeing (including for persons deprived of liberty). Its conditions for existence include everyday activities, which change according to the context and are structured as a function of a person's external conditions.

The authors assert that occupational science conceptualizations are relevant to occupational therapy practice. Theoretical occupational science foundations can be applied to interventions, including in the population of persons deprived of liberty. The authors suggest that these conceptualizations can be used to establish foundations for interventions. Outlining the stages of the intervention based on occupational science concepts ensures that the process will reflect a focus on occupational elements.

Rodríguez and Gajardo [37], in their research into the perceptions of elderly people about their use of public transport, note that occupation provides structure to life, drives habit development, and regulates affective relationships both with others and with the context. Occupation also offers a means to address psychological and behavioral symptoms. Therefore, its conditions for existence are the demands of the environment and the conditions of the person. The relevance of therapeutic intervention in this context is crucial to increase the quality of life of elderly people.

Torrico et al. [38] in their study on the occupational performance of a group of women note that occupations are affected by the rhythms of daily life and are expressed in both work and family contexts. The authors reflect on whether occupation arises from an individual or is determined by historical or cultural context. Occupation consists of form, function, and meaning.

In the intervention process, the occupation increases productivity; affects a person's life satisfaction; satisfies basic survival needs (self-care, shelter, safety, and sustenance); supports social structures (defense against predators and the environment); develops personal abilities; and affects health. Occupations may also generate or be influenced by risk factors including hardship, marginalization, alienation, and inequality [41], as well as gender prejudices that limit the occupations of women.

The principal condition for existence of occupation is the person, that is, the human as an occupational being in a sociocultural context. Occupational choices are determined by economic, political, social, and cultural conditions and are associated with social justice and equality.

To summarize, authors in this category consider occupation and occupational science in terms of therapeutic interventions with specific groups of users or patients. Like category (1a), this category uses occupational terminology to account for a problem, but it differs by proposing a specific therapeutic intervention. Thus, occupational science constructs are present in the intervention processes.

(1c) Analysis of the Impact and Benefit of Occupation in Daily Life. This category is used by a group of authors who address the benefits of occupation in general rather than for a particular population. These authors include Gómez [42]; Da Silva et al. [43]; Muñoz and Salgado [44]; and Rueda et al. [45].

In terms of the definition and conceptualization of occupation, Gómez [42] argues that occupation is a powerful agent capable of driving significant life changes. Occupations organize life, create a day-to-day identity, and provide existence with meaning.

Occupation has both a purpose and meaning. Purpose initiates the activity of occupation, and meaning is a complex, unconscious process mediated by affective and social elements.

Gómez notes that the study of occupation reveals the practical dimension of individuality that emerges through performing an occupation. That is, the concept of individuality is fundamental to the theoretical foundation of occupational science. The author emphasizes that the practice of individual occupations overlaps and intersects with other occupations, making it impossible to understand an occupation as an isolated entity. The intersections between occupations are evident in family, social, and work environments.

Da Silva et al. [43] understand occupation as a therapeutic strategy and central element in the development of occupational therapy. They note that the meaning of occupation changes according to the cultural context. For example, roles that are significant in occidental societies may have no meaning in nonoccidental societies. The authors point out that participating in occupations positively impacts a person's health.

In terms of the conceptualization and definition of occupational science/occupation, Muñoz and Salgado [44] propose that occupation includes a person's everyday tasks and may include activities performed during one's free time, such as relaxation, recreation, or leisure. Occupation has form, function, and meaning. In this approach to understanding occupation, the physical context is crucial and an object of occupational science investigation.

For Rueda et al. [45], occupation differentiates persons from other living beings and is constitutive of humanity. Participation in occupations can (a) generate an occupational equilibrium or disequilibrium; (b) emerge as the product of the time and place in which a person performs his or her activities; (c) provide an individual and collective sense to human groups; and (d) promote social belonging and strengthen the bonds among persons. In conclusion, occupations help to make sense of the project of life.

Authors in this category evaluate occupational context from various perspectives. They address the benefits of occupation in general. Thus, this category provides universal characteristics of the occupation applicable to every person. It does not focus on a specific population, as in category (1b), nor does it only explain a phenomenon such as in category (1a).

This approach, which views occupation and occupational science from a practical perspective or as a means to explain human behavior, differs from the next approach, which employs epistemological and theoretical elements to explain and analyze occupation and occupational science.

(2) Occupation and Occupational Science as an Object of Study. This approach is characterized by (1) reflection on occupational science/occupation concepts; (2) discussion of the approaches used to analyze these constructs; and (3) analysis of theoretical positions that impact practical occupational therapy knowledge and theory. These reflections are second-order analyses, associated with philosophy or epistemology.

This approach can be divided into the following categories: (a) reflections on theoretical occupational science/occupation constructs and (b) local theories on occupational science/occupation as an object of study.

(2a) Reflections on Theoretical Constructs of Occupation or Occupational Science. Authors in this category offer ways to understand occupational science/occupation from a reflective and epistemological perspective.

Morrison [46] offers a conceptual foundation based on philosophical methods which challenges occupational science to engage in a speculative and metareflective process. This philosophy of human occupation (Spanish acronym FOH, for *filosofía de la ocupación humana*) links rhetoric with science to analyze the development, structure, and dissemination of occupational science/occupational therapy knowledge, from an interpretive and critical position.

For Morrison, occupation is a phenomenon amenable to philosophical analysis, a component of clinical occupational therapy practice, a subject of occupational science investigation, and a political element. Morrison cites authors such as Wilcock [41], emphasizing her theory of the occupational nature of human beings, developed through reflections on policies, ecosystems, and relationships between the person and the environment; Kronenberg et al. [47], emphasizing their political-social perspective; and Carrasco and Olivares [2], noting that the construct of occupation implies interdependence between the subject and the constructed reality.

Morrison et al. [48] also conceptualize FOH as a discipline that studies the structure of occupational therapy/occupational science knowledge, developing metatheories that allude first to scientific knowledge and then to scientific practice. The authors support their propositions by citing Díez and Moulines [49], Echeverría [50], Longino [51], and Marcos [52].

FOH addresses knowledge, learning, and internalization of information. The process allows for a critical approach towards the acquisition of occupational therapy knowledge and its translation into actions within the context of professional practice.

Paradigms, therefore, operate within both theory and practice. Paradigms facilitate articulation of key occupational therapy/occupational science concepts and illustrate the evolution of scientific knowledge within the social context of the professionals who generate the findings.

The article also applies Morín's complexity paradigm [53] to the study of occupational therapy/occupation. The advantage of this approach is its divergence from linear, mechanistic paradigms [54]. The notion of complexity liberates the authors from the health-sickness dichotomy and accommodates the totality of factors affecting quality of life. Conceptualizations derived from the complexity paradigm can be applied to occupational science, including multidimensionality and the impulse towards multidimensionality and critical thinking that leads to the problematization of previously taken-for-granted concepts.

Finally, the authors propose a social paradigm of occupation, based on Kuhn [19]. This paradigm considers the evolution of scientific knowledge within the social context of the professionals who generate the findings. The paradigm remains in constant development, positioning occupation as a complex, systematic concept with economic, political, health-related, cultural, and social dimensions that affect the equity and wellbeing of communities.

Ramírez and Schliebener [55] propose the use of dialectics to generate occupational science research and analysis methods. These authors examine occupation in relation to existing narratives, including the occupational reflections of characters found in classical Chilean literature.

The authors consider occupation to be a complex phenomenon that undergoes constant transformation, as its medium (the environment and the person) also experiences continual change. Occupations are understood in the local context and performed by people in the here and now, but each occupation also has a history, essence, and distinctive character that differentiate it from other occupations. The concept, therefore, possesses both an objective dimension, based on reality, and a subjective dimension, based on individual learning. The occupational action executed by a person represents the synthesis of both factors. This action consists of individual elements, which have distinctive features, and common elements, which remain constant in different places and times.

Ramírez and Schliebener posit that occupations create and transform society, changing recursively in the face of emerging requirements. Occupations also influence personal identity, thereby changing the way that a person performs other occupations. Occupations are based on material and historical conditions but are also influenced by the ideas of the performer. That is, occupations are performed in given a space and time in a way that involves both objective (social) and subjective (individual) elements. Certain conditions are required for each occupation, which are determined by other, previously performed occupations, implying a historical development of occupation.

The authors also argue for the utility of historical materialism to justify interventions in a specific population (historical materialism is an epistemological explanation that accounts for how human history has developed. Based on the ideas of Karl Marx and Friedrich Engels, historical materialism positions material conditions of existence as a basis for understanding juridical relationships and forms of state and of all civil society [56]. Thus, to think of human occupation from this perspective implies understanding the material historicity of occupations and how this explains, for example, occupational performance). These authors use dialectics as a foundation to study occupation, noting that its complexity makes it useful for elucidating this multifaceted concept. The authors view dialectics as the science of the general laws governing nature, avoiding the partialities associated with the subject performing the occupation. The authors consider a materialist perspective to be essential for comprehending occupation and its inherently subjective elements from an objective standpoint [57].

Rueda [58] redefines the concept of occupation based on hermeneutic and phenomenological rules [59]. Hermeneutics is used to generate a new reading of occupation by examining previous texts from various authors. Phenomenology is used to understand occupation as a pivotal point of human experience as well as explore the significance of this experience.

The author interprets occupation as a concept that involves a speculative knowledge or an attempt to comprehend the world, including the facet of the world called occupation.

Based on historical texts, the author notes that occupational therapy brought together biomedical and humanist knowledge from different perspectives. These views included content from studies conducted outside of Chile, but applicable to the Chilean context through hermeneutics.

Rueda also considers occupation from a bioethical. The author underscores concepts essential to occupation as understood in occupational therapy: knowing, doing, formal education, professional practice, models, techniques, and praxis. These concepts are based on Lolas [60], who notes that some characteristics of professional practice are defined by society. Professional practice includes the translation of knowledge into action; moreover, the author distinguishes between those who create and those who apply knowledge. The latter group ultimately fulfills the goals of professional practice. Specific professional actions are expressed through models, which facilitate deeds well done that articulate the knowledge, techniques, and interests of a profession.

Rueda notes that, in generating a body of knowledge and validating scientific findings, it is important to remain conscious of the discipline's theoretical framework. Therefore, if occupational science is incorporated into occupational therapy, the development and evolution of the two fields go hand-in-hand.

Authors in this category use different theoretical and philosophical approaches to reflect on occupation and occupational science but do not propose a redefinition of concepts.

(2b) Local Theories on Occupation or Occupational Science as an Object of Study. This second category applies the study of occupational science/occupation to local realities and, unlike the previous category, proposes a redefinition of concepts. The authors that use this approach are Álvarez et al. [61], Carrasco and Olivares [2], and Da Silva and de Araújo [62].

Álvarez et al. (2010) propose a theoretical construction of occupation, with conceptual bases including (a) Latin American perspectives on knowledge and (b) the epistemology of historical consciousness, citing Zemelman in both instances [63, 64]. The first element suggests that Latin American concepts have developed out of investigations into the social world, incorporating components such as subjects, collective subjectivities, and social movements, and an awareness of history and politics. The second element focuses on the ethics and politics of generating knowledge, opening new, coherent horizons that contrast historically fragmented perspectives on knowledge.

The authors note that the reconceptualization of the term occupation provides opportunities for discussion and growth within the discipline. Recognizing that national conceptualizations are based largely on international works, they applied the international literature to the Latin American process, emphasizing the need to define occupational science in the national context. The authors propose a local definition that is the product of long-term reflection: occupation is a meaningful everyday activity, performed by a person and named by the culture.

Carrasco and Olivares [2] cite Kuhn's paradigm [19] to support the assertion that occupational science/occupational therapy professionals hold the concept of occupation central to their disciplines despite different nuances in interpretation. The authors propose that general systems theory (GST) [65, 66] supports a deep understanding of occupation, as it conceptualizes human beings as high-complexity systems and therefore drives articulation of social and natural scientific findings through multidisciplinary studies. They further suggest that dynamic systems theory (DST) [65, 67, 68] may facilitate a more comprehensive understanding of occupation. DST goes beyond the hierarchical relationships established by GTS to encompass heterarchical associations. Furthermore, DST captures the dynamic nature of complex systems. By citing the theoretical constructs used in the field, Carrasco and Olivares apply a constructivist approach [69], emphasizing the role of occupational therapists in developing the theoretical foundation of their discipline.

The authors approach occupation as an element that can be understood through human and social dimensions and as the object of occupational therapy investigations. Occupation is a phenomenon that can be studied and explained, as it is performed and observed in a given environment.

Carrasco and Olivares refer to authors who approach occupation as an object of occupational science investigations that consists of observable elements, such as form, as well as interpretable elements, such as meaning and purpose. The study of occupation promotes development of the academic discipline and clinical occupational therapy practice.

The authors also note that occupation is not synonymous with activity [28] as perceived by individuals or society in general. Occupation is a discrete act and experience perceived as distinct by the person who performs it. This experience is individual and singular. Occupations are different each time they are performed due to the interaction among the various components, evolving across the lifespan.

The authors reference Kielhofner [70] to illustrate that occupational therapy has a unique perspective shared across the discipline, despite nuances that surface in applications to different contexts. The authors also cite other sources that define occupation: (a) Nelson [71], who proposes that the significance of occupation lies in its symbolic meaning, which emerges in a given space and time, and is therefore singular, and (b) Iwama [72], who emphasizes the individual meanings of occupation that materialize in different cultural and social contexts.

Carrasco and Olivares conceptualize occupation as a result of dynamic interactions between activity, purpose, occupational form, and meaning.

In sum, the authors propose a concept of occupation based on three types of constructions: (a) the habitual and historic occupational therapy factors—that is, person, environment, and activity—which are not subject to direct observation or analysis, as it is impossible to separate the person from their environment or activity; (b) factors that can be perceived and analyzed by an observer, that is, the occupation's form, function, and meaning; and (c) factors only interpretable by the person performing the occupation.

Occupation also has certain conditions for existence, such as association with the human and social spheres. These factors are evident when occupation is approached from a subjective perspective. This means that there are many ways to understand occupation that depend on the observer's viewpoint and context and therefore many ways to explain reality. Categories, which emerge through interactions among people (intersubjectivity) in a given situation (context), can facilitate such understanding. These concepts explain "reality" but they are not reality.

The study by Da Silva and de Araújo [62] reflects on local contextualization of occupational science/occupation elements in the practice of occupational therapists working in the Amazon rainforest of Pará, Brazil. These authors cite Clark and Lawlor [73], noting that occupational science is an emerging discipline that understands human beings as occupational beings. The authors emphasize the associations between commitment in the context of occupation and the context of human life, especially the influence of this relationship on health, wellbeing, and social participation, citing Rudman et al. [74] to demonstrate the role of occupation in supporting health and participation.

These authors, therefore, view occupation as participation in everyday activities: self-care, leisure, work, and so forth. The definition of occupation is ambiguous within the discipline, and the term activity is sometimes used interchangeably with occupation. Occupation encompasses a diversity of actions carried out by people in a given context. It is a type of activity that occupies a person within a social context and integrates human expression.

Moreover, occupation includes the activities carried out by a person (who may vary according to age, race, sex, etc.) in the context of work, leisure, and social activities during one's everyday life (which in turn encompasses many contexts influenced by one's culture). Occupations are essential for a person's life, health, and wellbeing; they allow a person to organize his or her world; they are dynamic; and they evolve throughout the lifespan.

Occupation also has therapeutic value that transcends the everyday. Occupation in this sense can generate change, as it touches the social, cultural, economic, biological, and philosophical spheres. The authors approach occupation as a broad subject, noting that a clear description of occupation supports effective occupational therapy interventions.

Occupations consist of actions and meanings that evolve over a person's lifetime, generating change and transformation. Therefore, occupations have a meaning in a given context, provide structure, and endow a person with humanity; their social context is the condition for their existence.

Authors in this category, although employing a series of theoretical constructs that come from different fields of knowledge (especially in the United States), manage to reconstruct or contextualize the occupation for relevant perspectives with the local reality, which enriches regional theoretical and reflexive development.

4. Discussion and Conclusion

This study identified the main approaches to understanding and applying concepts of occupation and occupational science in the literature of the discipline as published in the RChTO between 2001 and 2012. These findings document the diversity of the discipline and contribute to the education of new occupational therapists.

This analysis made it clear that many positions can be used to study occupation. Approaches to understanding occupational science are informed by concepts of occupation, based on literature relevant to authors in occupational science and related fields. The analysis clearly revealed two different approaches. The first considers occupational science/occupation from a practical perspective and as a means to explain human behavior; the second considers occupational science/occupation as an object of study. These approaches were developed on a regional level and have been used as a foundation for local professional practice.

The first main approach is characterized by the application of occupational science/occupation constructions. This approach includes three categories: the use of an occupational perspective to explain particular phenomena; application of occupational science/occupation constructions to therapeutic interventions; and the study of the impact and benefits of occupational science/occupation in daily life.

The second main approach focused on occupational science/occupation as an object of study and can be divided into two branches. One is based on the global analysis of theoretical constructs while the other offers local perspectives on occupational science and occupation.

The latter refers rather to a reconstruction, contextualization, or adaptation of different international theoretical perspectives, and not to the creation of other theories to explain occupation. Thus, the value of this category is that it finds ways to apply international theories at a local level, making them culturally relevant.

A noteworthy finding of this study is that there were only two Latin American theoretical proposals offered in RChTO publications (2001–2012) [2, 55]. Likewise, only one original Latin American definition appeared [61].

In light of the above, we asked about the characteristics of the diffusion of knowledge of occupational therapy in Chile. In Chile and in neighboring countries, the theoretical contributions are generated by groups of academics from the main state universities. In the earlier publications, between the years 1960 and 1980 approximately, a reductionist biomedical paradigm is perceived, which has marked the pattern of practice of the profession in the region. However, the concern to include social participation spaces is not neglected. Later publications are concerned with the empowerment of individuals and groups in their own processes of health maintenance and recovery. In these later publications, the focus is not on the disease but on the person in his or her own context, and on the opportunities that context offers for activities that can be understood as healthy in terms of their meaning for the individual, linked to his or her history, beliefs, and life within a cultural environment.

These results lead to the following questions: What barriers to developing local knowledge do Latin American occupational therapists face? Do Latin American occupational therapists have the motivation, time, and training necessary to carry out research and publish manuscripts? Is the habit of reflecting on interventions an established part of professional practice? Does the discipline, on a Latin American level, place importance on the systematization of professional practices and development of evidence? On an institutional level, are there incentives and support to develop research competency and dissemination of knowledge?

Addressing these questions is crucial to supporting and promoting occupational science/occupational therapy research, a strong professional identity, evidence-based practice, continuing education, scientific societies, and application of research to professional practice. Academic staff responsible for developing occupational therapy curricula should review the competencies needed to improve the discipline and integrate research as a dimension of professional practice.

This study illustrates the recent directions of the discipline at the regional level, examining the written expressions in a particular Spanish-language occupational therapy journal. Therefore, the findings are applicable only to this specific geographic and cultural sphere. It would be interesting to ask the following question: What other fields and media develop and publish reflections and studies of occupational science/occupation?

It seems appropriate to investigate whether studies such as the present have been conducted in other Latin American countries since there are cultural similarities between them, due to their common history. In this way, it would contribute to a broader and deeper knowledge, possibly applicable to the reality of this region, in the areas of theory and practical knowledge. It is also clear, in our view, that the development of knowledge should consider the exercise of distinguishing local knowledge from universal disciplinary knowledge.

Thus, this study provides a new perspective on the way that authors in the field apply occupational science/occupation concepts. It is possible that other sources of literature would yield different approaches for understanding occupational science/occupation concepts.

This study focused on the historical context and temporal elements of the descriptions of occupation in each article. Research to address occupation from cross-sectional (social-historical-cultural) and longitudinal perspectives (current views, issues relevant to the "here and now," capturing unique and unrepeatable moments in time) would also be useful.

This article contributes to the systematization of data relevant to professional practice and provides insights on fundamental concepts such as occupation. The article illustrates current trends in the discipline in terms of research, practice, and education of occupational therapists.

New conceptualizations offered by Latin American authors enrich international development of occupational science and, therefore, the occupational therapy profession.

Acknowledgments

The present study is part of the research project "Updates in Occupational Science: A Contribution to Research-Based Teaching" and was funded by the "Fund for Applied Research in Occupational Therapy and Occupational Science of the Department of Occupational Therapy and Occupational Science of the University of Chile (2013)."

References

[1] M. Apablaza, "The challenge of training: a reflection from practice as trainer occupational therapists," *Chilean Journal of Occupational Therapy*, vol. 15, no. 2, 2015.

[2] J. Carrasco M and D. Olivares A, "Making way to go: construction and understanding of Occupation for research and practice in Occupational Therapy," *Chilean Journal of Occupational Therapy*, vol. 8, pp. 5–16, 2008.

[3] E. I. Blanche and E. Henny-Kohler, "Philosophy, science and ideology: a proposed relationship for occupational science and occupational therapy," *Occupational Therapy International*, vol. 7, no. 2, pp. 99–110, 2000.

[4] R. Morrison, "Pragmatist epistemology and Jane Addams: fundamental concepts for the social paradigm of occupational therapy," *Occupational Therapy International*, vol. 23, no. 4, pp. 295–304, 2016.

[5] P. Crist, M. Scaffa, and B. Hooper, "Occupational therapy education and the centennial vision: preface," *Occupational Therapy in Health Care*, vol. 24, no. 1, pp. 1–6, 2010.

[6] B. Hooper, "The occupation of teaching: elements of meaning portrayed through educators' teaching diagrams," *Journal of Occupational Science*, vol. 18, no. 2, pp. 167–181, 2011.

[7] B. Hooper, "On arriving at the destination of the centennial vision: navigational landmarks to guide occupational therapy education," *Occupational Therapy in Health Care*, vol. 24, no. 1, pp. 97–106, 2010.

[8] B. Hooper, "Shortening the distance between the 'i' and the 'it': a transformative approach to improving teaching," *Occupational Therapy in Health Care*, vol. 21, no. 1-2, pp. 199–215, 2007.

[9] B. Hooper and W. Wood, "Pragmatism and structuralism in occupational therapy: the long conversation," *American Journal of Occupational Therapy*, vol. 56, no. 1, pp. 40–50, 2002.

[10] C. Mattingly and M. H. Fleming, *Clinical Reasoning: Forms of Inquiry in A Therapeutic Practice*, Davis, F. A., Philadelphia, Pa, USA, 1994.

[11] E. J. Yerxa, "Infinite distance between the/and the it," *American Journal of Occupational Therapy*, vol. 63, no. 4, pp. 490–497, 2009.

[12] M. N. Ikiugu and H. M. Rosso, "Facilitating professional identity in occupational therapy students," *Occupational Therapy International*, vol. 10, no. 3, pp. 206–225, 2003.

[13] R. Bustos, "Chilean Journal of Occupational Therapy is the most consulted of Faculty of Medicine' jurnals in Internet," Faculty of Medicine, Universidad de Chile, http://noticias.med.uchile.cl/actividades-decanato/9588-revista-chilena-de-terapia-ocupacional-es-la-mas-consultada-en-internet-de-la-facultad-de-medicina.html.

[14] R. Zemke and F. Clark, *Occupational Science: The Evolving Discipline*, F. A. Davis Company, Philadelphia, Pa, USA, 1996.

[15] E. J. Yerxa, "Occupational science: a renaissance of service to humankind through knowledge," *Occupational Therapy International*, vol. 7, no. 2, pp. 87–98, 1998.

[16] G. Whiteford and C. Hocking, *Occupational Science: Society, Inclusion, Participation*, John Wiley & Sons, Milton, Australia, 2012.

[17] N. A. Casullo, R. Forster, and A. Kaufman, *Itineraries Modernity. Currents of thought and intellectual traditions from the Enlightenment to Postmodernism*, Eudeba, Buenos Aires, Argentina, 1999.

[18] J. García-Arias, "Could the theory of thought modes explain some of the differences between mainstream and keynesian/post-keynesian economics?" *Social Science Journal*, vol. 15, no. 4, pp. 573–585, 2010, http://www.redalyc.org/articulo.oa?id=28012285002.

[19] T. Kuhn, *The Structure of Scientific Revolutions*, University of Chicago Press, Chicago, Ill, USA, 2nd edition, 1970.

[20] G. Kielhofner, *Conceptual Foundations of Occupational Therapy Practice*, F. A. Davis, Philadelphia, Fla, USA, 4th edition, 2009.

[21] S. L. M. Letelier, M. J. J. Manríquez, and G. G. Rada, "Systematic reviews and metaanalysis: are they the best evidence?" *Medical Journal of Chile*, vol. 133, no. 2, pp. 246–249, 2005.

[22] A. L. Strauss and J. M. Corbin, *Bases of Qualitative Research: Techniques and Procedures for Developing Grounded Theory*, Univ. of Antioquia Press, Medellín, Colombia, 2002.

[23] D. Pierce, K. Atler, J. Baltisberger et al., "Occupational science: a data-based american perspective," *Journal of Occupational Science*, vol. 17, no. 4, pp. 204–215, 2010.

[24] R. Sautu, *Everything Is Theory: Research Objectives And Methods*, Lumiere, Buenos Aires, Argentina, 2005.

[25] Knowledge Master Corporation, "Conceptualization," http://conceptmaps.it/KM-Conceptualization-esp.htm.

[26] L. Leive, "Bedtime routine in the first years of life: first theoretical approach from an occupational Science perspective," *Chilean Journal of Occupational Therapy*, vol. 11, no. 2, pp. 70–83, 2011.

[27] P. A. Cabello, E. Henny, M. C. Hidalgo, and L. Vásquez, "The occupations of the children of parents with disabilities," *Chilean Journal of Occupational Therapy*, vol. 8, pp. 79–83, 2008.

[28] D. Pierce, "Untangling occupation and activity," *American Journal of Occupational Therapy*, vol. 55, no. 2, pp. 138–146, 2001.

[29] A. Esdaile and A. Olson, *Mothering Occupations. Challenge, Agency and Participation*, F.A. Davis, Philadelphia, 2004.

[30] J. Evans and S. Rodger, "Mealtimes and bedtimes: windows to family routines and rituals," *Journal of Occupational Science*, vol. 15, no. 2, Article ID 9686615, pp. 98–104, 2008.

[31] C. H. Christiansen, "Defining lives: occupation as identity: an essay on competence, coherence, and the creation of meaning [The Eleanor Clarke Slagle lecture]," *American Journal of Occupational Therapy*, vol. 53, no. 6, pp. 547–558, 1999.

[32] D. Nelson and J. Jepson-Thomas, "Occupational form, occupational performance, and a conceptual framework for therapeutic occupational," in *Perspectives in Human Occupation-Participation in Life*, P. Kramer, J. Hinojosa, and C. B. Royeen, Eds., pp. 87–155, Lippincott Williams and Wilkins, Baltimore, Md, USA, 2003.

[33] B. J. Drápela, G. M. d. Huidobro, S. J. Núñez, and T. M. Palacios, ""Meanings associated to criminal activities" in men who are deprived of their liberty in Centro de Detención Preventiva Santiago Sur," *Chilean Journal of Occupational Therapy*, vol. 8, pp. 47–58, 2008.

[34] M. M. E. Fernández, G. A. Gaviglio, and S. G. Adur, "An analysis on participation in productive enterprises in mental health area, in the context of social economy in Buenos Aires city-Argentina," *Chilean Journal of Occupational Therapy*, vol. 12, no. 2, 2012.

[35] E. Imperatore Blanche, "Deficit Sensory Integration: Long-term effects on occupation and play," *Chilean Journal of Occupational Therapy*, vol. 5, pp. 1–6, 2005.

[36] S. Mella, V. Villarroel, R. Sepúlveda, and G. Guzmán, "Occupation: a proposal for intervention with persons deprived of liberty based on occupation," *Chilean Journal of Occupational Therapy*, vol. 8, pp. 37–46, 2008.

[37] J. Rodríguez and J. Gajardo, "About the contribution of occupational therapy to non-pharmacologic approaches for the treatment of psychological and behavioral symptoms associated with dementia," *Chilean Journal of Occupational Therapy*, vol. 12, no. 2, 2012.

[38] P. Torrico, D. Urrutia, and M. Schliebener, "How meaningful is for the women themselves the activities they carry out?" *Chilean Journal of Occupational Therapy*, vol. 8, pp. 17–25, 2008.

[39] S.-P. C. Fanchiang, "The other side of the coin: growing up with a learning disability," *American Journal of Occupational Therapy*, vol. 50, no. 4, pp. 277–285, 1996.

[40] R. Zemke, *Time, Space and the Kaleidoscopes of Occupation*, The Eleanor Clarke Slagle Lecture, 2004 AOTA Conference, Minneapolis, MN, USA, 2004.

[41] A. Wilcock, *An Occupational Perspective of Health*, Slack Inc., Thorofare, NJ, USA, 2nd edition, 2006.

[42] L. S. Gómez, "The occupation and its significance as a factor of personal identity," *Chilean Journal of Occupational Therapy*, vol. 3, pp. 43–47, 2003.

[43] L. Da Silva Araújo, N. Fierro Jordán, P. Guitérrez Monclus, and O. Rodriguez, "Occupational science and occupational therapy: its relations and applications to clinical practice," *Chilean Journal of Occupational Therapy*, vol. 11, no. 1, pp. 79–87, 2011.

[44] E. I. Muñoz and G. P. Salgado, "Leisure occupations: approach from a perspective of development, life cycles and human needs," *Chilean Journal of Occupational Therapy*, vol. 6, pp. 39–45, 2006.

[45] L. Rueda, M. A. Montenegro, D. Poblete, and F. Traipe, "Post Traumatic Stress: interference and occupational adjustment," *Chilean Journal of Occupational Therapy*, vol. 8, pp. 27–35, 2008.

[46] R. Morrison J, "Rhetoric of science. Descriptions and critical reflection about creation of knowledge. Contributions to Occupational Therapy," *Chilean Journal of Occupational Therapy*, vol. 11, no. 1, pp. 89–101, 2011.

[47] F. Kronenberg, S. Simó Algado, and N. Pollard, *Occupational Therapy Without Borders: learning From The Spirit of Survivors*, Médica Panamericana, Buenos Aires, Argentina, 2006.

[48] R. Morrison, D. Olivares, and D. Vidal, "The Philosophy of Human Occupation and The Social Paradigm of the Occupation. Some reflections and suggestions on current epistemologies in Occupational Therapy and Occupational Science," *Chilean Journal of Occupational Therapy*, vol. 11, no. 2, pp. 102–119, 2011.

[49] J. Díez and C. Moulines, *Fundamentals of Philosophy of Science*, Ariel, Barcelona, Spain, 1997.

[50] J. Echeverría, *Philosophy of Science*, Akal, Madrid, Spain, 2nd edition, 1998.

[51] H. Longino, *The Fate of Knowledge*, Princeton University Press, NJ, USA, 2002.

[52] A. Marcos, *Science and Action. A Practical Philosophy of Science*, Fondo de Cultura Económica, Mexico City, Mexico, 2010.

[53] E. Morin, *Introduction to Complex Thought*, Gedisa, Barcelona, Spain, 1998.

[54] J. Solana, *With Edgar Morin, for a complex thought. Interdisciplinary implications*, Akal, Madrid, Spain, 2005.

[55] R. Ramírez P and M. Schliebener T, "Occupation and dialectics, an analysis from materialistic dialectic," *Chilean Journal of Occupational Therapy*, vol. 9, pp. 167–178, 2009.

[56] A. Giddens, *A Contemporary Critique of Historical Materialism*, vol. 1, Stanford University Press, Broadway, Calif, USA, 1995.

[57] A. Spirkin and O. Yajot, *Fundamentals of dialectical and historical materialism*, Austral, Santiago, Chile, 1972.

[58] L. Rueda Castro, "Occupation: science and technique of occupational therapy," *Chilean Journal of Occupational Therapy*, vol. 3, pp. 1–5, 2003.

[59] J. Acevedo, *Heidegger and the Technical Era*, Universitaria, Santiago, Chile, 2nd edition, 1999.

[60] F. Lolas, *Bioethics and Medical Anthropology*, Mediterráneo, Santiago, Chile, 2000.

[61] E. Álvarez, S. Gómez, I. Muñoz et al., "Concept of occupation: definition and development. Essay about an experience of theoretical construction from a local identity," *Chilean Journal of Occupational Therapy*, vol. 7, pp. 76–82, 2007.

[62] L. Da Silva and O. de Araújo, "Human occupation and occupational therapist practice's in Pará Amazon: a phenomenological perspective," *Chilean Journal of Occupational Therapy*, vol. 10, pp. 99–110, 2010.

[63] H. Zemelman, *The Horizons of Reason*, Anthropos, Madrid, Spain, 1992.

[64] H. Zemelman, *Subject: Existence and Power*, Anthropos/UNAM, Barcelona, Spain, 1998.

[65] M. Arnold and F. Osorio, *Introduction to Basic Concepts of General Systems Theory*, Möbius strip, 1998, http://www.redalyc.org/articulo.oa?id=10100306.

[66] L. Bertalanfly, *The General Systems Theory*, Fondo de Cultura Económica, Mexico City, Mexico, 1976.

[67] F. Capra, *The Web of Life*, Harper Collins, London, UK, 1997.

[68] J. A. S. Kelso and B. Tuller, "A dynamical basis for action systems," in *Handbook of Cognitive Neuroscience*, M. S. Gazzaniga, Ed., Plenum, New York, NY, USA, 1984.

[69] T. Ibáñez, *Social Psychology Constructionist*, Univ. de Guadalajara Press, Jalisco, México, 1994.

[70] G. Kielhofner, *Model of Human Occupation*, Médica Panamericana, Buenos Aires, Argentina, 3rd edition, 2004.

[71] D. L. Nelson, "Occupation: form and performance," *American Journal of Occupational Therapy*, vol. 42, no. 10, pp. 633–641, 1988.

[72] M. Iwama, *The Kawa Model, Culturally Relevant Occupational Therapy*, Churchill LivingstoneElsevier, New York, NY, USA, 2006.

[73] F. Clark and M. Lawlor, "The Making and mattering of occupational science," in *Willard and Spackman. Occupational Therapy*, E. Crepeau, E. Cohn, and B. Schell, Eds., pp. 14-11e, Wolters Klover Lippincott Williams and Wilkins, Philadelphia, Pa, USA, 2009.

[74] D. L. Rudman, J. V. Cook, and H. Polatajko, "Understanding the potential of occupation: a qualitative exploration of seniors' perspectives on activity," *American Journal of Occupational Therapy*, vol. 51, no. 8, pp. 640–650, 1997.

18

A Qualitative Study to Explore Ways to Observe Results of Engaging Activities in Clients with Dementia

Masahiro Ogawa,[1] Seiji Nishida,[2] and Haruna Shirai[3]

[1] *Department of Human Health Sciences, Graduate School of Medicine, Kyoto University, Kyoto, Japan*
[2] *Faculty of Health and Welfare, Prefectural University of Hiroshima, Hiroshima, Japan*
[3] *School of Health Sciences, Bukkyo University, Kyoto, Japan*

Correspondence should be addressed to Masahiro Ogawa; ogawa.masahiro.4w@kyoto-u.ac.jp

Academic Editor: Lynette Mackenzie

Background. Many occupational therapists face the challenge of helping clients with dementia to select and perform meaningful occupations, which may be difficult due to cognitive impairment. Understanding tacit knowledge of well-experienced occupational therapists could positively affect occupational therapy practice for clients with dementia. *Objectives of Study.* To explore the observations of experienced occupational therapists when evaluating the effects of activities in clients with dementia. *Methods.* Ten occupational therapists with over 10 years of clinical experience participated in this qualitative study. In-depth interviews were conducted to ask the question, "What do you observe in clients with dementia when you assess the effectiveness of activities among these clients?" *Findings.* From 47 cases, we found five major themes and 18 subthemes. Main themes were "engaging activity," "emotional expression during activity," "verbal expression during activity," "social interaction through activity," and "something obtained as outcome of activity." *Relevance to Clinical Practice.* The 18 subthemes could be used as viewpoints to observe engagements of activity in clients with dementia. *Limitations and Recommendations for Further Research.* Future studies could examine which viewpoints were utilized for each type of activity and/or severity of dementia as this was not investigated in the current study.

1. Introduction

The primary goal of occupational therapy is to engage people in occupation [1]. Successful occupation in an engaging activity by individuals with dementia is associated with positive affective outcomes [2, 3]. For example, observation of nursing home residents with dementia revealed that greater well-being was associated with positive and enjoyable engagement in activities [4]. Perrin [5] indicated that the loss of ability to engage in occupation occurring in progressive dementia is a powerful sign of unmet human needs and a major threat to the health and well-being of clients with dementia. These problems were caused by the difficulty of clients with dementia to choose and engage in occupations. In particular, dementia often deprives individuals of the ability to engage in occupations because of difficulty in occupational choice and linguistic representation about feeling and emotion. This is due to both lack of awareness and cognitive impairments such as memory disturbance, orientation disturbance, loss of decision-making capacity, and lack of language comprehension or expression [6]. Therefore, in occupational therapy, many occupational therapists face the challenge of helping clients to select and perform meaningful occupations.

In clinical settings, well-experienced occupational therapists competently select and facilitate their patients' occupational engagement. They empirically seem to have unconscious viewpoints when observing the subjective experiences, feelings, and emotions expressed by a client while engaging in an activity. Understanding occupational therapists' unconscious judgement could positively affect occupational therapy practice for clients with dementia. Therefore, the question arises: "What are the observations of experienced occupational therapists when evaluating the effects of activities in people with dementia?"

During the past decade, understanding the subjective experience of well-being and quality of life has been recognized to be important when observing people with dementia. [7, 8]. Because clients with dementia have difficulty expressing their feelings and experiences while performing activities, they might also struggle with formal self-report measures that examine the effects of engaging occupations, such as the Canadian Occupational Performance Measure (COPM) [9] and the Aid for Decision-Making in Occupation Choice (ADOC) [10].

Studies analyzing interviews conducted with people with dementia have recommended a combination of observations and interviews [11, 12]. Observational assessment for clients with dementia can be crucial, especially for those with severe dementia. Tomori et al. [13] reported that when using the ADOC, an iPad application allowing the user to choose meaningful activities could not in fact identify meaningful activities for clients with severe dementia because of their inability to express opinions. Therefore, certain observational assessment tools, such as Dementia Care Mapping (DCM) [14, 15], have been developed to improve the well-being of individuals with dementia. Brooker and Duce [16] reported that DCM could be used to assess the impact of therapeutic activity in individuals with dementia. It has been reported that meaningful activities for people with dementia are crucial to their well-being, but it is currently unknown which viewpoints of the therapists' observation enable them to determine clients' well-being. Obtaining clearer and more explicit viewpoints could help us in explaining how clients with dementia engage in activities and to judge whether these activities are meaningful. Therefore, this study examined the observations made by experienced occupational therapists while evaluating the effects of activities in clients with dementia.

As a research methodology, the phenomenological approach focuses on the world of everyday life and pays special attention to the careful description of how the ordinary is experienced and expressed in the consciousness of individuals [17, 18]. Moreover, when collecting data on the experiences of occupational therapists, in-depth interviews can be useful to gain a window into the subjective human experience and to develop insight into how individuals think about the world [19]. Given the characteristics of these methods, the phenomenological approach and in-depth interviews are suitable to examine the observations of occupational therapists when evaluating the effects of activities in clients with dementia.

The objective of this study was therefore to explore the observations of experienced occupational therapists when evaluating effects of activity in clients with dementia using the aforementioned methodology. By clarifying the viewpoints, we aimed to design an observational assessment framework for clients with dementia.

2. Methods

2.1. Participants. Study participants were experienced occupational therapists who were proficient at verbally expressing their experiences. Participants were recruited via purposive sampling based on the following inclusion criteria: having more than 10 years' clinical experience and having given lectures or published articles regarding occupational therapy for people with dementia. We deliberately selected participants with various backgrounds to obtain a wide range of items for observing occupational engagement in theoretical sampling [20].

Prior to the interview, participants received written and oral explanations of the research purpose, research method, and protection of personal information. The explanation was carefully performed to ensure participant understanding, and written consent was obtained from each participant. The study was approved by the Ethics Committee of the Medical Department of Kyoto University (approval number: 1126).

2.2. Data Collection. Data were collected in a quiet room where the interview could be recorded face-to-face; only the participant and the interviewer were present. All interviews were audio-recorded with a voice recorder.

Interviews were conducted using an in-depth interview as a reference, according to the method outlined by Lyscak et al. [21]. The interview comprised open-ended questions in which information was solicited relating to the question, "What do you look for in clients with dementia when you assess effects of activity for them?" The primary goal of in-depth interviewing is to delve deeply into a particular event, issue, or context [21].

An unstructured, conversational data collection approach was used. During the interview, participants were asked to recall specific cases in which clients with dementia had experienced positive effects after having engaging in activities. In addition, it was explained to participants that activities were provided by occupational therapists to facilitate their clients to perform or participate in activities. Participants were encouraged to talk about and observe activities they performed with clients and how clients responded. Participants were also asked to explain how they determined that a specific activity was meaningful or effective for the client.

In cases where a participant could not recall a phenomenon, the interviewer asked additional questions to clarify what was observed. For example, the interviewer prepared specific prompts that were asked if necessary, such as "Please recall a situation where you tried to continue to provide a client with an activity. How did the client respond and why did you decide to provide that activity?"

Furthermore, to identify clients' concrete (i.e., objective) actions without the observer's subjective interpretation, follow-up questions were used to delve more deeply into participants' unconscious viewpoints regarding the observation. For instance, after a participant stated that a client's response had been different than his/her usual response when performing a specific activity, the interviewer asked, "How did he/she concretely respond in a manner different from the usual response?" The interviewer worded this question even more specifically if necessary.

Participants recalled and described one client until they could not recall anything further about him or her. Most participants recalled five clients. Each client's severity of

Table 1: Participant characteristics.

Participant number	Clinical workplace	Gender	Years of experience
1	Nursing home	Female	19
2	Nursing home	Female	27
3	Care prevention	Male	13
4	Home-visiting rehabilitation	Female	14
5	Subacute rehabilitation hospital	Male	11
6	The hospital specializing in dementia	Female	20
7	Home-visiting rehabilitation	Female	30
8	Hospital for the elderly	Female	10
9	Home-visiting rehabilitation	Male	15
10	The hospital specializing in dementia	Male	11

dementia was assessed by having participants classify them into three categories: mild, moderate, or severe.

2.3. Data Analysis. Data analysis was performed according to Moustakas' modification of the Stevick-Colaizzi-Keen method for the analysis of phenomenological data [22]. All recorded interviews were transcribed verbatim. First, verbatim transcripts were read to gain a better understanding of the content, including which effects of activity were observed. In the next step of data analysis, participants' experiences of expressing effects of the activity were highlighted and key sentences were underlined and coded to extract invariant meaning units. From these units, similar codes were combined to generate higher-level abstracted themes. Data analysis was conducted using MAXQDA 10 (VERBI, GmbH, Berlin, Germany) qualitative data analysis software.

During data analysis, three researchers—who were experienced in qualitative analysis and were occupational therapists themselves—were asked to provide supervision on a regular basis and provide a second opinion to ensure the reliability and validity of the study. Themes, invariant meaning units, and the content of each theme were repeatedly checked until a consensus was reached.

3. Results

Participants consisted of 10 occupational therapists (6 males, 4 females) with an average clinical experience of 17.0 (±6.9 SD) years. Their primary clinical workplaces consisted of three nursing homes, three home-visiting rehabilitation centers, two hospitals specializing in dementia, one subacute rehabilitation hospital, one hospital for the elderly, and one preventive care service. Participant characteristics are shown in Table 1. Interview duration lasted between 42 and 67 min. From these interviews, 47 client stories were obtained and 154 labels were created. Of the 47 clients, 12 were classified as having mild dementia, 18 as moderate, and 17 as severe.

The viewpoints of occupational therapists while observing activities of patients with dementia were classified into five major themes and 18 subthemes. The major themes were "engaging activity," "emotional expression during activity," "verbal expression during activity," "Social interaction through activity," and "something obtained as outcome of activity." Major themes, subthemes, and brief explanations are shown in Table 2. In the following section, subthemes are in italic font for clarity.

3.1. Major Theme 1: Engaging Activity. Participants observed clients' *directing attention to activity* and *initiating activity* as an effect of activities. Moreover, *continuing activity* and *concentrating on activity* led clients to devote themselves to activities. During activities, clients *expressed their skills and knowledge* or *tried new things during activity*, such as playing a role in an activity or trying new things until a solution was found.

3.1.1. Directing Attention to Activity. Gazing at targets (e.g., book, TV, photo, and iPad) and responding to stimuli from an activity were observed as meaningful actions by some participants. For example, one client who had been previously inactive was watching images on television when her hometown was suddenly shown. When a location that was profoundly memorable to her appeared on the screen, she responded by opening her mouth and saying, "Ah!" The occupational therapist observed the client directing attention to the pictures and thus decided to show them to her once per week as an activity. Gazing at and responding to an activity stimulus indicated that the client was directing attention to an activity, leading therapists to judge that the activity was meaningful.

3.1.2. Initiating Activity. Some participants noted whether a patient initiating an activity was important in assessing the patient. For example, a participant placed a magazine near an inactive client with severe dementia, and said to her, "This picture is so cute! This food looks yummy!" In response, the client willingly turned the page. The therapist was thus able to recognize the client's interest and ability for the first time. In another case, a client who usually roam around joined the group after a therapist called him saying, "It's time for art." The participant observed an effective change in the client from a previously inactive condition to the initiation of activity (drawing a picture).

3.1.3. Continuing Activity. Participants remarked that participation in activities often led patients to repeat the same

Table 2: Major themes, subthemes, and brief explanations for each subthemes.

Main themes	Subthemes	Brief explanations for each subthemes
Engaging activity	Directing attention to activity	To direct one's attention and to show an interest to activity from a gaze, utterance, and an expression
	Initiating activity	To initiate an activity of one's own will or to initiate it after invitation without refusal to an activity
	Continuing activity	To continue an activity for a long time
	Concentrating on activity	To concentrate on an activity with serious expression and innocence
	Expressing skill and knowledge	To express knowledge or to explain it to others
	Trying new things during activity	To change the posture, or make a task and a role in an activity and to try a new thing during an activity
Emotion during activity	Expressing delight during activity	To smile or be glad without severe expression
	Being calm through activity	To be clam or relaxed without anxiety or poise
Expression during activity	Increasing utterance	To increase amount of words or to speak fluently
	Reminiscing	To recall the past and to do a reminiscence
Social interaction through activity	Starting social interaction	To be interested in others, for example, to gaze others and to try to communicate with them
	Sharing an activity with other people	To do something with others or to share place or activity with others
	Teaching other people	To engage in an activity as a role of teaching someone knowledge and skills
	Considering other people	To consider others, to do something for them, and to thank others during activity
	Expressing themselves to other people	To express one's feeling or opinion in words to others
Something obtained as outcome of activity	Expressing a sense of capability	To confirms one's own ability or to show sense of capability about results of the activity
	Expressing satisfaction	To indicate satisfaction to a result of the activity and praise from others
	Attracting next activities	To show the sign which looks forward to the next activity, to plan the next activity, or to begin different activity of one' will continuously

activity and/or continue an activity. For instance, one participant found that an incommunicable client was interested in gardening. Therefore, the participant facilitated him in watering flowers. The participant could not determine whether the client was satisfied but observed that he kept watering for a long time, which seemed to be an effect of the activity. In this manner, repeating an activity or repeatedly spending a long time on an activity was often facilitated by engagement in the activity.

3.1.4. Concentrating on Activity. Concentrating on an activity consisted of patients displaying serious facial expressions and settling down to do an activity without losing concentration. Participants observed clients' serious facial expressions during an activity, such as playing the samisen (a traditional Japanese musical instrument), cooking, and sewing. Furthermore, clients who were usually restless could participate in activities such as crafts and cooking. Based on their experiences, participants considered these activities to be effective.

3.1.5. Expressing Skills and Knowledge. Expressing knowledge meant to naturally facilitate skills or knowledge that clients had acquired in the past. For example, one client weaved a basket out of willow shoots. The therapist considered her manipulation of the materials to be very skillful and therefore inferred that the client had prior experience weaving. Another example was when clients discussed knowledge of farm products while farming. Participants observed that expressing knowledge and skills often resulted from engaging in related activities.

3.1.6. Trying New Things during Activity. Participants considered it meaningful when clients tried new things during activities. In one instance, a client was gardening while sitting in his wheelchair. He was unable to reach a seed and consequently stood up to reach it, demonstrating that he was trying something new. In another example, a client started drawing a picture using only one color but then noticed a case of colored pencils and started to use several colors. When clients solved problems and/or changed methods as per their own desires or necessity, therapists regarded this as a meaningful event.

3.2. Major Theme 2: Emotional Expression during Activity. Participants considered an activity to be effective when clients with dementia were found to *express delight* through smiling or acting/looking glad and *being calm*, for example, by appearing *relaxed* and anxiety-free.

3.2.1. Expressing Delight during Activity. Many participants had observed clients smiling and being glad. Smiling was one of the main indicators therapists used to judge the effectiveness of activities. Expressing delight was divided into expression due to activities and expression caused by social interactions. For instance, some activities, such as knitting, singing, and watering flowers, made clients smile. As an example of expression caused from social interaction during activities, a client expressed gladness after receiving praise for her outstanding work on an artistic handicraft.

3.2.2. Calm through Activity. Activities sometimes helped to soften clients' expression of emotion, especially for those who experienced anxiety, anger, restlessness, and desire to go home. The task of folding laundry was offered to a nursing home resident who frequently complained about wanting to go home and experienced restlessness, and the task of folding laundry became her purposeful activity in the nursing home. A staff in the nursing home thanked her and the resident then softened her expression. Gardening, cooking, and other activities helped to calm clients and ease their facial expression.

3.3. Major Theme 3: Verbal Expression during Activity. Participants suggested that verbal expression-related activities were meaningful as a viewpoint. This major theme was composed of two subthemes: *increased utterance* and *reminiscing.*

3.3.1. Increased Utterance. Some participants paid attention to quantitative aspects of utterances when clients participated in activities. For example, a client with severe dementia who was otherwise nonverbal uttered one word (the name of her hometown) when she was asked about it during a group conversation. As another example, clients fluently mentioned their past experiences or confident topics. Participants regarded activities as effective when they led to increased numbers of positive utterances.

3.3.2. Reminiscing. When performing an activity, patients sometimes recalled old memories. Some participants explained that reminiscing changed clients' facial expressions (e.g., leading them to smile) led them to feel satisfaction and/or to talk about something on their own accord. Although reminiscence itself was considered an activity, other activities led to reminiscing, which participants considered a result of participating in these activities.

3.4. Major Theme 4: Social Interaction through Activity. Social interaction resulting from engaging activities was considered crucial as a viewpoint. Five subthemes arose from this major theme: *initiating social interaction, sharing an activity with other people, teaching other people, considering other people,* and *expressing themselves to other people.*

3.4.1. Initiating Social Interaction. Participants reported that engaging in an activity often led to the initiation of social interaction. For instance, while playing a game in a group, one client called out to another and encouraged her. Similarly, a client who was not interested in others gazed at another individual and started social interaction with them; this interaction had been inspired by a conversation that interested her. Initiating social interaction was thus regarded as an effect of participation in activities.

3.4.2. Sharing an Activity with Other People. Sharing an activity with others was often observed during performing an activity. While participating in a game as part of a group, a client saw another member succeed and these two clients jointly experienced the joy of this individual's success. In another case, while painting a large picture, two clients shared roles with each other. Sharing something, such as a role, goal, feeling, instrument, or place, induced by performing activities with other people, was observed by some participants as an effect of participation in activities.

3.4.3. Teaching Other People. One participant noted that an important aspect sometimes resulting from activities was that clients would pass on their knowledge or teach skills to others. For example, a nursing home client who had previously enjoyed sewing no longer engaged in this activity. The participant showed the client tools and materials for sewing and asked her, "Please, teach me to sew." The client then began to sew and in doing so, the participant observed her talking, changing facial expressions, and laughing. Teaching an activity therefore provided patients with purpose and helped them to form social relationships. As such, this represented a positive effect of participation in an activity.

3.4.4. Considering Other People. When clients performed activities, participants saw them consider the feelings of others. Clients were observed to worry about others, thank them, tell them a joke to calm them, or invite them to participate in activities. Some clients also gave others something they had made during an activity; for example, after cooking a meal, one client invited her friend to eat it. In sum, considering other people during or as a result of an activity was perceived as meaningful behavior by the participants.

3.4.5. Expressing Themselves to Other People. Expressing clients' own opinions to others was regarded as being as important as considering other people. One participant mentioned that a client had insisted to others, "I want to paint red here. This part should be blue" and so forth. The participant believed that the activity held a special meaning for the client in this situation because he shared with others his own objectives and opinions regarding the activity.

3.5. Major Theme 5: Something Obtained as Outcome of Activity. The majority of participants observed that doing and finishing activities led to various outcomes for clients, enhancing their capability, satisfaction, and motivation to complete the following activity. This major theme was divided into three subthemes: *expressing a sense of capability*, *expressing satisfaction*, and enhancing appeal of *future activities*.

3.5.1. Expressing a Sense of Capability. The verbal and facial expressions of participants were seen to indicate their capability after assessing the outcome, for example, to confirm the existence of themselves and to feel confident about their ability during and after an activity. For example, after completing a craft a patient took pride, saying to others, "This is my work." As another example of confirmation of their own ability, after cooking one client verbally acknowledged, "There are things I can still do." These behaviors were considered to represent a sense of capability as a result of participating in activities.

3.5.2. Expressing Satisfaction. One effect that was reported by participants was that clients expressed satisfaction through their behavior as an outcome of activities and/or in response to praise from other people. In various activities, clients seemed to appreciate participating in a housekeeping activity such as folding laundry, were pleased by praise for their handmade crafts, and were delighted at winning a game.

3.5.3. Enhancing Appeal of Future Activities. Participants considered it meaningful when clients engaged in planning future activities or started a new activity after the end of another. A successful activity empowered clients to start the next activity. In one example, a client looked forward to joining the same group to participate in a cooking activity the next week.

4. Discussion

The finding of this study summarized viewpoints expressed by occupational therapists to evaluate the effects of activities in clients with dementia. Referring to these subthemes could provide us with clear analytical viewpoints regarding engaging activities and help us to verbally interpret clients' meaningful behaviors. Categorizing these viewpoints was unconsciously used by well-experienced occupational therapists, which could be an important aspect in this study. Moreover, this framework which consisted of the subthemes has the potential to be used to assess clients' needs to engage in an activity and to examine the effects of an activity in people who cannot verbally express their needs or feelings, such as patients with dementia.

A novel aspect of this study was that well-experienced occupational therapists observed various aspects of interaction among people, activities, and the social environment. Certain observational assessments exist for individuals who cannot complete self report questionnaires, such as the Volitional Questionnaire (VQ) [23]. The VQ provides the occupational therapist with insight into a person's inner motives related to participation in meaningful occupations. The VQ assesses individuals' volition, whereas the viewpoints gathered in this study involved individual strategies for managing an activity as well as feelings, emotions, and social interactions evoked by the activity. Engagement in activities requires that connectedness among self, others, and the environment is considered important to the individual [24]. Therefore, the viewpoints analyzed in this study could be used to widely assess and classify the effects of activity and to indicate to what degree a client can engage in an activity. These findings could be used to formulate new observational assessments of occupational engagement.

Two subthemes found in this study, reminiscing and calming though activity, could be specific to clients with dementia since reminiscence therapy is often used in this population. Calming is often required for individuals who display behavioral and psychological symptoms of dementia. Considering these subthemes, these viewpoints might be particular to clients with dementia. In other words, the other subthemes could be used to observe other clients without dementia. In particular, it might be useful to assess clients with cognitive disorder, such as children with severe dysfunction and people with stroke.

Hasselkus [25] performed a quantitative study to understand the experience of daycare staff for clients with dementia. This study found that daycare staff observed various indicators of clients' well-being, including smiling, laughing, being friendly, showing affection, not getting up consistently, not repeatedly asking questions, socializing with others, singing with "gusto," and talking a lot. These indicators seemed to be effects of the activities performed by clients. For example, "smiling" in the previous study seems to be similar to "expressing delight during activity" as a subtheme in this study and "socializing with others" could be "social interaction through activity" as a major theme of this study. In other words, the subthemes found herein would be similar to and perhaps even more structured than these indicators of the previous study. Therefore, the viewpoints developed in the present study could be useful for understanding the perspective of individuals with dementia in regard to engagement in activities.

The occupational participation of nursing home residents with dementia has been found to be sporadic and passive [26]. A marked poverty of occupational engagement also exists in hospital and other care settings among clients with severe dementia. Occupations, which clients could self-choose, would provide them with feelings of autonomy, support identity, expression, and create personal space [27]. Therefore, if care staff and other rehabilitation staff share the viewpoints expressed by occupational therapists in the present study, healthcare staff in various domains could offer meaningful activities. This would in turn facilitate clients with dementia to increase occupational engagement and lead to a greater quality of life.

Additional Points

Study Limitations. This study was the first attempt to gather viewpoints of well-experienced occupational therapists when observing clients engaged in activity. In this study, we interviewed occupational therapists regarding observational viewpoints for any activities in which their clients had participated, without identifying specific activities a priori. Occupational therapists utilize various activities in clinical settings. Therefore, certain subthemes were applicable to one activity but not another (e.g., an activity performed alone may not include social interaction). For these reasons, future studies will need to examine occupational therapists' observations according to purpose, form, or content of activity. Moreover, future studies could examine which of these viewpoints were suitable for each type of activity. Likewise, the viewpoints related to engaging activities are dependent on the severity of dementia. A client with severe dementia may not have many thoughts or ideas about carrying out an activity; he/she would be mainly concerned with sensation and with moving his/her body in response to those sensations [28]. The purpose of performing an activity is affected by the cognitive ability of the client. Therefore, future research is needed to clarify the relationship between the viewpoints and the severity of dementia. Finally, the study design purposefully included a variety of clinical settings and severities of dementia in order to encompass various viewpoints. Although 47 cases are not considered small for qualitative research, the sample consisted of only ten participants. Thus, all occupational therapists might not agree with the findings of this study. Future studies must examine the opinions of other occupational therapists regarding the viewpoints collected herein, which will in turn lead to the validation of these viewpoints.

Acknowledgments

This work was supported by a JSPS KAKENHI Grant-in-Aid for Research Activity Start-Up (Grant no. 26893132) from the Japan Society for the Promotion of Science.

References

[1] World Federation of Occupational Therapists, Position statement on client-centredness in occupational therapy, 2010, http://www.wfot.org/ResourceCentre.aspx.

[2] L. N. Gitlin, L. Winter, J. Burke, N. Chemett, M. P. Dennis, and W. W. Hauck, "Tailored activities to manage neuropsychiatric behaviors in persons with dementia and reduce caregiver burden: a randomized pilot study," *The American Journal of Geriatric Psychiatry*, vol. 16, no. 3, pp. 229–239, 2008.

[3] M. J. Graff, M. J. Vernooij-Dassen, M. Thijssen, J. Dekker, W. H. Hoefnagels, and M. G. OldeRikkert, "Effects of community occupational therapy on quality of life, mood, and health status in dementia patients and their caregivers: a randomized controlled trial," *The Journals of Gerontology: Series A*, vol. 62, no. 9, pp. 1002–1009, 2007.

[4] J. C. C. Chung, "Activity participation and well-being of people with dementia in long-term-care settings," *OTJR Occupation, Participation and Health*, vol. 24, no. 1, pp. 22–31, 2004.

[5] T. Perrin, "Occupational need in severe dementia: a descriptive study," *Journal of Advanced Nursing*, vol. 25, no. 5, pp. 934–941, 1997.

[6] K. A. Bayles, "Effects of working memory deficits on the communicative functioning of Alzheimer's dementia patients," *Journal of Communication Disorders*, vol. 36, no. 3, pp. 209–219, 2003.

[7] K. Algar, R. T. Woods, and G. Windle, "Measuring the quality of life and well-being of people with dementia: a review of observational measures," *Dementia*, vol. 24, pp. 1–16, 2014.

[8] J. C. Hughes, S. J. Louw, and S. R. Sabat, *Dementia: Mind, Meaning and the Person*, Oxford University Press, Oxford, England, 2005.

[9] M. Law, S. Baptiste, A. Carswell, MA. McColl, H. Polatajko, and N. Pollock, *Canadian occupational performance measure*, CAOT Publications, Toronto, Canada, 2005.

[10] K. Tomori, S. Uezu, S. Kinjo, K. Ogahara, R. Nagatani, and T. Higashi, "Utilization of the iPad application: aid for decision-making in occupation choice," *Occupational Therapy International*, vol. 19, no. 2, pp. 88–97, 2012.

[11] G. Hubbard, M. G. Downs, and S. Tester, "Including older people with dementia in research: challenges and strategies," *Aging and Mental Health*, vol. 7, no. 5, pp. 351–362, 2003.

[12] L. Nygård, "How can we get access to the experiences of people with dementia?" *Scandinavian Journal of Occupational Therapy*, vol. 13, no. 2, pp. 101–112, 2006.

[13] K. Tomori, H. Nagayama, Y. Saito, K. Ohno, R. Nagatani, and T. Higashi, "Examination of a cut-off score to express the meaningful activity of people with dementia using iPad application (ADOC)," *Disability and Rehabilitation: Assistive Technology*, vol. 10, no. 2, pp. 126–131, 2015.

[14] D. Brooker, "Dementia care mapping: a review of the research literature," *Gerontologist*, vol. 45, no. 1, pp. 11–18, 2005.

[15] T. Kitwood and K. Bredin, "A new approach to the evaluation of dementia care," *Journal of Advances in Health and Nursing Care*, vol. 1, pp. 41–60, 1992.

[16] D. Brooker and L. Duce, "Wellbeing and activity in dementia: a comparison of group reminiscence therapy, structured goal-directed group activity and unstructured time," *Aging and Mental Health*, vol. 4, no. 4, pp. 354–358, 2000.

[17] J. W. Creswell, *Qualitative Inquiry Research Design: Choosing among Five Approaches*, SAGE Publications, California, calif, USA, 2007.

[18] R. L. Luborsky and C. Lysack, "Overview of qualitative research," in *Research in Occupational Therapy: Methods of Inquiry for Enhancing Practice Account*, G. Kielhofner, Ed., pp. 326–340, 2006.

[19] D. Laliberte-Ruduman and S. Moll, "In-depth interviewing," in *Qualitative Research in Occupational Therapy: Strategies and Experiences*, J. V. Cook, Ed., Thomson learning, Inc, New York, USA, 2001.

[20] A. Strauss and J. Corbin, *Basics of Qualitative Research: Grounded Theory Procedures and Techniques*, SAGE, California, Calif, USA, 2nd edition, 1998.

[21] C. Lyscak, M. R. Luborsky, and H. Dillaway, "Gathering qualitative data," in *Research in Occupational Therapy: Methods of Inquiry for Enhancing Practice Account*, G. Kielhofner, Ed., vol. 74, pp. 341–357, 2006.

[22] C. Moustakas, *Phenomenological research methods*, SAGE Publications, Inc., 2455 Teller Road, Thousand Oaks California 91320 United States of America , 1994.

[23] J. Chern, G. Kielhofner, C. G. de las Heras, and L. C. Magalhaes, "The volitional questionnaire: psychometric development and practical use," *American Journal of Occupational Therapy*, vol. 50, no. 7, pp. 516–525, 1996.

[24] A. Han, J. Radel, J. M. McDowd, and D. Sabata, "Perspectives of people with dementia about meaningful activities: a synthesis," *American Journal of Alzheimer's Disease and other Dementias*, vol. 31, no. 2, pp. 115–123, 2015.

[25] B. R. Hasselkus, "Occupation and well-being in dementia: the experience of day-care staff," *American Journal of Occupational Therapy*, vol. 52, no. 6, pp. 423–434, 1998.

[26] T. Holthe, K. Thorsen, and S. Josephsson, "Occupational patterns of people with dementia in residential care: an ethnographic study," *Scandinavian Journal of Occupational Therapy*, vol. 14, no. 2, pp. 96–107, 2007.

[27] A. Öhman and L. Nygård, "Meaning and motives for engagement in self-chosen daily life occupations among individuals with Alzheimer's disease," *OTJR Occupation, Participation and Health*, vol. 25, no. 3, pp. 89–97, 2005.

[28] J. Pool, *The Pool activity level (PAL) instrument for occupational profiling*, Jessica Kingsley Publishers, London, 3rd edition, 2006.

19

Effectiveness of Information Processing Strategy Training on Academic Task Performance in Children with Learning Disabilities: A Pilot Study

Sutinun Juntorn, Sarinya Sriphetcharawut, and Peeraya Munkhetvit

Department of Occupational Therapy, Faculty of Associated Medical Sciences, Chiang Mai University, Chiang Mai, Thailand

Correspondence should be addressed to Peeraya Munkhetvit; peeraya.m@cmu.ac.th

Academic Editor: Jodie A. Copley

Learning disabilities (LD) can be associated with problems in the four stages of information processing used in learning: input, throughput, output, and feedback. These problems affect the child's ability to learn and perform activities in daily life, especially during academic activities. This study is a pilot study aimed at investigating the effectiveness of information processing strategy training using a combination of two approaches that address the ability to apply processing strategies during academic activities in children with LD. The two approaches are the Perceive, Recall, Plan, and Perform (PRPP) System of Intervention, which is a strategy training intervention, and the Four-Quadrant Model (4QM) of Facilitated Learning approach, which is a systematic facilitator technique. Twenty children with LD were assigned to two groups: the experimental group ($n = 10$) and the control group ($n = 10$). Children in the experimental group received the intervention twice a week for 6 consecutive weeks. Each treatment session took approximately 50 minutes. Children in the control group received traditional intervention twice a week for 6 consecutive weeks. The results indicated that the combination of the PRPP System of Intervention and the 4QM may improve the participants' ability to apply information processing strategies during academic activities.

1. Introduction

Learning disability (LD) is a neurological disorder that affects the brain's ability to process, store, and respond to information [1]. According to the Diagnostic and Statistical Manual of Mental Disorders, Fourth Edition, Revised (DSM IV-TR) [2] the term "LD" is a label given to a person who obtains considerably low scores on individually applied standardized tests appropriate for his/her chronological age, grade, and intellectual level. The tests cover reading, mathematics, and written expression skills [2]. Presently, LD is seen as one of the most significant limitations that obstructs participation in school and particularly in learning activities. In the USA, children with LD are the largest category of students receiving special education services. In Thailand, the latest study on children with LD reported that five percent of Thai children aged between six and 12 years (approximately 777, 250 children) have learning disabilities [3].

Occupational therapists use various models to inform intervention with the aim of improving the performance of children with LD. The information processing theoretical model is one model of cognition used by occupational therapists to guide education programing for the children in this group. Information processing is concerned with the stages of processing that supports learning throughout child development and contributes to purposeful and effective sensing and thinking skills, making performance quick and easy [1]. The first stage of processing comprises registration and attention to sensory information which is important to task performance [4, 5]. The second stage in processing is memory. Working memory (short-term memory) and long-term memory strategies are used to assign meaning to sensory information registered from the environment together with a store of knowledge from past experiences to enable children to predict what will happen next and direct the appropriate action. Children with LD are thought to have delayed processing capacity leading to reduced memory, characterized by inefficient storage and retrieval strategies [6]. They have a reduced ability to quickly recognize the sensory data such as objects, letters, words, and procedures previously learned and therefore require more repetition than their typical peers. The following stage of the information processing includes planning, organizing, and problem solving. This process is required for organizing multiple tasks and parts of tasks into a seamless whole [4]. More importantly, it also allows them to respond to new information or engage in new and complex learning to solve problems and to evaluate thinking, leading to independent learning. Children with LD often have problems with planning and problem solving. They often have difficulty in preparation and planning, even if they have good memory [7]. Research demonstrates that children with LD are unable to self-instruct as well as their typical peers [1]. The last stage of information processing is processing output and feedback. Independent learning is dependent not only upon efficient processing throughout the system, but also on the capacity to process the feedback information regarding their performance. Children who have reduced planning have trouble judging and monitoring responses resulting in difficulties in independent learning [1]. Previously, research has been conducted into effective ways to assist children with LD to perform in school learning. The methods used to help children process information for learning involves teaching them to use specific thinking strategies while engaged in sophisticated novel tasks. Many problem solving approaches have been used to develop the ability of information processing while children perform tasks. The unique characteristic of this approach shifts from direct instruction to the instruction of processing strategies during task performance [8].

Information processing employs a number of different processing strategies that are organized, integrated, and adapted to allow occupational performance. Efficiency depends on the ability to select the most appropriate processing strategies that result in "efficient use" of information processing [9]. Cognitive strategies are ways of thinking or the ability to organize thoughts in a goal-directed way in order to accomplish a goal [10]. Cognitive strategy use implies salience or use of known cognitive strategies in the "here and now." It is the ability to choose and apply the "best" strategy to fit a particular situation. Effective cognitive strategy use has been defined as the simplest and most efficient means of processing information relative to a situation and enables a person to participate in every activities without having to "think too hard" [11]. Reduced cognitive strategy use is different to implying the presence of reduced cognition per se in children with LD. While the majority of children with LD have typical cognitive capacity, their ability to "use" their cognition for function is thought to be compromised by their learning disorder [12]. Cognitive strategy training approaches are one of the ways that have been used to promote the capabilities associated with the use of processing strategies or cognitive strategies to improve academic performance [13]. This approach focuses on the acquisition and application of strategies to process information more efficiently. While performing the task, the children need cognitive strategies to perceive the nature of a task in the context of the environment, the recognition of similarities between the present tasks and past experiences. They must also be aware of task relationships and jobs, must direct goal expansion, engage in goal formation, and make decisions on their performance. The skill acquisition that resulted from the intervention in the form of strategy training approach helps children's ability to generalize functional performance in other environments [14]. Besides cognitive strategy training, systematic instruction approach can also enhance occupational performance by focusing on developing specific skills required for occupational performance [15]. Systematic instruction is one of the techniques of the functional task or behavioral approaches; it is a top-down approach similar to strategy training. The intervention used in this approach focuses on task analysis, cueing, prompting and chaining, support, and guiding task performance [16, 17]. These are consistent with an acquisition frame of reference based on learning theory [18]. The primary goal of this manner of intervention is to focus on the learner's ability to function according to the steps of the specific task to achieve skill acquisition in selected tasks during the treatment [16].

Most recently, Chapparo and Ranka [8] have developed an intervention approach that integrates strategy training, systematic instruction, learning theory, and information processing theory calling it the Perceive, Recall, Plan, and Perform System of Intervention (or PRPP System of Intervention). The PRPP System of Intervention was developed from the PRPP System of Task Analysis, which is a dynamic assessment. The uniqueness of this intervention is that it is an occupation-based practice. The PRPP System of Intervention aims to improve task performance mastery by addressing the specific cognitive strategy application behaviors identified through the PRPP System assessment that most impacts successful mastery. Strategy instructional methods used to address these behaviors incorporate cues and prompts that align with specific Perceive, Recall, Plan, and Perform processing operations and preferences. During the PRPP System of Intervention, the prompts of "Stop, Attend, Sense, Think, and Do" are initially used as content-free "metaprompts" to alert children to process information required for task performance. These global prompts are followed up with more specific content based behavioral prompts based on findings from the assessment component of the system [4]. The "Attend/Sense" strategy instruction addresses the perception problem that comes from poor attention to sensory images and lack of focus on the tasks. The children are stimulated to receive and encode information of activities until completed. The "Think" strategy instruction can help children enhance recall skills when they could not recognize sensory images or made mistakes with recognition, naming things incorrectly, or forgetting about the object's instruction. This strategy instruction focuses on repetition and organization which are important strategies for keeping information in working memory [4]. Moreover, the "Think" strategy instruction also addresses the planning strategy problem by letting intervention focus on the child's ability to construct and evaluate their own goal-oriented strategies for action before performing tasks, especially the more novel or complex ones. When children use thinking strategy effectively, they can generalize performance to another situation. The "Do" strategy instruction helps children to start and stop. Moreover, this strategy is able to stimulate continuing, persisting, and flowing with the task until it is finished [4]. The efficacy of this approach has been observed in children and adults with a variety of diagnoses and conditions that impact everyday cognition [4] and also has been demonstrated through research with adults with traumatic brain impairment [19] and children with social and behavioral difficulties [20]. However, in order to effectively use the strategy training in the PRPP System of Intervention, the therapist needs to respond to the needs of each student and adjust the strategies to be in line with those needs. Moreover, one application of evidence based principles for systematic instruction of the PRPP System of Intervention involves ensuring that therapists consider the prompts, which are more behavioral and specific content based, by using the least to most prompt hierarchy [4]. Therefore, it is necessary for the therapists to have a guideline of systematic facilitation to serve as a scaffold for organizing the selection and implementation of effective teaching and learning strategies relevant to the needs of each child. In the past a study was conducted by Vygotsky [21], which found that children could develop advanced abilities through guidance from a facilitator to achieve autonomy through the use of systematic facilitation called "scaffolds." This concept involves the therapists being the motivators to the children who then motivate themselves. Additionally, the use of a prompts starts in the overt to covert manner. That aim is consistent with a study conducted by Mosston and Ashworth [22] that proposed that the nature of teaching will start from command style to self-teaching. The command style is a direct style that aims to teach learners about the key elements or how to respond to the demands of the task. The self-teaching style encourages learners to consider the barriers to performing the activity and how to best deal with them. This allows learners to use better decision-making processes.

The Four-Quadrant Model (4QM) of Facilitated Learning [18] is another approach that allows therapists to understand, plan, and coordinate the use of specific teaching and learning strategies by means of systematic facilitation. The 4QM was considered to be a suitable framework that could be used together with the PRPP System of Intervention in this study. The 4QM groups the various cognitive and physical learning strategies that children can apply to perform occupation tasks more autonomously. The use of prompts in the 4QM moves from the facilitator to the child. Also, the strategies that are more direct and allow learning about the characteristics of the task or the responses required combined with the indirect strategies enable learners to improve decision-making processes for better results. In this group the students are active in planning, executing, and evaluating performance. The 4QM would be relevant to occupational therapists that regularly facilitate skill acquisition as part of their service offering. It has been suggested as one way of informing the selection of effective learning strategies based on the changing needs of the learner when acquiring a new skill. Two continua integrations are used with the 4QM: (i) strategy directness and (ii) clustering the initiation source to prompting to group learning strategies according to the learner's needs. Numbers are used to identify the clusters. Quadrant 1 directly facilitates the prompting initiation that specifics the task and/or response, and indirect facilitator-initiated prompts encourage decision-making. In Quadrant 2, the learners recall that the use of overt self-prompt is encouraged. In Quadrant 3 autonomous performance is supported by the learners through self-regulatory cognitive and metacognitive strategies grouped in Quadrant 4 [23]. The Four-Quadrant Model of Facilitated Learning is shown in Figure 1.

The 4QM strategies had been used in a case study on four children and the PRPP System of Task Analysis was used to a measure the outcomes. The results showed that after the intervention the PRPP scores increased by 58–76% [24]. Moreover, the study of perspectives of the occupational therapists who had experience in working for seven or more years on the clinical utility of the 4QM process through focus groups found that participants can be made aware of the advantages of the 4QM. This helps guide therapist to respond to the needs of the learner with regard to their personal abilities and learning styles [25].

To apply the 4QM coupled with the PRPP System of Intervention, the PRPP System of Task Analysis was used by therapists in finding problematic descriptors across all PRPP System Quadrants. Next, the problematic descriptors were chunked to set a goal and plan the intervention. Afterwards, the 4QM, which focuses on using a systematic prompting appropriate for each child, was used in combination with the PRPP System of Intervention. This focuses on children learning to use a sequence of processing strategies to "Stop/Attend, Sense, Think, Do" so that children can use more efficient strategies to improve performance and autonomy.

However, the PRPP System of Intervention and the 4QM have never been used in children with LD. Thus, the aim of this study was to investigate the effects of information processing strategy training using a combination of two approaches for children with LD.

2. Methodology

2.1. Participants. Twenty children with LD were recruited from schools in Chiang Mai province, Thailand, by purposive sampling method, and were allocated to the experimental group ($n = 10$) or the control group ($n = 10$). All of them had reading disabilities and had received traditional intervention such as visual perception activities, visual-motor activities, sensory-motor activities, cognitive activities, and handwriting activities twice a week. The age range of the participants in the study was from 10 to 12 years. Participants were attending fourth to sixth grade in six inclusion schools in the broader area of Chiang Mai province, Thailand, which had children diagnosed with learning disabilities. The inclusion criteria were as follows: firstly, children could communicate without visual, hearing, and speaking impairments that could be traced back to the children's personal clinical profile. Secondly, parents had to agree to sign an informed consent to participate in the study. The participants who could not complete the intervention program were excluded.

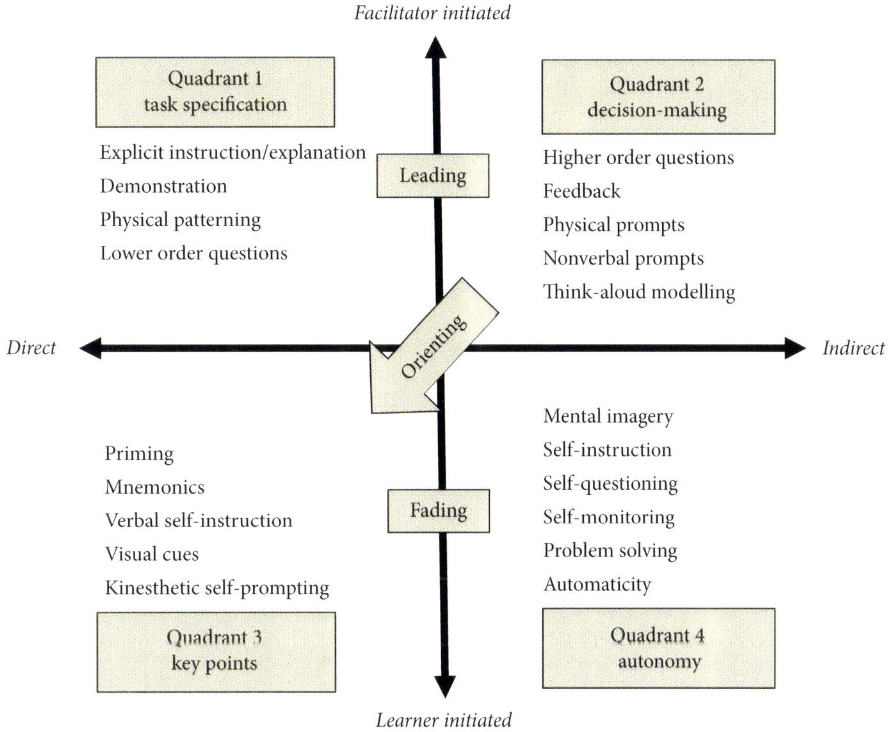

FIGURE 1: The Four-Quadrant Model of Facilitated Learning [modified from [18]].

2.2. Outcome Measures. The outcome measure used in this study was the Perceive, Recall, Plan, and Perform System of Task Analysis: Thai Version or PRPP System: Thai Version. The PRPP System: Thai Version is the Thai version of the original Perceive, Recall, Plan, and Perform (PRPP) System of Task Analysis which was developed by Chapparo in 2010 [4]. It is one of the occupation-focused assessments that measures cognitive strategy use in a specific context [8]. It is composed of two assessment stages. Stage One Analysis employed a standard behavioral task analysis to indicate the person's mastery for specific and relevant occupations. Stage Two Analysis adopts a cognitive task analysis which identifies the effectiveness of cognitive strategy use during task performance. This stage of the PRPP System of Task Analysis is conceptually divided into four quadrants: Perceive, Recall, Plan, and Perform. Each quadrant is broken down into three subquadrants and several underlying information processing strategies termed "Descriptors" as shown in Figure 2. Descriptor behaviors are rated by an observer on a 3-2-1 scale as follows [8]: 3 scores = a participant will receive 3 scores when the task is completed safely without assistance and prompts and using reasonable time; 2 scores = a participant will receive 2 scores when the task is completed safely, but some concern and deficit in this behavior are noted. Prompts may be needed and time is not restricted to receive this score. Last, a participant will receive a score of 1 when the task is uncompleted and student has demonstrated a behavioral deficit. Participants may act unsafely during completing the tasks, taking too much time or requiring too many prompts to receive this score.

The PRPP System of Task Analysis has standardized administrative procedures relative to language of the assessment, method of observation, and scoring. It has reported content, discriminant, cultural and concurrent validity, internal consistency, interrater reliability (occupational therapist-occupational therapist), and test-retest reliability [26–32]. For use in the PRPP System, the Thai Version was examined for its reliability and validity in Thai patients with acquired brain injury and showed high test-retest and interrater reliability [33]. The PRPP System: Thai Version was preliminarily used with Thai patients with stroke [34] and persons with schizophrenia [35].

2.3. Intervention Program. The intervention program in this study was based on the integration of the concept of the PRPP System of Intervention and the 4QM of Facilitated Learning program. As the PRPP System of Intervention broadens the traditional focus of programmed learning and behavioral task analysis by augmenting information processing strategies upon the cognitive process being employed while learning, the intervention sessions specifically targeted application of information processing strategies using graded prompts, progressing from content-free metaprompts to more specific content based behavioral prompts. The participants learn to apply *Stopping, Sensing, Thinking,* and *Doing* strategies to their performance during performing tasks. The PRPP Core Intervention Strategies are explained in Table 1.

The PRPP System of Intervention integrates aspects of a systematic instruction and information processing theory. It is a task-oriented information processing approach that

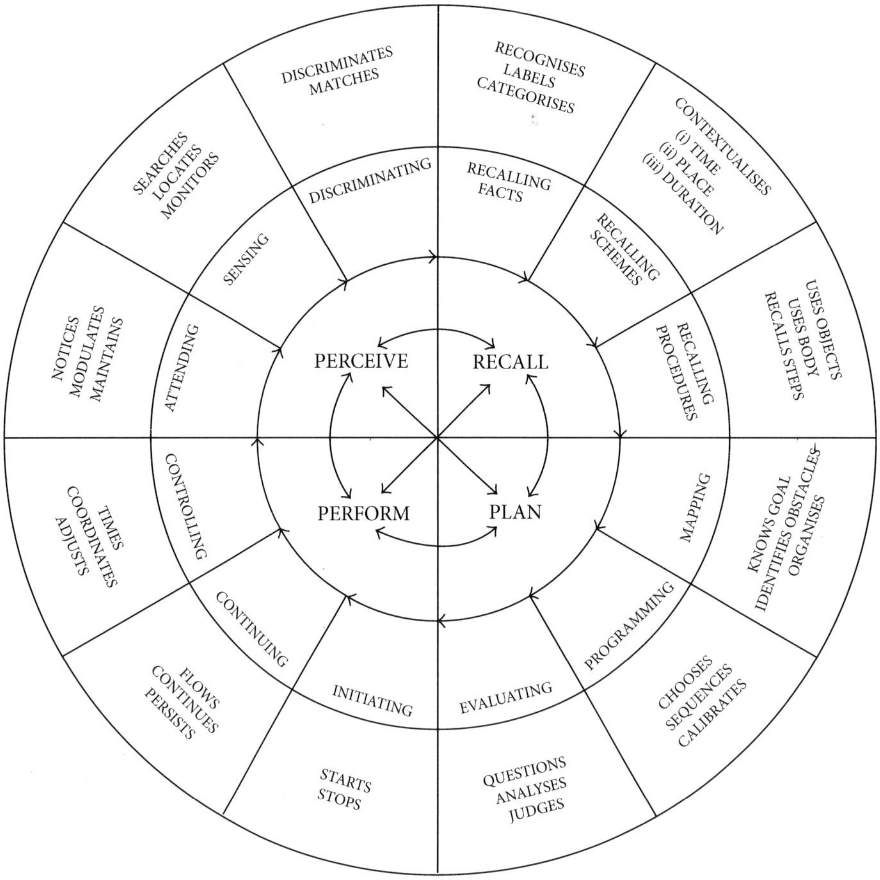

FIGURE 2: The PRPP System of Task Analysis: conceptual model of information processing behaviors [cited in [14]].

simultaneously focuses on task training, strategy training, and strategy application within the context of everyday performance [8]. To enable children to apply a sequence of processing strategies orders, which are "Stop, Sense, Think, and Do," they have to use prompts in the correct sequence. The suitable prompts can stimulate information processing required for task performance. The 4QM of Facilitated Learning is a program to provide a framework for therapists to understand teaching and learning processes. To use this model the therapists choose a strategy for using prompts, which matches the learners' requirements. It enables them to show their skills and improve performance in an autonomous way [23]. Each of the strategies in the 4QM involves methods that enable learning by using the backward method to find the beginning of the intervention. Although each of the participants in this study started by using different ways to initiate the process of the activity, ultimately after finishing the intervention program, most of the participants could use the strategies autonomously. Therefore to integrate these two approaches, the therapist needs to detect the impairment of the information processing strategy application during the activity by using the PRPP System of Task Analysis. After the therapist detects the dominant deficiency in the descriptors of each quadrant of the PRPP System in each child, the problematic descriptors would be set as a goal for intervention. Next, the 4QM strategies, which focus on using a systematic prompt appropriate on each child, were used together with the PRPP System of Intervention. This focuses on children learning to use a sequence of processing strategies to "Stop, Attend, Sense, Think, and Do" so that children can use more efficient strategies to autonomously perform tasks.

To understand how the combination of the PRPP System of Intervention and the 4QM approach was implemented in this study, an example of how to use this program is shown in Table 2.

The following are examples of how the 4QM and the PRPP System of Intervention work together in one case study. After evaluating the abilities of the child using the PRPP System of Task Analysis, it was found that the child had problems on descriptors such as Modulates, Maintains, Searches, Locates, Recalls Steps, Analyses, Judges, Flows, and Continues. The intervention for improving "Modulates" strategy involves the therapist holding the child's finger to help the child move to the text word by word. This is a physical patterning strategy in Quadrant 1 of the 4QM. At the same time, the therapist used a verbal prompt "Stop, Look at your page, Focus on the first word. . .Shift your eyes to the second word!" This is a strategy used in the process "Stop/Attend" in the PRPP System of Intervention. Such techniques can help children when reading and learning new vocabulary change their focus to the next word. Later, when the children can slide a finger to terminology correctly, the therapist then reduces

Table 1: PRPP Core Intervention Strategies [8].

Strategy	Definition
Intervention goal is task mastery	(i) Expected outcome is improved functional performance in everyday tasks required by the person's occupational roles and context. (ii) Intervention success is measured by increased functional performance.
Application of evidence based principle of systematic instruction	(i) Goal of intervention is clear to client. (ii) Least to most prompt hierarchy is used. (iii) Multiple opportunities for practice of the task and target cognitive strategy are offered and performance errors are prevented. (iv) Learning occurs across natural contexts to promote generalization. (v) Feedback is specific to task mastery and the cognitive strategy that is the target of intervention.
Cognitive strategies are behaviorally defined and measurable	(i) Strategies required for task performance are identified using the PRPP System of Task Analysis and their effectiveness measured before and throughout intervention.
"Chunking" of strategies across all PRPP Quadrants is planned	(i) Starting with "*Stop*," one or two strategies are targeted from each processing quadrant for "*Sense*" (Perceive Quadrant), "*Think*" (Recall and Plan Quadrants), and "*Do*" (Perform Quadrant). (ii) Single descriptors are not used. (iii) A line of processing required for the task mirrors the definition of arrows in the center of the PRPP System of Task Analysis.
Focus of intervention is on application of cognitive strategies (descriptors) to real-world performance	(i) The descriptor behaviors form the verbal, physical, or visual prompts given during performance. (ii) The therapist acts as a cognitive mediator. (iii) The patient is taught to self-instruct in the strategies.

Table 2: The example of using the combination of the PRPP System of Intervention and the 4QM approach for academic activity (reading comprehension and written expression).

Target descriptors/subquadrants/quadrants of PRPP System	Strategies of PRPP System of Intervention	Prompting of PRPP System of Intervention (verbal)	Prompting of 4QM
Modulates/Attending/Perceive	Stop/attend	"Focus on the first word, now shift your eyes to the second word"	(i) Physical patterning, Q1 (ii) Feedback, Q2 (iii) Visual cue, Q3 (iv) Self-monitoring, Q4
Maintains/Attending/Perceive		"Keep concentrating until you have finished the sentence"	(i) Nonverbal prompts, Q2 (iii) Kinesthetic self-prompting, Q3 (iii) Self- monitoring, Q4
Searches/Discriminating/Perceive Locates/Discriminating/Perceive	Sense	"Get your eyes ready to look for your page"	(i) Visual cues, Q3 (ii) Self-instruction, Q4
Recalls Steps/Recalling Procedures/Recall Analyses/Evaluating/Plan Judges/Evaluating/Plan	Think	"Remember what you did yesterday" "Ask your self does this look right? Which the word is more proper to be filled in the blank?"	(i) Mnemonics, Q3 (ii) Self-instruction, Q4 (ii) Explicit instruction/explanation, Q1 (iv) Verbal self-instruction, Q3 (v) Self-questioning & self-monitoring, Q4
Flows/Continuing/Perform Continues/Continuing/Perform	Do	"Keep going until you reach the last sentence"	(i) Nonverbal prompt, Q2 (ii) Visual cue, Q3 (iii) Self-monitoring, Q4

the aid by using a feedback strategy in Quadrant 2 of the 4QM with the comment "You slide too early!" This technique allowed the child to use self-regulatory procedures. Next, the child applied a visual cue strategy in Quadrant 3 of the 4QM by using a red pen to divide the word in order to see it more clearly. Finally, the child uses a self-monitoring strategy in Quadrant 4 of the 4QM to determine whether or not they read the words.

The intervention used in the "Maintains" strategy involves the therapist using verbal prompts such as "Keep concentrating until you have finished the sentence!" which is a strategy used in the process of "Stop/Attend" of the PRPP System of Intervention. At the same time, the therapist tapped on the line where the child read, which is a nonverbal prompt strategy found in Quadrant 2 of the 4QM, designed to keep kids focused on the task. Later, when the child is more focused, the therapist guides the child to use a kinesthetic self-prompting found in Quadrant 3 of the 4QM by tapping along the line while browsing to redirect eye gaze. Doing so helps enhances direct attention of the reader. Ultimately, the child could use a self-monitoring strategy found in Quadrant 4 of the 4QM to enhance constant attention to task.

During the "Searches" and "Locates" strategies, the therapist uses verbal prompt such as "Get your eyes ready to look for your page!" which is a strategy used in the process of "Sense" of the PRPP System of Intervention. Afterward, the therapist guides the child to highlight vocabulary which is a keyword in the question to find the answer in the article. This strategy is a visual cue mentioned in Quadrant 3 of the 4QM. Lastly, the child could use a self-instruction strategy found in Quadrant 4 of the 4QM to find the answer.

The intervention of "Recalls Steps" strategy starts with a verbal prompt "Remember what you did yesterday!" This is a strategy used in the process of "Think" of the PRPP System of Intervention. Next, the therapist guides the child to use a mnemonics strategy in Quadrant 3 of 4QM where the child reminds herself to recall the steps involved in performance by saying the keywords in the task steps. It starts with reading the passage and choosing a word to fill in the blanks. Afterward, the question is read and the answer is written. Ultimately, the child engages in covert self-instruction in Quadrant 4 of the 4QM until the task was completed.

The intervention of "Analyses" and "Judges" strategies starts from an explicit instruction and explanation in Quadrant 1 of the 4QM by writing the words on the board, along with reading and explaining the meaning of the word. This strategy can then involve filling in gaps to make a complete sentence. This method can teach the child to learn the right information. Next, the therapist uses a verbal prompt such as "Ask yourself, does this look right?" and "Which word should be filled in the blank?" This strategy is used in the process of "Think" of the PRPP System of Intervention. After that, the therapist guides the child to use a verbal self-instruction strategy found in Quadrant 3 of the 4QM to make decisions necessary to write the right word. The child says to herself "Is this word correct?" "Can another word be used instead?" Lastly, the child uses self-questioning and self-monitoring strategies found in Quadrant 4 of the 4QM to critique their plan of action.

The intervention of "Continues" and "Flows" strategies starts with a verbal prompt "Keep going until you reach the last sentence." This is a strategy used in the process of "Do" in the PRPP System of Intervention with a finger pointing to the line that the child is reading, a strategy of nonverbal prompt found in Quadrant 2 of the 4QM. After the child could operate continuously, she reminded herself by marking at the end of the line where she had completed the self-instruction to start a new line. This method is a visual cue strategy in Quadrant 3 of the 4QM. At the end, the child could use a self-monitoring strategy in Quadrant 4 of the 4QM until the task is completed.

2.4. Procedure. The proposal was sent to the Ethics Committee of the Faculty of Associated Medical Sciences, Chiang Mai University, Thailand, for approval. Then researcher asked for permission from the directors of each school and contacted teachers who worked with special needs children. Twenty children with learning disabilities were then recruited according to the predetermined criteria. After informed consent was obtained from participants' parents, all participants in the experimental group and the control group were asked to perform academic activities (reading comprehension and written expression). Each child was asked to read the passages which were designed for students at the fourth- to sixth-grade reading level. Next, the child filled in the appropriate words in the blanks to complete the sentences and article. Finally, the child was asked to answer the questions that followed. The criteria for specifying these activities were based on the PRPP System of Task Analysis: Thai Version [9]. The reading comprehension and written expression tasks were selected in the assessment process as they were considered important and meaningful for the participants' roles as students. The PRPP System of Assessment: Thai Version was done by a trained occupational therapist who was a blind assessor. Scores obtained from this stage were pretest scores.

All participants were then randomly assigned to the experimental (intervention) group ($n = 10$) or the control group ($n = 10$). The experimental group received the intervention program in addition to the traditional program twice a week for 6 consecutive weeks. Each session in the intervention program took approximately 50 minutes. The control group received traditional intervention twice a week from occupational therapists in the Rajanagarindra Institute of Child Development, Chiang Mai province, Thailand, only. The traditional programs of the control group kept the focus on the deficits of components of function. These programs were not aspects of occupation-based practices. The traditional programs focused on the activities of visual perception activities, visual-motor activities, sensory-motor activities, cognitive activities, and handwriting activities. Examples of activities used in the practice of the control group based on traditional programs are shown in Table 3.

After the intervention period was over, all participants in both groups were reassessed using the PRPP System: Thai Version by the same assessor. Scores obtained from this stage were posttest scores.

TABLE 3: Example of activities in the traditional program for the control group.

Visual perception activities	Visual-motor integration activities	Sensory-motor activities	Cognitive activities	Handwriting activities
(i) Finding the letters hidden in a ball bowl (ii) Doing pegboard (iii) Connecting the dots to complete the picture (iv) Finding the differences between two pictures	(i) Throwing the ball into the target vowel (ii) Rolling bowls to the target word (iii) Jumping on foam boards as instructed	(i) Moving body parts as the model (ii) A crawl through, climb over obstacles (iii) walking the balance beam (iv) Animal walk	(i) Matching card game (ii) Sequencing card game (iii) Categorize objects	(i) Writing letters on sand (ii) Sculpturing clay in to characters

2.5. Data Analysis

(1) The pretest and posttest scores obtained from Stage Two Analysis of the PRPP System: Thai Version were computed to compare scores between the intervention and the control group using the Mann–Whitney *U* Test. The significant level was set at .05.

(2) The pretest and posttest scores obtained from Stage Two Analysis of the PRPP System: Thai Version were computed to compare scores within the group using the Wilcoxon signed-ranks test. The significant level was set at .05.

(3) Effect sizes (ES) for mean differences were calculated by calculating for nonparametric tests [36]:

Mann –Whitney:
$r = Z/$square root of N, where N is total number of cases that will have Z values reported.
Wilcoxon signed-ranks test:
$r = Z/$square root of N, where N is number of observations of two times points.

3. Results

3.1. Demographic Data. The demographic characters of the samples are presented in Table 4. In the control group, the average age was 11.33 years. For the experimental group, the average age of the participants was 11.06 years. The majority of the participants in both groups were male.

3.2. The Comparison of Quadrant and Subquadrant Pretest Scores between the Control and Experimental Group. From Table 5, the Mann–Whitney *U* test analysis results indicated that the pretest scores of all quadrants and subquadrants showed no significant difference between the control and the experimental group except in the Mapping Subquadrant of the Plan Quadrant ($p > .05$).

3.3. The Comparison of Quadrant and Subquadrant Pretest and Posttest Scores between the Control and Experimental Group. From Table 6, for the control group, the pretest and posttest scores in all quadrants and subquadrants (except the Sensing Subquadrant in the Perceive Quadrant) demonstrated no significant difference ($p > .05$). For the experimental group, the pretest and posttest scores in all quadrants and subquadrants (except the Attending and Discriminating Subquadrants in the Perceive Quadrant, Recalling Schemes Subquadrant in the Recall Quadrant, and Initiating and Controlling Subquadrants in the Perform Quadrant) demonstrated significant difference ($p < .05$).

TABLE 4: Demographic variables of the control and experimental group.

Demographic characteristics	Control group ($n = 10$)		Experimental group ($n = 10$)	
	N	%	*N*	%
Gender				
Male	8	80	8	80
Female	2	20	2	20
Age				
10.0–10.11	4	40	5	50
11.0–11.11	3	30	5	50
12.0–12.11	3	30	—	—
Grade				
4	2	20	4	40
5	3	30	4	40
6	5	50	2	20

3.4. The Comparison of Quadrant and Subquadrant Posttest Scores between the Control and Experimental Group. From Table 7, the analysis results from the Mann–Whitney *U* test indicated that the scores of the Perceive, Plan, and Perform Quadrants showed a significant difference between the control and the experimental group at posttest ($p < .05$, $p < .001$). The Recall Quadrant showed no significant difference ($p > .05$). However, there were two subquadrants in the Recall Quadrant (Recalling Facts and Recalling Procedures) that demonstrated a significant difference between the two groups ($p < .05$).

4. Discussion

The purpose of the present study was to investigate the effectiveness of the combination of the PRPP System of Intervention and the 4QM approach on the academic activities (reading comprehension and written expression) of children with LD. The overall finding of the study demonstrated that after the intervention program the experimental group significantly improved in the mean scores of all PRPP System

Table 5: The comparison of the quadrant and subquadrant pretest scores between the control and experimental group on the academic activity (reading comprehension and written expression).

PRPP System: Thai Version		Mean rank				
Quadrant	Subquadrant	Control group (n = 10)	Experiment group (n = 10)	Z	Asymp.Sig (2-tailed)	Effect size (r)
Perceive		12.45	8.55	−1.49	.136	.33
	Attending	11.20	9.80	−.54	.59	.12
	Sensing	12.85	8.15	−1.91	.06	.43
	Discriminating	11.45	9.55	−.82	.41	.18
Recall		12.30	8.70	−1.38	.17	.31
	Recalling Facts	12.75	8.25	−1.84	.07	.41
	Recalling Schemes	11.05	9.95	−.43	.66	.10
	Recalling Procedures	9.10	11.90	−1.14	.25	.26
Plan		11.50	9.50	−.77	.44	.17
	Mapping	13.25	7.75	−2.19	.03*	.49
	Programming	11.20	9.80	−.59	.56	.13
	Evaluating	11.20	9.80	−.58	.57	.13
Perform		11.05	9.95	−.43	.67	.10
	Initiating	11.75	9.25	−1.10	.27	.25
	Continuing	10.40	10.60	−.09	.93	.02
	Controlling	10.50	10.50	.00	1.00	.00

Note. * $p < .05$.

Table 6: The comparison of the quadrant and subquadrant pretest and posttest scores on the academic activity in the control group and experimental group.

PRPP System: Thai Version		Control group (n = 10)			Experimental group (n = 10)		
Quadrant	Subquadrant	Z	Asymp.Sig (2-tailed)	Effect size (r)	Z	Asymp.Sig (2-tailed)	Effect size (r)
Perceive		−1.69[b]	.09	.38	−2.56[a]	.01*	.57
	Attending	−.62[b]	.54	.14	−1.85[a]	.07	.41
	Sensing	−2.69[b]	.01*	.60	−2.72[a]	.007*	.61
	Discriminating	−1.52[b]	.13	.34	−1.30[a]	.19	.29
Recall		−.42[a]	.67	.09	−2.39[a]	.02*	.53
	Recalling Facts	−1.88[b]	.06	.42	−2.54[a]	.01*	.57
	Recalling Schemes	−1.51[a]	.13	.34	−1.44[a]	.15	.32
	Recalling Procedures	−.85[a]	.40	.19	−2.46[b]	.01*	.55
Plan		−1.18[b]	.24	.26	−2.50[a]	.01*	.56
	Mapping	−.67[b]	.51	.15	−2.84[a]	.004*	.64
	Programming	−.86[b]	.39	.19	−2.58[a]	.01*	.58
	Evaluating	−1.67[b]	.10	.37	−2.51[a]	.01*	.56
Perform		−.69[b]	.50	.15	−2.68[a]	.007*	.60
	Initiating	−.27[b]	.79	.06	−1.41[a]	.16	.32
	Continuing	−1.00[b]	.32	.22	−2.72[a]	.007*	.61
	Controlling	−.45[a]	.66	.10	−1.60[a]	.11	.36

Note. [a]Based on negative ranks. [b]Based on positive ranks. * $p < .05$.

Quadrants (Perceive, Recall, Plan, and Perform), whereas the control group did not show a significant improvement in all quadrants. There may be several reasons for this finding. Firstly, the intervention program focused on facilitating multiprocess sequences of strategies. Since the nature of information processing is dynamic and employs a number of different cognitive strategies [9], the cognitive strategy training that is effective must stimulate multiple cognitive processes rather than individual cognitive skills without focusing on the interrelationships between specific cognitive skills for performing tasks [37]. The intervention program in this study focuses on the optimization of the problematic

Table 7: The comparison of quadrant and subquadrant posttest scores between the control and experimental group on the academic activity (reading comprehension and written expression).

PRPP System: Thai Version		Mean rank				
Quadrant	Subquadrant	Control group ($n = 10$)	Experiment group ($n = 10$)	Z	Asymp.Sig (2-tailed)	Effect size (r)
Perceive		15.50	5.50	−3.80	.000**	.85
	Attending	13.40	7.60	−2.24	.03*	.50
	Sensing	15.50	5.50	−3.93	.000**	.88
	Discriminating	12.65	8.35	−1.85	.06	.41
Recall		10.25	10.75	−.19	.85	.04
	Recalling Facts	13.65	7.35	−2.46	.01*	.55
	Recalling Schemes	9.55	11.5	−.75	.46	.17
	Recalling Procedures	7.70	13.30	−2.22	.03*	.50
Plan		14.75	6.25	−3.24	.001*	.72
	Mapping	14.50	6.50	−3.09	.002*	.69
	Programming	14.50	6.50	−3.47	.000**	.78
	Evaluating	14.80	6.20	−3.39	.000**	.76
Perform		14.75	6.25	−3.26	.001*	.73
	Initiating	10.50	10.50	.000	1.00	.00
	Continuing	15.40	5.60	−3.93	.000**	.88
	Controlling	12.50	8.50	−1.62	.11	.36

Note. $^{**}p < .001$. $^{*}p < .05$.

strategies that have been "chunked" together in each quadrant of the PRPP System of Task Analysis. The therapists teach children to learn and apply a sequence of processing strategies to "Stop/Attend, Sense, Think, and Do" with the systematic prompt of the 4QM by the process of attention and sensory perception (Perceive Quadrant), memory (Recall Quadrant), response planning and evaluation (Plan Quadrant), and performance monitoring (Perform Quadrant) to have the flow of information processing from initial input to response output. The effective intervention program of each stage of information processing may occur through the system in the following manner.

In order for the stimulating attention and sensory perception (Perceive Quadrant) to be more efficient, the prompt of "Stop/Attend/Sense" and systematic prompt of the 4QM were used to encourage children to modulate arousal and reallocate attention. This includes the modulation of attention (Attending Subquadrant) and discrimination of sensory information (Discriminating Subquadrant). Improvement of each problematic descriptor score in Perceive Quadrant was due to facilitation on the function of the problematic descriptors during performance of the task. For example, if the children have a problem on "Modulates" strategy, prompting was used to help children shift their eyes in order to encourage them to change the focus of their attention to suit the reading task. The verbal prompt "Focus on the first word!...Shift your eyes to the second word!" which is in the PRPP System of Intervention and the prompting hierarchy of the 4QM were used to enhance the ability to get the appropriate scope for task performance and to allocate the attention to different parts of the tasks. These help children to focus on specific and significant elements of task performance within specific boundaries. The effective "Modulates" strategy improves attention ability (Attending Subquadrant) since it is a part of attention mechanisms, which is the main element of the perceive process. The result is that these intervention programs help children be more effective at gathering sensory behaviors while performing academic activities.

To promote memory (Recall Quadrant), the prompt of "Think to remember" and systematic prompt of the 4QM were used to encourage children to store, retrieve, and use the information necessary to perform tasks effectively. For example, if the children have a problem on the "Recalling Steps" strategy, all of prompts were focused on encouraging the children to remember the sequence of task. The verbal prompt "Remember what you did yesterday," which is in the PRPP System of Intervention, and the mnemonics strategy of the 4QM were applied to improve the ability to recall information about how to sequence steps needed for task. These techniques are confirmed by Thagard (2005), who described how repetition and organization of instruction can help children to get information into working memory [6]. The effective "Recalling Steps" strategy improved recalling procedures ability (Recalling Procedures Subquadrant), which is the one element of the recall process. Therefore, the intervention program can enhance the recall ability while performing academic tasks.

To promote response planning and evaluation (Plan Quadrant), the prompt of "Think to problem-solve" and the systematic prompt of 4QM were used to encourage children to construct and evaluate their own goal-oriented strategies for action before performing tasks. For example, if the children have difficulties with "Analyses" and "Judges" strategies application, all prompts were employed to help the children to analyze real and potential constraints and act accordingly and to make safe and informed decisions. The verbal prompt "Ask your self does this look right. . .Which word is more proper to be filled in the blank?" which is in the PRPP System of Intervention and prompting hierarchy of the 4QM should be used to help the children to learn the right information about tasks, evaluate the outcome, and decide how to accomplish the tasks in the most complete manner. The effective "Analyses" and "Judges" strategy improves evaluating ability (Evaluating Subquadrant), reflecting a monitoring and appraisal process. The children can use thinking strategies for planning and problem solving of complex and novel occupational tasks by being able to self-evaluate and decide the need to change or adapt. Finally, children may have a complete idea of the expected outcomes and prepare to put a plan into action.

To promote performance monitoring (Perform Quadrant), the prompt of "Do" and the systematic prompt of the 4QM were used to encourage children to actively respond and process information that requires the ability to plan and initiate the start and stop of action. For example, if the children demonstrate problems with "Flows" and "Continues" strategies, any prompting improves the children's ability to persist in carrying out a plan in a smooth, flowing manner until the step or task is completed. The verbal prompt "Keep going until you reach the last sentence," which is in the PRPP System of Intervention, and the prompting hierarchy of the 4QM were used to facilitate the children to transfer between tasks and parts of tasks and to complete tasks. In doing so, the continuing process (Continuing Subquadrant) in the performing procedure was developed, as well.

Next, prompting that starts from the therapist to the child is a special feature that is used in the intervention program. This approach was used to minimize reliance on therapists and to promote a quicker transition to independent performance [18]. While implementing intervention, the therapist must find a way to direct a pathway toward autonomy and, at the same time, be flexible concerning the child's response time and the context of the task to be performed. The intervention program that uses scaffolding or a systematic facilitator support is a guideline to help therapists choose the appropriate prompt to enhance occupational performance and to help the student to be able to complete the performance autonomously. Facilitator-initiated methods were used in the early stages for the children to understand the characteristics of the task and the performance required and to help them make decisions about the task. Afterward, the therapist encourages the child to engage and use learner-initiated strategies to select the target recall key points essential to task performance. At this point, the child is able to perform the task autonomously.

Finally, the main characteristic of the intervention program is that it is a top-down approach. Thus, the therapist always responds to any changes in the learner's requirements and initiates an adapting strategy in order to make sure the children can do specific work which is important for them. There are decisions to be made about the development of efficient performance and responses to errors. When the child develops their performance by themselves, they can better transfer knowledge to real-life situations. Furthermore, the child's motivation is the most important factor that affects the child's ability to engage in tasks. Since this combined intervention is client-centered, the expected outcomes are determined by considering the child's occupational roles and context of the learning situation. Children are likely to be more motivated to engage in improving their performance when they identify goals to work on by themselves [38].

In summary, targeting cognitive strategies, facilitating multiprocess sequences of strategies that moved away from therapist to child, and the client-centered nature of the intervention were thought to be the reasons for the success achieved using the combination of the PRPP System of Intervention and the 4QM approach on the academic activities.

Limitations and Suggestions for Future Studies. This study showed that applying the combination of the PRPP System of Intervention and the 4QM approach was an effective treatment method to be used with the sample of children with LD. The success of the systematic strategy instruction program was found in the effective information processing strategy applications for treading comprehension and written expression tasks. These findings are worthy of further investigation. However, there are some limitations inherent in this study. First, the sample size was small and the participants were recruited from only Thai schools that supported children who had disabilities. Future research is recommended to apply this intervention program on a larger sample size and from a variety of backgrounds. Lastly, the participants were diagnosed with learning disabilities in reading (dyslexia). Future research should include children with different types of LD. Moreover, studies in the future should apply this program to other sample groups who have problems with information processing application such as ADHD and DCD. Future research that examines the combination of the PRPP System of Intervention and the 4QM approach program should focus on continuing the techniques of this study and a long-term follow-up study should be done on the children who received the intervention program. Since the combination of the PRPP System of Intervention and the 4QM approach is a client-centered approach, analyzing qualitative data of information processing strategy application ability of activities in the samples should be explored before and after receiving intervention from both children and their parents.

5. Conclusion

This study evaluated the effectiveness of the combination of the PRPP System of Intervention and the 4QM approach. The combination of these two approaches was shown to be effective in improving learning strategies during the academic activity in Thai children with LD. The experimental group had significantly improved in the mean scores of all quadrants of the PRPP System: Thai Version.

Acknowledgments

The researchers gratefully acknowledge the support of the Faculty of Associated Medical Sciences, Chiang Mai University, Thailand, for providing the funding and opportunity to conduct this research project. They are also extremely grateful to the participants who took the time to participate in the study.

References

[1] C. Chapparo and S. J. Lane, "Learning disabilities and intellectual disabilities: why is this so hard for me?" in *Kids Can Be Kids: A Childhood Occupations Approach*, S. J. Lane and A. C. Bundy, Eds., pp. 525–548, F.A. Davis Company, Philadelphia, Pa, USA, 2012.

[2] American Psychiatric Association, *Diagnostic and Statistical Manual of Mental Disorder (DSM IV-TR)*, American Psychiatric Association, Washington, DC, USA, 2000.

[3] P. Khaimook, "The development of children aged 6–12 years who have learning problems in school," 2014, http://rajanukul.go.th/main/index.php?mode=news&group=2&submode=news&idgroup=678.

[4] C. Chapparo, "Perceive, Recall, Plan and Perform (PRPP): occupation-centered task analysis and intervention system," in *Occupation-Centered Practice with Children: A Practical Guide for Occupational Therapists*, S. Rodger, Ed., pp. 183–203, Wiley-Blackwell, Chichester, UK, 2010.

[5] C. M. Schneck, "A frame of reference for visual perception," in *Frame of Reference for Pediatric Occupational Therapy*, P. Kramer and J. Hinojosa, Eds., pp. 349 389, Lippincott Williams & Wilkins, Philadelphia, Pa, USA, 3rd edition, 2009.

[6] P. Thagard, *Mind: Introduction to Cognitive Science*, MIT Press, Cambridge, Mass, USA, 2005.

[7] B. Wong, *Learning about Learning Disabilities*, Elsevier Academic Press, Boston, Mass, USA, 3rd edition, 2004.

[8] C. Chapparo and J. Ranka, *The PRPP System: Intervention*, The University of Sydney, Lidcombe, Australia, 2007.

[9] C. Chapparo and J. Ranka, *The PRPP System of Task Analysis: User's Training Manual: Available from the Discipline of Occupational Therap*, Faculty of Health Sciences, University of Sydney, Lidcombe, Australia, 2005.

[10] C. Chinn and L. Chinn, "Cognitive Strategies," 2009, https://www.education.com/reference/article/cognitive-strategies/.

[11] M. Pressley and J. R. Levin, *Cognitive Strategy Research: Educational Applications*, Springer, New York, NY, USA, 1983.

[12] M. Pressley and J. R. Levin, *Cognitive Strategy Research: Psychological Foundations*, Springer, New York, NY, USA, 1983.

[13] H. L. Swanson, P. Kehler, and O. Jerman, "Working memory, strategy knowledge, and strategy instruction in children with reading disabilities," *Journal of Learning Disabilities*, vol. 43, no. 1, pp. 24–47, 2010.

[14] M. T. Nott, *Occupational Performance and Information Processing in Adults with Agitation Following Traumatic Brain Injury*, Discipline of Occupational Therapy, Faculty of Health Sciences, University of Sydney, Lidcombe, Australia, 2008.

[15] M. M. Sohlberg, L. Ehlhardt, and M. Kennedy, "Instructional techniques in cognitive rehabilitation: a preliminary report," *Seminars in Speech and Language*, vol. 26, no. 4, pp. 268–279, 2005.

[16] G. M. Giles, "Management of behavioral disregulation and noncompliance in the post-acute severely brain -injured adult," in *Rehabilitation of the Severely Brain-Injured Adult: A Practical Approach*, G. M. Giles and J. Clark-Wilson, Eds., pp. 81–96, Stanley Thornes, Cheltenham, UK, 2nd edition, 1999.

[17] M. E. Snell and T. J. Zirpoli, "Intervention strategies," in *Systematic Instruction of Persons with Severe Handicaps*, M. E. Snell, Ed., pp. 110–149, Merill Publishing, Columbus, Ohio, USA, 3rd edition, 1987.

[18] C. Greber, J. Ziviani, and S. Rodger, "The four-quadrant model of facilitated learning (Part 2): strategies and applications," *Australian Occupational Therapy Journal*, vol. 54, supplement 1, pp. S40–S48, 2007.

[19] M. T. Nott, C. Chapparo, and R. Heard, "Effective occupational therapy intervention with adults demonstrating agitation during post-traumatic amnesia," *Brain Injury*, vol. 22, no. 9, pp. 669–683, 2008.

[20] J. Challita, C. Chapparo, J. Hinitt, and S. Lowe, "The effectiveness of the perceive, recall, plan, perform (PRPP) System of Intervention on the social skills of children with learning difficulties. Published Abstract: Occupational Therapy Australia, 25th National Conference and Exhibition, July," *Australian Occupational Therapy Journal*, vol. 60, supplement 1, article 43, 2013.

[21] L. S. Vygotsky, "Mind in society: the development of higher psychological processes. Translated by Cole M, Scribner S, John-Steiner V, Souberman E," in *The Essential Vygotsky*, R. W. Reiber and D. K. Robinson, Eds., pp. 345–400, Kluwer Academic, New York, NY, USA, 1978.

[22] M. Mosston and S. Ashworth, *Teaching Physical Education*, Benjamin Cummings, San Francisco, Calif, USA, 2002.

[23] C. Greber and J. Ziviani, "A frame of reference to enhance teaching-learning: the four-quadrant model of facilitated learning," in *Occupation Center Practice with Children: A Practical Guide for Occupational Therapists*, S. Rodger, Ed., pp. 234–263, Blackwell, Oxford, UK, 2010.

[24] C. Greber, J. Ziviani, and S. Rodger, "The four quadrant model of facilitated learning: a clinically based action research project," *Australian Occupational Therapy Journal*, vol. 54, no. 2, pp. 149–152, 2007.

[25] C. Greber, J. Ziviani, and S. Rodger, "Clinical utility of the four-quadrant model of facilitated learning: perspectives of experienced occupational therapists," *Australian Occupational Therapy Journal*, vol. 58, no. 3, pp. 187–194, 2011.

[26] G. Aubin, E. Stip, I. Gelinas, C. Rainville, and C. Chapparo, "Assessment of information-processing skills during daily task performance in persons with schizophrenia: usefulness of the Perceive, Recall, Plan, and Perform (PRPP) System of Task Analysis," in *Proceedings of the 15th World Conference of the Federation of Occupational Therapists*, Santiago, Chile, 2010.

[27] K. Boland, *Assessing information processing in the context of pretend play [Ph.D. thesis]*, Discipline of Occupational Therapy, Faculty of Health Sciences, University of Sydney, Lidcombe, Australia, 2004.

[28] C. Chapparo and J. Ranka, *Development of an Information Processing Task Analysis to Identify Errors in Self-Maintenance Performance of Brain Injured Clients: Final Category B Grants Research Report*, University of Sydney. Faculty of Health Sciences, Lidcombe, Australia, 1992.

[29] M. Fordham, *Perceive, Recall, Plan, Perform (PRPP) rating scales (parent and teacher): reliability and validity [Ph.D. thesis]*,

Discipline of Occupational Therapy, Faculty of Health Sciences, University of Sydney, Lidcombe, Australia, 2001.

[30] J. Lohri, *Information and sensory processing abilities of young children with autism spectrum disorder [thesis]*, Discipline of Occupational Therapy, Faculty of Healthy Sciences, University of Sydney, Lidcombe, Australia, 2005.

[31] J. Pulis and C. Chapparo, "Assessment of children with information processing deficits: the PRPP system of task analysis," in *Proceedings of the 2nd Paediatric Conference. What Works with Kids hosted by OT Australia-QLD*, Occupational Therapy Australia, Brisbane, Australia, 2002.

[32] M. Still, R. Beltran, S. Catts, and C. Chapparo, "Cognitive and functional assessment of patients with early psychosis," *Acta Psychiatrica Scandinavica. Supplementum*, vol. 413, pp. 40–41, 2002.

[33] P. Munkhetvit, *Cognitive assessment in patients with acquired brain injury in Thailand [Ph.D. thesis]*, Discipline of Occupational Therapy, Faculty of Health Sciences, University of Sydney, Lidcombe, Australia, 2005.

[34] P. Munkhetvit, "Types of cognitive deficits during the performance of ADL and IADL in persons with CVA," *The Journal of Occupational Therapist Association of Thailand*, vol. 11, no. 1, pp. 19–30, 2008 (Thai).

[35] S. Bunyachatakul, P. Munkhetvit, T. Srikamjak, and A. Sarakam, "Cognitive deficits during the performance of activities of daily living in Schizophrenic patients," *Bulletin of Suan Prung*, vol. 26, no. 2, pp. 15–24, 2010.

[36] L. Woodrow, *Writing About Quantitative Research in Applied Linguistics*, Palgrave Macmillan, New York, NY, USA, 2014.

[37] J. P. Toglia, "A dynamic interactional approach to cognitive rehabilitation," in *Cognition and Occupation across the Life Span: Models for Intervention in Occupational Therapy*, N. Katz, Ed., pp. 29–72, The American Occupational Therapy Association, Bethesda, Md, USA, 2nd edition, 2005.

[38] H. J. Polatajko, A. D. Mandich, C. Missiuna et al., "Cognitive Orientation to daily Occupational Performance (CO-OP): Part III-The protocol in brief," *Physical and Occupational Therapy in Pediatrics*, vol. 20, no. 2-3, pp. 107–123, 2001.

20

Effects of Oral Stimulation Intervention in Newborn Babies with Cri du Chat Syndrome: Single-Subject Research Design

Mi Kyung Kim[1] and Deok Ju Kim[2]

[1]*Department of Occupational Therapy, Sanggye Paik Hospital, Seoul, Republic of Korea*
[2]*Department of Occupational Therapy, Health Science College, Cheongju University, Cheongju, Republic of Korea*

Correspondence should be addressed to Deok Ju Kim; dj7407@hanmail.net

Academic Editor: Claudia Hilton

The purpose of this study is to treat dysphagia in a newborn baby with cri du chat syndrome using an oral stimulation intervention and to examine its effects. The subject of this study was a baby born 2 weeks prematurely. Since birth, his oxygen saturation (SaO_2) decreased while feeding, and he had difficulty with mouth feeding. Thus, an NG feeding tube was inserted, and dysphagia treatment was initiated on the sixth day after birth. A baseline phase and an intervention phase were performed using an AB design. The oral stimulation intervention was not performed in the baseline phase, as only nonnutritive sucking training using a rubber pacifier was used during the baseline phase. During the intervention phase, nonnutritive sucking training and oral stimulation intervention were simultaneously conducted. After the intervention period, daily oral milk intake and intake per feeding of the subject noticeably increased. The oxygen saturation while feeding rose over 90% on average, and the baby did not present with hypoxia. The oral stimulation intervention provided prior to feeding resulted in highly positive effects, including induced normal development of the baby, stimulation of his transition from the NG feeding tube to bottle feeding, increased oxygen saturation, and a shortened hospital stay.

1. Introduction

Cri du chat syndrome is a congenital genetic disorder resulting from the deletion of different sizes of the short arm of chromosome 5 (5p). It was first reported in 1963 by French doctor Jerome Lejeune who is renowned for his discovery of Down syndrome. One of the remarkable clinical symptoms of cri du chat is a characteristic cat-like cry. Affected children cry with a weak one-octave-higher minor key. Some cases reported an anomaly in a deformed larynx or tracheobronchomalacia. The crying sound barely changes through growth, but the frequency of the cry may decrease [1].

Clinical features vary considerably from patient to patient but childhood and distinct facial dysmorphism. Malocclusion, hyper- and hypotonia, and delayed motor development are also common as well as microcephaly. Affected children also present with hypertelorism, micrognathia, epicanthal folds, deformed low-set ears, palate problems x(high arch or very wide and flat in shape), hypotonia, abnormal palm lines, and intellectual disability. Birth weight is markedly low, the face is round, and the eyes are wide-set in these subjects. The prevalence is 1 in 15,000 to 50,000 births, and the rate is known to be higher in females than in males [2]. The age of the mother is not associated with the presence of the syndrome, but several studies reported that a history of radiation in prepregnancy, infection of influenza or mumps in early pregnancy, and medication used before or during the pregnancy may be the cause [3]. Many patients die during their early childhood. Most patients surviving to adulthood demonstrate an IQ level lower than 20. Typical characteristics include eating problems due to difficulty in swallowing and sucking from early childhood. Most children with the syndrome are born with a low weight at birth, showing poor growth. Their cognitive and linguistic abilities and development of motor nerves are significantly delayed. They demonstrate behavioural problems, including attention deficit hyperactivity disorder (ADHD), aggressiveness, and repetitive behaviour [4].

In the cri du chat syndrome, dysphagia is frequently observed in young children occurring since their neonatal period. The term dysphagia comprehensively includes all problems that can occur during the process in which food travels from the mouth to the stomach [5]. Patients with dysphagia mainly show functional disabilities in the oral and pharyngeal phases, such as residues in the pharynx and aspiration. This causes various complications including malnutrition, aspiration pneumonia, and dehydration, which can even cause death in some severe cases [6]. Dysphagia not only interrupts growth of the child but is also an important issue that might threaten one's survival.

Amongst premature and newborn babies, some show problems in oral feeding due to various causes, including a weakened cardiorespiratory system and oral muscles, problems in anatomical jaw structure, and overreaction to touching the mouth. In this case, a nasogastric feeding tube (NG feeding tube) is usually applied to initiate feeding. An NG feeding tube is a device used to improve the nutritional status of undernourished patients and to provide effective nutritional support. However, babies may be exposed to risks of side effects such as complications like aspiration, diarrhoea, and abnormal oral reflexes, as the period of using the NG feeding tube increases [7]. The transition to oral feeding is not easy for premature and newborn babies with weak swallowing abilities; thus, great time and sophisticated nursing care are required until they can handle oral feeding. Studies to investigate nonnutritive sucking and oral stimulation intervention, aiming at shortening the period of hospital stay by improving the oral feeding ability, should be conducted. In particular, oral stimulation intervention is an effective solution to improve dysphagia in premature and newborn babies [8, 9]. Oral stimulation therapy has been proposed as an effective measure in improving dysphagia of premature infants and newborns, but few studies reflect actual cases of interventions for premature infants and newborns that employ this method. This study is intended to help clinical therapists by providing guidelines for oral stimulation therapy and the effects of treatment.

There are only a handful of cases in existing studies that have investigated clinical cri du chat syndrome cases, due to its characteristic as a rare disorder. A few studies treated ophthalmological opinions and deformities to the genitourinary system. However, unfortunately, no study was found on neonatal dysphagia treatment. We reasoned that an occupational therapist is the most fitting therapist than any other specialists in treating dysphagia, and their role and intervention methods are absolutely critical. According to this law, "Dysphagia rehabilitation is calculated as training by one occupational therapist of a dysphagia patient in one-on-one sessions lasting at least 30 minutes" [10]. Therefore, this study presents the treatment and results of dysphagia in cri du chat syndrome patients by an occupational therapist using oral stimulation intervention.

2. Methods

2.1. Participants

2.1.1. Medical History. The baby patient included in this study was born at 37 weeks + 5 days weighing 3120 g via C-section according to the parents' requirements at P obstetrics on March 14, 2017. The oxygen saturation (SaO_2) of the baby reduced at every feeding from the morning of his birth. His physical characteristics included a similar single palm line on both palms (Figure 1), a protruding short fourth toe (Figure 2), both hands rotated inwards, both ears showed a skin tag (Figure 3), a left club foot (Figure 4), and a high-arched palate (Figure 5). The baby was moved to S Hospital based in Seoul for more in-depth examinations. After the transfer, he was diagnosed with cri du chat syndrome based on his cat-like cry and physical defects. Cyanosis occurred while feeding due to shortness of breath, so an NG feeding tube was inserted. Swallowing therapy was requested to the department of rehabilitation medicine on March 20, 2017.

2.1.2. Swallowing Function. Dysphagia was first evaluated 6 days after birth. In the initial evaluation, the baby received an NG feeding tube while on ventilator support. In oral motor function, the oral sensory ability was normal. However, his ability to close his lips and cheek and jaw stability were low due to weak facial muscle tone. Rooting reflex and bite reflex were intact, but his suck-swallow reflex was impaired. Sucking power was weak. Sucking, swallowing, and breathing were not smoothly coordinated. This reduced the oxygen saturation while feeding down to 72%. When the aspirator oxygen concentration was maintained at 21% (oxygen: 2 L/min, oxygen aspiration path: high flow), the oxygen saturation was recovered back to 90%. The possible amount per feeding was 5 cc per time.

2.2. Study Environment and Design

2.2.1. Study Environment. The treatment of dysphagia was performed while the baby was inside the incubator in the Neonatal Intensive Care Unit (NICU) of the S Hospital. The environment was equipped with baby bottles for feeding, instruments for the NG feeding tube, in case of difficulty in mouth feeding, and a device to measure oxygen saturation. The subject of this study is a premature baby in the NICU. Hospitals do not use FEES and VFES because they can be dangerous to premature infants in the NICU. Although more objective evaluation results could be obtained using FEES or VFES, we could not use either given the condition of our subject.

2.2.2. Study Design. This study is based on a single-subject research design and applied AB design. The study period was from March 15 to April 7, 2017. Twenty sessions were performed in total. During the baseline phase, nonnutritive sucking training (with a rubber pacifier) was initiated. A nurse provided nutrition using oral feeding or the NG feeding tube. During the intervention phase, 30 minutes of nonnutritive sucking training and another 30 minutes of oral stimulation intervention were performed, followed by oral

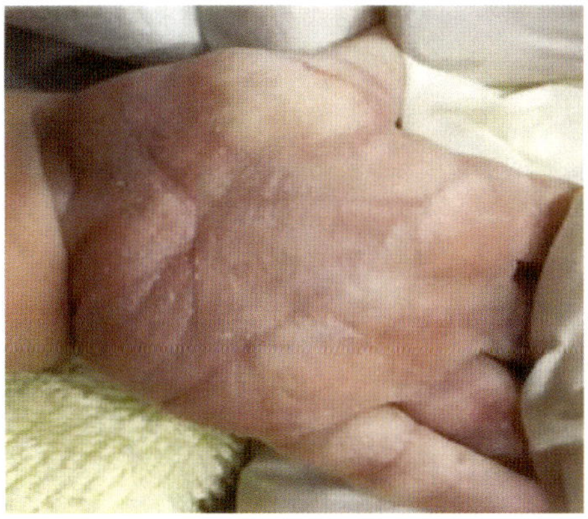

Figure 1: Single palm lines on both hands.

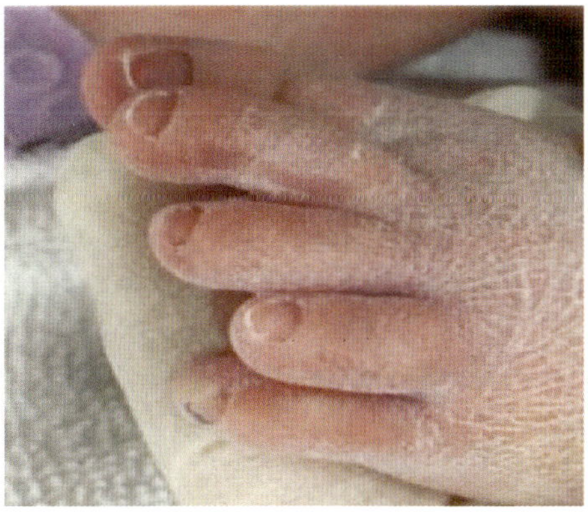

Figure 2: Protruding short fourth toe.

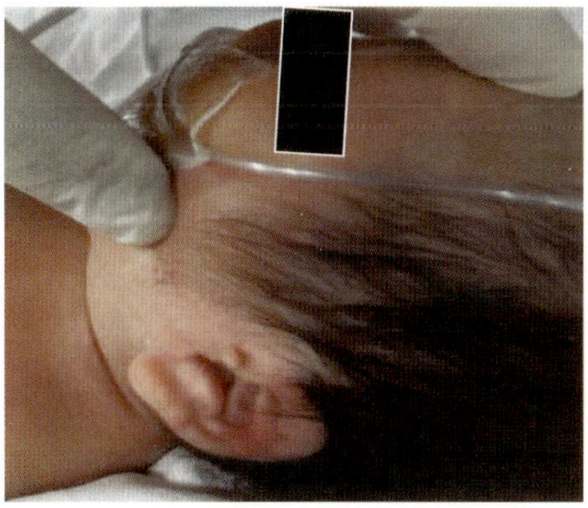

Figure 3: Both ears with a skin tag.

or use of the NG feeding tube, which were equally performed at the baseline phase.

2.3. Instruments

2.3.1. Evaluation of Feeding Amount: Baby Bottle. A Green mom PP bottle of 140 mL for newborn babies was used to measure the feeding amount in this study. The minimum unit of the bottle was 10 mL.

2.3.2. Evaluation of Oxygen Saturation: Masimo Radical 7. To measure the oxygen saturation of the subject, a Signal

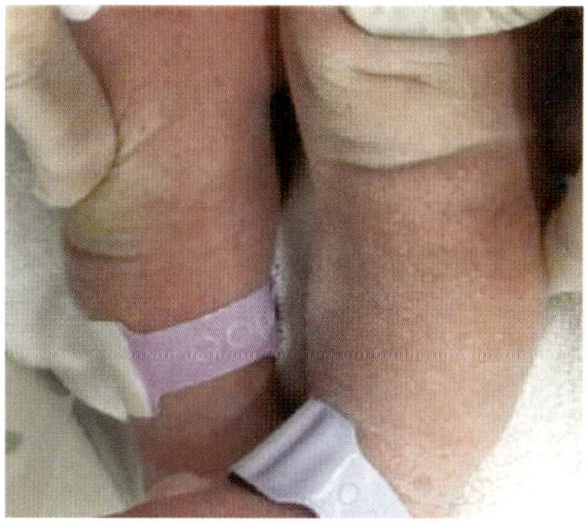

Figure 4: Left leg with a club foot.

Extraction Pulse CO-Oximeter manufactured by Masimo Radical 7 was used (Figure 6). Many studies found that this equipment significantly reduced false alarms and accurately detected actual warning signs. Its reliability was proven in more than 100 independent and objective studies. It is estimated to have been used for more than 100 million patients in major hospitals and medical institutions around the world. For measurement, the equipment records the evolution of oxygen saturation of the subject while feeding. An oxygen saturation falling below 80% indicates reduced ability to suck, swallow, and breathe, which is considered as hypoxia [11].

2.4. Study Procedure

2.4.1. Baseline Phase. During the baseline phase, the baby was fed 40 cc every 3 hours. Oral feeding was first attempted with a baby bottle, and the remaining feeding sessions were provided by the use of the NG feeding tube. During this period, only nonnutritive sucking training was performed without oral stimulation intervention. The amount of oral milk intake fed with a bottle and the evolution of oxygen saturation while feeding were measured once a day, 5 times per week. To minimise error in measurement, no treatment stimuli were provided during this measurement. The same nurse fed the baby with milk inside the incubator at a specific hour to minimise any environmental factors that may have affected the baby's swallowing.

2.4.2. Intervention Phase. During the intervention phase, nonnutritive sucking training and oral stimulation intervention were performed for 30 minutes each, and feeding was provided equally as during the baseline phase. The oral stimulation intervention was performed 5 times a week for 3 weeks (15 times in total). During this period, the feeding amount and oxygen saturation were measured daily after the oral stimulation intervention.

2.4.3. Details of Intervention. The objective of dysphagia treatment is to help preterm infants' transition from feeding tube use to oral feeding. The stimulation program was designed in reference to the "oral stimulation program" conducted by Fucile et al. [12] and Choi et al. [13]. The program

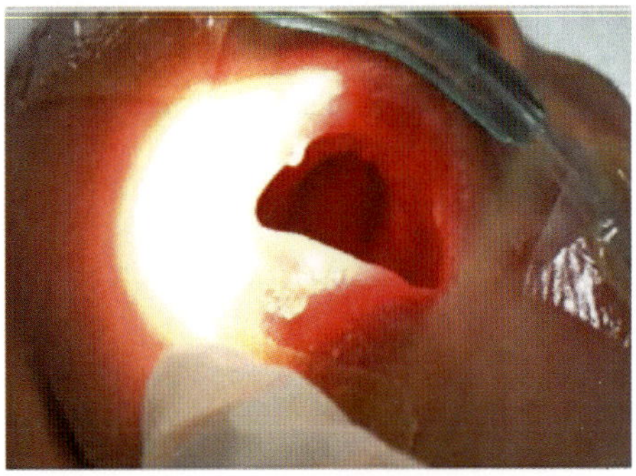

FIGURE 5: High-arched palate.

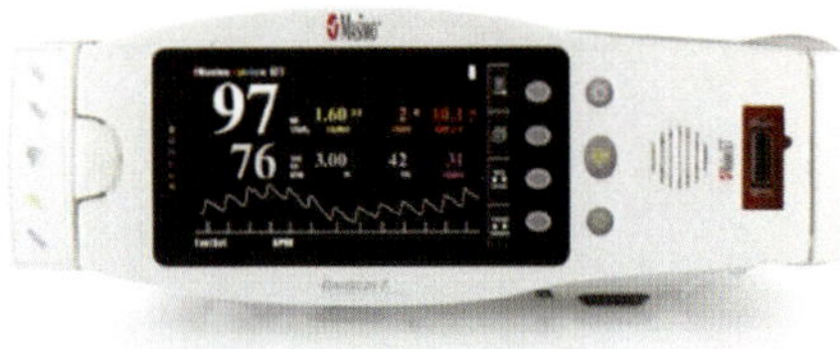

FIGURE 6: Masimo Radical 7.

is performed for 30 minutes in each session and consists of stimulating the cheeks, upper and lower lips, upper and lower gums, internal cheeks, and the edge of the tongue, in that order (Table 1). Treatment of this program was performed by an occupational therapist with more than 10 years of experience in child dysphagia treatment and education. The activity level was adjusted during the program according to the condition of the baby.

2.5. Analysis Methods. Collected data were analysed with Microsoft Office Excel 2007. The feeding amount and oxygen saturation were checked daily during both the baseline and intervention phases. A frequency analysis was performed on the results. Measured values obtained during these phases were comparatively analysed with visual graphs and descriptive statistics to observe the evolution.

3. Results

3.1. Evolution of the Daily Oral Feeding Amount. The visual evolution of the daily oral feeding amount is presented in Figure 7. During the baseline phase, the mean and standard deviation values (mean ± SD) were 11.6 ± 2.0 mL. Nonnutritive sucking training and a 30-minute oral stimulation therapy were performed during the 15th session of the intervention phase. The mean ± SD values of the intervention phase were found to be 43.8 ± 22.5 mL, whereas the average value of the intervention phase increased by about 32.8 mL.

During the intervention phase, 13 of the 15 sessions showed results greater than +2 standard deviations of the baseline on average, except for the sixth and eighth sessions. This indicates that oral stimulation intervention had a positive effect on changes in the oral feeding amount.

3.2. Evolution of the Amount per Oral Feeding. The progress of each oral feeding is presented in the graph in Figure 8. The mean ± SD of the baseline phase was 7.0 ± 2.5 mL, and the mean ± SD in the intervention phase was 27.1 ± 13.1 mL. That of the latter increased by 20.1 mL. During the intervention phase, 13 of the 15 sessions showed results greater than +2 standard deviations from the baseline on average, except for the sixth and eighth sessions. This shows that oral stimulation intervention had a positive effect on changes in the oral feeding amount.

3.3. Evolution of Oxygen Saturation. The evolution of oxygen saturation while feeding is presented in Figure 9. The mean ± SD of the baseline phase was 72.4 ± 3.0%, and that of the intervention phase was 90.7 ± 10.9%, whereas the latter increased by 18.3%. During the intervention phase, all 15 data values were greater than +2 standard deviations of the baseline on average, which indicates that the oral stimulation intervention had a positive effect on the increase of oxygen saturation while feeding. The resulting values demonstrate that those of oxygen saturation from the tenth to fourteenth sessions fell lower than the average value. This is because the baby went through difficulties in adaptation as the aspirator was completely removed, and he breathed on his own while fed after the tenth session. Afterwards, the baby gradually adapted to self-breathing. The oxygen saturation increased while feeding because of the oral stimulation intervention program.

4. Discussion

Cri du chat syndrome is a disorder caused by the loss of the chromosome 5p's short arm, which causes characteristics physical birth defects and the typical cat-like cry. In the neonatal period, neonates with cri du chat syndrome present difficulty in feeding and shortness of breath. In the childhood stage, they may present with frequent upper airway infection, otitis media, and diarrhoea, often requiring internal medicine treatment [14]. The feeding problem, which is particularly frequent during the neonatal period, is a serious problem that can even threaten the survival of the baby; therefore, dysphagia treatment during this phase is highly critical.

The subject of this study showed dysphagia and decreased oxygen saturation while feeding since the early neonatal period, and dysphagia treatment was initiated on the sixth day after birth. In particular, reduced oxygen saturation while feeding can cause instability in the cardiovascular system, respiratory system, and central nervous system, formation of an immature oral structure, and other problems [15]. An uncoordinated suck-swallow-breath pattern hinders safe and successful oral feeding. If proper breathing is not maintained in between sucking, owing to the dysfunctional coordination of sucking, swallowing, and breathing, the infant may suffer reduced oxygen saturation. Repeated hypoxia can damage the cerebrum by reducing blood flow to the cerebrum. Delayed development of the oral feeding ability can lead to growth retardation [14].

Various studies on oral stimulation intervention for improving oral feeding ability have been conducted [8, 9].

Table 1: Oral stimulation program.

Structure	Stimulation steps	Frequency	Duration
Cheek	(1) Place the index finger at the base of the nose. (2) Compress the tissue, move finger toward the ear, then down, and toward the corner of the lip (in a C pattern). (3) Repeat for the other side. (i) Purpose: improve the range of motion and strength of cheeks and improve lip seal	4x each cheek	2 min
Upper lip	(1) Place the index finger at the corner of the upper lip. (2) Compress the tissue. (3) Move the finger away in a circular motion, from the corner toward the centre, and to the other corner. (4) Reverse direction. (i) Purpose: improve the lip range of motion and seal	4x	1 min
Lower lip	(1) Place the index finger at the corner of the lower lip. (2) Compress the tissue. (3) Move the finger away in a circular motion, from the corner toward the centre, and to the other corner. (4) Reverse direction. (i) Purpose: improve the lip range of motion and seal	4x	1 min
Upper and lower lip curls	(1) Place the index finger at the centre of the upper lip. (2) Apply sustained pressure and stretch downward toward the midline. (3) Repeat for the lower lip, apply sustained pressure, and stretch upward toward the midline. (i) Purpose: improve the lip strength, range of motion, and seal	2x each cheek	1 min
Upper gum	(1) Place a finger at the centre of the gum, with firm sustained pressure slowly move toward the back of the mouth. (2) Return to the centre of the mouth. (3) Repeat for the opposite side. (i) Purpose: improve the range of motion of the tongue, stimulate swallowing, and improve sucking	2x	1 min
Lower gum	(1) Place a finger at the centre of the gum, with firm sustained pressure slowly move toward the back of the mouth. (2) Return to the centre of the mouth. (3) Repeat for the opposite side. (i) Purpose: improve the range of motion of the tongue, stimulate swallowing, and improve sucking	2x	1 min
Internal cheek	(1) Place a finger at the inner corner of lips. (2) Compress the tissue, move back toward the molars, and return to the corner of the lip. (3) Repeat for the other side. (i) Purpose: improve the cheek range of motion and lip seal	2x each cheek	2 min
Lateral borders of the tongue	(1) Place a finger at the level of the molar between the side blade of the tongue and the lower gum. (2) Move the finger toward midline, pushing the tongue toward the opposite direction. (3) Immediately move the finger all the way into the cheek, stretching it. (i) Purpose: improve the tongue range of motion and strength	2x each cheek	1 min
Midblade of the tongue	(1) Place an index finger at the centre of the mouth. (2) Give sustained pressure into the hard palate for 3 seconds. (3) Move the finger down to contact the centre blade of the tongue. (4) Displace the tongue downward with a firm pressure. (5) Immediately move the finger to contact the centre of the mouth at the hard palate. (i) Purpose: improve the tongue range of motion and strength, stimulate swallowing, and improve sucking	4x	1 min
Elicit a suck	(1) Place a finger at the midline, centre of the palate, gently stroke the palate to elicit a suck. (i) Purpose: improve sucking and soft palate activation	N/A	1 min
Pacifier	(1) Place a pacifier in the mouth. (i) Purpose: improve sucking and soft palate activation	N/A	3 min

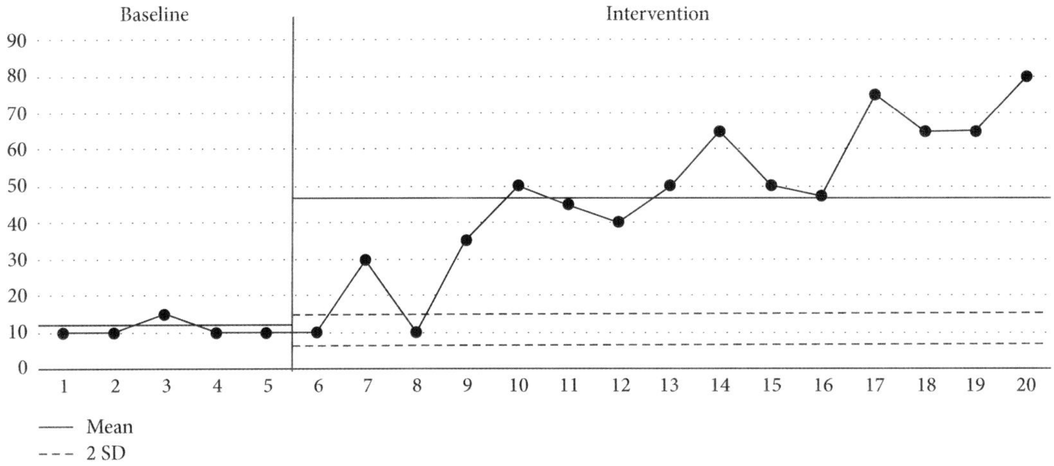

FIGURE 7: Evolution of the total amount of oral feeding.

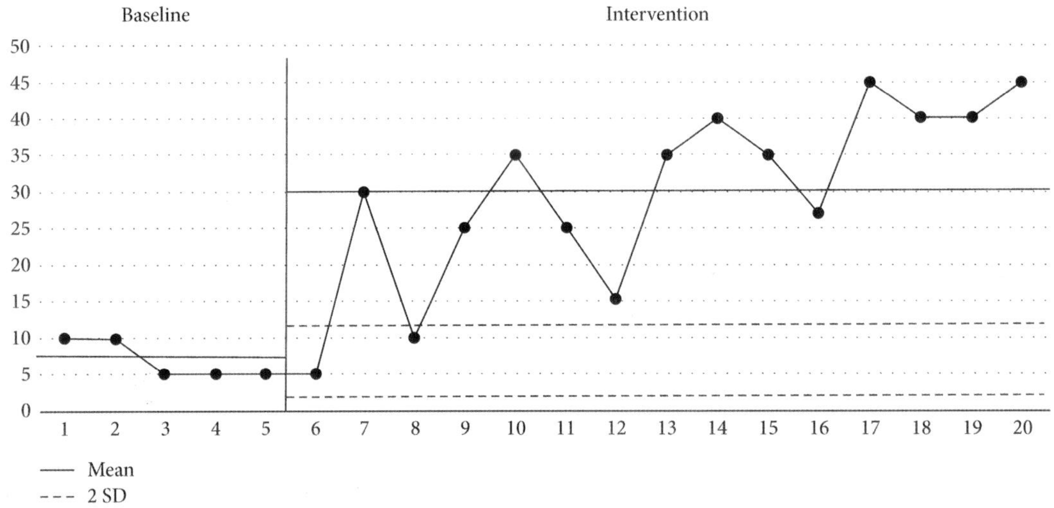

FIGURE 8: Evolution of the amount per oral feeding.

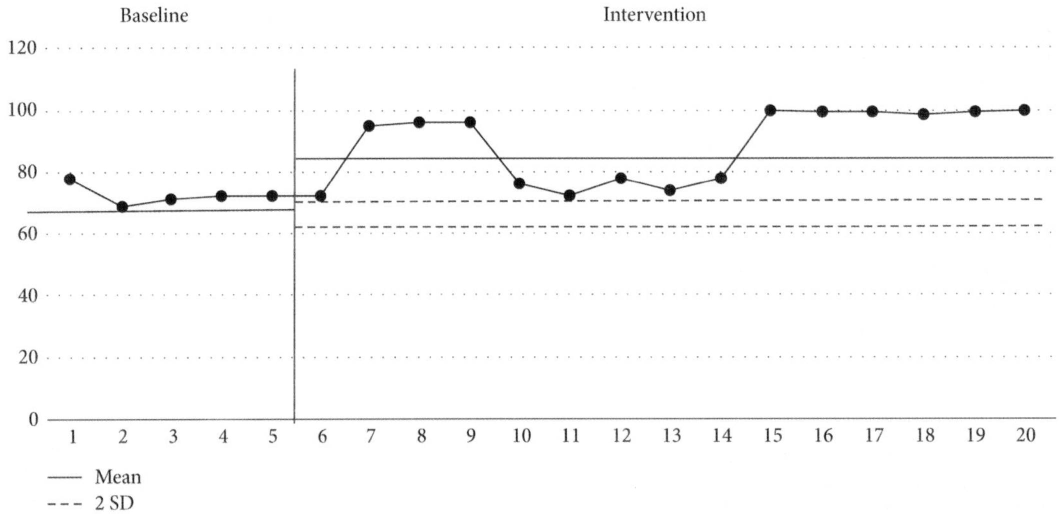

FIGURE 9: Evolution of oxygen saturation.

This study also employed an oral stimulation program to verify whether such programs are truly effective for dysphagia. This method stimulated the cheeks, upper and lower lips, upper and lower gums, internal cheeks, and the edge of the tongue to treat dysphagia in premature and neonatal babies. The duration and frequency of stimulation was properly adjusted for each phase. This study conducted an oral stimulation intervention program to a baby with cri du chat syndrome for 4 weeks according to our manual. The study was a single-subject research design and applied AB design. Only nonnutritive sucking training was performed during the baseline phase. During the intervention phase, nonnutritive sucking training and a 30-minute oral stimulation intervention were simultaneously performed.

The average daily intake of the subject was 11.0 ± 2.0 mL in the baseline phase and 43.8 ± 22.5 mL in the intervention phase, in which the latter increased by 32.8 mL. As for evolution of intake per feeding, the average of the baseline phase was 7.0 ± 2.5 mL, and that of the intervention phase was 27.1 ± 13.1 mL, which increased by 20.1 mL. Fucile et al. [16] conducted an experiment on 32 premature babies to investigate the effect of oral stimulation intervention. The experimental group moved on to bottle feeding from an NG feeding tube 7 days earlier with a greater feeding amount compared to the control group, showing a positive effect. Boiron et al. [17] found that the feeding amount increased when oral stimulation intervention was performed immediately before feeding. The increased amount of feeding led to an increased body weight, and the in-hospital period shortened. Their results support those of this study. In respect to the evolution of oxygen saturation, the average of the baseline phase was 72.4 ± 3.0%, and the intervention phase showed 90.7 ± 10.9%, with the latter increasing by 18.3%. Feeding is a complex process that requires exact harmonization of sucking, swallowing, and breathing, and it is difficult to increase the feeding amount steadily if breathing is not good. This has been proven in several studies. The increase in the subjects' feeding amount in this study indicates that the functions of sucking, swallowing, and breathing have improved in the end, which is attributed to the effects of oral stimulation. [18]. Choi et al. [13] reported that sucking frequency increased when the mouth area was stimulated during oral feeding. They also observed that this increased oxygen saturation stabilized the patient's behavioural status.

Finger sucking strength of the baby gradually increased compared to the beginning, as the intervention frequency increased. Amaizu et al. [19] observed that the complete bottle feeding was attained earlier when the first bottle feeding was started earlier. The bottle feeding amount increased as the baby's sucking ability developed. This probably functioned as positive feedback to the baby and improved the sucking ability even further. Intervention occurring on a continued and regular manner particularly stimulates more positive results [12]. This study regularly provided stimulation at a specific hour every day, which enabled us to observe the baby more closely.

The limitations of this study are as follows. First, this study was limited as a single-subject design due to the characteristics of the cri du chat syndrome, which is a rare disease. This makes it difficult to generalise the effects of intervention to all babies with cri du chat syndrome. Second, this study does not include a follow-up period that allows continued examination of the treatment effect after the end of the intervention phase. It is recommended that future studies shall investigate the continuity of treatment effects using an ABA research design. This study is meaningful because it conducted an oral stimulation intervention program on a baby affected by the cri du chat syndrome. Currently, there are few domestic and international cases of feeding intervention to premature and neonate babies to assist with their normal development. The study offers meaningful implications as it stimulated the transition from the NG feeding tube to bottle feeding and confirmed that the program was a highly effective treatment intervention that augmented oxygen saturation.

5. Conclusion

This study presented the process and results of dysphagia treatment to a baby with cri du chat syndrome through an oral stimulation intervention program led by an occupational therapist. We employed an AB design and determined a baseline phase and an intervention phase. The oral stimulation intervention was not provided during the baseline phase, and nonnutritive sucking training using a rubber pacifier was performed. During the intervention phase, the nonnutritive sucking training and the oral stimulation intervention were conducted simultaneously.

In terms of the intervention results, the daily intake and the intake per feeding noticeably increased in the intervention phase compared to the baseline phase. The oxygen saturation from the morning of the day of birth to the baseline phase decreased at every feeding (the rate was lower than 80% on average, and the baby presented with hypoxia). After the intervention phase, this value rose to over 90% on average. The oral stimulation intervention conducted prior to feeding promoted normal development of the baby, demonstrating highly positive effects, including stimulation of the transition from the NG feeding tube to bottle feeding, increased oxygen saturation, and reduced hospital stay.

References

[1] C. Zamfir, M. Dassonville, G. Rodesch, and H. Steyaert, "A rare malformation: double duodenal atresia associated with malrotation in a patient with "Cri du chat" syndrome," *Journal of Pediatric Surgery Case Reports*, vol. 12, pp. 3–5, 2016.

[2] S. Erlenkamp and K. E. Kristoffersen, "Sign communication in cri du chat syndrome," *Journal of Communication Disorders*, vol. 43, no. 3, pp. 225–251, 2010.

[3] D. Z. S. Furtado, F. B. V. de Moura Leite, C. N. Barreto et al., "Profiles of amino acids and biogenic amines in the plasma of cri-du-chat patients," *Journal of Pharmaceutical and Biomedical Analysis*, vol. 140, no. 5, pp. 137–145, 2017.

[4] S. N. Kim, Y. A. Kim, M. H. Jeon, D. S. Kim, and H. I. Kim, "A systematic review and meta-analysis on the effects of oral stimulation interventions on the transition from tube to oral feeding in premature infants," *Journal of Korean Clinical Nursing Research*, vol. 23, no. 2, pp. 151–160, 2017.

[5] A. C. V. Silva, S. R. C. Fabio, and R. O. Dantas, "A scintigraphic study of oral, pharyngeal, and esophageal transit in patients with stroke," *Dysphagia*, vol. 23, no. 2, pp. 165–171, 2008.

[6] G. Mann, G. J. Hankey, and D. Cameron, "Swallowing disorders following acute stroke: prevalence and diagnostic accuracy," *Cerebrovascular Diseases*, vol. 10, no. 5, pp. 380–386, 2000.

[7] Y. J. Kim and J. S. Seo, "Nutritional assessment of ICU inpatients with tube feeding," *Journal of the Korean Dietetic Association*, vol. 21, no. 1, pp. 11–24, 2015.

[8] L. M. Einarsson-Backes, J. Deitz, R. Price, R. Glass, and R. Hays, "The effect of oral support on sucking efficiency in preterm infants," *American Journal of Occupational Therapy*, vol. 48, no. 6, pp. 490–498, 1994.

[9] M. K. Lee, *Effect of Oral Stimulation on Feeding Performance, Growth, Length of Hospital Stay in NICU Korea Preterm Infants*, Samyook University, Gyeonggi-do, Republic of Korea, 2017.

[10] Occupational Therapy Compilation Committee, *Health and Medical Low*, Seoul, Republic of Korea, Edu factory, 2017.

[11] *Operator's Manual. EU Authorized Representative for Masimo Corporation*, Masimo Corporaton, Hannover, Germany, 2017.

[12] S. Fucile, E. Gisel, and C. Lau, "Oral stimulation accelerates the transition from tube to oral feeding in preterm infants," *The Journal of Pediatrics*, vol. 141, no. 2, pp. 230–236, 2002.

[13] H. W. Choi, H. W. Park, H. Y. Kim et al., "Feeding desaturation and effects of orocutaneous stimulation in extremely low birth weight infants," *Journal of the Korean Society of Neonatology*, vol. 17, no. 2, pp. 193–200, 2010.

[14] J. Y. Im, *Effect of Argumentative and Alternative Communication Intervention on Initial Communicative Ability of Children with Nonverbal Cat's Cry Syndrome*, Daegu University, Daegu, Republic of Korea, 2013.

[15] S. L. Gardner and M. I. Hagedorn, "Physiologic sequelae of prematurity: the nurse practitioner's role. Part V. Feeding difficulties and growth failure (pathophysiology, cause, and data collection)," *Journal of Pediatric Health Care*, vol. 5, no. 3, pp. 122–134, 1991.

[16] S. Fucile, E. G. Gisel, and C. Lau, "Effect of an oral stimulation program on sucking skill maturation of preterm infants," *Developmental Medicine & Child Neurology*, vol. 47, no. 3, pp. 158–162, 2005.

[17] M. Boiron, L. D. Nobrega, S. Roux, A. Henrot, and E. Saliba, "Effects of oral stimulation and oral support on non-nutritive sucking and feeding performance in preterm infants," *Developmental Medicine & Child Neurology*, vol. 49, no. 6, pp. 439–444, 2007.

[18] I. H. Gewolb, J. F. Bosnia, E. W. Reynolds, and F. L. Vice, "Integration of suck and swallow rhythms during feeding in preterm infants with and without bronchopulmonary dysplasia," *Developmental Medicine & Child Neurology*, vol. 45, no. 5, pp. 344–348, 2003.

[19] N. Amaizu, R. J. Shulman, R. J. Schanler, and C. Lau, "Maturation of oral feeding skills in preterm infants," *Acta Paediatrica*, vol. 97, no. 1, pp. 61–67, 2008.

21

Occupational Therapy for Adults with Overweight and Obesity: Mapping Interventions Involving Occupational Therapists

Svetlana Solgaard Nielsen[1] and Jeanette Reffstrup Christensen[1,2]

[1]The Research Initiative of Activity Studies and Occupational Therapy, Research Unit of General Practice, Department of Public Health, The University of Southern Denmark, J.B. Winsløws Vej 9a, 5000 Odense C, Denmark
[2]The Research Unit for Physical Activity and Health at Work, Department of Sports Science and Clinical Biomechanics, The University of Southern Denmark, Campusvej 55, 5230 Odense M, Denmark

Correspondence should be addressed to Svetlana Solgaard Nielsen; ssolgaard@health.sdu.dk

Academic Editor: Lynette Mackenzie

Background. Worldwide obesity rates are increasing. The effectiveness of occupational therapy in overweight and obese adults has not yet been clarified. *Objectives.* The scoping review aimed at examining the evidence on interventions involving occupational therapists in the treatment of adults with overweight and obesity. *Methods.* Data on interventions involving occupational therapists and reporting on lifestyle-related outcomes in overweight and obese adults was extracted from the databases Cochrane, PubMed, CINAHL, and Embase, including hand and reference search. The scoping review methodology of Arksey and O'Malley was used. Conclusions were based on numerical and narrative analysis. *Results.* Thirteen articles reporting on eleven studies met the inclusion criteria. Several studies showed significant weight loss. However, the studies possessed high heterogeneity and showed insufficient explication of the role and contribution of occupational therapy to the outcomes. *Conclusions.* The interventions with involvement of occupational therapists were suggested to help short-term weight loss. Occupational therapists contributed to the outcomes with a holistic approach, educating on the role of activity, providing technological support, and promoting enjoyment of being active. There is a need for further documentation of the effectiveness, role, and contributions of occupational therapy in the treatment of overweight and obese adults in all settings.

1. Introduction

The prevalence of obesity has increased continuously since 1980 and has even doubled in more than 70 countries [1]. Obesity relates to numerous health issues, such as cardiovascular disease, several types of cancer, and diabetes mellitus [2]. Besides resulting in health problems, obesity can impede engagement in meaningful daily activities and lower one's opportunities in education, leisure time, and work [3–5].

Lifestyle interventions, dieting, pharmacology, and bariatric surgery have been named as the methods typically used today in the treatment of adults with overweight and obesity [6–9]. The evidence has recommended combining a calorie-reduced diet (with the energy deficit of at least 500 kcal/day) and physical activity increased to 30 min in most weekdays, as the first-line option in obesity treatment [6–8]. An intervention ought to include behavioral treatment as the third component facilitating adherence to diet and physical activity recommendations, to be called "a lifestyle intervention" [6].

There is strong evidence for intensive lifestyle interventions which vary up to 6 months, for clinically significant weight loss (5–10% of initial weight, approximately 8 kg) [6]. There is moderate evidence for lifestyle interventions in intermediate-term weight loss (weight reduction with another 8 kg during the next 6 months of intervention) [6]. Although lifestyle interventions of duration $\geq$ 1 year have been associated with weight regain, they have shown a higher effect on weight loss compared to standard care, e.g., advice [6]. The interventions of high-frequency contacts with health professionals ($\geq$14 contacts in total for the first 3 to 6 months) have achieved the best effect [6].

Single-component approaches have been found less effective than multicomponent approaches [6, 7]. The optimal duration of lifestyle interventions leading to clinically significant weight loss and optimal strategy for additional weight loss beyond the initial 6 months of intervention, as well as long-term approaches (2–5 years) to the maintenance of lost weight, are still to be clarified [6, 8, 10].

Researchers point at the need for all health professionals to be upskilled for effective management of the "obesity epidemic" [11, 12]. Occupational therapists possess key skills that help to promote health and to establish persistent lifestyle changes through participation in activities of choice, prevention of occupational deprivation, and increase in the perceived quality of life [3, 13]. However, the evidence of the effectiveness of occupational therapy in overweight and obese clients is scarce [14–17]. Several nonsystematic reviews have outlined the role, main target populations, domains, and strategies for occupational therapy addressing individuals with overweight and obesity [14, 17, 18]. Neither a systematic review nor a systematic investigation of the scope of occupational therapy interventions in the field has yet been conducted [14, 17, 18]. This study aimed at examining the evidence from studies evaluating the effectiveness of interventions involving occupational therapists in the treatment of adults with overweight and obesity.

2. Materials and Methods

2.1. Design. The current review followed Arksey and O'Malley's five steps of scoping review procedure with the advantage of methodological improvements done by Davis et al., Levac et al., Colquhoun et al., Tricco et al., and Peters et al. These are (1) defining the research question; (2) identifying relevant studies; (3) study selection and inclusion; (4) data charting; and (5) collating, summarising, and reporting of the results [19–25]. The 6th step of Arksey and O'Malley's scoping review procedure, consultation with stakeholders as a required knowledge translation component, will be reflected in Discussion. This study followed the principles of the Declaration of Helsinki [26].

2.2. Defining the Research Questions

(i) What characterizes the interventions involving occupational therapists identified in the current evidence?

(ii) Which significant improvements in lifestyle and health behavior were made by adults with overweight and obesity who participated in interventions involving occupational therapists?

The search strategy with inclusion and exclusion criteria was developed using the PCC model (population, concept, and context) [24]. The three-fold focus in the search strategy was related to the following: adults with overweight or obesity, interventions that involved occupational therapists, and intervention outcomes showing changes in lifestyle and health behavior.

2.3. Identifying Relevant Studies. A three-step literature search was performed from February to April 2017 (last search: 22 April 2017) to identify studies that reported outcomes of interventions for adults with overweight or obesity, where occupational therapists were involved. Firstly, an initial literature search was made in PubMed to identify relevant keywords, synonyms, word modifications, and thesaurus terms, according to the PCC criteria in this study [24]. Secondly, the database-specific searches were conducted in the databases PubMed, Embase, CINAHL, and the Cochrane library using block search strategy. The thesaurus terminology of each database and words, e.g., "occupational therapy", "occupational therapists", "obesity", "obese", "overweight", "bariatric", "lifestyle", "health behaviour", "habits", and "activities of daily living", as well as their terminological variations, were included. Truncations were used when relevant. No time restrictions were used. Thirdly, additional publications of relevance were searched manually in reference lists. Google Scholar and Bibliotek.dk were inspected using the terms "occupational therapy" and "obesity" and "occupational therapy" and "overweight". Unpublished items on interventions of interest were searched in ClinicalTrials.gov and WHO International Clinical Trials Registry Platform (ICTRP). Websites of organisations with expert knowledge in the field, the University of Southern California (USA), and Ergoterapeutforeningen (the Labour-Union for Occupational therapists in Denmark) were inspected. The second search was done in OTseeker on 22 April 2017. No further articles were found. The software reference program Endnote X8 was used to organise search results.

2.4. Study Selection and Inclusion. Selection of articles eligible for inclusion was guided by inclusion and exclusion criteria according to the research questions. The articles were selected in agreement with the authors. The inclusion criteria were as follows: (i) interventions in all settings addressing lifestyle in overweight or obese adults > 18 years; (ii) identified occupational therapists' involvement in the interventions; (iii) reported outcomes on the effectiveness of the interventions between participants before and after or between groups; and (iv) both articles published in peer-reviewed scientific journals and "grey literature," e.g., treatment reports, evaluations, and public presentations. The exclusion criteria were as follows: (i) parents to children with overweight or obesity problems; (ii) pregnant women; (iii) articles written in languages other than English, Danish, Swedish, Norwegian, or German; and (iv) expert opinions, editorials, commentaries, interviews, conference thesis, lectures, periodicals, or abstracts.

A selection form was developed to reduce the risk of selecting bias and support the iterative approach to the selection process [21] (Figure 1). The selection form assisted the decision-making process upon data screening. The articles that did not fit into the selection form were excluded. Both authors were involved in all parts of the review process. An agreement was achieved upon discussion between the authors.

Study__________

Reference____________

1. Is this an intervention study?
   Yes (go to the next step) Unclear (go to the next step) No (stop)
2. Were the participants at least 18yo?
   Yes (go to the next step) Unclear (go to the next step) No (stop)
3. Were the participants overweight and/or obese?
   Yes (go to the next step) Unclear (go to the next step) No (stop)
4. Were the participants pregnant?
   No (go to the next step) Unclear (go to the next step) Yes (stop)
5. Were occupational therapists involved in the intervention?
   Yes (go to the next step) Unclear (go to the next step) No (stop)
6. Was the study a primary study?
   Yes (go to the next step) Unclear (go to the next step) No (stop)
7. Was the study experimental or observational?
   Yes (go to the next step) Unclear (go to the next step) No (stop)
8. Did the study reported on treatment outcomes?
   Yes (go to the next step) Unclear (go to the next step) No (stop)
9. Was the study written in English, German, Danish, Norwegian or Swedish?
   Yes (include) No (stop)

FIGURE 1: Selection form.

2.5. Data Charting. The data charting form was developed and pilot-tested on a sample of three of the included articles in terms of further justifications. The final data charting form included information on the first author, year of publication, country of origin, publication source, study design, methods, sample size, the participants' age and gender, intervention's duration and content, comparator, and the role and contributions of occupational therapy to outcomes. Descriptive statistics on study results and effects at baseline, post intervention, and follow-up (when available) and p values were extracted and provided in the data extraction form.

2.6. Collating, Summarising, and Reporting the Results. Analysis of the extent, nature, and composition of the included studies was conducted. Infographics were applied to illustrate the results, supported by narrative comments. Nonnumerical findings were subject to qualitative thematic analysis. A tabular summary of the results across the reviewed studies was made in terms of mapping the evidence for answering the research question.

3. Results

The process for literature search, assessment, and selection is specified in the flowchart [27] (Figure 2). Initially, 582 records were sourced from the database search. Additional articles ($n = 69$) were found through reference lists ($n = 651$). After removing the duplicates ($n = 79$), the inclusion of the articles ($n = 572$) was made in two steps. All titles and abstracts were screened for relevance on the topic and excluded if they were not relevant for occupational therapy and obesity or overweight in the title, abstract, or keywords ($n = 418$). The remaining articles ($n = 154$) were inspected in full-text.

A total of 13 articles representing 11 studies describing interventions addressing adults with overweight and obesity, where occupational therapists were involved, were found eligible for this review.

The articles ($n = 4$) representing different phases of the same study ($n = 2$) were considered one study, in terms to avoid repetitive descriptions of the identical approach [28–31].

3.1. The Sample Characteristics. Three of the identified studies were RCT's [28–32], and three were quasiexperiments [33–35]. The rest ($n = 5$) were pre-/posttest studies of single cohorts [36–38] or single cases [39] or case groups [40] (Table 1).

Over the half of the included studies ($n = 6$) addressed individuals with mental problems (range 22–71 years old) [28, 29, 33–36, 39]. One study addressed diabetes patients (age range 37–87) [32] and another cancer patients (age range 42–79) [38]. Study samples of the participants who completed the interventions varied from 2 to 91 participants [28–31, 39, 40]. Many studies had high dropout rates 30–38% [28, 29, 32, 33, 37]. However, one study had only a few dropouts [30, 31], and another no dropout at all [35]. The interventions were composed of the following: 1-phase intervention ($n = 4$), 2-phase intervention ($n = 6$), and 3-phase intervention ($n = 1$) (Figure 3). Of the 2-phase intervention, two studies had an active maintenance phase that included ongoing treatment [30, 31, 35]. Thus, there were short-term (≤6 months of active treatment) ($n = 8$),

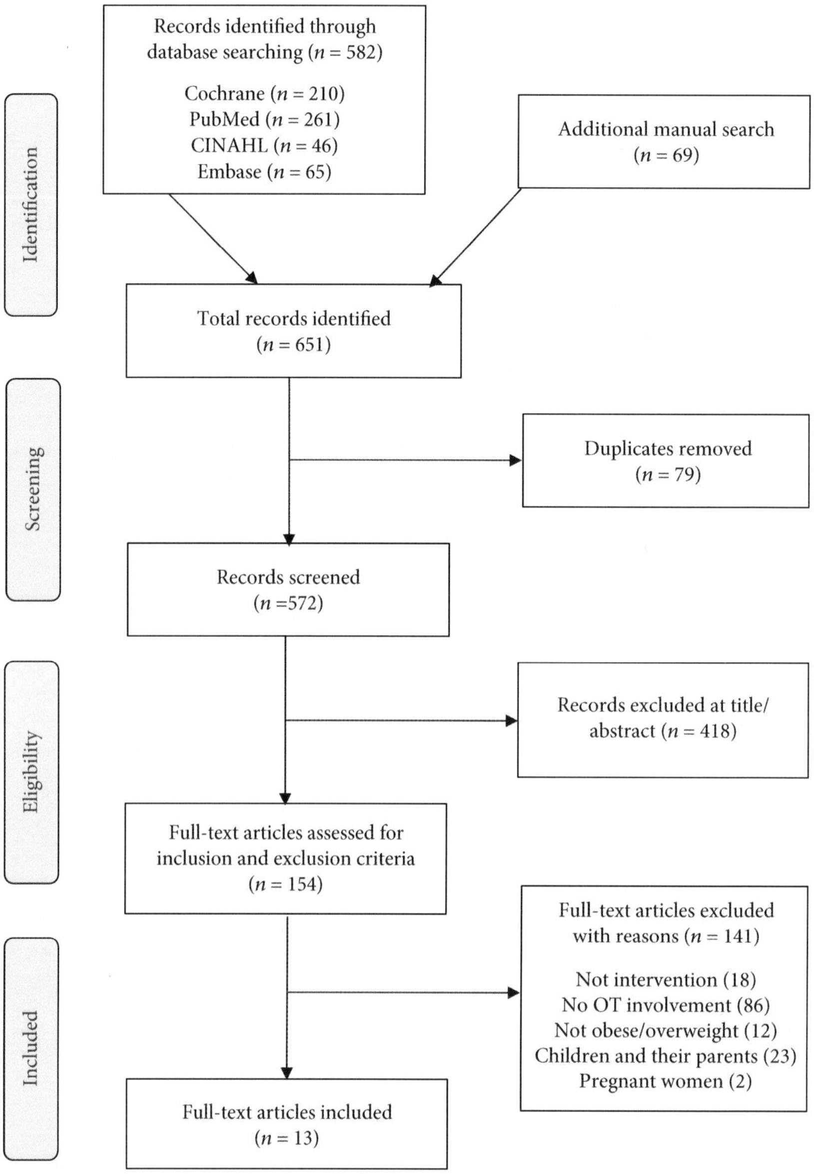

Figure 2: Flowchart, according to PRISMA [27].

intermediate-term (>6 months and ≤12 months of active treatment) ($n = 1$), and long-term weight loss interventions (>1 year of active treatment) ($n = 2$) in the sample [6].

The extent of occupational therapy involvement varied across the identified interventions. Two studies were solely occupational therapist-led [36, 39]. In another two studies, occupational therapists collaborated with other health professionals, either psychiatric nurses [34] or physical therapists [37]. The remaining studies ($n = 7$) were multidisciplinary interventions. The multidisciplinary profile in five studies included nurses, psychologists, dietitians, podiatrists, fitness instructors, sports scientists, or social workers [28–31, 33, 35, 38]. In two studies, the professionals involved, besides the occupational therapists, remained unspecified [32, 40]. The levels of transparency of occupational therapy engagement varied from reporting on the involvement of occupational therapists in several intervention processes, e.g., planning, execution, team supervision, and intervention management [28–31, 33–36, 38–40], to limited involvement, e.g., executing or team supervision only [32, 37].

Various attempts to promote the healthy lifestyle and health behavior changes in overweight and obese adults were described in the identified studies. Several studies from the sample did not declare any specific occupational therapy role and contribution. However, the studies operated with methods relevant to occupational therapy. Intervention components (as focus fields in an intervention) and intervention strategies (as methods of impact on the focus fields) across the studies were synthesized and differentiated according to the level of transparency in the declaration of the occupational therapy role and contribution (Table 2).

TABLE 1: Data extraction form.

Author (year), country [ref.], journal, purpose	Design, sample, age	Duration/ frequency	Intervention/controls	OT role and contribution to outcomes	Outcomes	Results at discharge	Results at follow-up
Rynne & McKenna (1999), Australia [38] The British Journal of OT (BJOT), The Royal College of Occupational Therapists (UK) To evaluate an outpatient diabetes education program	Cohort One group Pre–/posttest Adults with non-insulin-dependent diabetes mellitus ($n = 26$) Females: 27% Mean age 74 yo (range 37–87 yo)	3 mths in total 1 mnth/1 hr á wk 2 mths follow-up	IG (participants and their relatives/ friends) (groups at max. 10): information on the basic physiology of diabetes; management of hypoglycemia and sick days; medications and blood glucose testing; dietary management; weight control; role of PA; foot care; motivation; Diabetes Australia services	OT as part of multidisciplinary team Planning and executing, in line with a nurse, dietitian, psychologist, podiatrist and a representative of an NGO for diabetes Client-centered approach to the intervention; planning teaching-learning process; education on the role of activity and self-management of diabetes; training in managing weight control based on exercise recommendations from the national clinical guidelines (USA); supporting clients' self-management of lifestyle and adaptive behavior; systemic and holistic rehabilitation process; co-operation with community services	Diabetes knowledge	NS (unspec.)	NS (unspec.)
					Self-management behavior in diet	NS (unspec.)	NS (unspec.)
					Self-management behavior in exercise	($p < 0.001$)*	($p < 0.01$)*
					Perceptions of wellness	NS (unspec.)	NS (unspec.)
					BMI	NS (unspec.)	NS (unspec.)
					Metabolic control	NR	($p < 0.01$)*
Haber et al. (2000), USA [37] Family & Community Health journal, The Journal of Health Promotion and Maintenance (USA) To examine the impact of a health promotion program on the health behavior of older adults	Cohort One group Pre–/posttest Mixed-methods Older inactive, overweight and physically limited adults recruited from two sites IG included ($n = 42$) IG completed ($n = 35$) Mean age: 71 yo, range 64–89 yo Female 83%	9.75 mths in total 7 wks (=1.75 mths)/14 hr (1 hr twice a wk) Follow up: 8 mths post intervention	IG: 40 min PA; heart rate/PA intensity calculation; information on nutrition and stress management; 20 min group discussion on social, cognitive, and behavioral issues; social skills and environmental control training; realistic and measurable health goal setting; listing health benefits and motivational inspiration; self-affirmations; linking new health behavior with existing habits; homework assignments to increase PA time and healthy nutrition; phone calls between sessions	OT as part of OT/PT undergraduate team Executing, in co-operation with PT Active collaboration with clients; time administration; realistic and measurable health goals; supervised discussion in small groups; rethinking of existing habits, planning of new health behaviors, and environment control and modifications; adaptation of new exercise behavior; patient education and practice in progressive muscle relaxation; estimation of training intensity and heart-rate; individual diet calculation, in co-operation with dietitians; self-assessment on exercise and nutrition (additional fruit and vegetable consumption); information and experiential learning on stress management; using social support to motivation, listing health benefits and motivational inspiration, and repeating affirmations to oneself; improving memory function with social support	Brisk walk exercises	($p = 0.02$)*	NS (unspec.)
					Flexibility exercises	($p = 0.0001$)*	NS (unspec.)
					Strength exercises	($p = 0.01$)*	NS (unspec.)
					Association for health behavior change vs the following:		
					(i) Participants' educational level	NR	NS (unspec.)
					(ii) PT's involvement	NR	NS (unspec.)
					(iii) Participants' race	NR	NS (unspec.)
					Regular PA (min. of 3 t./wk at ≥20 min)	NR	NS (unspec.)
Voruganti et al. (2006) Canada [35] The Canadian Journal of Psychiatry (Canada) To assess the feasibility of clinical implementation and evaluate the effectiveness of a novel adventure- and recreation-based group intervention	Quasiexperiment Pilot, pre–/posttest Case–control Two groups Adults with schizophrenia IG ($n = 23$) CG ($n = 31$) Treatment adherence = 97%, no dropouts Mean ± SD age IG: 32 ± 7.5 yo Mean ± SD age CG: 41 ± 9.4 yo	20 mths in total 8 mths intervention (2 modules at 8 wks = 8 sessions) 12 mths of maintenance phase	IG: summer and winter modules with various outdoor activities. Participants encouraged to maintain weekly contacts with the treatment team between modules. CG: recruited from wait list, received standard clinical care included some recreational activities	OTs as part of multidisciplinary team Planning, executing, and supervising, in line with a nurse and a social worker No specific OT contributions declared OTs were involved in the multidisciplinary novel adventure-based intervention including outdoor activities for psychiatric rehabilitation			[Maintenance phase]
					Weight loss	NR	($p < 0.05$)*[a]
					Self-esteem	($p < 0.05$)*	($p < 0.05$)*
					Global functioning	($p < 0.05$)*	Marginally improved
					Self-appraised cognitive abilities	Marginally improved	NR

Table 1: Continued.

Author (year), country [ref.], journal, purpose	Design, sample, age	Duration/ frequency	Intervention/controls	OT role and contribution to outcomes	Outcomes	Results at discharge	Results at follow-up
Brown et al. (2006), USA [33] Psychiatric Rehabilitation Journal, the American Psychological Association (USA) To examine the efficacy of psychiatric rehabilitation weight loss program	Quasiexperiment Two groups Pre–/posttest, pilot Adults with serious mental illnesses, BMI ≥ 25 Recruited ($n = 59$) Completed ($n = 36$) Dropout IG ($n = 7$); CG ($n = 16$) Completed IG ($n = 21$); CG ($n = 15$) Female IG: 71% Female CG: 60% Mean age IG: 47 yo, range 30–61 yo Mean age CG: 41 yo (range 30–61 yo)	3 mths in total 2 hr/wk	IG: weight loss and psychiatric rehabilitation principles; diet, frequent contact with professionals, dietary education, 30–45 min moderate PA 3–5 days/wk, goal setting, social and instrumental support, skill and transfer training (dining out), granted materials (calorie counts, cooking utensils etc.) CG: no treatment	OTs as part of multidisciplinary team Planning and executing, in line with a dietician and exercise psychologist No specific OT contributions declared OTs were represented in the multidisciplinary program aimed to utilize the psychiatric rehabilitation principles and weight loss strategies	Between-group diff.: (i) Weight (ii) BMI (iii) Waist circumference (iv) Diastolic BP (v) Systolic BP (vi) Total lifestyle profile (vii) Lifestyle profile nutrition subscale (viii) Lifestyle profile PA subscale (ix) Energy intake In-group diff. (IG): (i) Total lifestyle profile (ii) Lifestyle profile nutrition subscale (iii) Lifestyle profile PA subscale (iv) Energy intake (v) Fat intake	 $(p = 0.009)^*$ $(p = 0.008)^*$ $(p = 0.021)^*$ $(p = 0.32)$ $(p = 0.23)$ $(p = 0.51)$ $(p = 0.35)$ $(p = 0.037)^*$ $(p = 0.45)$ $(p = 0.05)^*$ $(p = 0.023)^*$ $(p = 0.022)^*$ $(p = 0.045)^*$ $(p = 0.09)^*$	
Pendlebury et al. (2007), UK [34] International Journal of Neuropsychopharmacology (JNP), Oxford Academic (UK) To evaluate long-term changes in weight and patient attendance based on the outcomes from the first 4 years of a behavioral treatment program	Quasiexperiment Multiple treatment reversal designs, time-series, longitudinal Repeated pre–/posttest Adults with schizophrenia and affective disorder, on psychotropic medication, wishing to lose weight ($n = 93$) Total patient episodes ($n = 103$), incl. Reenrollments ($n = 10$) Females: 61% Age mean 43.7 ± 1.2 yo (range 22–71 yo)	4 years in total One session/wk	IG (open drop-in program): measuring weight; group discussion on dietary experiences; group discussion on 8 informal rotational topics (to solve any actual issues on weight loss)	OTs as part of multidisciplinary team Planning and executing, in line with a psychiatric nurse No specific OT contributions declared OTs were represented in the multimodal program that incorporated nutrition, exercise and behavioural intervention, providing a holistic lifestyle approach to weight loss	7% body weight and BMI change at 3–6–9 mths; 1–1, 5–2–3–4 y Normal BMI achieved Weight loss Weight loss correlation with young age Weight loss correlation with adherence to the program Weight loss correlation with diagnosis Weight loss correlation with mono- or multimedication	 23% [at the end of each patient episode] $(p = 0.031)^*$ $(p < 0.0001)^*$ $(p = 0.02)^*$ NR	 NR Sign. NR[b] NS (unspec.) NS (unspec.) NS (unspec.) $(p = 0.26)$
McClure et al. (2010) USA [32] The American Journal of OT (AJOT), The American OT Association (USA) To report a randomised controlled study of a program, designed to achieve improvements in physical and emotional breast cancer–related lymphedema (BCRL) symptoms.	RCT Two groups Individuals with BCRL, BMI ≥ 29.8 ($n = 32$) IG ($n = 16$) CG ($n = 16$) Dropout ($n = 11$) Mean ± SD age IG: 57.0 ± 2.9 yo (30.7; 78.0) Mean ± SD age CG: 59.7 ± 2.1 yo (42.2; 78.7) Female: 100%	17 wks/4.25 mths in total 5 sessions at 2 hr/5 wks/1.25 mths and a self-monitored home program (3 mths)	IG (The Breast Cancer Recovery Program): of The FLOW video (McClure & Bittman, 2003) and relaxation techniques at home daily; verbal instructions and written educational material on lymphedema coping and relaxation techniques (deep diaphragmatic breathing, progressive muscle relaxation and facial massage); a question-and-answer component and group discussion at every session CG: professional advice/usual practice	OTs as part of multidisciplinary team (team composition not declared) Supervising the assessors; guiding the assessment process Mood and quality of life monitoring	Bio-impedance z (arm swelling) Arm flexibility Volume Weight loss Quality of life in norm-based physical function Quality of life in general health Quality of life in vitality Mood	$(p = 0.049)^*$ $(p = 0.19)$ NS (unspec.) $(p = 0.038)^*$ $(p = 0.02)^*$ $(p = 0.03)^*$ $(p = 0.05)^*$ $(p = 0.03)^*$	NR $(p = 0.10)$ NS (unspec.) Maintained sign. (unspec.) NR NR NR $(p = 0.017)^*$
Jacobs et al. (2011), UK [40] British Journal of OT (BJOT), the Royal College of	Cohort Three groups Pre–/posttest	3 mths	IG 1: the solo Wii group ($n = 2$): individual Wii exercise, yoga, balance, and strength activities 4 t/wk, 30–	OTs as main interventionists Planning, executing Integral approach to PA, diet and	Weight: (i) IG1 (ii) IG2 & IG3	 $(r^2 = 0.53)^*$ NS (unspec.)	

Table 1: Continued.

Author (year), country [ref.], journal, purpose	Design, sample, age	Duration/ frequency	Intervention/controls	OT role and contribution to outcomes	Outcomes	Results at discharge	Results at follow-up
Occupational Therapists (UK) To investigate effect of Nintendo Wii Fit as an occupation to promote weight loss in students.	A-B design, explorative 1-year university students ($n = 5$) Dropout: 1 out of 6 Age> 18 yo Females: 100%		45 min IG 2: the double Wii group ($n = 2$): the same training as group 2, but with a partner IG 3: the typical activity group ($n = 1$): moderate intensity physical activity (e.g., walking to class)	activity participation; motivating for increase in PA; incorporating PA into daily routines; decreasing negative impact of obesity; promote participation in meaningful roles; using VR technology as a therapeutic tool for exercise; instructing in use of VR technology; encouraging to exercise with VR technology in leisure time	BMI: (i) IG1 (ii) IG2 & IG3 Motivation for PA: (i) IG1 (ii) IG2 & IG3 PA level: (i) IG1 (ii) IG2 & IG3	 ($r^2 = 0.78$)* NS (unspec.) NS, sugg. Improved NS (unspec.) NS, remained moderate NS (unspec.)	
Bacon et al. (2012), Australia [39] The British Journal of OT (BJOT), the Royal College of Occupational Therapists (UK) To evaluate the Nintendo Wii Fit use in changing engagement in PA	Pre-exp. explorative Single-case design Mixed methods Adults with mental illness ($n = 2$)	8 wks	IG: Wii Fit in individual or group sessions	OTs as main interventionists Planning, executing Providing access to meaningful PA PA participation on collaboration with the participants; positive role modelling; establishing positive activity behaviors and lifelong habits; instrumental support with VR technology for PA as part of the intervention and in leisure time; instruction in use of VR technology; making activity enjoyable	Total daily PA time Attitudes towards PA Use of Wii Fit	NS, increased More positive attitudes towards PA Increased PA, provided meaningful occupation and showed potential use of the technology	
Christensen et al. (2011), DK [30], and Christensen et al. (2012), DK [31] BMC Public Health (USA) To evaluate the effects of the first 3 mths and 12 mths of follow-up of a 1-year long lifestyle intervention aimed to achieve weight loss among health care workers	Cluster RCT To groups Single-blinded Overweight health care workers ($n = 98$) IG ($n = 55$) CG ($n = 44$) Females: 100% Divided into 7 groups Dropout phase 1 ($n = 7$) Dropout phase 2 ($n = 8$) Mean age 45.5 yo (range 36–55 yo)	12 mths in total 1 hr/wk during working time Two phases: weight loss-phase (3 mths), weight loss maintenance phase (9 mths)	IG: individually dietary plan with energy deficit of 1200 kcal/day (15 min/hr); strengthening exercises (15 min/hr) and CBT (30 min/hr); leisure time aerobic fitness: 2 hr/wk; additional reducing of energy intake; 15 min circuit training during the 6th–9th mth of intervention; local sport activities and jogging outdoor during the 9th–12th mth of intervention; motivation to use training log books for home exercises; composition of one's own diet; setting realistic easy-to-implement goals based on participants' preferences and perception of meaningfulness; coping with cravings and practicing the intervention principles in everyday life CG: monthly oral presentations at 2 hr during working time.	OTs as part of multidisciplinary team Planning/managing, executing, supervising No specific OT contributions declared OTs were represented in the multidisciplinary program that incorporated nutrition, exercise and behavioral intervention and applied to the clients' workplace and local environments	Body weight BMI Body fat percentage Waist circumference BP Musculoskeletal pain Maximal oxygen uptake Isometric maximal muscle strength of 3 body regions	($p < 0.001$)*[c] ($p < 0.001$)* ($p < 0.001$)* ($p < 0.001$)* ($p < 0.001$)* NS (unspec.) NS (unspec.) NS (unspec.)	[Maintenance phase] ($p < 0.001$)*[d] ($p < 0.001$)* ($p < 0.001$)* ($p < 0.001$)* ($p < 0.001$)* NS (unspec.) NS (unspec.) NS (unspec.)
Brown et al. (2011), USA [28], and Brown et al. (2014), USA [29] Psychiatric Services, the	RCT Two groups Adults with serious mental illness IG ($n = 47$)	12 mths in total Intervention: 3 mths (3 hr/wk) Maintenance: 3	IG (RENEW): energy intake reduction min. 500 kcal/day; education on nutrition; PA min. of 30 min/day; individualized goal setting; eating	OTs as part of multidisciplinary team Planning, executing, in line with a nurse, dietician and fitness instructor No specific OT contributions declared	Weight loss 5% (clinically sign.) at 3 mths Weight loss 10% (weight loss maintenance) at 6 mths	($p = .01$)*[e] ($p = .22$)[f]	NR NR

TABLE 1: Continued.

Author (year), country [ref.], journal, purpose	Design, sample, age	Duration/ frequency	Intervention/controls	OT role and contribution to outcomes	Outcomes	Results at discharge	Results at follow-up
American Psychiatric Association (USA)/ Schizophrenia Research, the Schizophrenia International Research Society (USA) To access RENEW (recovering energy through nutrition and exercise for weight loss) program in individuals with serious mental illness at four mental health centers	CG ($n = 42$) Enrolled ($n = 136$) Completed, at follow-up ($n = 89$) Females 61% Mean ± SD age 44.6 ± 10.9 yo	mths (3 hr/mth) Support: 6 mths	together; 2 meal replacements a day; weekly phone support in maintenance phase, no contact in support phase CG: usual treatment (medication, case management, voluntary participation in day programs); no restrictions from attending wellness elsewhere	OTs were represented in the multidisciplinary program that incorporated psychiatric rehabilitation principles and evidence-based weight loss strategies; providing education and practice in modifying nutrition and PA; incorporated social and instrumental support, goal setting, skills and transfer training, and cognitive compensation.	Weight regain at 12 months (follow up)		($p = .47$) [g]
					Differences by weight changes by site	At 3 vs 6 months: ($p = .017$) * vs ($p = .043$) *	At 12 months: ($p = .076$)
Brown et al. (2015), USA [36] Psychiatric Rehabilitation Journal, The American Psychological Association (USA) To evaluate the Nutrition and Exercise for Wellness and Recovery (NEW-R) weight loss intervention.	Cohort Pilot pre–/posttest One group Adults with severe mental illness ($n = 18$) and a BMI> 25 Dropout: 2 out of 18 Females 89% Age range 23–64 yo Mean ± SD age 47.3 ± 10.5 yo	6 mths in total Intervention: 2 mths (16 hr, 2 hr./wk) Follow-up: 4 mths	IG: Education; PA (20–30 min. Moderate intensity); healthy meals; provided printed materials (recipes and books with guidelines for eating out) and exercise bands	OTs as main interventionists Planning, executing Increasing PA participation (moderate); practicing healthy eating in groups; instrumental support to healthy eating (recipes and guidelines for eating out) and exercise (elastic bands); encouraging positive cognition; motivating for sustainable health behavior changes in long term; planning daily behaviors with impact on weight; focusing on active learning and small changes	An average weight loss	($p = 0.12$)[h]	($p = 0.03$)*[i]
					Increased knowledge about nutrition	($p = 0.05$)*	NR
					Increased PA	($p = 0.09$)	NR
					Association between attendance and body weight	NS (but tended towards significance)	NR

BP = blood pressure; CBT = cognitive behavioral therapy; CG = control group; hr = hour; diff. = difference; IG = intervention group; n = number analysed; mth/mths = month/months; NGO = nongovernment organisation; NR = p value not registered; NS = not significant; OT = occupational therapy; OTs = occupational therapists; PA = physical activity; PTs = physical therapists; RCT = randomized controlled trial; sign. = significant; sugg. = suggested; unspec. = unspecified; VR = virtual reality; wk/wks = week/weeks; yo = years old. * indicates statistically significant effect at 95% CI. [a,b,c,d,e,f,g,h,i] Mean weight loss in the intervention group: [a] −5.4 kg; [b] −6.2 kg; [c] −3.6 kg; [d] −5.8 kg; [e] −2.2 kg; [f] −1.9 kg; [g] −0.7 kg; [h] −1,4 kg; and [i] −4.3 kg.

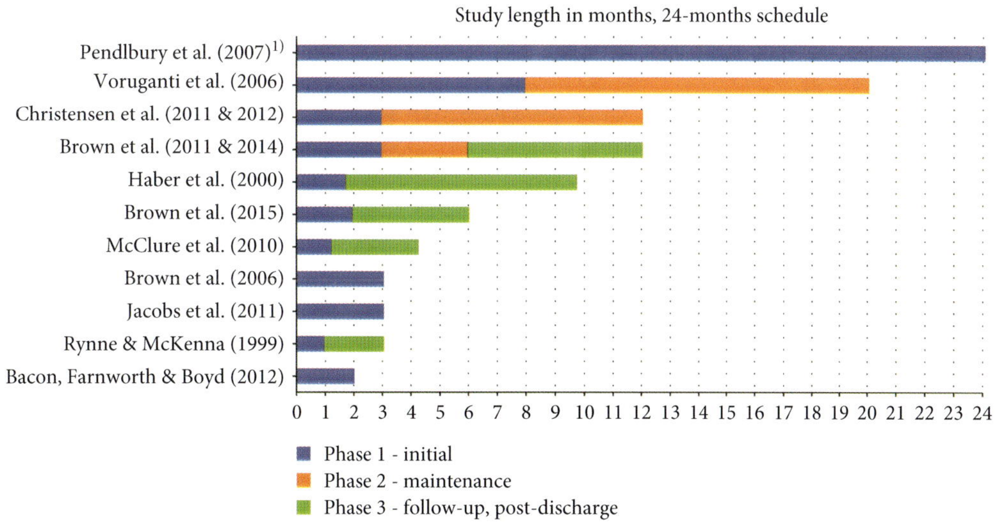

FIGURE 3: Interventions' phases and length.

Regarding the major components of lifestyle interventions in obesity treatment described in the international guidelines in treatment of overweight and obesity, one-component (physical activity, $n = 3$) [35, 39, 40], two-component (physical activity and cognitive techniques, $n = 1$) [32], and three-component (diet, physical activity and CBT-elements, $n = 7$) [28–31, 33, 34, 36–38] studies were represented in the included articles.

3.2. The Reported Outcomes. All the studies aimed at making an impact on body weight in populations with obesity and/or risk of metabolic complications. Six studies (55%) were directly addressing weight change, while the rest focused on change in overall health behavior ($n = 1$) [37], self-management of disease symptoms ($n = 2$) [32, 38], or sedentary lifestyle ($n = 2$) [35, 39]. Weight loss, body mass index (BMI), and waist circumference were the most commonly used outcomes across the sample (Table 3).

3.2.1. Weight Loss. Eight studies from the sample used weight loss to evaluate the intervention effect, and all found improvements [28–36, 40]. Significant body weight reductions were identified in short- [28–30, 32, 33, 36, 40], intermediate- [31], and long-term [34, 35]. The weight loss was most frequently achieved through a comprehensive approach combining physical activity, dieting and behavioral treatment [28–31, 33] compared to controls or in-group [36]. However, the combination of physical activity and behavioral treatment [32], as well as stand-alone physical activity or behavioral treatment [34, 35, 40], could also result in significant weight loss.

3.2.2. BMI. BMI was assessed in five of the included in this research studies [30, 31, 33, 34, 38, 40]. Three studies identified a significant effect on BMI at intervention discharge [30, 33, 40], and one at the end of the maintenance phase [31]. Thus, one RCT found significant effects on BMI in short-term and intermediate-term [30, 31]. However, mixed results in different subgroups [40] and no significant results on BMI [38] were also found.

3.2.3. Waist Circumference. A significant effect on waist circumference was experienced by the participants in two studies, one RCT and one quasiexperiment [30, 31, 33]. Waist circumference as an effect measure was chosen less frequently than changes in weight across the sample. The effects on waist circumference were maintained up to one year.

3.2.4. Other Outcomes. Most studies used multiple outcome measures, such as a combination of objective anthropometric, biochemical, and physical variables and self-reported psychosocial variables. Both significant and nonsignificant findings were represented.

4. Discussion

The current study aimed at examining the evidence from studies evaluating the effectiveness of interventions involving occupational therapists in the treatment of adults with overweight and obesity. The most reviewed interventions were composed as multicomponent and multidisciplinary, involved graduated health professionals, offered frequent client contacts, and used elevated daily physical activity combined with better nutrition control, as recommended by the evidence on managing lifestyle changes in overweight and obese adults [11–14]. However, only seven interventions would fully match the definition of "comprehensive lifestyle interventions" having three components—physical activity, dieting, and cognitive behavioral therapy (or its elements) [11]. The sample did not sufficiently match the clinical recommendations to intervention length and reduction of energy intake, while the daily range of physical activity planned was not apparent [6, 8, 9].

Table 2: Intervention components (a) and intervention strategies (b) presented in the included studies.

(a)

Intervention component categories	Intervention component modalities	Declared OT role in the sample [ref.]	The roles not specifically assigned to OT in the sample [ref.]
Physical activity (PA)	Interventionist-led	Promoting participation in moderate exercise [36]; assisting participation in exercise supported with VR technology [39, 40]	Promoting participation in PA [28, 29]; providing strengthening exercises at workplace, graduating PA progression [30, 31]; practicing PA in groups [33]; inclusion of feasible, available, assessable, affordable, and likely effective outdoor activities that are time-limited and suitable for evaluation, replication, and implementation into mental health services [35]
	In leisure time/self-managed	Providing access to exercise, e.g., with elastic bands [36] and VR technology [39, 40]; encouraging behavior changes by self-assessment of PA [37]	Encouraging continued strengthening exercises and initiating aerobic exercises at home [30, 31]
Relaxation techniques	Interventionist-led	Practicing progressive muscle relaxation [37]	Use of relaxation techniques [32]
	In leisure time		Encouraging home relaxation practice [32]
Nutrition	Dieting	Encouraging behavior changes by self-assessment of additional fruit and vegetable consumption [37]	Encouraging calorie reduction [28, 29]; composing individual dietary plan based on the Danish dietary recommendations, dietary records, and identification of dietary preferences, using evidence-based guidelines for calorie reductions [30, 31]; using recommendations from the clinical guidelines in treatment of overweight and obesity in adults (USA) and encouraging proper fluid intake [33]
	Meal replacement and meal preparation		In combination with identification of food preferences and ideas to preparation of favorite foods in a healthy way, moving from meal replacement to purchasing food at the grocery store [28, 29]; teaching to move from meal replacements to purchasing food at the grocery store, improving food purchasing habits and meal preparation techniques minimizing the need for extensive menu planning and cooking [33]
	Social eating	Providing healthy meal experience as part of group sessions [36]	Providing experiences in eating together [28, 29] and dining out [33]
Cognitive techniques	CBT elements	Encouraging positive cognition [36]	Using CBT elements in promoting health behavior changes at workplace, encouraging positive thinking [30, 31]
	Coping		Reflecting dysfunctional attitudes and coping behaviors [30, 31]; instructing in coping techniques [32]
	Memory support	Guidance in improving memory function with social support [37]	Teaching compensatory strategies for cognitive impairments [28, 29], i.e., as part of psychiatric rehabilitation strategies [33]
	Motivational support	Guidance in using social support to motivation, listing health benefits and motivational inspiration, repeating affirmations to oneself, and environment modifications [37]; making activity enjoyable [39]; positive role modelling [39]	Using simplification of material, active learning, repetition, flexible methods of presenting information, visual aids and reinforces [33]; improvement of motivation, self-esteem, and sense of belonging [35]
Disease-specific topics		Mood and quality of life monitoring in postsurgical breast cancer survivors [32]	Diabetes management in relation to hypoglycemia, sick days, medication, blood glucose testing, foot care, and psychological issues [38]

(b)

Intervention strategies	Intervention strategy modalities	Declared OT role in the sample [ref.]	The roles not specifically assigned to OT in the sample [ref.]
Assessment		Supervising the assessors and guiding the assessment process [32]	
Education	On nutrition		Instructing in nutrition [28, 29]; teaching the importance of regular eating [34]; teaching identification of energy values, use of food labels, food composition, and appropriate portion sizes, with focus on experiential learning [33]
	On exercise	Providing exercise recommendations based on clinical guidelines (USA) within a multidisciplinary intervention [38]	Recommending moderate PA 3–5 times a week [33]
	On the role of activity	Education on the role of activity [38]	Teaching the importance of daily activity scheduling [34]
	On disease		Teaching self-management of diabetes [38]
	On stress management	Providing information and experiential learning on stress management [37]	
	Unspecified	Having focus on active learning [36]	Providing information on various rotational topics in relation to healthy lifestyle [34]
Individual goal setting		Promoting individual choice and assistance in setting daily and weekly goals [36]; helping in setting realistic and measurable goals [37]	Help in setting individualized goals [28, 29, 33], i.e., individual weight loss goals [30, 31]
Group discussion	Interventionist-led	Providing supervised discussion in small groups [37]	Building up team spirit to prevent dropout [30, 31]; promoting of sharing experiences, question-and-answer approach for providing modified learning opportunities for an individual [32]; providing social support through group interaction [33]; encouraging patients to help each other through voluntary experience exchange [34]
Phone call support		Providing encouragement and support to health behavior changes [37]	Weekly phone calls during maintenance phase aimed problem solving and goal setting, monthly phone calls in follow-up phase to promote sustainability [28, 29]
Instrumental support	Printed/written materials	Supporting behavioral changes with recipes and guidelines for eating out [36]	Providing disease-related printed materials [32]; weekly newsletter in maintenance phase monthly mails in follow-up phase with tips and reminders encouraging healthy lifestyle [28, 29]; promoting calorie count guides [33]
	Video guiding		Video guide for self-monitoring of disease-related health issues in breast cancer survivors [32]
	Exercise tools	Promoting accessibility to exercise through providing elastic bands [36]; supporting exercise with VR technology [39, 40]	Providing training tools, e.g., pedometers, weights, stretch bands, heart rate monitors, and workout videotapes [33]
	Cooking utensils		Providing cooking utensils to promote proper nutrition [33]
	Unspecified		Instrumental support given/unclear [28, 29]
Skill training	Weight control	Training in managing weight control [38]	
	Exercise self-management	Teaching to estimate own training intensity and heart-rate [37]	
	Relaxation techniques	Teaching progressive muscle relaxation [37]	Instruction in relaxation techniques [32]
	One's own diet composition	Co-operating with dietitians in helping clients to calculate an individual diet [37]	
	Use of technology	Instructing in use of VR technology in exercise [39, 40]	
	Self-control for sustainable health behavior changes	Planning daily behaviors that can impact weight with focus on small changes [36]; inspiration for rethinking of existing habits, planning of new health behaviors and environment control [37]	Focusing on transferring behavioral changes into habit patterns in maintenance phase, identifying small successes and issues in daily living [28, 29]; Using a fast food guide on a dining out session [33]
	Social skills		Improvement of social skills [35]

TABLE 2: Continued.

Intervention strategies	Intervention strategy modalities	Declared OT role in the sample [ref.]	The roles not specifically assigned to OT in the sample [ref.]
Homework assignments	On exercises	Encouraging behavior changes by self-assessment [37]	Encouraging positive thinking with homework between sessions [30, 31]; daily PA log [33]
	On nutrition	Encouraging behavior changes by self-assessment [37]	Nutrition log [33]
Community involvement	Patient organisation	Promoting co-operation with community services [38]	Co-operating with a community support program to provide support between group sessions [33]
	Family and friends	Prompting systemic and holistic rehabilitation process [38]	
	Local sport and leisure facilities		Encouraging using local sport facilities to increase daily PA [30, 31]; planning and promoting participation in adventure outdoors activities [35]

BP = blood pressure; CBT = cognitive behavioral therapy; OT = occupational therapy; PA = physical activity.

4.1. Treatment Effects

4.1.1. Weight Loss. Comprehensive lifestyle interventions having an impact on physical activity, diet, and behavior are recognized in other evidence as the most effective treatment aimed at weight loss in overweight and obese adults [6]. Overall evidence found three-component lifestyle interventions resulting in significant weight loss at the average follow-up of three years, with an average weight reduction of −2.2 kg [41]. Dieting in combination with physical activity brought better results in weight loss than physical activity alone [42, 43].

The current research found no significant improvement in weight from education as the only intervention form, which partly supports the importance of the comprehensive approach [38]. However, a number of interventions from the sample showing significant improvements in weight were not comprehensive per definition, as they had no dietary component included. The only intervention from the sample comparable in its duration (min. of 3 years) with the other evidence showed weight reduction above the average for lifestyle interventions in general [34].

The long-term (>1 year) effect on weight loss was found in two one-component interventions from the sample [34, 35]. They both had a high level of user-involvement and flexibility in planning, according to the participants' actual needs. We believe that the core principles of occupational therapy, such as client-centeredness and promotion of active participation, as well as the setting of realistic goals and using of meaningful occupations, might be the factors that allowed significant weight loss, despite less comprehensive intervention composition. As the two studies were both based on long-term contacts with occupational therapists and their collaborators, the results also supported the positive impact on weight loss of prolonged and frequent contacts with educated healthcare professionals [6, 7].

Only three interventions operated with the clinically significant weight loss measure (≥5% of the initial body weight) [28, 29, 34, 36]. Clinically significant weight loss was considered moderate and realistic to achieve, as well as being an important indicator for the satisfactory level of weight loss concerning human metabolic function and ability to prevent diabetes and hypertension [6, 7, 9]. Being aware of that would prevent unrealistic goals and underpin the favourable effects of weight loss starting with low weight loss levels [44]. Many other health science studies assessed clinically significant weight loss, and the parameter became an inclusion criterion for a systematic review on the topic [42].

The little focus on clinically significant weight loss in the identified interventions could be the consequence of the paucity in quantitative research on the topic, particularly RCTs, in the field of occupational therapy. We suppose that attention to clinically significant weight loss in occupational therapy interventions will become more common, as soon as further investigations of strong methodology emerge in the field, urging higher comparability of the results.

4.1.2. Weight Regain. One study from the sample (an RCT with active treatment period = 6 months) showed nonsignificant weight regain in the intervention group at follow-up (12 months post recruitment/6 months post intervention) [29]. On the other hand, three interventions with active treatment duration ≥ 1 year were effective in the maintenance of the initial weight loss at the final assessment [30, 31, 34, 35]. The current research showed that sufficient weight maintenance can be achieved by 1-year continuous treatment, inclusive maintenance phase [30, 31].

Lifestyle interventions longer than 1 year were associated with weight regain [6]. Weight maintenance phases were recommended not to be ended earlier than ≥1 year from baseline [42]. However, maintenance phase duration > 1 year was not associated with a better effect on maintenance of the initial weight loss and its percentage [42]. Weight regain to preintervention level at 5 years post intervention was considered common for weight loss interventions and independent of BMI or metabolic status [7]. Weight regain could though be prevented by adapting individual weight maintenance strategies including continued healthy eating, high-level physical activity on regular basis, continued contacts with healthcare professionals (in any format), self-monitoring of body weight (e.g. once a week), and environmental support [7]. Additionally, maintenance of lost weight was found to require another approach, different from that for the initial weight loss [45].

Table 3: Summary of the reported outcomes.

Outcomes reported		Significant at discharge, studies (n)	Significant at follow-up, studies (n)	Nonsignificant at discharge, studies (n)	Nonsignificant at follow-up, studies (n)
Anthropometrics	Weight loss	6	4	3	1
	Weight regain	—	—	—	1
	BMI	3	1	3	1
	Body fat percentage	1	1	—	—
	Waist circumference	2	1	—	—
Biochemical and physical	Blood pressure	1	1	1	—
	Metabolic control measure	—	1	—	—
	Max oxygen uptake	—	—	1	1
	Isometric max muscle strength	—	—	1	1
	Flexibility, arm	—	—	1	1
	Bio-impedance z (arm swelling)	1	—	—	—
	Increased physical activity (alone or in small, or bigger groups)	—	—	3	1
	Brisk walk	1	—	—	1
	Flexibility	1	—	—	1
	Strength	1	—	—	1
	Lifestyle profile, physical activity subscale (between groups)	1	—	—	—
	Lifestyle profile, physical activity subscale (in-group)	1	—	—	—
	Lifestyle profile, nutrition subscale (in-group)	1	—	—	—
	Lifestyle profile, nutrition subscale (between groups)	—	—	1	—
	Musculoskeletal pain	—	—	1	1
Psychosocial	Global functioning	1	—	—	1
	Quality of life, in norm-based physical function	1	—	—	—
	Quality of life, in general health	1	—	—	—
	Quality of life, in vitality	1	—	—	—
	Mood	1	1	—	—
	Motivation	—	—	1	—
	Self-esteem	1	1	—	—
	Perception of wellness	—	—	1	1
	Self-management behavior in exercise	1	1	—	—
	Attitudes towards exercise	—	—	1	—
	Increased knowledge about nutrition	1	—	—	—
	Energy intake (in-group)	1	—	—	—
	Energy intake (between groups)	—	—	1	—
	Fat intake (in-group)	1	—	—	—
	Self-management behavior in diet	—	—	1	1
	Diabetes knowledge	—	—	1	1
	Differences by weight changes by site	1	—	—	1

Not identified outcome reports are marked with "—."

While our findings supported the evidence, no interventions from the sample assessed the effect at 5 years post intervention. However, the two studies with the longest treatment durations (20–48 months) proved to achieve sufficient weight maintenance at the final assessment showing occupational therapy potentially capable of weight maintenance up to 4 years of treatment [34, 35]. The interventions were mainly based on either behavioral treatment or recreational outdoor physical activities.

From the above-named treatment elements important for weight maintenance, the two studies had their regularity, continued contact with occupational therapists, and environmental support (during the treatment sessions) in common. The presence of the other elements seemed more uncertain. Prolonged contacts with occupational therapists and supportive in-treatment environments might build up the sense of belonging through occupation in the participants and thus support weight maintenance after the initial weight loss. The positive correlation between belonging and well-being was found previously [46].

4.1.3. BMI. BMI is a commonly used and recommended variable in weight loss interventions [6, 7]. However, the variable requires attention to possible assessment issues [7]. BMI may vary in different populations, because of differences in body fat and lean mass ratio depending on age, sex, race or nationality, or occupation, e.g., in athletes [47–49]. Other methods, e.g., measuring waist circumference, can be recommended to support BMI assessments in estimating the overweight and obesity burden on health [6].

4.1.4. Waist Circumference. Similar to the sample studies, measuring of waist circumference was rather rare in other lifestyle interventions for adults with overweight and obesity [41]. However, lifestyle interventions may significantly reduce waist circumference compared to standard care, as well as maintain the effect for up to three years [41]. It is not known yet, whether the reported effects on waist circumference will sustain beyond one year of active treatment. Further investigations with at least three years of follow-up will also improve the comparability of occupational therapy results with other evidence on the reduction of waist circumference.

4.2. Occupational Therapy Role and Contribution to the Outcomes. As seen in the previous evidence, the identified interventions involving occupational therapists belonged to the secondary and tertiary health promotions, i.e., addressing adults in the risk of impairments or with present diagnoses [17, 50]. However, this review showed that the involvement of occupational therapists may also be relevant in primary health promotion of overweight and obesity, e.g., among healthcare workers and university students. As seen in the included interventions, occupational therapists appeared competent in the planning and execution of weight loss interventions, whether of mono- or multidisciplinary study setup. However, monodisciplinary occupational therapy interventions gave more space for an explication of the occupational therapy role and contributions to positive outcomes. However, we believe that multidisciplinary interventions involving occupational therapists offered a more specialized impact on lifestyle in overweight and obese adults as recommended in the international clinical recommendations. The occupational therapy impact declared in the included interventions did not include either education on nutrition and diabetes nor meal replacement. Since the topics on nutrition and disease may require specialized knowledge and skills, we found it appropriate that occupational therapists co-operated with dietitians, nurses, etc. in these fields. The multimodal and multidisciplinary approach to overweight and obesity has its advantages and is supported by evidence [51]. Thus, occupational therapy will consequently face the demand on an explication of its role, especially in multidisciplinary approaches.

We experienced that the current occupational therapy involvement was not comprehensively explicated and transparent in the reviewed interventions. The occupational therapy role and approach to treatment were reflected in a few articles from the sample. At the same time, the intervention components and strategies described in the articles with less transparency of occupational therapy involvement were close to those with clearly declared occupational therapy involvement, independently of mono- or multidisciplinary intervention character. Both types of interventions named above had similar components, e.g., physical activity practice, nutrition adjustments, relaxation techniques, cognitive techniques, and disease-specific elements. Both used collaborating with clients, education, setting individual goals, delivering instrumental, and social support, promoting active learning and sharing experiences, and supporting skill transfer to everyday life. However, education on the role of activity, focus on enjoyment from being active, and holistic approach to rehabilitation involving family and friends were only mentioned in the articles that delivered more comprehensive descriptions of occupational therapy contribution. Those qualities may be highlighted as the professional occupational therapy contribution in the interventions for overweight and obese adults. Additionally, occupational therapists contributed to the outcomes with a more rigorous use of VR (virtual reality) technology for exercise. Surprisingly, meal preparation and coping were only mentioned in the articles with no reports on a defined occupational therapy role. Meal preparation as a therapeutic tool would often be considered by occupational therapists in treatment planning [52]. Coping strategies, e.g., strengthening self-efficacy in an individual, would rather be in the occupational therapy scope as well [53]. We suppose that some core parts of the occupational therapy scope were lacking in this review due to the rather small sample size.

On the basis of the identified intervention components and strategies, all the reviewed studies could to a certain extent be linked to the previously outlined occupational therapy focus domains (e.g., "health promotion and prevention, increasing physical activity participation, modifying dietary intake, and reducing the impact of obesity") and strategies (e.g., "assessment, modifying the environment, education, and introducing and adapting occupations") [17]. All the interventions were promoting participation in adapted activities for weight loss to improve health and well-being and prevent disability [18]. However, the levels of adaptation and voluntary choice, as well as the scope of activities used within the interventions, varied across the sample. The fact of occupational therapists' involvement in the included studies contrasted with a poor specification of occupational therapy impact in the intervention descriptions. On the other hand, the similarities in the intervention components and strategies declared across the sample, including few monodisciplinary occupational therapy interventions, allowed us to suppose that occupational therapy impact in vivo might be greater than it was possible to detect in the current review.

The identified interventions link to occupational therapy also due to their focus on implementing of the new healthy lifestyle and sustainable changes in everyday practice related to physical activity, nutrition, and cognition, rather than only on weight-related outcomes. The evidence has described the occupational therapy role in lifestyle approaches as the mediator between some new wanted and needed healthy behaviors and an individual's habitual conditions [18]. Changing lifestyle and health behavior demands improvements in occupational performance through a holistic approach, which cannot be reduced solely to better physical fitness in an individual [54]. Thus, occupational therapy interventions may operate with a broader understanding of lifestyle, not limited to the presence of the three components (physical activity, nutrition, and cognitive treatment) mentioned in clinical recommendations to overweight and obesity treatment. We believe that every true occupational therapy intervention would potentially be "a lifestyle intervention" due to its focus on the whole person, knowledge transfer, and skills' adaptation into real life. Consultations with stakeholders, such as former and potential study participants, occupational therapy practitioners, other healthcare professionals from the multidisciplinary intervention teams, and researchers in the field of overweight and obesity may prove our assumptions and deepen the definition of the role and the impact of the OT in this area.

Occupational therapy contributed to the outcomes in the reviewed interventions with a holistic approach, sharing knowledge on the role of activity in people's life, supporting the new exercise routines with technology and encouraging enjoyment from being active. Further explication of the occupational therapy role and contribution in overweight and obesity treatment would deepen the understanding of occupational therapy potential in the field and let occupational therapists be involved in the future interventions for overweight and obese individuals at all levels of health promotion. For example, the use of assessment tools and indicators for changes in lifestyle and health behavior that are relevant for occupational therapy would open the door for more comprehensive descriptions of occupational therapy impact in future overweight and obesity interventions involving occupational therapists. We hope that the current review will inspire occupational therapy researchers to improve the quality and transparency of the evidence on the topic.

4.3. Study Limitations. Limitation of the methodological approach in this study is that scoping reviews provide an in-breadth overview on the topic, and not in-depth. This scoping review was not aimed to map all the literature on occupational therapy in the field of overweight and obesity but only focused on experimental studies from selected databases and with the identifiable involvement of occupational therapists. The selection strategy included keywords assigned by authors and may cause some of the relevant studies to be missing. Both primary and secondary articles usually are in focus of scoping reviews [55]. This review differentiated between these two categories, referring to the secondary evidence in the background and discussion sections of this study. Only primary publications were subject to analysis. Therefore, the scope of interventions addressing individuals with overweight and obesity and involving occupational therapists may be not accurately reflected in this scoping review.

5. Conclusion

The current review suggested that the interventions involving occupational therapists may help overweight and obese adults to achieve a significant change in weight loss in the short-term. Additional studies are still needed to confirm the suggestion. Whether occupational therapy can help the achievement of clinical significant intermediate- and long-term weight loss is still to be investigated.

This study found a little improvement in the evidence quality since Haracz et al. underscored insufficiency of the evidence in this field of research in 2013–14. A few randomized controlled blinded trials were identified in this study, which was indicating ongoing development in this area of practice and research. The review showed occupational therapists being competent actors in different parts of the intervention process in both the mono- and multidisciplinary overweight and obesity interventions. We found that occupational therapists contributed to the intervention outcomes with a holistic approach, providing knowledge on the role of activity in humans, supporting changes in health behavior with technology and promoting the enjoyment from being active.

We recommend the initiation of further comprehensive lifestyle interventions, e.g., randomized clinical trials, with the involvement of occupational therapists in the treatment of overweight and obese adults in all settings. The international clinical recommendations in the field, the OT-relevant assessment methods, and long-term follow-up phases ought to be considered for inclusion in the future interventions. Further evaluations of the effectiveness of the overweight and obesity interventions for adults involving occupational therapists together with a more comprehensive explication of the OT role and contributions to the intervention outcomes will improve the current evidence in this area.

Disclosure

The authors are responsible for the content and writing of this paper.

References

[1] GBD 2015 Obesity Collaborators, A. Afshin, M. H. Forouzanfar et al., "Health effects of overweight and obesity in 195 countries over 25 years," *The New England journal of medicine*, vol. 377, no. 1, pp. 13–27, 2017.

[2] World Health Organization, "Obesity and overweight, fact sheet," January 2017, http://www.who.int/mediacentre/factsheets/fs311/en/.

[3] F. Clark, F. S. Reingold, and K. Salles-Jordan, "Obesity and occupational therapy (position paper)," *The American Journal of Occupational Therapy*, vol. 61, no. 6, pp. 701–703, 2007.

[4] P. M. Ilvig and J. R. Christensen, "Degree of disability among female healthcare workers who are overweight or obese," *Cogent Medicine*, vol. 4, no. 1, article 1282032, 2017.

[5] S. S. Wang, K. D. Brownell, and T. A. Wadden, "The influence of the stigma of obesity on overweight individuals," *International journal of obesity and related metabolic disorders*, vol. 28, no. 10, pp. 1333–1337, 2004.

[6] National Health, Lung, and Blood Institute, *Managing overweight and obesity in adults: Systematic evidence review from the Obesity expert panel. Evidence report*, National Health, Lung, and Blood Institute (NHLBI), U. S. Department of Health and Human Services (USDoHaH), National Institutes of Health (NIH), 2013, November 2013, https://www.nhlbi.nih.gov/sites/default/files/media/docs/obesity-evidence-review.pdf.

[7] National Health and Medical Research Council, *Clinical Practice Guidelines for the Management of Overweight and Obesity in Adults, Adolescents and Children in Australia*, National Health and Medical Research Council, Melbourne, 2013, January 2017, https://www.nhmrc.gov.au/_files_nhmrc/publications/attachments/n57_obesity_guidelines_140630.pdf.

[8] D. C. Lau, J. D. Douketis, K. M. Morrison et al., "2006 Canadian clinical practice guidelines on the management and prevention of obesity in adults and children [summary]," *CMAJ*, vol. 176, no. 8, pp. S1–13, 2007.

[9] V. Yumuk, C. Tsigos, M. Fried et al., "European guidelines for obesity management in adults," *Obesity Facts*, vol. 8, no. 6, pp. 402–424, 2015.

[10] The Danish Health Authority, *Overweight – The Prevention Pack*, The Danish Health Authority, Copenhagen, 2018, https://www.sst.dk/da/udgivelser/2018/~/media/92E34F6D5D94489F803C677FE757C3C2.ashx.

[11] W. P. James, "WHO recognition of the global obesity epidemic," *International Journal of Obesity*, vol. 32, no. S7, pp. S120–S126, 2008.

[12] J. Lang, C. James, S. Ashby et al., "The provision of weight management advice: an investigation into occupational therapy practice," *Australian Occupational Therapy Journal*, vol. 60, no. 6, pp. 387–394, 2013.

[13] M. Forhan, "Obesity and healthy occupations," in *Discussion Document*, Professional issue forum, CAOT, Whitehorse, Yukon, 2008.

[14] M. Forhan and S. Gill, "Cross-border contributions to obesity research and interventions: a review of Canadian and American occupational therapy contributions," *Occupational Therapy In Health Care*, vol. 27, no. 2, pp. 129–141, 2013.

[15] M. Forhan, "Weight loss interventions for rehabilitation patients with obesity," *Current obesity reports*, vol. 3, no. 3, pp. 330–335, 2014.

[16] J. Heslop, "A critical review into the role of occupational therapy in promoting the quality of life for people with bariatric needs," *British Journal of Occupational Therapy*, vol. 72, no. 4, p. 173, 2009.

[17] K. Haracz, S. Ryan, M. Hazelton, and C. James, "Occupational therapy and obesity: an integrative literature review," *Australian Occupational Therapy Journal*, vol. 60, no. 5, pp. 356–365, 2013.

[18] F. S. Reingold and K. Jordan, "Obesity and occupational therapy," *The American Journal of Occupational Therapy*, vol. 67, pp. S39–S46, 2013.

[19] H. Arksey and L. O'Malley, "Scoping studies: towards a methodological framework," *International journal of social research methodology*, vol. 8, no. 1, pp. 19–32, 2005.

[20] K. Davis, N. Drey, and D. Gould, "What are scoping studies? A review of the nursing literature," *International journal of nursing studies*, vol. 46, no. 10, pp. 1386–1400, 2009.

[21] D. Levac, H. Colquhoun, and K. K. O'Brien, "Scoping studies: advancing the methodology," *Implementation Science*, vol. 5, no. 1, p. 69, 2010.

[22] H. L. Colquhoun, D. Levac, K. K. O'Brien et al., "Scoping reviews: time for clarity in definition, methods, and reporting," *Journal of Clinical Epidemiology*, vol. 67, no. 12, pp. 1291–1294, 2014.

[23] A. C. Tricco, E. Lillie, W. Zarin et al., "A scoping review on the conduct and reporting of scoping reviews," *BMC Medical Research Methodology*, vol. 16, no. 1, p. 15, 2016.

[24] M. D. Peters, C. M. Godfrey, H. Khalil, P. McInerney, D. Parker, and C. B. Soares, "Guidance for conducting systematic scoping reviews," *International journal of evidence-based healthcare*, vol. 13, no. 3, pp. 141–146, 2015.

[25] H. Khalil, M. Peters, C. M. Godfrey, P. McInerney, C. B. Soares, and D. Parker, "An evidence-based approach to scoping reviews," *Worldviews on evidence-based nursing.*, vol. 13, no. 2, pp. 118–123, 2016.

[26] World Medical Association, "Declaration of Helsinki: ethical principles for medical research involving human subjects," *JAMA*, vol. 310, no. 20, pp. 2191–2194, 2013.

[27] D. Moher, A. Liberati, J. Tetzlaff, D. G. Altman, and The PRISMA Group, "Preferred reporting items for systematic reviews and meta-analyses: The PRISMA Statement," *PLoS medicine*, vol. 6, no. 7, article e1000097, 2009.

[28] C. Brown, J. Goetz, and E. Hamera, "Weight loss intervention for people with serious mental illness: a randomized controlled trial of the RENEW program," *Psychiatric services*, vol. 62, no. 7, pp. 800–802, 2011.

[29] C. Brown, J. Goetz, E. Hamera, and B. Gajewski, "Treatment response to the RENEW weight loss intervention in schizophrenia: impact of intervention setting," *Scizophrenia Research*, vol. 159, no. 2-3, pp. 421–425, 2014.

[30] J. Christensen, A. Faber, D. Ekner, K. Overgaard, A. Holtermann, and K. Søgaard, "Diet, physical exercise and cognitive behavioral training as a combined workplace based intervention to reduce body weight and increase physical capacity in health care workers - a randomized controlled trial," *BMC Public Health*, vol. 11, no. 1, p. 671, 2011.

[31] J. R. Christensen, K. Overgaard, I. G. Carneiro, A. Holtermann, and K. Søgaard, "Weight loss among female health care workers - a 1-year workplace based randomized controlled trial in the FINALE-health study," *BMC Public Health*, vol. 12, no. 1, p. 625, 2012.

[32] M. K. McClure, R. J. McClure, R. Day, and A. M. Brufsky, "Randomized controlled trial of the breast cancer recovery program for women with breast cancer-related lymphedema," *The American Journal of Occupational Therapy*, vol. 64, no. 1, pp. 59–72, 2010.

[33] C. Brown, J. Goetz, A. Van Sciver, D. Sullivan, and E. Hamera, "A psychiatric rehabilitation approach to weight loss," *Psychiatric Rehabilitation Journal*, vol. 29, no. 4, pp. 267–273, 2006.

[34] J. Pendlebury, R. Holt, H. Wildgust, and R. I. G. Holt, "Long-term maintenance of weight loss in patients with severe mental illness through a behavioural treatment programme in the UK," *Acta Psychiatrica Scandinavica*, vol. 115, no. 4, pp. 286–294, 2007.

[35] L. Voruganti, J. Whatham, E. Bard et al., "Going beyond: an adventure- and recreation-based group intervention promotes well-being and weight loss in schizophrenia," *The Canadian Journal of Psychiatry*, vol. 51, no. 9, pp. 575–580, 2006.

[36] C. Brown, H. Read, M. Stanton, M. Zeeb, J. A. Jonikas, and J. A. Cook, "A pilot study of the nutrition and exercise for wellness and recovery (NEW-R): a weight loss program for individuals with serious mental illnesses," *Psychiatric Rehabilitation Journal*, vol. 38, no. 4, pp. 371–373, 2015.

[37] D. Haber, C. Looney, K. Babola, M. Hinman, and C. J. Utsey, "Impact of a health promotion course on inactive, overweight, or physically limited older adults," *Family & Community Health*, vol. 22, no. 4, pp. 48–56, 2000.

[38] A. Rynne and K. McKenna, "Evaluation of an outpatient diabetes education programme," *British Journal of Occupational Therapy*, vol. 62, no. 10, pp. 459–465, 1999.

[39] N. Bacon, L. Farnworth, and R. Boyd, "The use of the Wii fit in forensic mental health: exercise for people at risk of obesity," *British Journal of Occupational Therapy*, vol. 75, no. 2, pp. 61–68, 2012.

[40] K. Jacobs, L. Zhu, M. Dawes et al., "Wii health: a preliminary study of the health and wellness benefits of Wii fit on university students," *British Journal of Occupational Therapy*, vol. 74, no. 6, pp. 262–268, 2011.

[41] C. Galani and H. Schneider, "Prevention and treatment of obesity with lifestyle interventions: review and meta-analysis," *International Journal of Public Health*, vol. 52, no. 6, pp. 348–359, 2007.

[42] S. Ramage, A. Farmer, K. Eccles, and L. McCargar, "Healthy strategies for successful weight loss and weight maintenance: a systematic review," *Applied Physiology, Nutrition, and Metabolism*, vol. 39, no. 1, pp. 1–20, 2014.

[43] J. Batsis, L. E. Gill, R. K. Masutani et al., "Weight loss interventions in older adults with obesity: a systematic review of randomized controlled trials since 2005," *Journal of the American Geriatrics Society*, vol. 65, no. 2, pp. 257–268, 2017.

[44] L. Womble, S. Wang, D. Sarwer et al., "Do patients adjust weight loss expectations?," *Obesity Research*, vol. 8, no. 1, p. 41, 2000.

[45] C. Sciamanna, M. Kiernan, B. J. Rolls et al., "Practices associated with weight loss versus weight-loss maintenance: results of a national survey," *American Journal of Preventive Medicine*, vol. 41, no. 2, pp. 159–166, 2011.

[46] K. R. Whalley Hammell, "Belonging, occupation, and human well-being: an exploration: Appartenance, occupation et bien-être humain: Une étude exploratoire," *Canadian Journal of Occupational Therapy*, vol. 81, no. 1, pp. 39–50, 2014.

[47] H. Bambrick, "Relationships between BMI, waist circumference, hypertension and fasting glucose: rethinking risk factors in indigenous diabetes," *Australian Indigenous Health Bulletin*, vol. 5, no. 4, p. 1, 2005.

[48] P. Deurenberg, M. Deurenberg-Yap, and S. Guricci, "Asians are different from Caucasians and from each other in their body mass index/body fat per cent relationship," *Obesity Reviews*, vol. 3, no. 3, pp. 141–146, 2002.

[49] W. James, R. Jackson-Leach, C. NiMhurchu et al., "Overweight and obesity (high body mass index)," in *Comparative Quantification of Health Risks: Global and Regional Burden of Disease Attributable to Selected Major Risk Factors*, M. Ezzati, A. Lopez, A. Rodgers, and C. Murray, Eds., pp. 497–596, World Health Organization, Geneva, 2004.

[50] A. Scriven and A. Atwal, "Occupational therapists as primary health promoters: opportunities and barriers," *British Journal of Occupational Therapy*, vol. 67, no. 10, pp. 424–429, 2004.

[51] K. Z. Brewster, B. Nowrouzi, and L. Davis, "The role of occupational therapy in obesity management," *University of Toronto Medical Journal*, vol. 91, no. 1, pp. 33–35, 2014.

[52] W. Bryant and E. McKay, "What's cooking? Theory and practice in the kitchen," *British Journal of Occupational Therapy*, vol. 68, no. 2, pp. 67–74, 2005.

[53] M. Gage, "The appraisal model of coping: an assessment and intervention model for occupational therapy," *The American journal of occupational therapy*, vol. 46, no. 4, pp. 353–362, 1992.

[54] E. Orellano, W. I. Colón, and M. Arbesman, "Effect of occupation- and activity-based interventions on instrumental activities of daily living performance among community-dwelling older adults: a systematic review," *The American journal of occupational therapy*, vol. 66, no. 3, pp. 292–300, 2012.

[55] J. Grimshaw, L. McAuley, L. Bero et al., "Systematic reviews of the effectiveness of quality improvement strategies and programmes," *Quality & safety in health care*, vol. 12, no. 4, pp. 298–303, 2003.

22

Enhancing a Client-Centred Practice with the Canadian Occupational Performance Measure

A. Enemark Larsen,[1] B. Rasmussen,[1] and J. R. Christensen[2,3]

[1]*Department of Occupational Therapy, Institute of Medwifery and Therapy, University College Copenhagen, Sigurdsgade 26, DK-2200 N Copenhagen, Denmark*
[2]*Department of Public Health, University of Southern Denmark, JB Winsløwsvej 9A, 5000 Odense, Denmark*
[3]*Department of Sports Science and Clinical Biomechanics, University of Southern Denmark, Campusvej 55, 5230 Odense, Denmark*

Correspondence should be addressed to A. Enemark Larsen; anel@phmetropol.dk

Academic Editor: Mélanie Levasseur

Background. The active participation of clients is an important aspect of rehabilitation quality as conceptualized in client-centred practice (CCP). A recommended outcome measure for enhancing CCP is the Canadian Occupational Performance Measure (COPM). However, the relationship between COPM use and CCP enhancement has not been documented. *Aim.* The aim of this study was to examine whether the use of the COPM enhanced CCP. *Methods.* We performed a scoping review in five steps: (1) *identifying* a search strategy with inclusion and exclusion criteria; (2) *screening* relevant databases for published and unpublished studies by using selected keywords and by manually scrutinizing reference lists; (3) agreeing on *eligible* papers between authors in terms of inclusion and exclusion criteria; (4) charting *included* data; and (5) *analysing* data using qualitative content analysis. *Results.* Twelve studies were included in the review. The results indicated enhanced CCP in two themes when using the COPM. These themes appeared to influence each other; therefore, the first theme, *Conditions for enhancing CCP when using the COPM*, represented the circumstances needed for the second theme, *Enhancing CCP when using the COPM*, to be fulfilled. *Conclusion.* The use of the COPM seems to enhance CCP if certain conditions are present.

1. Introduction

The active participation of clients is an important aspect of the quality of rehabilitation processes and the aim in healthcare institutions around the world [1, 2]. Similar in Denmark, since 2013, the hospital staff have endeavoured the active involvement of clients through a systematic collection of information from clients about their experiences during rehabilitation [3]. The information has been collected within the Danish Model of Quality in the Healthcare System (DDKM) and used to improve the quality of hospital services [3]. Thus, active participation of clients is included as a key component in the 2020 visions of healthcare systems in many countries [4]. The 2020 visions aim to create a healthcare system that is suited to each individual and more responsive to each client's preferences, needs, and values [4]. However, fulfilling this aim is difficult [5, 6]. A recent study showed that although the aim is the active participation of clients in the rehabilitation process, the process often does not truly reference the client's wishes and goals and is not collaborative [7]. Another study showed that clients experienced inadequate rehabilitation that did not emphasize their individual and emotional needs [8]. Furthermore, clients who require help to manage uncertainties have experienced unaddressed problems [8, 9]. All this evidence illustrates the need to optimize efforts to enhance client participation in the rehabilitation process [10].

One conceptual framework that includes the active participation of clients is "client-centred practice" (CCP), described by Carl Rogers as practice that is nondirective and focuses on the concerns expressed by the client [6, 11]. In occupational therapy (OT), CCP has always been an integrated value and a fundamental element [12]. Research on CCP has increased over the last few decades [6, 13–15]. A systematic review revealed five thematic conceptual elements that should be addressed when working with CCP, namely, power, listening and communicating, partnership, choice, and hope [6].

A recommended method believed to enhance CCP in the rehabilitation process is the use of the Canadian Occupational Performance Measure (COPM) [16]. The COPM is designed to identify changes in the client's personal perceptions of occupational performance over time, and studies show that the identification of self-perceived occupational performance problems (OPPs) seems to enhance client motivation and the relevance of the individualized goals in rehabilitation [16–20]. The COPM consists of the following five steps and three scores: (1) the clients identify their OPPs within the areas of self-care, productivity, and leisure and score their *importance* on a scale ranging from 1, not important, to 10, extremely important. (2) The clients prioritize up to five OPPs on which to focus during the intervention. (3) The clients rate their *performance* and (4) their *satisfaction with performance* of the identified OPPs. Both scales range from 1 to 10, with higher values indicating better performance and greater satisfaction. (5) Performance and satisfaction with performance are reassessed after an appropriate interval of time, normally between three to six months, and changes in the clients' perceptions of their occupational performance can be calculated [16].

Generally, studies on concurrent and content validity that included a variety of clients and OT practitioners show that the COPM is a valid measure of occupational performance [20]. Studies have also documented the COPM's utility in providing an individualized perspective of the client's values, judgements, and preferences regarding occupational performance and thus its ability to facilitate clinical decision-making and monitor functional progress [19, 20].

Given that the aim of the COPM interview is not only to identify, prioritize, and score the OPPs but also to enhance CCP, it seems important to evaluate whether the latter aim is actually fulfilled. Studies of the COPM have also reported the ability of the COPM interview to enhance CCP [17–20]. Additionally, in the systematic review by Parker and Sykes, the COPM interview enabled clients to name and frame their problems, allowed them to be experts on their own circumstances, and empowered them to be more critical of their own performance, that is, the use of the COPM seemed to support CCP [21]. However, a review from 2011 that examined the COPM and other measurements identified a paucity of literature concerning the client's experiences with the COPM, leaving the question of whether the use of the COPM can enhance CCP [22]. Thus, the aim of the current study was to examine the literature and determine whether the use of the COPM can enhance CCP.

2. Materials and Method

2.1. Design. The current scoping review followed the recommendations from the commentary of Colquhoun et al. [23], which advised the use of the following methodological steps outlined in the Arksey and O'Malley framework [24] and further enhanced by Levac et al. [25]: (1) identification: identify the research questions. (2) Screening: find the relevant studies. (3) Eligibility: select the studies relevant to the question. (4) Inclusion: chart the data. (5) Analysis: collate, summarize, and report the results. Because our aim was to examine the *literature* on the COPM, the optional 6th step of the scoping review procedure, consultation with stakeholders as a required knowledge translation component, was not applied in this review [23–25].

2.2. Procedure

2.2.1. Identification. We developed a search strategy with inclusion and exclusion criteria and used the PICO (population, intervention, comparison, outcome) model to identify keywords relevant to our research question [26] as we wanted to examine whether the COPM (the 'I') would enhance CCP (the 'O'). Thus, in our search strategy, we included all kinds of populations from all kinds of settings (the 'P's), but we did not include any comparisons (the 'C').

2.2.2. Screening. The literature search was performed in two steps between September and December 2016 (last search: 18.12.2016). First, an initial literature search in PubMed and CINAHL was performed to identify relevant keywords, synonyms, word modifications, and thesaurus terms to use to adjust the O criteria—the clarification of the term "client-centred" [26]. Several searches using different word combinations were performed until we found a search strategy that seemed to identify studies on the COPM and CCP. Keywords were narrowed to the framework of "client-centred" as this is the term used in the COPM and the OT profession, for which the COPM was developed. Other concepts such as "patient-centred" or "patient-focused care" were not included, because although similar, they define an organizational process rather than a conceptual approach to ensure the participation and engagement of clients. Thus, we used the following keywords: ((COPM) OR "Canadian Occupational Performance Measure") AND ((client-center*) OR client-centre*)).

Second, database-specific searches using PubMed, CINAHL, OTseeker, PEDro, Web of Science, and SCOPUS were conducted using the thesaurus terminology for each database. Truncations were used when relevant. The above-mentioned keywords were also used to search for unpublished items on interventions of interest in SwePub and NORA. Google Scholar was also examined using the terms "COPM" and "CCP".

2.2.3. Eligibility. The selection of papers eligible for inclusion was guided by inclusion and exclusion criteria based on the research question. The papers were selected by agreement among the authors. The *inclusion criteria* were the following: (I) studies of all kinds of interventions in all settings, addressing all adult clients ≥ 18 years to whom the COPM had been administered. (II) Studies that revealed the OTs' or their clients' experiences with the use of the COPM to enhance CCP. (III) Published and unpublished qualitative and quantitative studies. (IV) Studies published from January 2005 to August 2016 as the research on the COPM and CCP has increased over the past decade. The *exclusion criteria* included the following: (I) studies in which the COPM only was used as an outcome measure, without data on the participants perception of the use of the COPM. (II) Studies focussing on children. (III) Studies written in languages other than English, Danish, Swedish, or Norwegian. (IV) Editorials, commentaries, interviews, lectures, periodicals, and abstracts.

The two first authors conducted the study selection. Agreement was reached by discussion between the authors, and the third author was consulted if unresolved disagreements occurred. All studies were entered into an Excel sheet to identify and exclude duplicates. The titles and abstracts of the remaining studies were assessed for the inclusion and exclusion criteria, thus facilitating the exclusion of studies that did not fit the research question. The remaining studies were read in full, and studies that were unfit to answer the research question were excluded. Finally, the reference lists of the studies that were read were examined to identify additional studies eligible for inclusion in the scoping review.

2.2.4. Inclusion. As recommend by Levac et al. [25], the authors collectively conducted first assessment of the included studies to determine which descriptive variables to extract to answer the research question. Because the included studies were mostly qualitative, we followed the recommendations of Levac et al. and used a qualitative content analysis approach [25, 27].

2.2.5. Analysis. The qualitative content analysis was based on the recommendations of Graneheim and Lundman, focussing on latent context analysis centred on an in-depth interpretation of the underlying meaning of the text [27]. The two first authors performed the analysis. The included studies were read independently to obtain a general sense of the entire pool of included studies. Then, each author performed a systematic identification of textual information, located the important structures and information from each study, and entered these textual units into a table to identify how these "constellation of words" related to the central meaning. The two tables were compared, and the differences were discussed to subsequently form a common table of significant "meaning units" that had been identified and agreed upon. To ensure that all relevant content was identified, the authors reread all studies while searching for text in accordance with the identified "meaning units" and entered new findings into the table. The content of the meaning units was condensed and abstracted to identify adequate labels, or codes, to represent each condensed meaning unit. The authors compared the codes to identify differences and similarities and sorted the codes into themes and subthemes related to the research question. Finally, all studies were reread to ensure that all the information had been extracted into the themes and subthemes, and dialogues with the third author ensured that nothing in the studies contradicted the themes [27].

3. Results

As presented in Figure 1, we identified 174 studies, and 90 studies remained after duplicates were removed. After the titles and abstracts were screened, 22 studies remained for full-text readings. The authors independently read the 22 studies and discussed their inclusion and exclusion, which left eight studies. After a careful examination of the reference lists of the eight studies, four studies were added.

The twelve studies included one systematic review [28], one opinion paper [29], one quantitative study [30], four qualitative studies [1, 31–33], and five mixed-method studies [19, 34–36], including one unpublished PhD dissertation [11]. The contents of each study, including their aims, methods, samples, and settings, are summarized in Table 1.

The analysis of the literature on the ability of the COPM to enhance CCP revealed two main themes, with five subthemes in the first theme and four subthemes in the second. The two main themes seemed to influence and affect each other; thus, the first theme represented the circumstances required for the second theme to be fulfilled. The first theme considered the prerequisite conditions for CCP when conducting a COPM interview. Some of these conditions related to the OTs' skills and attitudes, specifically in relation to *communication* and *willingness to listen to the clients' points of view*. Others related to how *the environment* seemed to affect the ability of the COPM interview to enhance CCP, particularly in terms of the institutional *commitment to CCP* and the willingness to *share the power with the client*.

The second theme concerned the aspects of CCP that a COPM interview seemed to enhance. These aspects included how the interview could lead to an increase in the OT's awareness of the client's preferences, needs, and values, such as that the OT *got to know the client* and was able to *enhance the client's self-awareness*. Additionally, the use of the COPM interview seemed to enable the processes of *forming a partnership* and *develop collaborative goals*. When these aspects of CCP occurred, they seemed to positively strengthen and increase the OT's behaviours and the environmental conditions under which the COPM was administered. The themes are narratively presented, and an example of the analysis and translation from meaning units to themes is shown in Table 2.

3.1. Conditions for Enhancing CCP When Using the COPM. Our analysis of the included studies indicated that certain conditions should be met if CCP is to be enhanced by the use of the COPM. The OTs' skills and their willingness to *communicate with* and *listen to* the clients' points of view are necessary for the COPM to enhance CCP [11, 19, 30, 31, 33, 36]. A statement by one of the OTs in one of the studies supported the importance of these factors: "It takes very expert communication skills to use [the COPM] in the way it is designed and for it to actually have a therapeutic benefit" [33]. Tuntland et al. reported that personnel without bachelors-level qualification felt a need for additional training in the COPM interview and CCP, indicating that they regarded their expertise as insufficient [30]. Stevens et al. focused on the OTs' communication skills: "It's about the skillful interview in the initial stages and communication to establish what the client is having difficulties with and negotiate with them the areas they want to work on... being honest with them ... [and] provide and renegotiate ... goals..." [28].

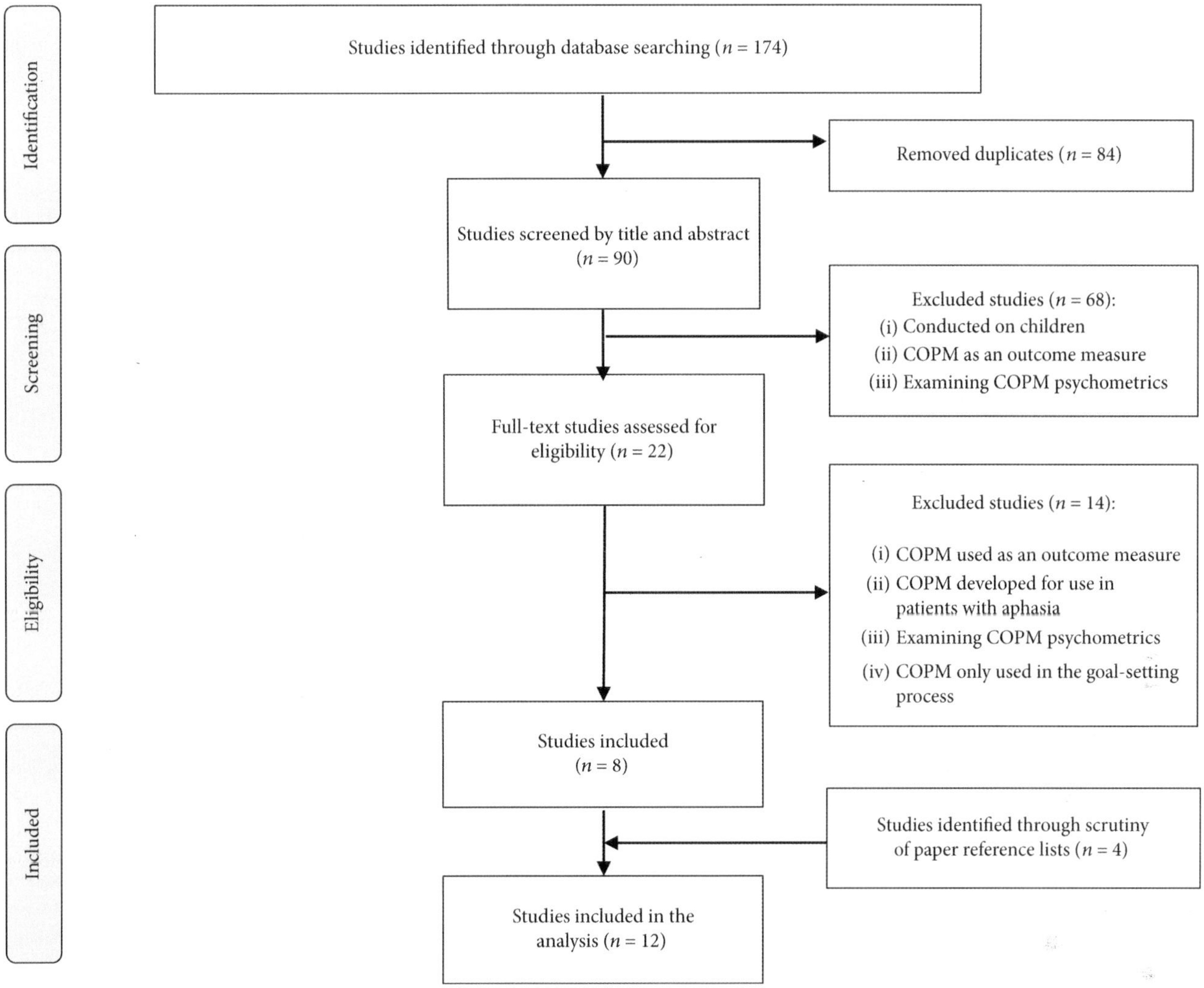

FIGURE 1: Study flow.

Other studies indicated that for the COPM interview to facilitate CCP, a *commitment to CCP* that included an acceptance of the client's opinion, that is, *sharing the power*, was important [1, 11, 19, 28, 29, 33, 36]. Further, the OT's reluctance to use the COPM and his or her commitment to CCP could be interpreted as depending on *the environment* in which the rehabilitation occurred. For instance, if the OT focused on restoring physical function while working in a hospital, contradictory paradigms such as the traditional biomedical model would be inconsistent with the use of the COPM, which is based on a holistic approach [1, 19]. It seemed that therapy was influenced by the environmental conditions of the respective institutions and that this could lead to differences in expectations between clients and OTs [1, 19, 28, 36]. The OTs felt uncomfortable having to listen to and go along with their clients and expressed ambivalence when dealing with the clients' wishes if these wishes differed from the OTs' own [1, 19, 28]. This process was difficult if the OTs found the clients' goals unrealistic as the OTs felt they had the expertise to know what was best for the client [1, 28]. Stevens et al. found that "Some [OTs] indicated that involving patients even undermined the therapy and reduced the patient's motivation, reporting that they [the patients] set unrealistic goals or had unrealistic expectations" [28]. Thus, in some settings, an OT's reluctance to use the COPM to determine the client's point of view and to power were identified as impediments [1, 28], and discrepancies between client aspirations and OT expectations were observed [1, 19, 32, 36]. In a survey on CCP, Parker found that although only 6% of participating OTs agreed with the statement that "the therapist should set the treatment goals," 27% of the OTs agreed that "the therapist has different goals than those of the client" [11]. In the studies by Richard and Knis-Matthews [1] and Engelbrecht et al. [36], differences in the goals of the therapy were observed. The clients identified goals outside the context of the residence programme, such as returning to work or school, whereas the OTs focused on achieving goals within the residence programme [1]. In these studies, the OTs' ideas of feasibility seemed to limit collaborative goal setting [1, 36]. These limitations were related to the clients' constitutions, for example, if the clients had just become ill or did not have the cognitive ability to conduct a COPM

TABLE 1: An overview of the included papers ($n = 12$).

Reference name/ number	Goal/aim	Study design	Method	Materials (sample and context)
Bjørkedal et al. [31]	To qualitatively evaluate the feasibility of client-centred OT intervention focused on enabling meaningful occupations and supporting the recovery process for individuals with schizophrenia in the early phases of recovery.	Qualitative study.	A qualitative study comprising an eight-week client-centred OT intervention and semistructured interviews with five of the six clients out of 10 who completed the intervention. The COPM was used to initiate and guide the intervention, and the Canadian Model of Client-Centred Enablement was used for the client-therapist relationship.	Ten participants with schizophrenic disorders, five of whom (three women and two men) participated in postintervention semistructured interviews. They were recruited from the community and lived in their own apartments.
Colquhoun et al. [34]	To survey OTs currently using the COPM to gather their perceptions about the use of the COPM on a routine basis. A secondary objective was to propose a meaningful template for summarizing routine COPM data.	Mixed method study.	The OTs were given a short-answer written questionnaire that focused on the key areas, derived from the literature, in the routine outcome measures used. These questions related to the feasibility of the COPM and the value of the data. In addition, the resulting five months of COPM data were summarized into a proposed template based on what the OTs found meaningful.	Three female OTs, with six, eight, and 31 years of practice. They had been working in the geriatric unit for one year, five years, and one year, respectively.
Colquhoun et al. [35]	To determine whether COPM administration was associated with changes in eight dimensions of OT practice.	Mixed-method study.	A before-and-after study with repeated tests. The eight practice dimensions were assessed after three months of usual care (no COPM use) and after three months of intervention (COPM use) using chart-stimulated recall (CSR) interviews and chart audit.	24 OTs working in eight inpatient geriatric rehabilitation facilities across two large urban centres. Potential sites were identified by geographic area and the presence of inpatient geriatric rehabilitation units.
Donovan et al. [32]	To describe the occupational concerns and goals of mothers who care for children with disabilities.	Qualitative study.	A qualitative design analysing retrospective data collected using the COPM.	38 mothers of children with disabilities.
Enemark Larsen and Carlsson [19]	To evaluate the utility of the COPM in an interdisciplinary geriatric rehabilitation context (RCC) in Copenhagen in terms of (a) its utility to both OTs and physiotherapists, (b) its utility to document change, and (c) the therapists' experiences with the administration and usability of the COPM.	Mixed-method study.	Data were collected from a pre- and postassessment with the COPM and a questionnaire answered by all participating therapists.	18 therapists (11 physiotherapists and seven OTs) participated in the project group. 185 elderly clients referred to the RCC by home care personnel or general practitioners participated in the study through consecutive sampling over a period of eight months.
Engelbrecht et al. [36]	To determine whether healthcare workers could successfully identify the occupational performance priorities of adult people with disabilities (PWD) living in a Kwaguqa community in the Mpumalanga province of South Africa.	Mixed-method study.	A nonexperimental descriptive design using descriptive survey questionnaires, for example, the COPM, which captured quantitative and qualitative data.	25 adults (17 men and 8 women) from the Thembelihle Self Help Centre and the Kwaguqa Association for the Disabled Workshop with mobility or dexterity problems, aged 18 to above 60 years of age, plus seven female healthcare workers responsible for the service in the Kwaguqua area.

Table 1: Continued.

Reference name/ number	Goal/aim	Study design	Method	Materials (sample and context)
Gustafsson et al. [33]	To investigate the goal-setting process and clinical utility of the COPM from the perspective of OTs within a spinal cord injury unit (SIU).	Qualitative study.	A focus group interview was conducted with seven OTs working in an SIU to explore their experiences and use of goalsetting and the COPM. Inductive thematic analysis identified key themes from their comments.	Seven female OTs, with a mean age of 29.7 (SD 8.38) years. Their clinical experience working in the hospital SIU ranged from less than 6 months to more than 20 years.
Hannah [29]	To summarize the psychological impact of severe hand injuries, to discuss coping strategies for the social impacts of severe hand injuries, and to outline assessments and strategies that can be used by hand therapists to treat the whole person, develop patient-centred goals, and improve therapy outcomes.	An opinion study based on a literature review.	Opinion based on a literature review.	No material included as due to the study format.
Parker [11]	To determine clients' and OTs' perceptions of the CCP in OT in the UK	PhD dissertation. Different studies—a review, a survey, and a qualitative design.	A mixed-method study examining the views of clients and therapists was undertaken using a systematic review to examine global evidence of client-centred outcome measures, a survey of the experiences of a sample of therapists and individual client and OT interviews.	Study (1): 25 OTs opted to attend the focus group. The gender profile of the group was 3 males and 22 females. Study (2): 230 questionnaires were sent to OTs, and 25% were returned. Study (3): four OTs with 4–30 years of education and four clients aged 35–81 years.
Richard and Knis-Matthews [1]	To compare the intervention goals identified by clients and an OT using the COPM.	Qualitative study.	In-depth interviews were conducted with an OT and her clients in conjunction with the use of the COPM.	Seven clients living in a long-term residential programme and diagnosed with schizophrenia and one OT who had worked at the programme for three years at the time of the study.
Stevens et al. [28]	To identify the currently available patient-specific measurement instruments used in the process of goalsetting and to assess their feasibility.	A qualitative systematic review.	After a systematic search in PubMed, EMBASE, CINAHL, PsychINFO, and REHABDATA, patient-specific instruments were included, structured within a goal-setting practice framework and subjected to a qualitative thematic analysis of feasibility.	25 patient-specific instruments were identified, and 11, one of which was the COPM, were included.
Tuntland et al. [30]	To investigate the validity, responsiveness, interpretability, and feasibility of the COPM when used by various health professions in home-dwelling older adults receiving assistance.	A quantitative study on psycometrics.	A quantitative study following the COSMIN guidelines and recommendations for evaluating methodological quality.	The sample included 225 participants, mean age 80.8 years, in need of rehabilitation for various health conditions. Data collection was conducted at baseline and at a 10-week follow-up. The assessments were conducted by 12 nurses, 33 OTs, 27 physiotherapists, five auxiliary nurses, and one social educator.

interview, or the environmental conditions, for example, what the OTs were expected to address or the available facilities [19, 28, 30, 35, 36]. However, if the environmental values aligned with CCP, the OTs seemed to translate the client requirements into goals based on the COPM interview [19].

Table 2: Meaning units, condensed meaning units, subthemes, and themes from the content analysis.

Examples of meaning units	Condensed meaning unit/interpretation of the underlying meaning	Subthemes	Theme
The participants found that the COPM made the challenges and barriers that they experienced in their everyday lives tangible, helping them set suitable personal goals and initiate the intervention ([31], p. 102).	The COPM helped the clients to comprehend their everyday lives and set suitable goals for intervention.		
The COPM proved to be a suitable measure for determining occupational performance priorities from the perspectives of both the PWD and the healthcare workers (HCWs), although this initially resulted in diverse lists of priorities ([36], p. 13).	The COPM helped the clients and the OTs identify OPPs. The identified OPPs differed between clients and OTs.		
The OTs felt that the COPM facilitated discussions with clients about functional independence and the formulation of OT-related goals. They felt that until they actually performed the COPM with a person, they did not really have a sense of the person's needs. The COPM was also thought to aid in increasing client motivation and the client's sense of control over their rehabilitation; it made the rehabilitation process meaningful for the client and provided OTs with client-centred directions and priorities for therapy. An OT stated, "[The COPM] also assists in your assessment of knowing the person's insight and adjustment to their disability" ([33], p. 340).	The COPM helped the OTs get to know their clients. The COPM also helped the clients and facilitated insights for both the OTs and the clients.	*Getting to know the client* and *Enhancing clients' self-awareness*	*Enhancing CCP with the COPM.*
The participants felt that the COPM interview led to greater awareness of their daily lives and to a feeling of being seen and listened to. They also reported that the interview enhanced their motivation to focus on improving occupational performance and that the information brought forward during the interview and scoring process was useful as a basis for developing rehabilitation goals ([30], p. 419).	The COPM led the clients to a greater awareness of their daily lives and enhanced motivation and development of goals.		

3.2. Enhancing CCP When Using the COPM. In all the studies, there was agreement regarding the benefits of using the COPM, most frequently expressed as the ability that the COPM provided for the OTs *to get to know the client.* This awareness was two sided; the OTs familiarized themselves with the clients and their aspirations, and *the clients gained better insight* and awareness of what they wanted and what to expect from the intervention. This often *facilitated partnerships* in the CCP through *collaborative goals.*

It seemed that the use of the COPM provided a positive starting point for CCP because it improved the OT's knowledge of the client's everyday life and aspirations and encouraged the collaborative formation of goals based on the identified OPPs [19, 28, 30–33]. Apparently, using the COPM could emphasize the importance of clinical judgement for guidance [31, 33]. In the study by Donovan et al., the use of the COPM increased equality in the therapeutic relationship by enhancing the understanding of individual clients' perspectives and shifting perceptions, attitudes, and behaviours towards occupations that are meaningful in the clients' lives [32]. In the study by Tuntland et al., the OTs considered the COPM to be very useful in planning and evaluating the intervention [30]. The majority (82%) of the clients stated that they felt the COPM interview and scoring were useful [30].

In addition to the OT's positive experiences with the COPM, the COPM also seemed to improve interdisciplinary teamwork around the client, providing broader information regarding the client, increased information on occupational performance, and a greater emphasis on team goal setting [11, 19, 28, 30].

Colquhoun et al. found evidence that OT knowledge of what matters to the client shows statistically significant improvements when using the COPM [34]. In hand therapy, the use of the COPM was thought to help the therapists focus on issues and goals that would assist the client in fulfilling important life roles [29].

Tuntland et al. found that the COPM was useful for determining goals, and clients felt that the COPM contributed information about "what is important to me" [30]. The COPM interview encouraged the clients to increase their attentiveness to their problems and enhanced their motivation, cooperation, and responsibility for their own therapy [28, 31], thus facilitating a process of self-awareness [19, 32]. The COPM interview seemed to improve the clients' understanding of their own issues, making difficult experiences in everyday life tangible, and thereby facilitated the client-centred partnership [31, 33]. As the COPM interview increased awareness of daily life and acknowledged the clients [30], it helped improve the degree to which the rehabilitation was client centred [33]. The importance of being acknowledged was also supported by Parker, in whose study clients expressed the overwhelming importance of how they were treated [11]. The clients expressed a fundamental need to be valued as individuals, indicating that the attitudes of the OTs in these relationships are more important than their actions [11].

4. Discussion

The assumption that the use of the COPM facilitates CCP led to the objective of this study to examine the literature to determine whether CCP is enhanced when the COPM is used. The scoping review found that the use of the COPM seemed to enhance CCP and that certain conditions were necessary for the COPM interview to have this desired effect.

4.1. The Use of the COPM Seemed to Enhance an Awareness That Goes beyond Assessments. The process of identifying OPPs seemed to change the clients' awareness of their self-perceived needs, which further appeared to affect the client's motivation, cooperation, and responsibility through the subsequent rehabilitation. The COPM interview seemed to influence the clients' attentiveness to and understanding of their problems, which seemed to facilitate a process of self-awareness, making difficult experiences in everyday life more tangible. Thus, starting a rehabilitation process with a COPM interview might help the client begin to come to terms with life. In this way, the COPM interview appeared to initiate a process similar to what Antonovsky called a "sense of coherence" (SOC) [37]. Studies have shown that a SOC contributes to a client's quality of life, health, and satisfaction with daily occupations [37, 38]. Provided that the COPM interview has this positive influence on the client's self-awareness, the COPM interview might facilitate CCP beyond the assessment by influencing the rehabilitation outcome itself.

4.2. The Use of the COPM Helped with Forming a Partnership and Making Collaborative Goals. The COPM interview led to an increased awareness of the client's preferences, needs, and values and helped the OT and the client form a partnership with meaningful and collaborative goals [11, 19, 28, 29, 31–33]. An important aspect of CCP is the establishment of a client-centred partnership in which the client plays an active role in defining goals [6]. Forming a partnership with clients and collaborating in goal setting have always been valued processes in OT [5, 6, 11, 12, 39, 40] that are described as ethical values in both national and international OT associations [41, 42]. Because partnerships and collaborative goalsetting have a positive effect on the outcomes of rehabilitation [15, 43], these aspects are important parts of healthcare politics and have formed the basis for many government policies in recent years [4, 44].

This scoping review revealed that using the COPM to examine client perceptions might help to minimize the OTs' misinterpretation of client needs, goals, and wishes [1, 32]. The included studies showed a discrepancy between goals of the OTs and those of their clients. Similar discrepancies between therapists and clients have been seen in other studies, for example, in stroke rehabilitation [15, 43]. Here, the OTs prioritized goals characterized by short timeframes, conservative estimates of outcomes, and physical function, that is, focused on impairments, independent self-care, and locomotion [15, 43], whereas the clients focused on resuming their predisease status and participating in social activities [15, 43].

4.3. Environmental and Therapeutic Factors Seemed to Affect If a COPM Interview Enhanced CCP. This review showed that the OTs' commitments to CCP, their willingness and ability to share power with the client, and the environment in which the rehabilitation occurred were important factors determining whether the COPM interview would positively affect CCP. Environmental factors affected the possibility of conducting a COPM interview as the OTs were reluctant to perform a COPM interview if the focus was on physical functions, that is, in settings where a medical paradigm was dominant [15, 19–21]. Some of the reluctance seemed to be an attempt to avoid the dilemma of different goals. This was also seen in the study of Mortenson and Dyck in which the OTs avoided the use of the COPM because they feared it would reveal differences between what the clients wanted to achieve and what the OTs were expected to deliver [45]. Other reasons for not using the COPM were that the clients had suddenly became ill or been hospitalized or that they did not have the cognitive ability to undergo a COPM interview [21]. When clients experience an acute disease, a preoccupation with the body's condition, symptoms, and prognosis may follow [46, 47], in addition to feelings of loss, decreased self-esteem, frustration, and anger [48]. Accordingly, in the early stages of a rehabilitation process, clients may ignore or be unaware of OPPs, which explains why it might be difficult to use the COPM under such circumstances [19, 21, 47]. However, the OTs' disinclination to use the COPM in the early stages of their clients' illnesses may reflect CCP in which the OTs acknowledged their clients' fragility and use of counselling for client-centred care [49]. Thus, although the COPM interview seems to enhance CCP, it can be argued that sometimes CCP is better provided without the COPM.

However, some OTs' reluctance to implement CCP could be due to the notion that the OTs considered themselves the experts and thus believed that they knew what was best for the clients. This illustrated a contradiction of paradigms, for example, the traditional biomedical model, with the therapist as the expert, versus the occupational model of the COPM, the Canadian Model of Occupational Performance (the CMOP), in which the client is considered the expert [12, 16]. It seems that the more therapists align with the medical paradigm for example, in hospitals, the lower their use of the COPM interview [15, 19]. This was also the case in a study of implementing the COPM in Taiwan. In that study, practice was driven by the biomedical model; thus, the concepts of COPM and CCP seemed unfamiliar and required adjustments from both therapists and their clients [49].

4.4. The COPM Interview Requires Advanced Communication Skills. Effective communication skills appeared to be vital to the successful use of the COPM and the enhancement of CCP. Corresponding findings have been reported in other studies on CCP, which describe a focus on interviewing skills, for example, the ability to listen actively, communicate in an appropriate language, and share information that aligns with the clients' needs [4–7, 20, 21, 38, 39]. Studies on how to support the successful implementation of the COPM have shown that introductory courses, ongoing support, and follow-up supervision during the implementation process are beneficial [19, 33–35]. Regular reviews might also be beneficial since Colquhoun et al. found that despite support, sustained use of the COPM was not observed [35].

4.4.1. Methodological Considerations. Despite rigorous measures, such as using two reviewers for all sources, this study has limitations that are inherent to scoping reviews in general, such as the synthesis of both published and unpublished studies and qualitative and quantitative research to balance broadness and depth. Since a scoping review is not meant to be exhaustive but rather to provide a good sense of the literature in a particular area, it is likely that some relevant publications were not included in this study. Moreover, given the global nature of the COPM, the exclusion of studies published in languages other than English or Scandinavian makes it unlikely that all relevant studies are included. The number of studies may also have been limited because we narrowed our keywords to the framework of "client-centred," the term used by the COPM and the OT profession. However, by screening the references of the included articles, we attempted to limit the number of missed articles.

5. Conclusion

This scoping review examined whether the use of the COPM could enhance CCP. Twelve studies were identified that used different designs and a range of clients in various settings. The review found that the use of the COPM seems to enhance CCP, specifically by improving awareness of client perspectives, wishes and hopes for the future, thereby reinforcing a partnership with collaborative goalsetting. However, to use the COPM interview to enhance CCP, professional communication skills, power sharing, and an institutional commitment are required.

References

[1] L. F. Richard and L. Knis-Matthews, "Are we really client-centered? Using the Canadian Occupational Performance Measure to see how the client's goals connect with the goals of the occupational therapist," *Occupational Therapy in Mental Health*, vol. 26, no. 1, pp. 51–66, 2010.

[2] D. T. Wade, "Editorial," *Clinical Rehabilitation*, vol. 21, no. 12, pp. 1059–1062, 2007.

[3] Institut for Kvalitet og Akkreditering i Sundhedsvæsenet (IKAS), *Den Danske Kvalitets Model. Akkrediteringsstandarder for Sygehuse, 2012*, Department of Quality and Accreditation in the health service. The Danish Quality Model. Accreditation Standards for Hospitals, 2012, Danish. http://www.ikas.dk/FTP/PDF/D12-6522.pdf.

[4] I. Kickbusch, T. Behrendt, and Organisation mondiale de la santé. Bureau régional de l'Europe, *Implementing a Health 2020 Vision: Governance for Health in the 21st Century: Making it Happen*, World Health Organization, Regional Office for Europe, 2013.

[5] G. Palmadottir, "Client-therapist relationships: experiences of occupational therapy clients in rehabilitation," *British Journal of Occupational Therapy*, vol. 69, no. 9, pp. 394–401, 2006.

[6] T. Sumsion and M. Law, "A review of evidence on the conceptual elements informing client-centred practice," *Canadian Journal of Occupational Therapy*, vol. 73, no. 3, pp. 153–162, 2006.

[7] M. Freil, A. Wandel, L. Pedersen, A. B. R. Jönsson, and M. NyborgLæger og sygeplejerskers forståelse af patientinddragelse, "En spørgeskemaundersøgelse blandt ansatte på hospitaler," in *Doctors and Nurses' Understanding of Patient Involvement. A Questionnaire Survey among Employees in Hospitals*, ViBIS (Knowledge Center for User Involvement in Health Care), 2014, Danish. http://www.danskepatienter.dk/sites/danskepatienter.dk/files/Rapporten.pdf.

[8] A. T. Johnsen, M. A. Petersen, L. Pedersen, L. J. Houmann, and M. Groenvold, "Do advanced cancer patients in Denmark receive the help they need? A nationally representative survey of the need related to 12 frequent symptoms/problems," *Psycho-Oncology*, vol. 22, no. 8, pp. 1724–1730, 2013.

[9] D. Blanch-Hartigan, N. Chawla, R. P. Moser, L. J. Finney Rutten, B. W. Hesse, and N. K. Arora, "Trends in cancer survivors' experience of patient-centered communication: results from the health information national trends survey (HINTS)," *Journal of Cancer Survivorship*, vol. 10, no. 6, pp. 1067–1077, 2016.

[10] A. A. Poulsen, J. Ziviani, K. Kotaniemi, and M. Law, "'I think I can': measuring confidence in goal pursuit," *British Journal of Occupational Therapy*, vol. 77, no. 2, pp. 64–66, 2014.

[11] D. M. Parker, *An Exploration of Client-Centred Practice in Occupational Therapy: Perspectives and Impact. A Thesis Submitted to the University of Birmingham for the Degree of Doctor of Philosophy*, School of Health and Population Sciences: University of Birmingham, 2013.

[12] K. G. Conceptual, *Foundations of Occupational Therapy Practice*, F.A. Davies, Philadelphia, 4th edition, 2009.

[13] E. M. Castro, T. Van Regenmortel, K. Vanhaecht, W. Sermeus, and A. Van Hecke, "Patient empowerment, patient participation and patient-centeredness in hospital care: a concept analysis based on a literature review," *Patient Education and Counseling*, vol. 99, no. 12, pp. 1923–1939, 2016.

[14] A. Kjellberg, I. Kåhlin, L. Haglund, and R. R. Taylor, "The myth of participation in occupational therapy: re-conceptualizing a client-centred approach," *Scandinavian Journal of Occupational Therapy*, vol. 19, no. 5, pp. 421–427, 2011.

[15] S. Rosewilliam, C. Sintler, A. D. Pandyan, J. Skelton, and C. A. Roskell, "Is the practice of goal-setting for patients in acute

stroke care patient-centred and what factors influence this? A qualitative study," *Clinical Rehabilitation*, vol. 30, no. 5, pp. 508–519, 2016.

[16] M. Law, S. Baptiste, A. Carswell, M. C. MA, H. Polatajko, and N. Pollock, *Canadian Occupational Performance Measure*, Ottawa, Ed., Ont.: CAOT Publications ACE, 5th edition, 2014.

[17] C. Donnelly, J. J. Eng, J. Hall et al., "Client-centred assessment and the identification of meaningful treatment goals for individuals with a spinal cord injury," *Spinal Cord*, vol. 42, no. 5, pp. 302–307, 2004.

[18] B. Kirsh and L. Cockburn, "The Canadian Occupational Performance Measure: a tool for recovery-based practice," *Psychiatric Rehabilitation Journal*, vol. 32, no. 3, pp. 171–176, 2009.

[19] A. Enemark Larsen and G. Carlsson, "Utility of the Canadian Occupational Performance Measure as an admission and outcome measure in interdisciplinary community-based geriatric rehabilitation," *Scandinavian Journal of Occupational Therapy*, vol. 19, no. 2, pp. 204–213, 2011.

[20] A. Carswell, M. A. McColl, S. Baptiste, M. Law, H. Polatajko, and N. Pollock, "The Canadian Occupational Performance Measure: a research and clinical literature review," *Canadian Journal of Occupational Therapy*, vol. 71, no. 4, pp. 210–222, 2004.

[21] D. M. Parker and C. H. Sykes, "A systematic review of the Canadian Occupational Performance Measure: a clinical practice perspective," *British Journal of Occupational Therapy*, vol. 69, no. 4, pp. 150–160, 2006.

[22] K. Fuller, "The effectiveness of occupational performance outcome measures within mental health practice," *British Journal of Occupational Therapy*, vol. 74, no. 8, pp. 399–405, 2011.

[23] H. L. Colquhoun, D. Levac, K. K. O'Brien et al., "Scoping reviews: time for clarity in definition, methods, and reporting," *Journal of Clinical Epidemiology*, vol. 67, no. 12, pp. 1291–1294, 2014.

[24] H. Arksey and L. O'Malley, "Scoping studies: towards a methodological framework," *International Journal of Social Research Methodology*, vol. 8, no. 1, pp. 19–32, 2005.

[25] D. Levac, H. Colquhoun, and K. K. O'Brien, "Scoping studies: advancing the methodology," *Implementation Science*, vol. 5, no. 1, p. 69, 2010.

[26] The Joanna Briggs Institute, "Joanna Briggs Institute Reviewers' Manual," in *Edition. The Joanna Briggs Institute*, The University of Adelaide, South Australia, 2014.

[27] U. H. Graneheim and B. Lundman, "Qualitative content analysis in nursing research: concepts, procedures and measures to achieve trustworthiness," *Nurse Education Today*, vol. 24, no. 2, pp. 105–112, 2004.

[28] A. Stevens, A. Beurskens, A. Köke, and T. van der Weijden, "The use of patient-specific measurement instruments in the process of goal-setting: a systematic review of available instruments and their feasibility," *Clinical Rehabilitation*, vol. 27, no. 11, pp. 1005–1019, 2013.

[29] S. D. Hannah, "Psychosocial issues after a traumatic hand injury: facilitating adjustment," *Journal of Hand Therapy*, vol. 24, no. 2, pp. 95–103, 2011.

[30] H. Tuntland, M. Aaslund, E. Langeland, B. Espehaug, and I. Kjeken, "Psychometric properties of the Canadian Occupational Performance Measure in home-dwelling older adults," *Journal of Multidisciplinary Healthcare*, vol. 9, pp. 411–423, 2016.

[31] S. T. B. Bjørkedal, A. M. B. Torsting, and T. Møller, "Rewarding yet demanding: client perspectives on enabling occupations during early stages of recovery from schizophrenia," *Scandinavian Journal of Occupational Therapy*, vol. 23, no. 2, pp. 97–106, 2015.

[32] J. M. Donovan, B. J. VanLeit, T. K. Crowe, and E. B. Keefe, "Occupational goals of mothers of children with disabilities: influence of temporal, social, and emotional contexts," *The American Journal of Occupational Therapy*, vol. 59, no. 3, pp. 249–261, 2005.

[33] L. Gustafsson, G. Mitchell, J. Fleming, and G. Price, "Clinical utility of the Canadian Occupational Performance Measure in spinal cord injury rehabilitation," *British Journal of Occupational Therapy*, vol. 75, no. 7, pp. 337–342, 2012.

[34] H. Colquhoun, L. Letts, M. Law, J. MacDermid, and M. Edwards, "Feasibility of the Canadian Occupational Performance Measure for routine use," *British Journal of Occupational Therapy*, vol. 73, no. 2, pp. 48–54, 2010.

[35] H. L. Colquhoun, L. J. Letts, M. C. Law, J. C. MacDermid, and C. A. Missiuna, "Administration of the Canadian Occupational Performance Measure: effect on practice," *Canadian Journal of Occupational Therapy*, vol. 79, no. 2, pp. 120–128, 2012.

[36] L. H. Engelbrecht, J. M. F. Casteleijn, and K. Uys, "Could health care workers determine the occupational performance priorities of people with disability living in a developing community?," *South African Journal of Occupational Therapy*, vol. 38, pp. 8–14, 2008.

[37] A. G. W. Anke and A. R. Fugl-Meyer, "Life satisfaction several years after severe multiple trauma–a retrospective investigation," *Clinical Rehabilitation*, vol. 17, no. 4, pp. 431–442, 2003.

[38] R. I. Cederlund, E. Ramel, H.-E. Rosberg, and L. B. Dahlin, "Outcome and clinical changes in patients 3, 6, 12 months after a severe or major hand injury - can sense of coherence be an indicator for rehabilitation focus?," *BMC Musculoskeletal Disorders*, vol. 11, no. 1, pp. 286–286, 2010.

[39] K. R. Whalley Hammell, "Client-centred practice in occupational therapy: critical reflections," *Scandinavian Journal of Occupational Therapy*, vol. 20, no. 3, pp. 174–181, 2013.

[40] M.-J. Drolet and M. Désormeaux-Moreau, "The values of occupational therapy: perceptions of occupational therapists in Quebec," *Scandinavian Journal of Occupational Therapy*, vol. 23, no. 4, pp. 272–285, 2016.

[41] Ergoterapeutforeningen [Danish Association of Occupational Therapy], "Professionsgrundlag for ergoterapi – En dokumentsamling om mission visioner værdier faglig etik og samarbejde," in *The Conceptual Foundation of the Occupational Therapy Profession - a Repository of Mission, Visions, Values, Professional Ethics and Collaoration*, Ergoterapeutforeningen, Denmark, 2015.

[42] World Federation of Occupational Therapists, WFOT, *Statement on Occupational Therapy*, 2010.

[43] W. M. M. Levack, S. G. Dean, R. J. Siegert, and K. M. McPherson, "Navigating patient-centered goal setting in inpatient stroke rehabilitation: how clinicians control the process to meet perceived professional responsibilities," *Patient Education and Counseling*, vol. 85, no. 2, pp. 206–213, 2011.

[44] D. Regioner and Den Tværregionale Task Force, "Styring efter værdi for patienten," *Danish Regions, the Interregional Task Force. Control by Value for the Patient*, 2015, http://regioner.dk/media/1313/afrapportering-styring-efter-vaerdi-for-patienten.pdf.

[45] W. B. Mortenson and I. Dyck, "Power and client-centred practice: an insider exploration of occupational therapists' experiences," *Canadian Journal of Occupational Therapy*, vol. 73, no. 5, pp. 261–271, 2006.

[46] M. Müller, R. Strobl, and E. Grill, "Goals of patients with rehabilitation needs in acute hospitals: goal achivement is an indicator for improved functioning," *Journal of Rehabilitation Medicine*, vol. 43, no. 2, pp. 145–150, 2011.

[47] M. K. Dekkers and K. Søballe, "Activities and impairments in the early stage of rehabilitation after Colles' fracture," *Disability and Rehabilitation*, vol. 26, no. 11, pp. 662–668, 2009.

[48] J. Tracey, "The emotional response to the injury and rehabilitation process," *Journal of Applied Sport Psychology*, vol. 15, no. 4, pp. 279–293, 2003.

[49] Y.-H. Chen, S. Rodger, and H. Polatajko, "Experiences with the COPM and client-centred practice in adult neurorehabilitation in Taiwan," *Occupational Therapy International*, vol. 9, no. 3, 184 pages, 2002.

Integrating Occupational Therapy Specific Assessments in Practice: Exploring Practitioner Experiences

Eric Asaba,[1,2,3] Mio Nakamura,[4] Akie Asaba,[5] and Anders Kottorp[1,6]

[1] *Department of Neurobiology, Care Sciences, and Society (NVS), Division of Occupational Therapy, Karolinska Institutet, Alfred Nobels Allé 23, B4, Huddinge, Sweden*
[2] *Unit for Research, Education, and Development (FoUU), Stockholms Sjukhem Foundation, Stockholm, Sweden*
[3] *Department of Occupational Therapy, Tokyo Metropolitan University, Tokyo, Japan*
[4] *Department of Occupational Therapy, International University of Health and Welfare, Narita, Japan*
[5] *Karolinska University Hospital, Occupational Therapy and Physiotherapy Practice Areas, Huddinge, Sweden*
[6] *Faculty for Health and Society, Malmö University, Malmö, Sweden*

Correspondence should be addressed to Eric Asaba; eric.asaba@ki.se

Academic Editor: Patricia Belchior

Background. Occupational therapists sometimes find it challenging to integrate client-centered and occupational therapy specific assessments in practice. *The aim* of this study was to explore the use of occupational therapy specific assessments such as the Assessment of Motor and Process Skills (AMPS) among occupational therapists in Sweden and Japan. *Methods.* Interviews and qualitative thematic analyses were utilized. *Findings.* Four themes are reported: (1) use it or lose it, (2) simply no space until after hours, (3) biggest barriers can be colleagues, and (4) being more specific: communication. *Conclusion.* In keeping with previous studies, occupational therapists often find it challenging to implement client-centered and occupation-based assessment tools into practice. However, more work is needed to understand how best practices can be incorporated into a changing occupational therapy daily practice.

1. Introduction

Occupational therapists have during many decades used a wide range of formalized assessment tools, including tools borrowed from other disciplines, in order to provide relevant services to clients. During the last 20 years, the profession has seen a steady increase in the development and validation of assessment tools that more distinctly reflect occupational therapy domains of practice such as quality of occupational performance [1, 2], occupational gaps [3], and quality of social interaction [4] to name a few. Occupational therapists use assessment tools with an intended purpose to better guide intervention planning and to provide baseline and outcome measures in order to track progress and/or change among clients. For the purposes of this study, the authors adopt Fisher's [5] differentiation between occupation-centered, occupation-based, and occupation-focused assessments. Occupation-centered assessment refers to the centrality of occupation in informing decisions and action, a perspective; occupation-based assessment refers to situations in which occupation is a fundamental ingredient. Occupation-focused assessment refers to keeping the focus on occupation, with an immediate impact on occupational performance. For instance, an assessment in which occupation is performed as an essential part would by this definition be occupation-based, while an assessment in which goals pertaining to occupational performance are discussed and set, but where the particular occupations are not performed, would be occupation-focused.

2. Background

In a study conducted in northern Sweden, occupational therapists working in an acute hospital facility were interviewed regarding their experiences with integrating client-centeredness and occupation-focus into their practice based on the use of the Occupational Therapy Intervention and Process Model (OTIPM) [6]. Unsurprisingly, occupational therapists experienced a transformation of thought and action as they explicitly worked with a model to critically reflect on their own practices. Their experiences were imbued with both relief from the increased clarity with which they were working and ambiguity from hinders in the healthcare systems and the difficulties in changing organizational culture.

Contrary to the above depiction of deeply engaged therapists spending substantial time in continuing education and reflecting on their practice, it has also been documented that occupational therapists might find it challenging to incorporate specific tools in practice. In one study, 260 occupational therapists were surveyed, finding that occupational therapists most often choose an assessment tool because of availability and ease of administering the assessment (including ease of scoring and time efficiency) or that the tool facilitated client-centeredness [7]. In another study utilizing a survey and follow-up interviews, 50 therapists who had taken an AMPS course in England were asked about incorporating a new assessment in practice. [8]. Barriers to incorporating new assessment skills in clinical practice included the following: lack of support at the workplace, difficulty selecting appropriate clients, time to complete the assessment, and difficulties getting started. It was concluded that the successful implementation of an assessment tool such as AMPS in clinical practice would hinge upon receiving support from managers in the form of time, space for reflection, and invested resources in a continuum of learning [8]. These studies suggest that the utility of occupational therapy assessments might be explained by availability and ease of incorporation in practice rather than the soundness of the psychometric qualities of the assessment [7, 8].

Although client-centeredness and occupation are not new to occupational therapy, occupational therapists still find it difficult to incorporate client-centered and occupation-based or occupation-focused assessments in practice [7–10], even though occupational therapists place value on this type of assessment when asked. It is of importance to study the potential gap between practices in which occupation for different reasons cannot be integrated and a vision in which the value of occupation is central.

It is also relevant from an international perspective. A critique to the importation/exportation of theories (and implicitly assessments grounded in such theories) from one country context to another is well known [11]. It continues to be relevant and important to explore how occupational therapists reflect on their practice [12, 13] in order to situate clinical reasoning in different country/practice settings. Because the utility of assessments from a country/practice perspective is constantly evolving, it is of relevance to periodically and systematically explore experiences of using assessments among occupational therapists in different country/practice contexts.

The aim of this study is to explore the use of occupational therapy specific assessments such as the Assessment of Motor and Process Skills (AMPS) among occupational therapists working in Sweden and Japan.

Table 1: Aggregated demographics.

Demographics	Characteristic	$n = 19$
(i) Sex	Female	14
	Male	5
(ii) Country context	Sweden	7
	Japan	12
(iii) Work experience	General hospital (incl. rehabilitation)	11
	Home visit rehabilitation	1
	Education	3
	Nursing home	2
	Psychiatry facility	2
(iv) Interview style	Individual	8
	Focus group	11

3. Methods

3.1. Design. This study was based on qualitative interviews with occupational therapists from Sweden and Japan who had received training in the Assessment of Motor and Process Skills (AMPS) as well as other occupational therapy specific instruments such as A3 [14]. Data were analyzed in accordance with qualitative thematic analysis [15, 16]. All participants gave informed consent prior to being interviewed. The local ethics committee approved the study.

3.2. Participants. Information about the study was sent to occupational therapists in the A3 course database. The participants (14 women and 5 men) in this study expressed interest by making contact through email or telephone (see Table 1 for overview). Between the years 2004 and 2014, the A3 (formerly AAD) course was held 7 times with a total of 81 course participants (39 men and 42 women) in Japan and 8 times in Sweden with a total of 85 course participants (2 men and 83 women). A3, like the AMPS, requires each occupational therapist to submit 10 cases for calibration upon completion of the course. The validity of the instrument in Japanese and Swedish contexts as well as studies incorporating the assessment has been reported elsewhere [14, 17–23]. Recruitment from the A3 database was seen as relevant because all therapists would have also attended an AMPS course and would have recently taken an initiative to update their knowledge by having attended an A3 course.

All participants were licensed to practice occupational therapy in Japan or Sweden. In addition, all Japanese participants were calibrated AMPS raters. The participants in Japan had between 1 and 7 years of experience using AMPS (mean = 3; SD = 1.95) and participants in Sweden had 4–15 years of experience using AMPS (mean = 9; SD = 3.53). Among the participants, there were both those who used assessments on a regular basis and those who did not. Participant practice areas included the following: physical rehabilitation, home rehabilitation, psychiatry, and education. In order to uphold confidentiality, participant demographics are given in aggregate.

3.3. Data. Data gathering and analysis were iterative. The two country contexts represented geographic areas where there has been a strong interest in AMPS. This was relevant because by identifying challenges and support in integrating assessments such as these in different contexts new knowledge is facilitated in terms of strategies for integrating critical clinical reasoning in practice across different contexts. Moreover, this type of exploration has not previously been conducted over national borders or in Japan and Sweden.

Focus group interviews were initially used to build on the collective experiences of the participants. The method allowed members within the group to build on or refute experiences based on their own practice. However, due to the challenge of finding a common time and place, individual interviews were added to include perspectives that might otherwise be lost. It was possible to probe with questions in both the individual interviews and focus groups in order to integrate and deepen the information gathered.

Semistructured interview questions in conjunction with follow-up questions following general principles of qualitative research were used to gain an understanding of participant experiences [24]. All participants were interviewed on one occasion at a place of their convenience, which included their workplace, a seminar room at a university campus, a conference venue seminar room, or a café. Questions included the following: "can you tell me about how you use client-centered assessments in your practice," "what do you experience as challenges using these assessments," "what has made it possible for you to use these assessments," and "can you describe how these assessments help you in your practice?" The interviewer sometimes used more direct probes such as "can you describe in more detail?" or, in the case of a group interview, "has anyone else shared this experience?" In this way, the interviews were structured to develop richness around particular topics generated by both interviewer and participants. Interviews lasted between 45 and 90 minutes and were digitally recorded and transcribed. All interviews were performed by the first author or a research assistant in the project.

3.4. Data Analysis. The data analysis was based on techniques using thematic analysis [16, 25] and grounded in concepts of analyzing verbal narratives [15]. In keeping with thematic analytic, a back-and-forth process between interviewing and analysis was performed. All audio materials were transcribed near verbatim, retaining pauses, laughter, and nuances of expressions through bracketed qualifiers. These transcripts were carefully read and coded in three steps. All quotations used in this article were translated by the coauthors and the original Japanese text was maintained during the course of the analysis. The software program, Atlas.ti [26], was used during the analysis phase to code and organize data.

The data was analyzed inductively and although this process involved overlapping between steps, the procedure is outlined stepwise here for the purposes of clarity. All Swedish data were independently coded by the first author and all Japanese data were independently coded by the second author. The first author independently coded some of the Japanese data, which served as a way for the first and second authors to discuss and calibrate the coding process. During the analysis, all data were maintained in the original language. The first and second authors had regular meetings to compare and discuss coding during this phase. All data material was finally reviewed by the first author. The translation of quotes was performed by the first, second, and third authors and compared for accuracy. All authors were part of a discussion and interpretations of the findings.

In the first step, open coding entailed identifying and breaking the text into manageable bits that were assigned codes. Codes captured phenomena in one or a few words and were later applied to more segments of the text. Examples of early codes were "no space," "difficult to explain," and "don't have time" to name a few. In the second step, codes were merged and previously coded transcripts were revisited; existing as well as new codes within and across participants were sought by comparison across the data. In this way, both open coding and focused coding were used. Codes such as "don't have time" and "it takes time to prepare" were merged and codes such as "changing the schedule" and "evaluations after hours" contributed to a broader abstraction of the data. In the third step, similar codes were consolidated and organized into coherent groupings, whereby 4 themes were identified. These themes represent possibilities and barriers in using client-centered and occupational therapy specific assessments in practice.

4. Findings

Findings from the thematic analysis are presented in four themes. The title for each theme is taken from participant quotes under each theme. Although the naming of each theme is intended to be representative, each theme encompasses more than the phrase: (1) use it or lose it, (2) simply no space until after hours, (3) biggest barriers can be the work culture, and (4) being more specific: communication. The occupational therapists interviewed in this study unanimously communicated an interest in informing their practice with client-centeredness and occupation-focused and/or or occupation-based assessments and interventions. Yet obstacles were also described. Barriers were consistent for occupational therapists in both Swedish and Japanese contexts; however, it is also important to note that some participants in both contexts did not experience these problems. Finally, an interesting finding was that several participants, when pushed to reflect on what they could do to change their situation, reflected that they probably could incorporate more client-centeredness and occupation-based and occupation-focused practice into their work.

5. Use It or Lose It

Something that influenced the choice in what assessments to use was the participant's own familiarity with the assessment as well as the extent to which a particular assessment was situated as routine within their practice. One participant said the following:

> *I simply think, with regard to evaluations, if you don't use it you loose [sic] it and you just don't get it.*

Along the same lines, another participant expressed the following:

But often I experience that it is a bit slow in the beginning, but then the more I do the assessments the faster I get...and it takes time to sit with the AMPS bible, one has to look things up, and learn things, if one should put a 4 or a 2 or a 1 for each item...but it takes time, but then when one masters it, then it doesn't take as long.

All the participants used various assessments in practice but were here referring to occupational therapy specific assessments such as AMPS, A3, and COPM. According to these participants, these occupational therapy specific assessments often required more time and effort to perform than using hospital or facility specific ADL or goal checklists. On the other hand, participants were motivated to use the occupational therapy specific assessments because they felt that using these assessments yielded relevant information and made intervention planning clearer. Another participant says the following:

If one does many, it is better to do many AMPS, because the more one does the easier it gets. Because one has all the criteria in ones head. And one, like now when I've been gone for a while, then it's going to take a longer time. But that doesn't mean that I am going to refrain from it...I'll just have to offset some extra time instead, so that I can do it.

In this way, participants expressed a strong sense of integrity in being able to work according to best practices. However, strategies and priorities in making this work were highly individual for the participants in this study. Moreover, all participants felt that routine was a necessity in making assessments go smoothly.

The daily routine is too busy, there are so many things to learn, before I know it I actually cannot use an assessment. If I don't use it I don't know how to do it anymore, especially AMPS I find difficult so I end up not using it as frequently and in the end I might not be using it at all, sort of my situation now.

Participants expressed a need to create a routine for the use of occupational therapy specific assessments in practice. Moreover, experiences shared here also allude to certain challenges in creating routines, something that is taken up in subsequent themes.

6. Simply No Space until After Hours

Among participants, time was experienced as a significant factor impacting upon choices in day-to-day practices as well as the integration of practices to routines. A scarcity in time to complete all expected tasks within their workloads was one aspect in addition to the amount of time it took to perform an assessment such as AMPS, A3, or COPM to name a few. However, these experiences also need to be nuanced.

Well, actually, the staff know about AMPS and A3 and—I'd like to say that I don't have time, but actually if I wanted to make the time I could.

Participants expressed a subtle reflection about the possibility to actually do more if initiative was to be taken. Yet a common experience and sentiment among the participants was that time was a scare commodity. One participant said the following:

So if I do an ADL assessment in preparation for a team planning meeting, so I often do, so I choose Suunnas, because it is quicker. Because if I would do an entire formal AMPS it requires so much more sort of.

Another participant said the following:

And we block, if the patient is in a 4-person room and one chooses to do a shower task and make the bed, well then it takes a long time and then one blocks the bathroom very long.

Participants illustrated in their shared stories about everyday practices that each day was filled with choices based on weighing the pros and cons of choosing a lengthier versus shorter assessment, perhaps based on requiring observations or longer interviews. In the above situation, the participant reflected no ethical contemplation about the choice but rather expressed this as a matter of practicality. Another therapist summarized the sentiment: "I am simply too busy." However, when therapists felt that they should choose an occupation-based assessment but could not due to time or space, then it introduced a significantly more difficult dilemma. One therapist shared her individual solution to this dilemma:

I have to do evaluations outside of working hours. We only have one small rehab room for staff and clients to share, and in the morning we see about 10 clients and in the afternoon about 7 clients. There is simply no space to do an AMPS evaluation until afterhours.

Strategies such as these can also be seen as reflecting a degree of consideration for peers as well as clients, in avoiding a too great burden. A therapist in another facility responded about how the team solved issues around physical space:

But the more we fix our physical spaces to look like home environments, the easier it gets to do assessments. There are ironing boards, a kitchen, a bathroom, a bed to make and so forth. One works actively here so that patients can access familiar occupations, vacuum and so on.

Similarly, another therapist concurred that environment was an important element in being able to perform assessments such as AMPS.

If I tell the kitchen staff 3 days in advance, um, and oh yeah they ask "what do you need," for instance how many slices of bread, and they will prepare it, and the hospital covers the costs, and so it is sort of that type of environment, it is easy to manage, it is how it is for me but I realize that I should be thankful for the environment.

All occupational therapists who were interviewed in both Japanese and Swedish contexts concurred that time was scarce in relation to the volume of work that they felt needed to be done. Moreover, the physical environment was also experienced as relevant; however, the environment was to different degrees a barrier or possibility depending on organization.

7. Biggest Barriers Can Be the Work Culture

The impact of the work culture on choice of assessments was expressed as a barrier. When participants worked in teams where they experienced consensus and clear leadership, social conformity was in many ways a positive factor. One participant says the following:

One should have consensus, we have two rehabilitation programs and that steers us, because since we work at xx facility, it is a requirement for us to use valid and reliable instruments.

Another participant says the following:

What is there, what we use here is also. . .it should not just depend on me, what one choses, that one does an assessment.

Surprisingly, however, some therapists expressed that when this sense of consensus works to create a majority culture that does not include the use of client-centered or occupation-based assessments, the greatest challenge is the team itself. One participant says the following:

The biggest barriers are my occupational therapy colleagues. They choose a very biomechanical approach and when their clients see me with my client, they wonder why we are doing things differently and seemingly more fun. Then my colleagues make me feel like I should just do as they do.

The culture of the work environment is vital for the choices made by therapists. In some cases, this culture serves to strengthen a notion of client-centered practice and in other cases it serves to exclude those that try to introduce these ideas.

8. Being More Specific: Communication

The positive aspect of working in a client-centered and occupation-based manner was the ability to effectively communicate with clients regarding concrete observations in situations where the client had carried out tasks and where there were concrete understandings about where the person might have done well or was in need of assistance. One participant says the following:

It used to be difficult for me to communicate about performance concretely, but when using AMPS I can be more specific about what the person did (needed help with) and how it specifically related to real examples from daily life.

In this way, the use of AMPS provided an added value that could justify the added time or efforts in performing the assessment.

To be able to communicate is one thing, not only with the family, but with other staff members, it is sort of easier to explain. Since an actual occupation is used, it is clear what aspects the person is able to do or what the person is not able to do and this is directly connected to everyday life. When someone asks me, before it was difficult to be concrete, but with AMPS data I can be very specific about what I saw and how this is related to the goals and plans. I think this is something important.

For participants in this study, using an occupation-based assessment such as AMPS required a time investment for both the client and therapist. However, this process also gave the occupational therapist a greater degree of detail on which to base his/her assessment. This in turn led the participants to raise positive experiences about being able to be more concrete about the results of an assessment with an individual client as well as having a richer context around reported outcomes and intervention goals in a team or patient/family setting.

9. Discussion

The main findings from the study highlight what can facilitate and hinder the use of occupational therapy specific assessments in the context of occupational therapy practice in two different country contexts. The findings reflect that incorporating formalized occupational therapy evaluations in practice is challenging on multiple levels. The challenge of integrating new assessments into everyday habits and routines in clinical practice was noteworthy. This is not surprising but it can be concerning that occupational therapists choose assessments based on personal convenience rather than relevance for the case at hand. Given the instruments in focus for recruiting participants to this study, we revisit the Model of Human Occupation.

The Model of Human Occupation (MoHO) [27] can perhaps be useful in informing the lens through which we look when analyzing occupational therapists' experiences. MoHO has been characterized as a body of theory that explains how occupation is motivated, performed, and integrated in daily life. MoHO has primarily been applied to "patient" groups, although by definition applications should be possible to people that for one reason or another experience challenges in performing and/or changing their occupations. Of particular interest, here is the idea of habits and routines. Habitual behavior generally has to do with how people organize occupations in stable and repeatable routines; there is a certain element of automaticity and familiarity which comprises human behavior as habitual within the MoHO. This is of interest because the occupational therapists interviewed in this study raised the dilemma of changing habits in relation to practices in assessment procedures. From the perspective of the human as an occupational being [28, 29], the dilemma raised by the participants in this study can be understood as resistance or as a need to maintain routines in order to be able to work. In the Assessment of Motor and Process Skills (AMPS) manual [2], the need for systematically checking scoring criteria and not relying on habit is desirable for the purposes of validity and reliability of such a standardized evaluation. On the other hand, it is possible as participants in this study purported to establish habits and routines in the use of AMPS, even though the use of AMPS requires the systematic use of a manual. This is a concrete example of the complexity surrounding human occupation when applied to the everyday work of occupational therapists. As illustrated in the findings of this study, on one hand, habit is a necessity for finding a just right challenge and building competencies in performance. On the other hand, habitual action can impact upon the soundness of the results from assessments within occupational therapy practice, thus risking poor outcomes, especially when occupational therapists are implementing changes in their own evaluation practices. Understanding the balance between these two aspects and the need for critical reflection about one's minute practices is of high relevance for evidence-based and person-centered practice.

If occupational therapists choose assessments based more on access than on the immediate needs for the client, there is a risk that the client-centered aspects of practice also are undermined. Shifting power away from the healthcare provider toward the client, prioritizing goals relevant for the client, and focusing on enabling participation in society through occupation are important aspects of client-centeredness here and require the active utilization of relevant assessment tools and intervention models that place the client and his/her needs through occupation into focus. The risk of losing client-centeredness can emerge from small compromises in which a less relevant assessment tool is prioritized because of convenience and in so doing leading to goal setting and intervention planning that neglects empowering the client or focusing on what is most important for him/her [9, 30, 31].

Our findings suggest that the perceptions of the work context largely influenced the choice of a specific assessment. The implementation of new methods is influenced by various social networks. Most of the influencing factors described in our findings are related to individuals or to the organizational environment. Perhaps social networks, when optimal in function, can reduce situations where therapists do not prioritize what they believe is best practice. The participant who said "I'd like to say that I don't have time, but actually if I wanted to make the time I could" reflects something of a dilemma in that the therapist shows a sense of awareness about something lacking in her practice and yet chooses not to prioritize what she considers best practice. Based upon the findings in this study, this phenomenon or trend is something that occupational therapists need to look more carefully at in order to improve possibilities for changing practices and for further work in the integration of research and clinical practice [6, 32]. Although being beyond the scope of this paper, it can also be of interest for occupational therapists to look at implementation science as a way to facilitate the integration of best practices [33].

This study also highlights a discrepancy between how occupational therapists think they should work and how they actually work. The difficulty of incorporating knowledge and changing practice has been reported elsewhere [7, 8, 34, 35]; however, it is interesting to note that incorporating thinking about one's practice seems to be characteristic of therapists who have engaged in continued education [36]. Initially, the authors expected notable differences in experience based on country context; however, the data does not support this assumption. Instead, more generic aspects of practice context and organizational culture appear to have a stronger influence on the implementation process. In order to find innovative strategies to bridge gaps between recommendations and usual practice within clinical settings, it is vital to know what factors impact upon implementation of new methods.

Limitations. There are several limitations to this study. It was not possible to conduct data gathering in two country contexts within the same period, which meant that interview guides could not be revised based on two country contexts. On the other hand, the aim of the study was not to compare country contexts but rather to use Sweden and Japan because both were contexts in which many occupational therapists with AMPS training were active and also were in an active process of learning and implementing additional client-centered and occupation-based or occupation-focused evaluations in practice. The two contexts were thought to contribute with different cultural dimensions. Interestingly, the findings would suggest that Swedish and Japanese contexts have less to do with occupational therapy specific assessments than the practice contexts.

A limitation was that only therapists with initial AMPS and A3 training were recruited. Since there is previous research suggesting that it is difficult to implement time-intensive tools such as AMPS in practice, despite extensive training and in fact also suggested in the findings from this study, then it is of relevance to look at occupational therapists that arguably have optimal conditions. Another limitation is that information about why potential participants did not participate is not available. Information about the study was circulated to course participants in the A3 course database. There can be several reasons for why people did not respond, including the fact that email addresses could have changed, lack of interest in the study, or other competing priorities to name a few. It is possible that those who took initiative to participate were particularly interested in actively pursuing the use of AMPS and A3 in their practices.

Another limitation is that some interview questions were formulated, such as "what do you experience as challenges using these assessments?" or "can you describe how these assessments were helpful in practice?" This can be seen as biasing in that the questions assume that something was challenging or helpful. On the other hand, it is natural in both Swedish and Japanese to talk about challenges and possibilities. If questions had only been about challenges, the bias might have been more limiting; however, in this case, the questions get at two sides of a phenomenon.

Finally, it can be a limitation to have combined individual and focus group interviews because the type of data generated is different. However, the benefits of enriching the data by including individual interviews were seen to outweigh the drawbacks. Some participants had little flexibility in their schedules and therefore found it difficult to participate at the set time and place for a focus group. By incorporating individual interviews, the data also reflects voices among those who would not otherwise have been included.

10. Conclusion

The aim of this study was to explore occupational therapists' experiences in implementing the AMPS in combination with other client-centered and occupation-based or occupation-focused assessments within various clinical practice settings in Sweden and Japan. In keeping with previous studies, occupational therapists in a myriad of clinical and country contexts find it challenging to implement client-centered and occupation-based assessment tools into practice. More work is needed to understand how best practices can be implemented and sustained through the whole continuum of occupational therapy practice.

Disclosure

The authors alone are responsible for the content and writing of the paper. The study was conducted as an add-on to follow up the first author's postdoc project referred to in the manuscript.

Acknowledgments

The authors would like to thank all the participants for sharing their experiences and time. The study was partly funded by a grant from Karolinska Institutet, Center for Caring Sciences (Grant no. 1220/05-226). Special thanks are extended to colleagues at the Division of Occupational Therapy at Karolinska Institutet who have been part of the process and also to those who assisted in the work along the way: Yu Ishibashi, Sanna Edensand, Annikki Jauring, and Peter Bontje. Furthermore, the completion of the manuscript was in part made possible through a mobility grant from Tokyo Metropolitan University where Mio Nakamura was a doctoral student at the time.

References

[1] M. Law, S. Baptiste, M. A. McColl, A. Opzoomer, H. Polatajko, and N. Pollock, "The Canadian occupational performance measure: an outcome measure for occupational therapy," *Canadian Journal of Occupational Therapy*, vol. 57, no. 2, pp. 82–87, 1990.

[2] A. G. Fisher, *Assessment of Motor and Process Skills: Development, Standardization and Administration Manual*, vol. 1, Three Star Press, Fort Collins, Colo, USA, 5th edition, 2003.

[3] G. Eriksson, K. Tham, and J. Borg, "Occupational gaps in everyday life 1–4 years after acquired brain injury," *Journal of Rehabilitation Medicine*, vol. 38, no. 3, pp. 159–165, 2006.

[4] A. G. Fisher and L. A. Griswold, *Evaluation of Social Interaction*, Three Star Press, Fort Collins, Colo, USA, 2009.

[5] A. G. Fisher, "Occupation-centred, occupation-based, occupation-focused: Same, same or different?" *Scandinavian Journal of Occupational Therapy*, vol. 20, no. 3, pp. 162–173, 2013.

[6] M. Sirkka, K. Zingmark, and M. Larsson-Lund, "A process for developing sustainable evidence-based occupational therapy practice," *Scandinavian Journal of Occupational Therapy*, vol. 21, no. 6, pp. 429–437, 2014.

[7] N. M. Alotaibi, K. Reed, and M. S. Nadar, "Assessments used in occupational therapy practice: an exploratory study," *Occupational Therapy in Health Care*, vol. 23, no. 4, pp. 302–318, 2009.

[8] G. Chard, "An investigation into the use of the Assessment of Motor and Process Skills (AMPS) in clinical practice," *The British Journal of Occupational Therapy*, vol. 63, no. 10, pp. 481–488, 2000.

[9] J. I. K. Öhman and E. Asaba, "Goal setting in occupational therapy: a narrative study exploring theory and practice in psychiatry," *World Federation of Occupational Therapists Bulletin*, vol. 60, no. 1, pp. 22–28, 2014.

[10] T. Kaneyama and K. Inoue, "A survey of ADL assessment approaches used by occupational therapists in practice," *Okayama Journal of Occupational Therapy*, vol. 19, no. 1, pp. 13–22, 2010 (Japanese).

[11] M. Iwama, "Toward culturally relevant epistemologies in occupational therapy," *American Journal of Occupational Therapy*, vol. 57, no. 5, pp. 582–588, 2003.

[12] C. Mattingly, "In search of the good: Narrative reasoning in clinical practice," *Medical Anthropology Quarterly*, vol. 12, no. 3, pp. 273–297, 1998.

[13] C. Mattingly, *Healing Dramas and Clinical Plots: The Narrative Structure of Experience*, Cambridge University Press, Cambridge, UK, 1998.

[14] E. Asaba, I. Petersson, P. Bontje, and A. Kottorp, "The assessment of awareness of ability (A3) in a Japanese context: A Rasch model application," *Scandinavian Journal of Occupational Therapy*, vol. 19, no. 4, pp. 370–376, 2012.

[15] D. E. Polkinghorne, "Narrative configuration in qualitative analysis," *International Journal of Qualitative Studies in Education*, vol. 8, no. 1, pp. 5–23, 1995.

[16] C. Pope, S. Ziebland, and N. Mays, "Analysing qualitative data," in *Qualitative Research in Healthcare*, C. Pope and N. Mays, Eds., Blackwell Publishing Ltd, Malden, Mass, USA, 3rd edition, 2006.

[17] E. Asaba and A. Asaba, "Towards client-centered and occupation-based evaluation and intervention: A case study," *Okayama Journal of Occupational Therapy*, 2010.

[18] A. G. Fisher, L. A. Griswold, M. Munkholm, and A. Kottorp, "Evaluating domains of everyday functioning in people with developmental disabilities," *Scandinavian Journal of Occupational Therapy*, vol. 24, no. 1, pp. 1–9, 2017.

[19] A. Kottorp, B. Heuchemer, I. P. Lie, and C. H. Gumpert, "Evaluation of activities of daily living ability and awareness among clients in a forensic psychiatry evaluation unit in Sweden," *The*

British Journal of Occupational Therapy, vol. 76, no. 1, pp. 23–30, 2013.

[20] A. Kottorp, L. Ekstam, and I. Petersson Lie, "Differences in awareness between persons with left and right hemispheric stroke," *Scandinavian Journal of Occupational Therapy*, vol. 20, no. 1, pp. 37–44, 2013.

[21] A. Kottorp and I. Petersson, "Psychometric evaluation of an assessment of awareness using two different Rasch models," *Scandinavian Journal of Occupational Therapy*, vol. 18, no. 3, pp. 219–230, 2011.

[22] A. Öhman, L. Nygård, and A. Kottorp, "The relationship between occupational performance and awareness of disability in older adults with cognitive impairment or dementia," *Scandinavian Journal of Occupational Therapy*, vol. 18, pp. 133–142, 2011.

[23] R. L. Anderson, S. E. Doble, B. K. Merritt, and A. Kottorp, "Assessment of awareness of disability measures among persons with acquired brain injury," *Canadian Journal of Occupational Therapy*, vol. 77, no. 1, pp. 22–29, 2010.

[24] I. Seidman, *Interviewing as Qualitative Research: A Guide for Researchers in Education and the Social Sciences*, Teachers College Press, New York, NY, USA, 2nd edition, 1998.

[25] L. Ayres, "Thematic coding and analysis," in *The SAGE Encyclopedia of Qualitative Research Methods*, L. Given, Ed., Sage Publications Inc, Thousand Oaks, Calif, USA, 2008.

[26] T. Muhr, *ATLAS.ti. WIN 4.2 Build 061*, Scientific Software Development, Berlin, Germany, 1997.

[27] G. Kielhofner, *Model of Human Occupation: Theory and Application*, Lippincott Williams & Wilkins, Balitmore, Md, USA, 4th edition, 2008.

[28] A. Wilcock, *An Occupational Perspective of Health*, SLACK Inc, Thorofare, NJ, USA, 1998.

[29] M. P. Cutchin, R. M. Aldrich, A. L. Bailliard, and S. Coppola, "Action theories for occupational science: The contributions of Dewey and Bourdieu," *Journal of Occupational Science*, vol. 15, no. 3, pp. 157–165, 2008.

[30] K. K. Maitra and F. Erway, "Perception of client-centered practice in occupational therapists and their clients," *American Journal of Occupational Therapy*, vol. 60, no. 3, pp. 298–310, 2006.

[31] E. Wressle and K. Samuelsson, "Barriers and bridges to client-centred occupational therapy in Sweden," *Scandinavian Journal of Occupational Therapy*, vol. 11, no. 1, pp. 12–16, 2004.

[32] M. Sirkka, M. Larsson-Lund, and K. Zingmark, "Occupational therapists' experiences of improvement work: A journey towards sustainable evidence-based practice," *Scandinavian Journal of Occupational Therapy*, vol. 21, no. 2, pp. 90–97, 2014.

[33] C. R. May, M. Johnson, and T. Finch, "Implementation, context and complexity," *Implementation Science*, vol. 11, no. 1, article 141, pp. 1–12, 2016.

[34] D. Upton, D. Stephens, B. Williams, and L. Scurlock-Evans, "Occupational therapists' attitudes, knowledge, and implementation of evidence-based practice: A systematic review of published research," *The British Journal of Occupational Therapy*, vol. 77, no. 1, pp. 24–38, 2014.

[35] E. A. Balas and S. A. Boren, "Managing clinical knowledge for health care improvement," in *Yearbook of Medical Informatics 2000: Patient-Centered Systems*, J. Bemmel and A. T. McCray, Eds., pp. 65–70, Schattauer Verlagsgesellschaft, Stuttgart, Germany, 2000.

[36] L. Nygård, A. Kottorp, and L. Rosenberg, "Making use of research: Clinical views on an evaluation of everyday technology use," *Scandinavian Journal of Occupational Therapy*, vol. 22, no. 1, pp. 24–32, 2015.

Effect of Community-Based Occupational Therapy on Health-Related Quality of Life and Engagement in Meaningful Activities of Women with Breast Cancer

Daiva Petruseviciene,[1] Deive Surmaitiene,[2] Daiva Baltaduoniene,[1] and Egle Lendraitiene[1]

[1] *Department of Rehabilitation, Medical Academy, Lithuanian University of Health Sciences, Kaunas, Lithuania*
[2] *Kulautuva Hospital of Rehabilitation, Hospital of Lithuanian University of Health Sciences Kauno Klinikos, Kaunas, Lithuania*

Correspondence should be addressed to Daiva Petruseviciene; daiva.petruseviciene@lsmuni.lt

Academic Editor: Mélanie Levasseur

We aimed to evaluate the short-term effects of community-based occupational therapy on health-related quality of life and engagement in meaningful activities among women with breast cancer. An open label randomized controlled trial study design was applied. The participants were members of various societies of women with cancer. In total, 22 women have participated in the study. Participants of the experimental group ($n = 11$) participated in a 6-week community-based occupational therapy program and the usual activities of various societies, whereas the control group ($n = 11$) women participated in the usual activities of the societies only. 1 of the participants withdrew during the course; therefore 21 completed the study successfully. Participants of both groups were assessed for health-related quality of life and the participants of the experimental group were assessed for engagement in meaningful activities. The evaluation was carried out during the nonacute period of the disease—at the beginning of the study and after 6 weeks. Women of the experimental group demonstrated statistically significantly better scores in the global quality of life, role functions, physical, emotional, cognitive, and social functions, fatigue, insomnia, financial impact, systemic therapy side effects, and breast symptoms scales compared to the control group participants ($p < 0.05$) after the 6 weeks, as measured by the *EORTC QLQ-C30* questionnaire and its breast cancer module *QLQ-BR23*. Furthermore, women of the experimental group demonstrated significant greater engagement in meaningful activities when applying community-based occupational therapy ($p < 0.05$), as measured by using the Engagement in Meaningful Activities Survey (EMAS). The evaluation of the associations between the women's engagement in meaningful activities and changes in health-related quality of life showed that greater engagement in meaningful activities was associated with better emotional functions and a lower level of insomnia ($p < 0.05$). Based on the results of our study, we recommend applying occupational therapy in the field of community healthcare in order to maintain or improve breast cancer patients' health-related quality of life and suggest involving women into meaningful activities during community-based occupational therapy after clarifying which activities are important to them.

1. Introduction

On the global scale, cancer causes one-seventh of all deaths. According to the most recent estimates, there have been over 14 million new cases of cancer and over 8 million deaths from cancer registered worldwide, and it is expected that, due to the increasing numbers and aging of the population, these numbers will increase to, accordingly, 21.7 million and 13 million by the year 2030 [1].

Breast cancer, defined by the National Cancer Institute as cancer forming in breast tissues, is the most common malignant tumor among women and in as many as 19 out of 21 regions it is the leading cause of death among women in both the developed and the developing countries [2–4].

Over 1.5 million new cases of invasive breast cancer are registered globally every year, and this is the single most common form of cancer among women that is prevalent in absolutely all regions of the world [2, 5]. In European countries, breast cancer is also the most frequently diagnosed malignant tumor in women, and the prevalence of this disease has been increasing in most countries over the last decades [3, 6]. Despite the continuous improvement in the diagnostic and treatment techniques, breast cancer remains one of the most common cancers among women in Lithuania as well as in the rest of the world (in Lithuania, breast cancer is currently the second most common cancer after skin cancer (melanoma) and is undoubtedly their most urgent health problem). Even though survival rates in Lithuania are among the lowest, the overall situation is improving: breast cancer is detected at increasingly earlier stages, and women's survival is improving [7].

Unfortunately, the completion of breast cancer treatment does not mean the end of the disease [8]. Healthcare institutions with all the necessary services and specialists ensure integrated assistance to breast cancer patients. However, after discharge, women frequently experience emotional stress because of short-term or long-term adverse effects of the therapy, the risk of recurrence, difficulty getting information about their health status and its possible changes, financial problems, difficulty getting back to work, impaired sexual life, and so forth. Improving survival rates and the risk of late-onset adverse reactions increase the need for healthcare and rehabilitation services on the community level [3, 9, 10]. Consequently, quality of life questions related to the financial impact of the disease, concern about the future of the family, fear of disease recurrence, insufficient preparation for possible late-onset adverse reactions to the treatment, and possible changes in social support become increasingly relevant [11].

Today, it is the field of health-related quality of life that is being most actively developed in Lithuania as well as abroad [12]. Over the last several decades, breast cancer treatment has become more effective, which resulted in a significant increase in patients' long-term survival. Schoormans et al. (2015) stated that because of this, researchers had to focus increasingly on long-term consequences of the disease or the treatment, which they related to the quality of life, thus developing the concept of breast cancer patients' health-related quality of life [13].

The impact of the diagnosis and treatment of breast cancer differs depending on the patient, resulting in varying numbers and degrees of physical and psychological sequelae. The consequences may significantly impair a woman's ability to participate in meaningful activities, including housework, return to work, and adequate performance of the main social roles and responsibilities. This, in turn, may negatively affect the economic status and disrupt interpersonal relations, thus further impairing the woman's engagement in meaningful activities as well as her psychoemotional status and the quality of life. Despite the fact that the combined effect of breast cancer and its treatment may manifest themselves at any moment and last for a very long time, it is essential for the patients to resume their daily roles as soon as possible after the completion of the treatment and this is where the role of the occupational therapist is especially important [14]. According to Pergolotti et al. (2016), the economic effectiveness of occupational therapy and its usefulness in reducing disease consequences have already been proven, and yet occupational therapy is still rarely applied in the rehabilitation of cancer patients [15].

The theory of occupational therapy states that human subsistence is a social process, and people need meaningful activity; its absence is a major threat to human health, and thus occupational therapists in their professional practice strive to achieve their patients' maximum capacity to increase their ability to engage in activities that they see as important and meaningful [16, 17]. According to Cook and Thompson (2015), the meaningfulness of life significantly affects a person's physical, mental, and social wellbeing. Engagement in purposeful activities contributes to the satisfaction of the need for the meaningfulness of life, but only if this activity motivates the person, is interesting, can be successfully completed, and helps to achieve other significant aims. Engagement in purposeful activities directly affects a person's emotional condition, self-esteem, and self-confidence. Purposeful activities have been recognized as directly affecting the quality of life, and thus an important task when working with a patient is to clarify which activities are important for him or her. When purposeful activity is selected in accordance with the person's interests and priorities, it becomes meaningful [18]. Occupational therapists strive to and can help cancer patients live a meaningful life, be self-sufficient, participate in activities, be able to manage themselves and others, engage in work, leisure, and health promotion activities, and be a part of social groups and the family [16]. Occupational therapists' holistic approach and creative decisions may improve breast cancer patients' cognitive and physical capacity, mental health, and the quality of life [15].

When working in communities, occupational therapists have to be familiar with the characteristics of community-based activity in order to be able to pursue meaningful activities based on the community members' priorities. Active participation in community activities, social support, and engagement in meaningful activities positively affect community members' health and the quality of life [19]. Based on this theory, we wanted to determine the influence of community-based occupational therapy on breast cancer patients' health-related quality of life and engagement in meaningful activities.

No similar research was found and we were the first in Lithuania who made a study analyzing changes in health-related quality of life, engagement in meaningful activities, and its associations among breast cancer patients when applying occupational therapy in the field of community healthcare. We hope that the results of our study will be useful for occupational therapists working with breast cancer patients' communities.

Consequently, all these reasons have affected the following aim of the study: to evaluate the short-term effects of community-based occupational therapy on health-related quality of life and engagement in meaningful activities among women with breast cancer.

2. Methods

This randomized controlled trial was conducted with the permission of the Bioethics Center of the Lithuanian University of Health Sciences (number BEC-SR(M)-186), the permission of the European Organization for Research and Treatment of Cancer (EORTC) Quality of Life Group to use the quality of life questionnaire EORTC QLQ-C30 and its module EORTC QLQ-BR23 in the study, and the permission of the Associate Professor A. M. Eakman from Colorado State University to use the Engagement in Meaningful Activities Survey (EMAS) in the study. The study was performed during May–June 2016 in Kaunas city, with the mediation of the chairwomen of two societies of women who either had overcome their breast cancer or were still fighting it on the community level.

Eligible women were adult (≥18 years of age) and Lithuanian-speaking, with diagnosed breast cancer and functional status being ≤2b according to the ECOG *(Eastern Cooperative Oncology Group)* scale of performance status, were able to understand the essence of the study and simple instructions, were familiarized with the aim of the study, and volunteered to participate. Exclusion criteria were the following: refusal to participate in the study, women with severe decompensated comorbidities and mental diseases, and being incapable of independently filling out the questionnaires, and whose functional status was >2b according to the ECOG scale of performance status.

All the participants who met the inclusion criteria were in advance familiarized with the study, its aims, objectives, and methods, the confidentiality of the data, and the possibility of withdrawing from the study at any time and provided a written consent to participate in the study.

In total, 22 members of breast cancer patients' societies met the inclusion criteria. All participants had been diagnosed with breast cancer (code C50 according to the ICD-10-AM). The participants were randomly distributed into two groups: the experimental group and the control group, following simple randomization procedure (computerized random numbers). The distribution of the participants was equal in both groups. The participants were also distributed into two groups based on the analyzed characteristics: age, employment status, the duration of the disease, the stage of the disease, the location of the tumor, metastases, and functional status according to the ECOG. Detailed characteristics of the participants are presented in Table 1.

There were no significant differences in the participants' distribution between the groups concerning their age ($\chi^2(1) = 0$, $p = 1$), employment status ($p = 1$), the duration of the disease ($\chi^2(1) = 0$, $p = 1$), the stage of the disease ($p = 0.311$), the location of the tumor ($\chi^2(1) = 0$, $p = 1$), metastases ($p = 1$), or functional status according to the ECOG ($p = 1$), $p > 0.05$.

During the study, we evaluated changes in women health-related quality of life and experimental group participants' engagement in meaningful activities during the nonacute period of the disease. The methods used in the study were the following: a survey using a questionnaire designed by the author, testing, experiment, and statistical data analysis. During the survey, we evaluated the participants' sociodemographic data (age and employment status) and clinical factors: the duration of the disease, the stage of the disease, the location of the tumor, metastases, and functional status according to the ECOG. Testing was conducted twice: at the beginning of the study and after 6 weeks. In order to evaluate changes in the participants' health-related quality of life, we used the EORTC QLQ-C30 questionnaire and its module QLQ-BR23. The principal questionnaire, EORTC QLQ-C30, consists of 30 questions forming the global health status and quality of life scale, five functional scales, three symptom scales, and six separately evaluated components. The EORTC module QLQ-BR23 is a more specific questionnaire designed for breast cancer patients and consisting of 23 questions forming four functional scales and four symptom scales. After the calculation of the results according to the formulas presented by the authors, the score intervals in all scales and separately evaluated components ranged from 0 to 100 points. The questionnaires have been translated and adapted in many languages including Lithuanian and are suitable for the evaluation of cancer patients' health-related quality of life. In Lithuania, Banienė and Šinkariova (2015) evaluated the internal consistency of the scales of those questionnaires ($0.6 \leq \alpha \leq 0.9$) and, based on the obtained results, stated that the questionnaires are suitable for studies of breast cancer patients [20].

The testing of the experimental group participants' engagement in meaningful activities was also conducted at baseline and at the end of the study, using the Engagement in Meaningful Activities Survey. This survey has not been translated into Lithuanian and has not been adapted in Lithuania. For this reason, studies for the evaluation of the reliability and validity of the survey should be conducted. The results of the survey on engagement in meaningful activities reflect the level of the subjects' engagement in meaningful activities. The survey consists of 12 statements, each of which has the minimal value of 1 point and the maximal value of 4 points, where 1 point means "rarely"; 2 points, sometimes; 3 points, often; and 4 points, always. Engagement in meaningful activities was evaluated by a sum score. There is a growing body of scientific literature validating the psychometric properties of this test. The association of the results of this test with those of the evaluation of satisfaction with life and health-related quality of life has already been proven. Eakman with coauthors (2010) have proven the test-retest reliability of this instrument ($r = 0.56$) and evaluated the internal consistency of the scale ($\alpha = 0.89$), using the English version of this test in adult population [21]. All study participants filled out the questionnaires independently.

During the course of the study, the women participated in a 6-week community-based occupational therapy program and the usual activities of various societies, whereas the control group women participated in the usual activities of the societies only.

The community-based occupational therapy program was designed taking into account the most common sequelae of breast cancer and its treatment identified in literature: arm swelling, reduced range of motion of the arm, fatigue,

Table 1: Participants' characteristics.

Characteristic	Total n (%)	Experimental group n (%)	p value ⟷	Control group n (%)
Age				
Young or middle-aged (18–59 years)	11 (50)	6 (54.5)	1*	5 (45.5)
Elderly or old (60–80 years)	11 (50)	5 (45.5)		6 (54.5)
Employment status				
Employed or a student	9 (40.9)	4 (36.4)	1**	5 (45.5)
Unemployed, housewife, retired, or not working because of disability	13 (59.1)	7 (63.6)		6 (54.5)
Duration of disease				
<5 years	11 (50)	5 (45.5)	1*	6 (54.5)
≥5 years	11 (50)	6 (54.5)		5 (45.5)
Stage of the disease				
0, I, or II	17 (77.3)	10 (90.9)	0.311**	7 (63.6)
III or IV	5 (22.7)	1 (9.1)		4 (36.4)
Location of the tumor				
Left	12 (54.5)	6 (54.5)	1*	6 (54.5)
Right	10 (45.5)	5 (45.5)		5 (45.5)
Metastases				
Present	3 (13.6)	1 (9.1)	1**	2 (18.2)
Absent	19 (86.4)	10 (90.9)		9 (81.8)
Functional status according to ECOG				
0 or 1 b.	17 (77.3)	8 (72.7)	1**	9 (81.8)
2 b.	5 (22.7)	(27.3)		2 (18.2)

*Statistical significance was determined according to the χ^2 criterion with Yates correction, no significant differences between the groups, $p \geq 0.05$. **Statistical significance was determined according to Fisher's exact criterion, no significant differences between the groups, $p > 0.05$.

and impaired quality of life. According to Scaffa and Reitz (2014), active participation in community activities, social support, and engagement in meaningful activities have a positive effect on community members' health and quality of life [19]. Cook and Thompson (2015) supported this opinion stating that meaningful activities improve the quality of life [18]. For this reason, by applying this program, we strived to improve not only the experimental group participants' health-related quality of life, but also their engagement in meaningful activities.

During the study, we applied occupational therapy in groups. During each session, purposeful activities were combined with creative techniques, and the sessions were made meaningful through voluntary assistance to others, that is, emotional help when communicating with other women who had the same problems and so forth. The experimental group participants also received individual consultations by an occupational therapist if needed.

Duration of the program consisted of six meetings. The description of the program is provided in Table 2.

Occupational therapy sessions in groups were organized four times: once weekly at an arranged time in the evening (after work), up to 1.5 hours/day.

Note that the sessions in occupational therapy groups took place in a cozy and comfortable environment, and all the tools and materials required for the activities were supplied and were of good quality. Prior to the sessions, the participants received all the necessary information, and the focus during the sessions was on the process rather than on the results.

Statistical data analysis was conducted using the *IBM SPSS Statistics 22* software. The data were described by using the standard numeral characteristics (min and max values, median, and mean). The distributions were compared by applying the nonparametric criteria. Two dependent samples before and after the intervention were compared by applying the nonparametric Wilcoxon criterion and two independent samples by using the Mann–Whitney-Wilcoxon criterion. In order to determine the presence of a relationship between engagement in meaningful activities and health-related quality of life, we calculated Spearman's correlation coefficient. The difference or the relationship between the indices were considered to be statistically significant when $p < 0.05$.

3. Results

After six weeks, of 22 women randomized into the study, 21 completed the trial. The experimental group consisted of 10 participants and the control group consisted of 11. One woman withdrew from the study because of breast cancer recurrence. During the study, when applying occupational

TABLE 2: Description of the application of the occupational therapy program in the community of women with breast cancer.

	Topic	Aims	Activities
Session I	The beginning of the study	Familiarization, presentation of the study and the planned program, and initiation of the study.	Self-introduction and presentation of the study, a report on the topic of the study, initial filing out of the questionnaires, questions, and answers.
Session *II*	*"Plant and Give"*	Socializing, cooperation, increasing the hand movement amplitude or prevention, development of positive emotions, and sharing positive experience and emotions with those facing the same or similar problems.	Sapling replanting (gardening therapy), advice and discussions about the hand movement amplitude, and donation of saplings to hospitalized women with breast cancer.
Session *III*	*"Origami Crane – the Gift of Hope"*	Experiencing relaxation and calmness, expression of emotions, socialization, prevention or reduction of lymphedema, and sharing positive experience and emotions with those facing the same or similar problems.	Folding paper cranes (art therapy) + a lecture, exercises, and discussions on lymphedema treatment and prevention, as well as on an occupational therapist's assistance.
Session *IV*	*"Sharing the Strength"*	Experiencing relaxation and calmness, expression of emotions, socialization, presentation of the energy conservation principles and their practical application, and sharing positive experience and emotions with those facing the same or similar problems.	Making an original picture postcard (art therapy) while listening to specially selected calm music (music therapy) + a lecture and discussions on fatigue and energy conservation techniques (planning, adjustment of the environment, biomechanics of the body, etc.).
Session *V*	*"Knitting for Preterm Newborns"*	Gratuitous assistance.	Knitting socks + a lecture on the need for socks and donation of socks to preterm newborns.
Session VI	The end of the study	Discussion on the work done, sharing impressions and results, and conclusion of the study.	Summing-up of the program, repeated filling out of the questionnaires, feedback, discussions, questions/answers, etc.

therapy in the community, we strove to improve the participants' engagement in meaningful activities and thus their health-related quality of life. For this reason, the women's active participation in the assignments was highly important for us, and thus, to determine the actual impact of the applied program on the aforementioned indices, we only calculated the results for women who were involved in the study.

The health-related quality of life of women with breast cancer was evaluated during the nonacute period of the disease by calculating the scores in separate scales of the EORTC QLQ-C30 questionnaire and its module QLQ-BR23. The score could range from 0 to 100 points. A higher score in the global quality of life scale indicated better quality of life, a higher score in the functional scales better functioning, and a higher score in the symptom scales a greater degree of the manifestation of the symptom.

The evaluation of the participants' health-related quality of life at baseline using the EORTC QLQ-C30 questionnaire and its module QLQ-BR23 showed that the groups were homogeneous, $p > 0.05$ (Table 3).

Prior to the application of the community-based occupational therapy, the poorest evaluations in the EORTC QLQ-C30 questionnaire among the experimental group participants were on the global quality of life (50 (33.33–83.33; 50.75)), emotional functions (50 (8.33–100; 52.27)), cognitive functions (50 (0–83.33; 54.55)), and social functions (50 (16.67–83.33; 48.49)). The participants were also found to demonstrate the highest degrees of the manifestation of insomnia (66.67 (0–100; 66.67)) and the financial difficulties (66.67 (33.33–100; 69.7)). The results of the EORTC QLQ-BR23 questionnaire showed that the participants gave the poorest evaluations of the future perspective (33.33 (0–66.67; 33.33)) and demonstrated the highest degrees of the manifestation of breast symptoms (41.67 (8.33–75; 38.64)) such as pain, edema, tenderness, or skin problems.

Among the control group participants, the poorest evaluations in the EORTC QLQ-C30 questionnaire at baseline

TABLE 3: Distribution of evaluation scores in health-related quality of life questionnaire scales in the groups at baseline.

Scales of the quality of life questionnaires	Experimental group n (11)	Experimental group $x_{me}(x_{min}-x_{max}; \bar{x})$	$U; p$ $\longleftrightarrow$	Control group n (11)	Control group $x_{me}(x_{min}-x_{max}; \bar{x})$
		EORTC QLQ C-30			
Global health status/QoL	11	50 (33.33–83.33; 50.75)	41.5; 0.217	11	58.33 (33.33–91.67; 59.85)
Functional scales					
Physical functioning	11	60 (40–86.67; 63.64)	50; 0.519	11	73.33 (46.67–86.67; 67.88)
Role functioning	11	66.67 (16.67–100; 68.18)	60; 1	11	66.67 (33.33–100; 69.7)
Emotional functioning	11	50 (8.33–100; 52.27)	36.5; 0.116	11	66.67 (8.33–100; 65.91)
Cognitive functioning	11	50 (0–83.33; 54.55)	35.5; 0.101	11	83.33 (50–100; 72.73)
Social functioning	11	50 (16.67–83.33; 48.49)	32; 0.065	11	66.67 (50–100; 69.7)
Symptom scales					
Fatigue	11	55.56 (33.33–77.78; 54.55)	54.5; 0.699	11	44.44 (11.11–88.89; 50.5)
Nausea and vomiting	11	0 (0–50; 7.58)	54.5; 0.699	11	0 (0–66.67; 12.12)
Pain	11	33.33 (0–83.33; 34.85)	56; 0.797	11	33.33 (0–83.33; 28.79)
Dyspnoea	11	0 (0–33.33; 15.15)	50; 0.519	11	33.33 (0–66.67; 24.24)
Insomnia	11	66.67 (0–100; 66.67)	39; 0.171	11	66.67 (0–66.67; 48.49)
Appetite loss	11	0 (0–33.33; 9.09)	44; 0.3	11	33.33 (0–33.33; 18.18)
Constipation	11	33.33 (0–100; 42.42)	48; 0.438	11	0 (0–100; 24.24)
Diarrhoea	11	0 (0–66.67; 9.09)	60; 1	11	0 (0–100; 12.12)
Financial difficulties	11	66.67 (33.33–100; 69.7)	42; 0.243	11	66.67 (0–100; 51.52)
		EORTC QLQ BR-23			
Functional scales					
Body image	11	58.33 (0–83.33; 51.51)	28.5; 0.562	11	41.57 (25–91.67; 48.48)
Sexual functioning	11	100 (0–100; 81.82)	60; 1	11	100 (33.33–100; 81.82)
Sexual enjoyment	5	66.67 (33.33–100; 73.33)	9; 0.548	5	66.67 (33.33–100; 60)
Future perspective	11	33.33 (0–66.67; 33.33)	51.5; 0.562	11	33.33 (0–66.67; 27.27)
Symptom scales					
Systemic therapy side effects	11	23.81 (4.76–61.90; 31.6)	58; 0.898	11	28.57 (4.76–57.14; 29)
Breast symptoms	11	41.67 (8.33–75; 38.64)	41; 0.217	11	25 (0–66.67; 28.79)
Arm symptoms	11	33.33 (0–77.78; 37.37)	63; 0.898	11	44.44 (0–88.89; 38.38)
Upset by hair loss	6	16.67 (0–33.33; 16.67)	28.5; 0.573	8	33.33 (0–100; 29.17)

Statistical significance was determined according to the nonparametric Mann–Whitney-Wilcoxon criterion, no significant differences between the groups, $p \geq 0.05$.

were on the global quality of life (58.33 (33.33–91.67; 59.85)), and the participants were found to demonstrate the highest degrees of the manifestation of insomnia (66.67 (0–66.67; 48.49)) and financial impact (66.67 (0–100; 51.52)). The results of the EORTC QLQ-BR23 questionnaire showed that the participants gave the poorest evaluations of the future perspective (33.33 (0–66.67; 27.27)) and demonstrated the highest degrees of the manifestation of arm symptoms (44.44 (0–88.89; 38.38)) such as pain and edema.

The evaluation of changes in the overall scores of the quality of life questionnaire EORTC QLQ-C30 scales between the groups showed that, compared to baseline data, after six weeks (at the end of the study), the experimental group demonstrated statistically significantly better results in the global quality of life ($U = 0$; $p = 0.001$; $r = 0.85$), physical functions ($U = 20$, $p = 0.013$; $r = 0.54$), role functions ($U = 25.5$; $p = 0.036$; $r = 0.46$), emotional functions ($U = 8.5$; $p = 0.001$; $r = 0.72$), cognitive functions ($U = 10$; $p = 0.001$; $r = 0.72$), social functions ($U = 13$; $p = 0.002$; $r = 0.66$), fatigue ($U = 5$; $p = 0.001$; $r = 0.78$), insomnia ($U = 19$; $p = 0.01$; $r = 0.59$), and financial impact ($U = 23.5$; $p = 0.024$; $r = 0.52$) scales, $p < 0.05$. The scores in other functional or symptom scales of the quality of life did not differ statistically significantly between the groups, $p \geq 0.05$ (Table 4).

The evaluation of changes in the overall scores in the scales of the quality of life questionnaire module EORTC QLQ-BR23 between the groups showed that, compared to baseline data, after six weeks (at the end of the study), the experimental group demonstrated statistically significantly better results in the systemic therapy side effects ($U = 11$; $p = 0.001$; $r = 0.68$) and breast symptoms ($U = 24.5$; $p = 0.029$; $r = 0.48$) scales, $p < 0.05$. The scores in other functional or symptom scales did not differ statistically significantly between the groups, $p \geq 0.05$ (Table 5).

Considering the calculated strength of the effect, when a moderate effect was ≥0.5 and a strong effect was ≥0.8, we found not only statistically, but also clinically significant changes ($p < 0.05$) in the scores of the global quality of life (0.85), physical (0.54), emotional (0.72), cognitive (0.72), and social (0.66) functions, fatigue (0.78), insomnia (0.59), financial impact (0.52), and systemic therapy side effects (0.68) scales.

Among the experimental group women with breast cancer, engagement in meaningful activities was evaluated during the nonacute period of the disease. The evaluation was performed based on the results of the Engagement in Meaningful Activities Survey (EMAS)—the sum score that could range from 12 to 48 points, where <29 points indicated insufficient engagement; 29–41 points, moderate engagement; and >41 points, good engagement.

During the evaluation of the participants' engagement in meaningful activities at baseline, the median score in the experimental group was 29 points, the lowest score being 24 points (insufficient engagement) and the highest score being 35 points (moderate engagement). At the end of the study, after the application of the 6-week community-based occupational therapy program, the evaluation scores of the participants' engagement in meaningful activities changed statistically significantly ($Z = -2.829$; $p = 0.005$): the median score was 36 points, the lowest score being 31 points (moderate engagement) and the highest score being 42 points (good engagement), $p < 0.05$ (Figure 1).

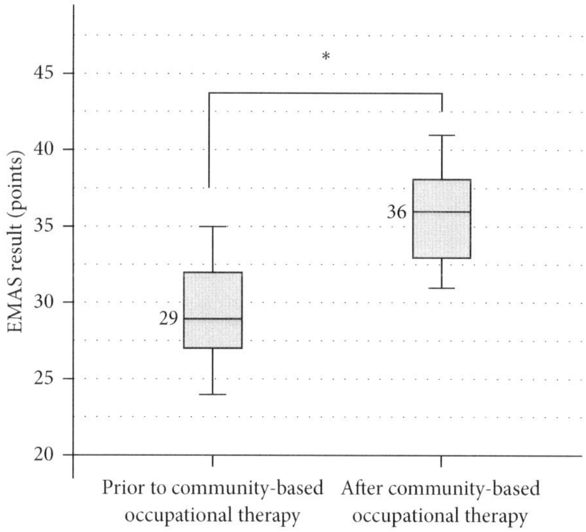

FIGURE 1: Changes in the engagement in meaningful activities in the experimental group participants, $^{*}p = 0.005$.

We also analyzed the relationship between breast cancer patients' engagement in meaningful activities and changes in their health-related quality of life. The results of the analysis showed that when evaluating the health-related quality of life on the EORTC QLQ-C30 questionnaire, the evaluation scores showed a statistically significant direct moderate relationship ($r(10) = 0.663$; $p = 0.037$) between engagement in meaningful activities and the score in the emotional functions scale: better results of the evaluation of the engagement in meaningful activities (i.e., a greater engagement in meaningful activities) were associated with higher evaluation scores of emotional functions, that is, better emotional functions, $p < 0.05$.

We also found a statistically significant inverse moderate relationship ($r(10) = -0.658$; $p = 0.039$) between engagement in meaningful activities and the evaluation scores in the insomnia scale: better results of the evaluation of the engagement in meaningful activities (i.e., a greater engagement in meaningful activities) were associated with lower evaluation scores of the insomnia scale, that is, a lesser degree of the manifestation of insomnia, $p < 0.05$.

We found a statistically significant inverse moderate relationship ($r(10) = -0.681$; $p = 0.030$) between engagement in meaningful activities and the evaluation scores in the constipation scale: better results of the evaluation of the engagement in meaningful activities (i.e., a greater engagement in meaningful activities) were associated with lower evaluation scores of the constipation scale, that is, a lesser degree of the manifestation of constipation, $p < 0.05$.

We did not find any statistically significant relationship for the evaluation scores of other functional or symptom scales of the quality of life questionnaire EORTC QLQ-C30 or any scale of the module EORTC QLQ-BR23, $p \geq 0.05$ (Tables 6 and 7).

Table 4: Characteristics of changes in the evaluation scores of the scales of the global quality of life questionnaire EORTC QLQ-C30 in the experimental and the control group women.

Scales of the quality of life questionnaire	EGr Before x_{me}	EGr After x_{me}	EGr change Z; p	CGr Before x_{me}	CGr After x_{me}	CGr change Z; p	Difference between the groups at the end U; p; r
			EORTC QLQ C-30				
Global health status/QoL	50	66.67	−2.829; 0.005*	58.33	50	−1.956; 0.05	0; 0.001**; 0.85
Functional scales							
Physical functioning	60	70	−2.384; 0.017*	73.33	60	−1.012; 0.311	20; 0.013**; 0.54
Role functioning	66.67	75	−1.023; 0.306	66.67	66.67	−1.409; 0.159	25.5; 0.036**; 0.46
Emotional functioning	50	62.5	−2.670; 0.008*	66.67	58.33	−1.480; 0.139	8.5; 0.001**; 0.72
Cognitive functioning	50	66.67	−2.060; 0.039*	83.33	50	−2.388; 0.017*	10; 0.001**; 0.72
Social functioning	50	66.67	−1.951; 0.051	66.67	50	−2.410; 0.016*	13; 0.002**; 0.66
Symptom scales							
Fatigue	55.56	44.44	−2.555; 0.011*	44.44	66.67	−2.568; 0.010*	5; 0.001**; 0.78
Nausea and vomiting	0	0	−1.089; 0.276	0	0	−1.289; 0.197	51; 0.809
Pain	33.33	16.67	−0.933; 0.351	33.33	33.33	−0.213; 0.832	41.5; 0.349
Dyspnoea	0	0	−1; 0.317	33.33	33.33	−1.382; 0.167	32.5; 0.114
Insomnia	66.67	33.33	−2.280; 0.023*	66.67	66.67	−1.890; 0.059	19; 0.01**; 0.59
Appetite loss	0	0	−0.707; 0.480	33.33	33.33	−1.633; 0.102	48; 0.654;
Constipation	33.33	16.67	−1.890; 0.059	0	0	−0.730; 0.465	48; 0.654;
Diarrhoea	0	0	−1; 0.317	0	0	−0.816; 0.414	40.5; 0.314;
Financial difficulties	66.67	66.67	−1.236; 0.216	66.67	66.67	−2.041; 0.041*	23.5; 0.024**; 0.52

*Statistical significance was determined according to the nonparametric Wilcoxon criterion; the differences between the groups were significant when $p < 0.05$. **Statistical significance was determined according to the nonparametric Mann–Whitney-Wilcoxon criterion; the differences between the groups were significant when $p < 0.05$. *Note.* EGr: experimental group; CGr: control group.

TABLE 5: Characteristics of changes in the evaluation scores of the scales of the global quality of life questionnaire module EORTC QLQ-BR23 in the experimental and the control group women.

Scales of the quality of life questionnaire	EGr Before x_{me}	EGr After x_{me}	EGr change $Z; p$	CGr Before x_{me}	CGr After x_{me}	CGr change $Z; p$	Difference between the groups at the end $U; p; r$
			EORTC QLQ BR-23				
Functional scales							
Body image	58.33	58.33	−0.512; 0.609	41.67	41.67	−1.2; 0.23	53; 0.918
Sexual functioning	100	66.67	−2.041; 0.041*	100	83.33	0; 1	32.5; 0.114
Sexual enjoyment	66.67	50	−1.604; 0.109	66.67	66.67	−0.816; 0.414	4.5; 0.095
Future perspective	33.33	33.33	−0.184; 0.854	33.33	33.33	−0.184; 0.854	55; 1
Symptom scales							
Systemic therapy side effects	23.81	23.81	−2.092; 0.036	28.57	38.1	−2.371; 0.018*	11; 0.001**; 0.68
Breast symptoms	41.67	25	−2.352; 0.019*	25	33.33	−0.511; 0.61	24.5; 0.029**; 0.48
Arm symptoms	33.33	23.61	−0.986; 0.324	44.44	44.44	−0.106; 0.915	48; 0.654
Upset by hair loss	16.67	33.33	−1.633; 0.102	33.33	33.33	−1.841; 0.066	22.5; 0.852

*Statistical significance was determined according to the nonparametric Wilcoxon criterion; the differences between the groups were significant when $p < 0.05$. **Statistical significance was determined according to the nonparametric Mann–Whitney-Wilcoxon criterion; the differences between the groups were significant when $p < 0.05$.

TABLE 6: Relationship between engagement in meaningful activities and evaluations scores of health-related quality of life (EORTC QLQ-C30) in women with breast cancer.

Scales of the quality of life questionnaire	Relationship with changes in the engagement in meaningful activities $r(n)$; p
EORTC QLQ-C30	
Global health status/QoL	$r(10) = -0.046$; $p = 0.899$
Functional scales	
Physical functioning	$r(10) = 0.26$; $p = 0.469$
Role functioning	$r(10) = 0.21$; $p = 0.561$
Emotional functioning	$r(10) = 0.663$; $p = 0.037^*$
Cognitive functioning	$r(10) = 0.041$; $p = 0.91$
Social functioning	$r(10) = -0.051$; $p = 0.888$
Symptom scales	
Fatigue	$r(10) = -0.316$; $p = 0.374$
Nausea and vomiting	$r(10) = 0.239$; $p = 0.506$
Pain	$r(10) = -0.039$; $p = 0.916$
Dyspnoea	$r(10) = 0.425$; $p = 0.221$
Insomnia	$r(10) = -0.658$; $p = 0.039^*$
Appetite loss	$r(10) = -0.619$; $p = 0.056$
Constipation	$r(10) = -0.681$; $p = 0.03^*$
Diarrhoea	$r(10) = -0.121$; $p = 0.739$
Financial difficulties	$r(10) = -0.326$; $p = 0.359$

* Statistical significance was determined according to Spearman's correlation coefficient; the association was statistically significant when $p < 0.05$.

TABLE 7: Relationship between engagement in meaningful activities and evaluations scores of health-related quality of life (EORTC QLQ-BR23) in women with breast cancer.

Scales of the quality of life questionnaire	Relationship with changes in the engagement in meaningful activities $r(n)$; p
EORTC QLQ-BR23	
Functional scales	
Body image	$r(10) = -0.048$; $p = 0.895$
Sexual functioning	$r(10) = -0.289$; $p = 0.418$
Sexual enjoyment	$r(10) = -0.079$; $p = 0.9$
Future perspective	$r(10) = -0.353$; $p = 0.317$
Symptom scales	
Systemic therapy side effects	$r(10) = 0.177$; $p = 0.624$
Breast symptoms	$r(10) = -0.423$; $p = 0.223$
Arm symptoms	$r(10) = -0.083$; $p = 0.819$
Upset by hair loss	$r(6) = 0.141$; $p = 0.79$

Statistical significance was determined according to Spearman's correlation coefficient; the association was statistically significant when $p < 0.05$.

4. Discussion

A review of both Lithuanian and foreign literature revealed a lack of research or any kind of projects in the context of applying community-based occupational therapy for women with breast cancer, which encouraged us to conduct this study where objectives were set: to evaluate the short-term effects of community-based occupational therapy on changes in health-related quality of life among women with breast cancer and on changes in the experimental group women's engagement in meaningful activities and to analyze the associations between engagement in meaningful activities and changes in health-related quality of life.

In Lithuania, over 1.5 thousand new cases of breast cancer are diagnosed annually [7]. Improving screening programs and modern therapeutic techniques as well as increasing life expectancy of cancer patients result in an increasing relevance of the quality of life questions related to late consequences of the disease and its treatment and this is where the holistic approach and creative decisions of occupational therapists may be of assistance [11, 15, 22]. Based on this idea, in our study we analyzed aforementioned indices among women with breast cancer during the nonacute period of the disease.

In total, 21 women participated in and successfully completed the study. Of these, 10 women participated in a 6-week community-based occupational therapy program consisting of 4 group sessions (once a week, ~1.5 hours/day). The program was designed according to the guidelines provided in the only source of literature describing a study similar to ours—a project by Robinson (2015). The basis for those guidelines was a community-based occupational therapy program for women with breast cancer, aimed at maximizing their capacity for daily activities after the completion of the treatment [23].

We evaluated health-related quality of life by using the questionnaires of the European Organization for Research and Treatment of Cancer (EORTC) Quality of Life Group—the global EORTC QLQ-C30 questionnaire and its module designed specifically for breast cancer, EORTC QLQ-BR23. These questionnaires have been translated into and adapted in many languages, including Lithuanian, and are suitable for the evaluation of health-related quality of life in individuals with breast cancer [24]. In our participants, we evaluated health-related quality of life twice—at baseline and after 6 weeks. The results of our study showed that, at the beginning of the study, the women's quality of life and emotional, cognitive, and social functions were impaired; they experienced stronger manifestations of insomnia and breast and arm symptoms and were concerned about their future perspectives and the financial impact of the disease. Meanwhile, upon completion of the 6-week community-based occupational therapy program, the evaluation results of these and other aspects of health-related quality of life—such as physical functions, role functions, and fatigue—improved statistically significantly, compared to the respective results in the control group participants who did not participate in the program.

EORTC questionnaires have been recommended by a number of foreign researchers [13, 22, 25–28]. The results of a systematic survey conducted by Ghislain et al. (2016) showed that a large proportion (44%) of their analyzed studies on health-related quality of life in women with breast cancer employed EORTC questionnaires. The aforementioned survey showed that the second most frequently used (39%) instrument for the evaluation of health-related quality of life was the FACT-B *(Functional Assessment of Cancer Therapy-Breast)* questionnaire [29]. Apart from those two questionnaires, other researchers applied FACT-G *(Functional Assessment of Cancer Therapy-General)*, FACT-BSC *(Functional Assessment of Cancer Therapy-Breast Cancer Specific Subscale)*, QLACS *(Quality of Life in Adult Cancer Survivors)'* SF-36 *(Medical Outcomes Short-Form Health Survey)*, and other instruments [11, 30, 31].

According to literature data, active engagement in meaningful activities positively affects the quality of life, and thus, in order to improve breast cancer patients' health-related quality of life, the women were involved in meaningful activities during the occupational therapy sessions [18, 19]. To evaluate changes in the study participants' engagement in meaningful activities and its relationship with health-related quality of life, we used the engagement in meaningful activities questionnaire during community-based occupational therapy. The women filled out this questionnaire at the beginning and at the end of the study. A survey of literature failed to identify any Lithuanian or foreign studies on the evaluation of breast cancer patients' engagement in meaningful activities. For this reason, we cannot compare our results, which showed that in the experimental group women who participated in the 6-week community-based occupational therapy program, engagement in meaningful activities improved significantly and that greater result was associated with a significant improvement in emotional functions and a reduction in the level of insomnia. We found only one study conducted by foreign researchers Pergolotti et al. (2015), where, based on the idea of participation in personally important activities for the improvement of the quality of life, the researchers analyzed participation in meaningful activities among older patients with cancer. Of the study subjects, 40% were breast cancer patients, whose participation in meaningful activities was evaluated by applying the MAPA *(The Meaningful Activity Participation Assessment)* test [32].

In this study, we strived to reveal the essence of occupational therapy in the community of women with breast cancer and the influence of this therapy on those women's health-related quality of life. The results of the study showed that occupational therapy significantly improves breast cancer patients' health-related quality of life and engagement in meaningful activities on the community level during the nonacute period of the disease.

One of the limitations of this study is a small number of participants in the groups, and thus in the future, this or a similar study should be performed with a larger sample. We also think that, in further studies, it would be expedient to evaluate whether a longer period of program application or a greater number of sessions would affect the results and improve the effectiveness of the program. In addition, future studies could be expanded by involving specialists of other areas (psychologists, art therapists, marketing specialists, etc.) because a successful implementation of the program requires not only the general competence of an occupational therapist, but also organizational skills, knowledge in marketing, and so forth in order to induce interest, attract, and invite the maximal possible numbers of women. The strong side of the study is that this was a new study in our country and that it provided positive emotions not only for the participants of the study, but also for hospitalized women who did not participate in the study, as voluntary assistance to others added meaningfulness to the sessions.

Authors' Contributions

All the authors have reviewed and approved the manuscript before submission.

Acknowledgments

The study was conducted with the permission of the Bioethics Center of the Lithuanian University of Health Sciences (no. BEC-SR (M)-186), the permission of the European Organization for Research and Treatment of Cancer (EORTC) Quality of Life Group to use the quality of life questionnaire EORTC QLQ-C30 and its module EORTC QLQ-BR23 in the study, and the permission of the Associate Professor A. M. Eakman from Colorado State University to use the Engagement in Meaningful Activities Survey (EMAS) in the study. The manuscript does not concern any commercial product.

References

[1] American Cancer Society, *Global Cancer Facts & Figures*, American Cancer Society, Atlanta, 3rd edition, 2015.

[2] National Cancer Institute, *NCI Dictionary of Cancer Terms*, https://www.cancer.gov/publications/dictionaries/cancer-terms?cdrid=444971.

[3] V. Ostapenko, A. Jackevičius, J. Didžiapetrienė, and V. Atkočius, *Lithuanian Breast Cancer: Scientific and Clinical Aspects. Scientific educational monograph*, National Cancer Institute, Vilnius, Lithuania, 2016.

[4] International Agency for Research on Cancer / World Health Organization, *Cancer Fact Sheet: Breast Cancer*, 2016, http://gco.iarc.fr/today/data/pdf/fact-sheets/cancers/cancer-fact-sheets-15.pdf.

[5] C. Conley, B. Bishop, and B. Andersen, "Emotions and Emotion Regulation in Breast Cancer Survivorship," *Healthcare*, vol. 4, no. 4, p. 56, 2016.

[6] European Network of Cancer Registries Factsheets, *Breast Cancer Factsheet*, European Union/ENCR, 2014, http://www.encr.eu/images/docs/factsheets/ENCR_Factsheet_Breast_2014.pdf.

[7] D. Gudavičienė, L. Steponavičienė, and N. Lachej, "Krūties vėžys Lietuvoje," *Acta Medica Lituanica*, vol. 22, no. 3, pp. 150–160, 2015.

[8] American Cancer Society, *Breast Cancer Facts & Figures 2015-2016*, American Cancer Society, Atlanta, 2015.

[9] E. Juozaitytė, A. Naudžiūnas, L. Valius, D. Krančiukaitytė-Butylkinienė, and et al., "Fundamentals of Family Medicine," in *Practical Skills. Tutorial*, pp. 13–70, UAB Vitae Litera, Kaunas, Lithuania, 2016.

[10] V. T. Devita, T. S. Lawrence, and S. A. Rosenberg, *Cancer: Principles & Practice of Oncology*, Lippincott Williams Wilkins, Wolters Kluwer, Philadelphia, USA, 8th edition, 2008.

[11] S. J. Sohl, B. Levine, and N. E. Avis, "Evaluation of the Quality of Life in Adult Cancer Survivors (QLACS) scale for early post-treatment breast cancer survivors," *Quality of Life Research*, vol. 24, no. 1, pp. 205–212, 2015.

[12] B. Gruževskis and U. L. Orlova, "Sąvokos Gyvenimo kokybė raidos tendencijos," *Socialinis darbas*, vol. 11, no. 1, pp. 7–18, 2012.

[13] D. Schoormans, K. Czene, P. Hall, and Y. Brandberg, "The impact of co-morbidity on health-related quality of life in breast cancer survivors and controls," *Acta Oncologica*, vol. 54, no. 5, pp. 727–734, 2015.

[14] Deluliis E. D. and Hughes J. K., *Occupational Therapy's Role in Breast Cancer Rehabilitation*, The American Occupational Therapy Association Fact Sheet, 2012.

[15] M. Pergolotti, G. R. Williams, C. Campbell, L. A. Munoz, and H. B. Muss, "Occupational therapy for adults with cancer: Why it matters," *The Oncologist*, vol. 21, no. 3, pp. 314–319, 2016.

[16] V. Repšaitė, *The effect of differential training on functional movements and autonomy of persons suffering from stroke*, Lithuanian University of Health Sciences, Medical Academy, 2015.

[17] American Occupational Therapy Association Fact Sheet, *The Role of Occupational Therapy With Health Promotion*, American Occupational Therapy Association, 2015.

[18] G. Cook and J. Thompson, "Purposeful activity," in *Nursing Case Studies on Improving Health-Related Quality of Life in Older Adults*, M. W. Kazer and K. Murphy, Eds., Gasch Printing, USA, 2015.

[19] M. E. Scaffa and S. M. Reitz, *Occupational Therapy in Community-Based Practice Settings*, F. A. Davis Company, Philadelphia, USA, 2th edition, 2014.

[20] I. Banienė and L. Šinkariova, "Relationship between the personality traits of women with breast cancer and the stress-related illness-related strategies for health-related quality of life," *Health Sciences*, vol. 25, no. 3, pp. 11–16, 2015.

[21] A. M. Eakman, M. E. Carlson, and F. A. Clark, "Factor Structure, Reliability, and Convergent Validity of the Engagement in Meaningful Activities Survey for Older Adults," *OTJR: Occupation, Participation, Health*, vol. 30, no. 3, pp. 111–121, 2010.

[22] P. O. Dialla, W.-O. Chu, P. Roignot et al., "Impact of age-related socio-economic and clinical determinants of quality of life among long-term breast cancer survivors," *Maturitas*, vol. 81, no. 3, pp. 362–370, 2015.

[23] H. Robinson, *A communitybased occupational therapy program for women afer breast cancer [Master, thesis]*, Afer Cancer Experience, 2015, http://utdr.utoledo.edu/cgi/viewcontent.cgi?article=1601&context=graduate-projects.

[24] N. K. Aaronson, S. Ahinedzai, B. Bergman et al., "The European Organization for Research and Treatment of Cancer QLQ-C30: a quality-of-life instrument for use in international clinical trials in oncology," *Journal of the National Cancer Institute*, vol. 85, no. 5, pp. 365–376, 1993.

[25] M. J. Yuste Sánchez, M. T. Lacomba, B. S. Sánchez et al., "Health related quality of life improvement in breast cancer patients: Secondary outcome from a simple blinded, randomised clinical trial," *The Breast Journal*, vol. 24, no. 1, pp. 75–81, 2015.

[26] K. Almutairi, E. Mansour, and J. Vinluan, "A cross-sectional assessment of quality of life of breast cancer patients in Saudi Arabia," *Public Health*, vol. 136, pp. 117–125, 2016.

[27] D. Moro-Valdezate, E. Buch-Villa, S. Peiró et al., "Factors associated with health-related quality of life in a cohort of Spanish breast cancer patients," *Breast Cancer*, vol. 21, no. 4, pp. 442–452, 2014.

[28] C. Rohani, H.-A. Abedi, R. Omranipour, and A. Langius-Eklöf, "Health-related quality of life and the predictive role of sense of coherence, spirituality and religious coping in a sample of Iranian women with breast cancer: a prospective study with comparative design," *Health and Quality of Life Outcomes*, vol. 13, article 40, 2015.

[29] I. Ghislain, E. Zikos, C. Coens et al., "Health-related quality of life in locally advanced and metastatic breast cancer: methodological and clinical issues in randomised controlled trials," *The Lancet Oncology*, vol. 17, no. 7, pp. e294–e304, 2016.

Occupational Therapy Practice in Sleep Management: A Review of Conceptual Models and Research Evidence

Eris C. M. Ho[1] and Andrew M. H. Siu[2]

[1]Occupational Therapy Department, Queen Elizabeth Hospital, Hospital Authority, Kowloon, Hong Kong
[2]Department of Rehabilitation Sciences, The Hong Kong Polytechnic University, Kowloon, Hong Kong

Correspondence should be addressed to Andrew M. H. Siu; a.siu@polyu.edu.hk

Academic Editor: Claudia Hilton

The effectiveness of sleep intervention developed by occupational therapists was reviewed, and a conceptual framework for organizing the developing practice of sleep management in occupational therapy was proposed in this paper. Evidence-based articles on sleep management practice in occupational therapy from 2007 to 2017 were retrieved. Four types of effective sleep management intervention were identified from the literature, including the use of assistive devices/equipment, activities, cognitive behavioral therapy for insomnia, and lifestyle intervention, and the use of assistive device was the most popular intervention. Applying the Person-Environment-Occupation Performance (PEOP) framework, we developed a conceptual framework for organizing occupational therapy practice in sleep management. The future development of occupation-based sleep intervention could focus on strategies to (1) minimize the influence of bodily function on sleep, (2) promote environment conducive to sleep, and (3) restructure daytime activity with a focus on occupational balance.

1. Introduction

Sleep problem is the difficulty in initiating or maintaining sleep or suffering from nonrestorative sleep accompanied by daytime functional impairment [1]. Sleep problems are a worldwide health issue, with an average prevalence rate ranging from 10% to 30% in developed countries [2, 3]. Hong Kong, a fast-paced city, has a relatively high prevalence (39.4%) of sleep problems [4]. Sleep is important for health and well-being. People with sleep problems are prone to suffer from serious medical conditions, such as obesity, heart disease, high blood pressure, and diabetes [5]. Sleep problems also affect cognitive performance, including alertness, reaction, memory, and learning [6]. Very often, sleep problems could impact on daily occupations such as work, daily activities, social performance, and well-being.

It is uncommon for people to seek help for insomnia [7, 8]. Instead of consulting health care professionals, many people use over-the-counter sleeping pills or use alcohol or substances to cope with sleep problems. Both methods can offer only a temporary or limited improvement of sleep quality, and the addictive and side effects may pose significant threats to health and well-being in the long run. In general, health care management of sleep problems involves pharmacological and/or nonpharmacological interventions [9]. Pharmacological intervention should be monitored by physicians, and medication is usually prescribed on a short-term basis, given the concerns of potential dependence and the side effects of medication on cognitive performance. Nonpharmacological sleep interventions often include sleep hygiene education, relaxation [10, 11], and cognitive-behavioral treatment for insomnia which targets the modification of maladaptive thoughts that perpetuate insomnia [12].

In occupational therapy theories, sleep is conceptualized as a restorative occupation with the goal of rest and recuperation, and good sleep and rest could support the formation of the occupation mix of self-care, work, and leisure during the day [13–15]. The concepts of occupational balance focus on time use and suggest that the balance between rest/sleep and daytime activity is important in promoting function and well-being [13, 16–18]. Sleep has a significant impact on functional performance in self-care, work, and leisure.

Thus, sleep and daytime functioning are closely interrelated, and excessive or insufficient sleep or daytime activities will contribute to occupational imbalance.

As a member of the primary care team, there is clearly a growing need for occupational therapists to provide interventions for patients with sleep problems and related mental health issues. To facilitate the development of sleep management practice in occupational therapy, there is a need to further conceptualize on how sleep and occupation are linked and identify evidence-based occupational-based interventions that could be used in clinical practice.

In sum, only a few conceptual models or frameworks, like the PEOP model or the concept of occupational balance, have attempted to discuss how sleep is related to occupation, and how it could fit into occupational therapy practice. While some evidence-based studies have been published on sleep interventions in occupational therapy practice, there appears to be great diversity in the target groups, objectives, and components of programs, and/or in methodology. There has been no formal review or analysis of the characteristics of intervention programs or their findings. This article aims to conduct a systematic review of the literature on occupational therapy theories and practice for patients with sleep problems and the research evidence published in the past ten years. The objectives are to (1) identify the key intervention approaches and the components of sleep management administered by occupational therapists, (2) examine the research evidence on the effectiveness of occupational therapy interventions for people with sleep problems, and (3) formulate a conceptual framework for sleep management in occupational therapy.

2. Review of Research Evidence

2.1. Literature Search. A literature search was performed according to the 2009 PRISMA Statement for systematic reviews [19]. Two researchers performed the review using the OneSearch search engine of the Hong Kong Polytechnic University, which integrated a number of research databases. The inclusion criteria were (1) sleep intervention developed by an occupational therapist, (2) sleep as primary outcome, (3) peer-reviewed articles, and (4) written in English. Papers only describing the role of occupational therapists in sleep management, theoretical papers, books, and editorial were excluded. The search included papers published between October 1, 2007, and October 1, 2017 (the previous ten years to the review). To ensure a comprehensive coverage of the literature, the search terms included "sleep," "rest," or "insomnia" and "occupational therapy," "occupational therapist," or "occupational therapy intervention." Keyword searches were performed in five key databases: Scopus (Elsevier), MEDLINE/PubMed, Science Citation Index (SCI), OneFile (GALE), and ScienceDirect. 256 articles were included, and after applying inclusion and exclusion criteria, 11 articles were retained for data synthesis [20–30]. Figure 1 shows the systematic search and review process.

2.2. Risk of Bias. Two assessors conducted the quality assessment of the articles. Level of evidence [31] was graded based on the research design. Eight out of the eleven articles were categorized as level III or above in terms of evidence, which indicates well-conducted studies with strong evidence including consistent results (Table 1). Three articles involved randomized controlled trials (RCT). Based on the *Cochrane Handbook of Reviews of Effectiveness of Interventions*, we evaluated the risk of bias in the three RCT studies (Table 2). The result showed that allocation sequence generation, concealment, and blinding were adequately performed in two out of the three studies. However, there are variations in detection and attrition bias among them. The design of the RCT studies are quite different: (1) there is broad variation in the duration of intervention (varied from three days to six months); (2) study samples include both adults and elderly; and (3) there is a lack of detail on the research methodology, for example, regarding randomization, baseline measurements, and blinding procedures. As the number of studies is small and there is inadequate information to conduct a formal meta-analysis of the interventions, a descriptive approach was used in the review of the research evidence.

Mixed Methods Appraisal Tool (MMAT) 2001 version [32] is adopted for quality assessment. This is a five-item checklist, designed for assessing the quality of the articles in relation to different types of research designs. Four areas focus on the methodology, outcomes, statistical process, and result interruption. Each item scored 0 or 1 and yield a maximum of 4 points (100%). The quality of 11 articles was examined, and the results are shown in Table 1. Overall speaking, 55% of the articles demonstrate satisfactory quality with rating 3/4 (75%) in MMAT and all level I and level II studies achieved satisfactory rating.

3. Analysis of Research Evidence

On the whole, occupational therapy-based sleep intervention was found to be effective in improving patients' sleep to different extents. Coverage of existing services and types of intervention were reviewed systematically to build up knowledge for further discussion. Three of the studies were level I RCTs [21, 23, 26], one was a level II nonrandomized study [25], three were level III one-group nonrandomized pretest and posttest studies (Eakman et al. 2016; [24, 30]), two were level IV descriptive studies that included analysis of outcomes (case series) [28, 29], and one was a level V case study [22]. Ten studies were from the United States, and one from Canada; no study on sleep intervention was published in an Asian country during the review period.

3.1. Characteristics of Target Population. To conduct an analysis of the articles, we summarized the study background (author, year of publication, and country), format (design and sample size), patients' characteristics (age range, sex, setting, and type of disease), and type of occupational therapy outcome and intervention (Table 3).

Sample size varies from two [28, 30] to 217 [26], and participants' age ranges from 30 days to 82 years old. The influence of participant group in sleep management is diverse. The diagnoses of participants include people with an autistic spectrum disorder (ASD) [22, 27, 29, 30], traumatic brain

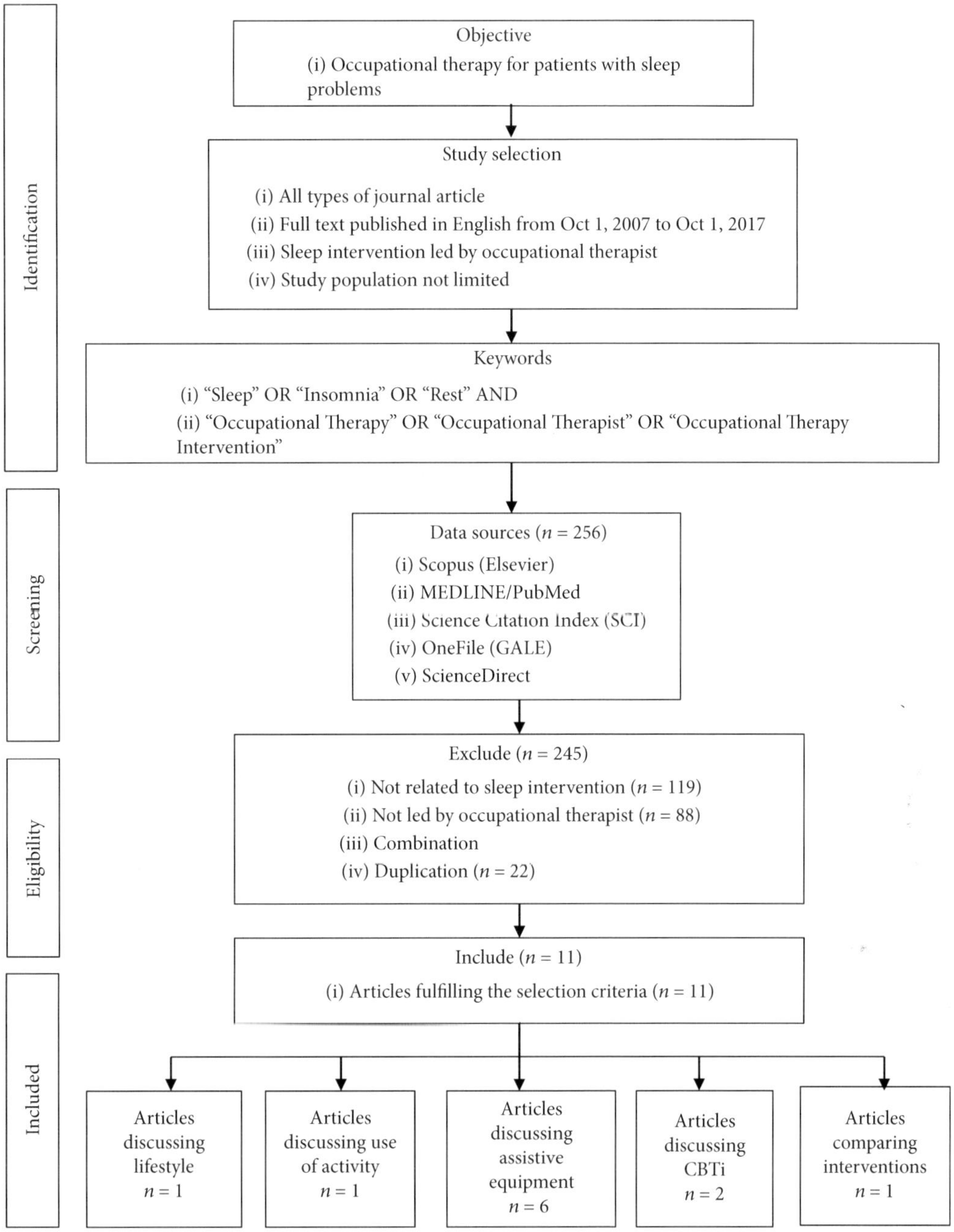

FIGURE 1: Flowchart of the literature search and selection process.

injury (TBI) [28], and posttraumatic stress disorder (PTSD) (Eakman et al. 2016). Other study participants include community-dwelling elderly, adults with sleep problems [23, 26], and in-patients [21, 24, 25]. Two studies focus on people with primary insomnia who had no medical or psychiatric problems, and whose insomnia was likely related to lifestyle and aging issues [23, 26].

3.2. Key Types of Sleep Intervention and Effectiveness. Four types of sleep intervention were identified: (1) use of assistive devices/equipment [21, 22, 24, 25, 27, 29]; (2) use of activities [28]; (3) cognitive behavioral therapy for insomnia (Eakman et al. 2016; [30]); and (4) lifestyle intervention [26]. Gutman et al. [23] compared the effectiveness of three different interventions: sleep aids, meditation activity, and sleep hygiene.

3.2.1. Use of Assistive Device/Equipment. Environment can significantly affect one's sleep, and a key occupational therapy intervention is the use of assistive aids or positioning to facilitate sleep onset. The six articles that used sleep aids evaluated the effectiveness of the Dreampad pillow, weighted blankets, and sleep tools including eye masks, earplugs, and white noise machines. The Dreampad pillow is a patented technology which conducts soothing music in the pillow that relaxes the body and mind, and it is supported with a music app of library of research-backed sleep-inducing music. The

Table 1: Quality assessment by Mixed Methods Appraisal Tool (MMAT) 2001 version.

Author, year	Research design	Type	Level of evidence (LoE)	Quality appraisal (MMAT)
Eakman et al., 2016	Single-arm feasibility pilot study	Quantitative descriptive	Level III	3/4
Farrehi et al., 2016 [21]	RCT	Quantitative randomization controlled (trials)	Level I	3/4
Gee et al., 2017 [22]	An ABA single-subject design	Qualitative	Level V	1/4
Gutman et al., 2016 [23]	RCT	Quantitative randomization controlled (trials)	Level I	3/4
Heidt et al., 2016 [24]	Experimental study design	Quantitative descriptive	Level III	4/4
Jarus et al., 2011 [25]	Waitlist control trials	Quantitative nonrandomization controlled	Level II	3/4
Leland et al., 2016 [26]	RCT	Quantitative randomization controlled (trials)	Level I	3/4
Schoen et al., 2017 [27]	A quasi-experimental, single-group, pretest/posttest design	Quantitative descriptive	Level III	2/4
Wen et al., 2017 [28]	Mixed-methods pilot study	Mixed methods	Level IV	1/4
Wolfhope et al., 2016	Mixed-methods pilot study	Mixed methods	Level IV	2/4
Wooster et al., 2015 [30]	A pretest-posttest, one group design	Quantitative descriptive	Level III	2/4

Table 2: Risk of bias table for the RCTs.

Author, year	Selection bias		Performance bias	Detection bias		Attrition bias		Reporting bias
	Random sequence generation	Allocation concealment	Blinding of participants	Patient-reported outcomes	All-cause mortality	Short-term	Long-term	Selective reporting
Farrehi et al., 2016 [21]	+	+	+	+	?	?	?	+
Gutman et al., 2016 [23]	?	?	?	?	?	+	?	+
Leland et al., 2016 [26]	+	+	+	?	?	+	+	+

Note. Categories for risk of bias are as follows: +: low risk; ?: unclear risk; −: high risk.

studies on the Dreampad pillow show that it could significantly improve sleep duration and latency [27, 29], improve sleep quality, and reduce nighttime awakenings [23]. It also helps to improve secondary outcomes, including autism-related behaviors and attention [27, 29] and quality of life and parent satisfaction (Schoen et al. 2016). Gee and colleagues (2007) found that the weighted blanket, a sleep aid developed for patients with ASD, could increase sleep duration and shorten latency.

Overall, there is much evidence supporting the effectiveness of sleep aids in promoting patients' sleep and reducing sleep disturbance during hospital stays [24] or reducing physical symptoms like pain [21] and fatigue [24]. Other than prescribing aids, there are also studies on how positioning could promote sleep in preterm babies. Jarus and colleagues [25] found that prone position showed more sleep pattern and less awake patterns than supine position.

3.2.2. Use of Activities. Two studies use mind-body activities to promote sleep, including iRest meditation, yoga, and breathing [23, 28]. It is generally believed that calming or mindful activity can improve sleep quality at night, but effectiveness varies in the articles reviewed. The use of meditation activity was found to result in statistically longer sleep time than sleep hygiene education alone [23]. Yoga and breathing techniques were not found to increase sleep duration, but could reduce depressive symptoms [28].

3.2.3. Cognitive Behavioral Therapy for Insomnia (CBTi). In recent years, increasing numbers of occupational therapists have undergone training in how to conduct CBTi for patients with sleep problems. CBTi is a structured program which aims to improve sleep by identifying and changing the negative thoughts and behaviors related to it, such as cognitive traps and beliefs concerning sleep restriction [10, 12]. CBTi

Table 3: Characteristics of included studies.

Author, year, country	Setting subject	Sample size (n), age, sex (M/F)	Level of evidence/clinical study design, inclusion/exclusion criteria (IC/EC)	Type of intervention	Outcome measure	Results
Eakman et al., 2016, USA	Various university campuses, 911 US Military veterans	$n = 8$, age 35.6 ± 7.4, sex 8/0	Level III Single-arm feasibility pilot study IC: post 911 military veteran attending college, service-connected injury, reported sleep difficulties, willing to complete daily diaries EC: diagnosis of epilepsy or bipolar disorder	Two months of sleep intervention: restoring effective sleep tranquility (REST) program 7 group sessions 8 individual sessions CBTi (i) Sleep restriction (ii) Stimulus control Sleep hygiene	(i) Sleep problems index II of the medical outcomes study sleep measure (MOS-sleep) (ii) Patient-reported outcomes measurement information system-sleep disturbance (PROMIS-SD) (iii) Pittsburgh Sleep Quality Index (PSQI) (iv) Dysfunctional Beliefs and Attitudes about Sleep Scale (DBAS) (v) Patient-reported outcomes measurement information system-ability to participate in social roles and activities (PROMIS-AP) (vi) Patient-reported outcomes measurement information system-satisfaction with participation in social roles (PROMIS-SP) (vii) Patient-reported outcomes measurement information system-pain interference (PROMIS-PI) (viii) Canadian Occupational Performance Measure (COPM)	(i) Reduced sleep difficulties ($t = 3.29$, $p = 0.02$) (ii) Reduced nightmares ($t = 2.79$, $p = 0.03$) (iii) Fewer dysfunctional sleep-related beliefs ($t = 3.63$, $p = 0.01$) (iv) Greater ability to participate in social roles ($t = -2.86$, $p = .03$) Trends toward improved satisfaction with participation and reduced pain interference
Farrehi et al., 2016, USA [21]	Hospital, aged 18–75	$n = 120$, age 56.22 ± 11.41	Level I RCT	(i) Intervention group: occupational therapy sleep tool intervention (eye mask, ear plugs, and white noise machine) sleep education on environment control (ii) Control group: sleep education	(i) COPM (ii) FIM (iii) Patient-Reported Outcome Measurement Information System Survey: fatigue, physical functioning, sleep disturbance, wake disturbance (iv) Brief Pain Inventory (short form) (v) Pain reduction associated with sleep deprivation	(i) Significant reduction of fatigue scores over 3 days, compared with controls ($p = 0.02$) (ii) Trend toward improvement in sleep disturbance, sleep-related impairment, physical functioning, pain severity, or paint interference ($p>0.1$) (iii) No difference in length of stay ($p = 0.9$) or use of opioids ($p = 0.7$)

Table 3: Continued.

Author, year, country	Setting subject	Sample size (n), age, sex (M/F)	Level of evidence/clinical study design, inclusion/exclusion criteria (IC/EC)	Type of intervention	Outcome measure	Results
Gee et al., 2017, USA [22]	Autism spectrum disorder	$n = 4$, age 3–6 years old	Level V An ABA single-subject design IC: children had a diagnosis of ASD, present with sleep problem, sensory over responsibility	Use of weighted blankets	(i) Sleep quality (ii) Time to fall asleep (iii) Sleep duration (iv) Behavioral ratings on waking	(i) Moderate improvement of the measured constructs related to sleep quality (ii) Increased in total amount of sleep per night (iii) Decrease in time to fall asleep (iv) Sleep between 1 and 3 hours a night more as a result of the weighted blanket
Gutman et al., 2016, USA [23]	Community living, adults aged 25–65	$n = 29$, age 43.2 ± 12.2, sex 9/20	Level I RCT IC: poor sleep for 2 months, agreed to follow sleep hygiene for 3 weeks EC: taking sleeping pills, suffered from pain, medical diagnosis causing sleep disruption, pets or family members causing sleep disruption, pregnant or smokers	Three weeks of sleep intervention of the following: (i) Dreampad pillow (ii) iRest meditation (iii) Sleep hygiene	(i) General Sleep Disturbance Scale (ii) Pittsburgh Sleep Quality Index (iii) Actigraph accelerometer (iv) Sleep diary	(i) iRest meditation group experienced statistically more time asleep than both the Dreampad pillow ($p < 0.006$) and sleep hygiene groups ($p < 0.03$) (ii) Dreampad pillow group experienced statistically fewer nighttime awakenings than iRest meditation ($p < 0.04$) and sleep hygiene groups ($p < 0.004$) (iii) No difference was found between groups in perceived sleep quality, length of time needed to fall asleep, or next-day fatigue level
Heidt et al., 2016, USA [24]	Hospital, aged 18–75	$n = 52$, age 57.5 ± 9.9, sex 29/23	Level III Experimental study design with single sample and pre-post testing	(i) Simple sleep-enhancing education (ii) Sleep-enhancing tools	(i) Patient-Reported Outcome Measurement Information System Survey: fatigue, physical functioning, sleep disturbance, wake disturbance	(i) Significant improvement in fatigue ($t = 5.5$, $p < 0.001$), sleep disturbance ($t = 3.9$, $p < 0.001$), and wake disturbance ($t = 3.8$, $p < 0.001$) (ii) No significant improvement in the physical function aspect ($p = 0.1$)

Table 3: Continued.

Author, year, country	Setting subject	Sample size (n), age, sex (M/F)	Level of evidence/clinical study design, inclusion/ exclusion criteria (IC/EC)	Type of intervention	Outcome measure	Results
Jarus et al., 2011, Canada [25]	Meir Medical Center, preterm infants	$n = 32$, postmenstrual age (days) 30.37 ± 2.57, sex 12/20	Level II RCT IC: birth weight less than 1750 g, stable in room air EC: major congenital anomalies or major neurological illness, using medication affects the infant's sleep-wake cycle	(i) Alternate position every 3-4 hours after feedings	(i) Actigraph measurement (ii) Naturalistic observations of newborn behavior (NONB)	(i) In the prone position, there were more approach reactions than withdrawal reactions ($p < 0.001$) while in the supine position (ii) In the prone position, more patterns were observed as opposed to more awake patterns
Leland et al., 2016, USA [26]	Various elderly community centers, age > 65	$n = 217$, age 74.2 ± 7.7, sex 65/141	Level I RCT	(i) Occupation-based intervention	(i) SF 36 (ii) Center for Epidemiologic Studies Depression Scale-Revised (iii) Sleep time (iv) Napping time	(i) The average time sleeping was 8.2 hours daily with SD 1.7 (ii) 29% of participants reported daytime napping at baseline, 35% of whom no longer napped at follow-up Among participants who stopped napping, those who received an occupation-based intervention replaced napping time with nighttime sleep, and those who did not receive an intervention experienced a net loss of total sleep ($p < 0.05$)
Schoen et al., 2017, USA [27]	South Shore Therapies and Knippenberg, Patterson, Langley, & Associates, children with autism spectrum disorder	$n = 15$	Level III A quasi-experimental, single-group, pretest/ posttest design IC: parents reported moderate to severe sleep disturbance EC: had stressful life circumstance that could account for new onset sleep difficulties, medical or psychiatric illness, medication known to cause insomnia or sedation, receiving medication or CBT for sleep disorder, could not comply with sleep diary or use of pillow	(i) iLs Dreampad pillow	(i) A sleep diary documented average sleep duration and average time to fall asleep during the preintervention phase and the last 2 weeks of the treatment phase (ii) The Children's Sleep Habits Questionnaire (CSHQ) (iii) The Pediatric Quality of Life Inventory (PedQL) (iv) The Parental Concerns Questionnaire (PCQ) (v) The Swanson, Nolan, and Pelham (SNAP-IV)	(i) Procedures were acceptable and feasible for families. All measures were sensitive to change. Children with ASD demonstrated significant change in sleep duration ($t = -3.01$, $p < 0.003$) and time needed to fall asleep ($t = -2.83$, $p < 0.005$) from pretest to intervention (ii) Improvements were noted in autism-related behaviors, attention ($t = -2.63$, $p < 0.009$), and quality of life ($t = -2.94$, $p < 0.003$), SNAP-IV ($t = -2.44$, $p < 0.015$); parent satisfaction was high

Table 3: Continued.

Author, year, country	Setting subject	Sample size (n), age, sex (M/F)	Level of evidence/clinical study design, inclusion/exclusion criteria (IC/EC)	Type of intervention	Outcome measure	Results
Wen et al., 2017, USA [28]	Traumatic brain injury	$n = 2$, age 31	Level IV Mixed-methods pilot study IC: diagnosis of chronic TBI (6-month postinjury), ability to stand/move, ability to follow a 3-step command, ability to read/speak English EC: neurological conditions like bipolar disorder and attention deficit hyperactive disorder	(i) Yoga (ii) Breathing exercise	(i) Pittsburgh Sleep Quality Index (ii) Neuropathy Pain Scale (iii) Behavior Rating Inventory of Executive Function (iv) Beck Depression Inventory	(i) One participant showed 25% reduction in depressive symptoms, and other improvements were found in the inhibition and emotional control scales of the BRIEF
Wolfhope et al., 2016, USA [29]	Saint Francis University, autism spectrum disorder	$n = 2$, age 3–6	Level IV A preexperimental single-case design and followed the OXO research design	(i) iLs Dreampad mini	(i) Self-created questionnaire (ii) FitBit Flex	(i) Increase in the number of hours of sleep received per night (ii) Increase in observed attention and focus (iii) Decrease in meltdowns
Wooster et al., 2015, USA [30]	Various community settings, children with autism spectrum disorder		Level III A pretest-posttest, one group design	(i) Occupational therapy-based parent educational program (ii) Sensory calming strategies, sleep hygiene xroutines, sleep schedules, bedtime routines, environmental modification, faded bedtime practices, and bedtime pass techniques	(i) Knowledge-basedpretest-posttest was designed and administered before and after the educational program (ii) Children's Sleep Habits Questionnaire (CSHQ): bedtime resistance, sleep anxiety, sleep onset delay, sleep duration, night waking, daytime sleepiness, sleep-disordered breathing, and parasomnias	(i) Significant increase in parental knowledge ($p = 0.003$) on the basis of the occupational therapy educational program provided

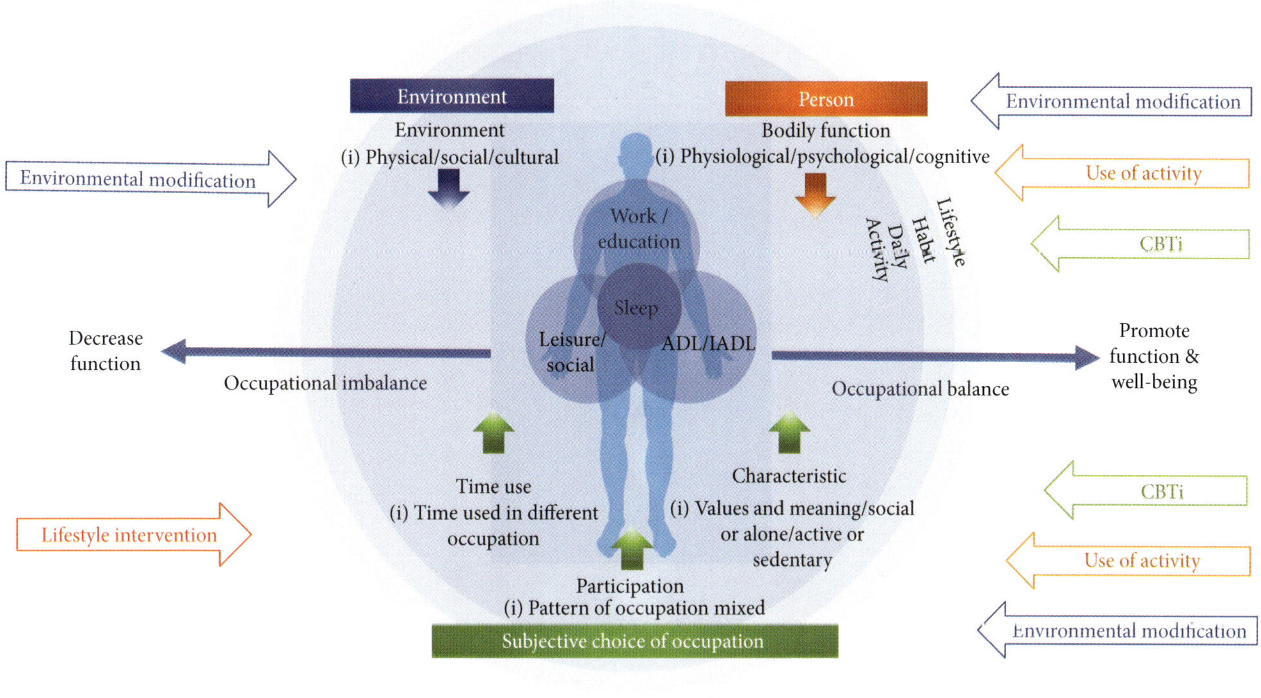

FIGURE 2: Occupational therapy on sleep management.

is usually conducted on a weekly basis and monitored via different assessments, like a sleep diary. Two of the studies adopted CBTi as the core of their sleep management program. They found that CBTi could significantly improve the ability to handle sleep issues in patients with PTSD [30], reduce their sleeping difficulties and nightmares, reduce dysfunctional sleep beliefs, and improve their ability to participate in social roles (Eakman et al. 2016).

3.2.4. Lifestyle Intervention. Among the selected articles, there is one large-scale RCT that focuses on lifestyle intervention to promote sleep among community-dwelling elderly [26]. The lifestyle intervention emphasizes the promotion of healthy sleep habits and activity rescheduling and facilitates role transition in aging through education, experience sharing, and goal setting. Too much or too little daytime activity is highly related to sleep pattern at night; rescheduling of daytime activity helps one in achieving a balanced lifestyle to facilitate sleep during night time. The program demonstrates positive changes in sleep behaviors, including increased sleeping hours, reduced sleep difficulties, and reduced nightmares [26]. Clients also reduced daytime napping and increased daytime engagement, especially social activities. This study suggests that sleep management does not only just concern sleep but also daytime functioning.

4. Conceptual Framework for Occupational Therapy Practice in Sleep Management

Few of the 11 articles explicitly mention the conceptual or theoretical framework used. Only two studies mention the use of cognitive behavioral therapy as a framework for guiding practice (Eakman et al. 2016; Wooster et al. 2016), while another refers to daytime engagement and how it is related to sleep based on a lifestyle redesign program [26]. In this part of the review, we would like to propose a conceptual model for organizing sleep interventions and occupational therapy practice based on the PEOP framework (Christiansen et al. 2011). Figure 2 shows how we could integrate the theory and practice of occupational therapy based on current research evidence and explains the unique role of occupational therapy in sleep management.

Based on the PEOP framework, occupation-based sleep management can focus on three levels: (1) person: minimizing the influence of bodily function on sleep (Eakman et al. 2016; [22, 25, 28, 30]); (2) environment: promoting environment conducive to sleep [21, 24, 27, 29]; and (3) occupation: restructuring daytime activity [26].

First, the "person" level relates to bodily function, which includes physiological, psychological, and cognition performance. Bodily function can affect one's sleep. People suffering from depression and pain and the elderly very often have sleep problems (Foley et al. 2004). Sleep interventions targeting bodily function could include the use of activity to promote calming effects on the body to shorten sleep latency [23, 28]; CBTi could be applied to manage the cognitive traps in PTSD (Eakman et al. 2016; [30]); or a weighted blanket could be used to address the overresponsivity of children with ASD [22] or to position a preterm baby [25]. Although bodily function cannot be improved quickly and is not totally reversible, this factor should also be considered with the aim of maximizing functioning.

Second, occupational therapists could use environmental interventions in the physical, social, or cultural domains to address sleep problems. This review shows that the control of environmental factors plays a significant role in sleep management [21, 24, 27, 29]. Examples of such an intervention include the use of the newly designed Dreampad pillow, weighted blankets, and sleep tools; controlling light, temperature, and humidity levels; and the use of body positions to tackle sleep problems caused by specific diseases. In Hong Kong, a densely populated city, living environment may create sleep barriers for patients. Circumstances permitting the use of sleep tools to reduce environmental stimuli may facilitate sleep. Besides physical environment, social environmental factors, such as sleep partner (both human and pets), also affect sleep and should be considered in an intervention.

Third, the subjective choice of daily activities is the most important area in future service development for sleep management. Everyone has the right to determine the combination of daily occupations to achieve occupational balance even when suffering from illness. However, one's daytime activity can clearly have an impact on one's sleep [26]. In sleep management programs, it is important for therapists to guide clients to choose daily activities and develop occupational balance (Figure 1), including how to organize daytime occupations (activity of daily living/household, work/education, and leisure/social), how to allocate time to daily occupations, and how to restructure activity patterns according to the meaning and purpose of activities.

The above analysis shows that occupational therapists provide sleep management guidance to patients from diverse disease groups in all age groups. Most of the programs presented in the literature were developed for a specific disease group, such as children with ASD ([22, 27, 29]; Wooster et al. 2016) or traumatic brain injury [28]. Although sleep is highly correlated with mental condition, the development of sleep programs in mental healthcare is relatively limited. Only one study among the 11 reviewed articles focuses on this (Eakman et al. 2016). The role of occupational therapists in sleep management in mental health settings has been explored over a long time (Faulkner et al. 2015), but the effectiveness of the proposed intervention has not been evaluated scientifically. A huge number of people suffering from insomnia in Hong Kong present with initial mood disturbance; early intervention plays an important role to prevent long-term healthcare burden.

5. Occupational Therapy-Based Sleep/Daytime Functional Assessment

This review has shown that occupational therapists should assess the occupational balance between daytime activities and sleep. Limited information on occupational therapy-related assessment was found in the literature. The Canadian Occupational Performance Measurement (COPM) (Eakman et al. 2016; [21]) and the Functional Independent Measure (FIM) [21] have been used in some sleep management studies to investigate daytime functioning. FIM focuses on one's functioning while COPM focuses on occupational performance and satisfaction, without fully exploring lifestyle. Dür et al. [33] developed an occupational balance questionnaire (OB-Quest) to further explore occupational balance, and it can be applied to assess the occupational balance of both patients and healthy individuals. More comprehensive occupation-based assessment will definitely advance the development of sleep management in occupational therapy.

6. Limitations

There are two key limitations of this study. First, only eleven studies were identified by the review. Although this reflects the lack of evidence-based studies of sleep intervention in occupational therapy, we may consider expanding the search and be more inclusive in the review. One such possibility is to widen the search criteria and include papers studying multidisciplinary sleep intervention programs in which the occupational therapists participate as a team member. The second limitation of this study is that it could not provide estimates on effect sizes of occupational therapy interventions in sleep management. Only three studies are level I clinical trials which could be used for meta-analysis. We decided not to proceed with meta-analysis based on a small number of studies, which are implemented using different intervention methods for different clients.

While studies on sleep in occupational therapy have become increasingly conspicuous, the number of relevant literature remains limited. It is necessary to extend the scope of research by including patients from different disease groups and types and patients with reported history of sleep problems. There is a great diversity in the methodologies adopted by the selected articles, including case-control trial, RCT, and case series. If only RCTs were to be reviewed here, only three articles would have been included, which would have limited the analysis. The heterogeneity of study designs may also have affected the analysis. Moreover, specific database in occupational therapy may be considered to include for revealing more related articles in occupational therapy such as OTseeker and OTsearch.

7. Conclusion

Sleep is a restorative occupation from the occupational therapy perspective. Its main function is to help us recover from daytime occupations, to build up energy to move forward. The selected literature provides an overview of the scope and types of sleep intervention. The findings, along with the rising incidence of sleep problems, indicate a need for further exploration in this topic. Occupational therapists could address the needs of people with insomnia, by developing sleep management programs using environmental intervention, assistive devices/equipment, the use of activity, CBTi, and lifestyle interventions. Based on the PEOP framework, occupation-based sleep interventions can aim to (1) minimize the influence of bodily function on sleep; (2) promote environment conducive to sleep; and (3) restructure daytime activity with a focus on occupational balance. Further development of sleep management from an occupational therapy perspective will strengthen the role of sleep within clinical practice, education, and research domains.

References

[1] American Academy of Sleep Medicine, "Insomnia," in *The international classifications of sleep disorders: Diagnostic and Coding Manual*, American Academy of Sleep Medicine, 2005, Westchester, IL, 2nd edition, 2005.

[2] D. Cunnington, M. F. Junge, and A. T. Fernando, "Insomnia: prevalence, consequences and effective treatment," *Medical Journal of Australia*, vol. 199, no. 8, pp. S36–S40, 2013.

[3] J. G. Ellis, M. L. Perlis, L. F. Neale, C. A. Espie, and C. H. Bastien, "The natural history of insomnia: focus on prevalence and incidence of acute insomnia," *Journal of Psychiatric Research*, vol. 46, no. 10, pp. 1278–1285, 2012.

[4] W. S. Wong and R. Fielding, "Prevalence of insomnia among Chinese adults in Hong Kong: a population-based study," *Journal of Sleep Research*, vol. 20, no. 1Part1, pp. 117–126, 2011.

[5] C. Wiseman-Hakes, A. Colantonio, and J. Gargaro, "Sleep and wake disorders following traumatic brain injury: a systematic review of the literature," *Critical Reviews in Physical and Rehabilitation Medicine*, vol. 21, no. 3-4, pp. 317–374, 2009.

[6] C. Alford and S. Wilson, *Sleep and Quality of Life in Medical Illnesses*, Humana Press, Totowa, NJ, 2008.

[7] J. M. Y. Cheung, D. J. Bartlett, C. L. Armour, N. Glozier, and B. Saini, "Insomnia patients' help-seeking experiences," *Behavioral Sleep Medicine*, vol. 12, no. 2, pp. 106–122, 2013.

[8] Y. Liu, J. Zhang, S. P. Lam et al., "Help-seeking behaviors for insomnia in Hong Kong Chinese: a community-based study," *Sleep Medicine*, vol. 21, pp. 106–113, 2016.

[9] D. J. Kupfer and C. F. Reynolds, "Management of insomnia," *The New England Journal of Medicine*, vol. 336, no. 5, pp. 341–346, 1997.

[10] C. M. Morin, R. R. Bootzin, D. J. Buysse, J. D. Edinger, C. A. Espie, and K. L. Lichstein, "Psychological and behavioral treatment of insomnia: update of the recent evidence (1998–2004)," *Sleep*, vol. 29, no. 11, pp. 1398–1414, 2006.

[11] C. M. Morin, P. J. Hauri, C. A. Espie, A. J. Spielman, D. J. Buysse, and R. R. Bootzin, "Nonpharmacologic treatment of chronic insomnia. An American Academy of Sleep Medicine review," *Sleep*, vol. 22, no. 8, pp. 1134–1156, 1999.

[12] M. D. Mitchell, P. Gehrman, M. Perlis, and C. A. Umscheid, "Comparative effectiveness of cognitive behavioral therapy for insomnia: a systematic review," *BMC Family Practice*, vol. 13, no. 1, p. 40, 2012.

[13] D. Howell and D. Pierce, "Exploring the forgotten restorative dimension of occupation: quilting and quilt use," *Journal of Occupational Science*, vol. 7, no. 2, pp. 68–72, 2000.

[14] M. Reilly, "Occupational therapy can be one of the great ideas of 20th century medicine," *American Journal of Occupational Therapy*, vol. 16, pp. 1–9, 1962.

[15] A. A. Wilcock and E. A. Townsend, "Occupational justice," in *Willard and Spackman's Occupational Therapy*, B. A. Boyt Schell, G. Gillen, and M. Scaffa, Eds., pp. 541–552, Lippincott Williams & Wilkins, Philadelphia, PA, 12th edition, 2014.

[16] C. L. Backman, "Occupational balance: exploring the relationships among daily occupations and their influence on well-being," *Canadian Journal of Occupational Therapy*, vol. 71, no. 4, pp. 202–209, 2004.

[17] K. W. Hammell, "Self-care, productivity, and leisure, or dimensions of occupational experience? Rethinking occupational "categories"," *Canadian Journal of Occupational Therapy*, vol. 76, no. 2, pp. 107–114, 2009.

[18] L. A. Llorens, "Changing balance: environment and individual," *The American Journal of Occupational Therapy: Official Publication of the American Occupational Therapy Association*, vol. 38, no. 1, pp. 29–34, 1984.

[19] D. Moher, A. Liberati, J. Tetzlaff, D. G. Altman, and for the PRISMA Group, "Preferred reporting items for systematic reviews and meta-analyses: the PRISMA statement," *British Medical Journal*, vol. 339, no. jul21 1, p. b2535, 2009.

[20] A. M. Eakman, A. A. Schmid, K. L. Henry et al., "Restoring effective sleep tranquility (REST): a feasibility and pilot study," *British Journal of Occupational Therapy*, vol. 80, no. 6, pp. 350–360, 2017.

[21] P. M. Farrehi, K. R. Clore, J. R. Scott, G. Vanini, and D. J. Clauw, "Efficacy of sleep tool education during hospitalization: a randomized controlled trial," *The American Journal of Medicine*, vol. 129, no. 12, pp. 1329.e9–1329.e17, 2016.

[22] B. Gee, T. McOmber, J. Sutton, and K. Lloyd, "Efficacy of weighted blankets for children with autism spectrum disorder, sensory over-responsivity, and sleep disturbance," *American Journal of Occupational Therapy*, vol. 71, article 7111515242p1, 4_Supplement_1, 2017.

[23] S. A. Gutman, K. A. Gregory, M. M. Sadlier-Brown et al., "Comparative effectiveness of three occupational therapy sleep interventions," *OTJR: Occupation, Participation and Health*, vol. 37, no. 1, pp. 5–13, 2016.

[24] S. Heidt, J. Ryan Scott, K. Clore et al., "Sleep-enhancing education intervention effect on patient-reported outcomes in hospitalized adults," *American Journal of Occupational Therapy*, vol. 70, article 7011510216p1, 4_Supplement_1, 2016.

[25] T. Jarus, O. Bart, G. Rabinovich et al., "Effects of prone and supine positions on sleep state and stress responses in preterm infants," *Infant Behavior and Development*, vol. 34, no. 2, pp. 257–263, 2011.

[26] N. E. Leland, D. Fogelberg, A. Sleight et al., "Napping and nighttime sleep: findings from an occupation-based intervention," *American Journal of Occupational Therapy*, vol. 70, no. 4, pp. 7004270010p1–7004270010p7, 2016.

[27] S. A. Schoen, S. Man, and C. Spiro, "A sleep intervention for children with autism spectrum disorder: a pilot study," *The Open Journal of Occupational Therapy*, vol. 5, no. 2, 2017.

[28] P.-S. Wen, I. Herrin, A. L. de Mola et al., "Yoga for sleep, pain, mood, and executive functioning in persons with traumatic brain injury," *American Journal of Occupational Therapy*, vol. 71, article 7111515267p1, 4_Supplement_1, 2017.

[29] K. Wolfhope and A. Hudkins, "Increasing quality of sleep utilizing the iLs Dreampad mini in children with autism spectrum disorder," *American Journal of Occupational Therapy*, vol. 70, article 7011515252p1, 4_Supplement_1, 2016.

[30] D. Wooster, H. Gwin, S. Gwin et al., "Efficacy of sleep education for parents with children with autism spectrum disorder," *American Journal of Occupational Therapy*, vol. 69, article 6911515153p1, Supplement 1, 2015.

[31] D. L. Sackett, W. M. C. Rosenberg, J. A. M. Gray, R. B. Haynes, and W. S. Richardson, "Evidence-based medicine: what it is and what it isn't," *British Medical Journal*, vol. 312, no. 7023, pp. 71-72, 1996.

[32] P. Pluye, E. Robert, M. Cargo et al., "Proposal: a mixed methods appraisal tool for systematic mixed studies reviews," 2011, http://www.webcitation.org/5tTRTc9yJ.

26

The Role of the Occupational Therapist in Disaster Areas: Systematic Review

M. Parente,[1] M. Tofani,[2] R. De Santis,[2] G. Esposito,[1] V. Santilli,[2] and G. Galeoto[2]

[1] *Sapienza Università di Roma, Rome, Italy*
[2] *Department of Anatomical, Histological, Forensic and Orthopaedic Sciences, Sapienza Università di Roma, Piazzale Aldo Moro 5, 00185 Rome, Italy*

Correspondence should be addressed to G. Galeoto; usifi.aifilazio@gmail.com

Academic Editor: Erna I. Blanche

Background. Disasters are increasingly more frequent events on our planet. During disaster the role of the occupational therapist will require a more specific operative framework within nongovernmental organizations and community health services. *Design.* Systematic review. *Objective.* The aim of this study is to evaluate the evidence that highlight occupational therapist's role in disaster area through a systematic review. *Materials and Methods.* Research on MEDLINE was performed. All articles from 2005 to 2015 concerning rehabilitation and occupational therapy in disaster areas were included. *Results.* Ten studies were selected to be included in this review. Four interesting points emerged: the importance of having rehabilitation intervention in postdisaster situations, the necessity to include a rehabilitation team in the early phase of disaster response, the need to provide a method to address the difficult evacuation, and finding the safest method of transport of people with preexisting disabilities and new injuries. *Conclusions.* The amount of evidence with respect to specific intervention of the occupational therapist's role in a disaster situation is limited. However some evidence suggests that it could be a good means for reducing the number of medical complications and deaths of persons with preexisting disabilities. The evidences found highlight the necessity to create a multidisciplinary team addressing needs in disasters situation, in which the occupational therapist could certainly contribute.

1. Introduction

Disasters are increasingly more frequent on our planet, even though their distribution is directly linked to the geophysical characteristics of the different regions.

According to the International Federation of Red Cross and Red Crescent Societies, disaster is a sudden, calamitous event that seriously disrupts the functioning of a community or society and causes human, material, and economic or environmental losses that exceed the community's or society's ability to cope based on its own resources [1]. Though often caused by nature, disasters can have human origins.

Usually, disasters are classified into two macrocategories: natural hazards and technological or man-made hazards. Natural hazards are naturally occurring physical phenomena caused either by rapid or slow onset events which can be geophysical (earthquakes, landslides, tsunamis, and volcanic activity), hydrological (avalanches and floods), climatological (extreme temperatures, drought, and wildfires), meteorological (cyclones and storms/wave surges), or biological (disease epidemics and insect/animal plagues). Technological or man-made hazards (complex emergencies/conflicts, famine, displaced populations, industrial accidents, and transport accidents) are events that are caused by humans and occur in or close to human settlements. These can include environmental degradation, pollution, and accidents. The combination of hazards, vulnerability, and inability to reduce the potential negative consequences of risk results in disaster.

From 1900 to 2014 natural hazard exponentially increased (Figure 1); in particular during the last decade these phenomena have often been registered in different parts of the world, as indicated by Centre for Research on the Epidemiology of Disasters (CRED) (Figure 2) [2].

The effects of each disaster do translate not only into numbers of deaths, but also mostly into long-term disabilities that result from it. The most frequent disabilities are spinal

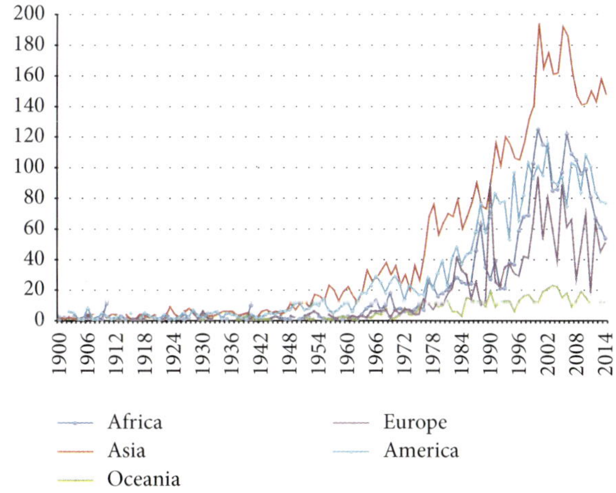

Figure 1: Number of natural disasters in the world from 1900 to 2014.

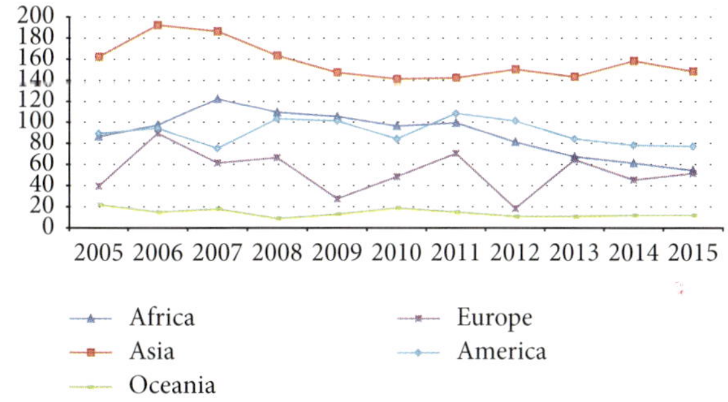

Figure 2: Number of natural disasters in the world from 2005 to 2015.

cord injury, traumatic brain injury, fracture, limb amputation, peripheral nerve injury, and crush injury [3].

In the early stages after a disaster, humanitarian organizations and community health services have to schedule aids in emergency conditions. Furthermore, both volunteers and those associated with humanitarian organizations actually prove to be able to manage complex circumstances [4].

For this reason, a multidisciplinary emergency team should include rehabilitation professionals: as their competences and expertise could be useful to recognize and manage similar disabilities while trying to reduce the high risk of medical complications and, in turn, a possible aggravation unstable situation during the acute phase [4, 5]. Indeed the most urgent priority is to save lives and help people with disabilities who are at greater risk of dying or being left behind during the evacuation [6, 7]. Special attention should be given to these vulnerable categories of persons by rehabilitation professionals.

2. Objective

The aim of this study is to evaluate the evidences available in the literature that highlight the occupational therapist's role in a disaster situation through a systematic review.

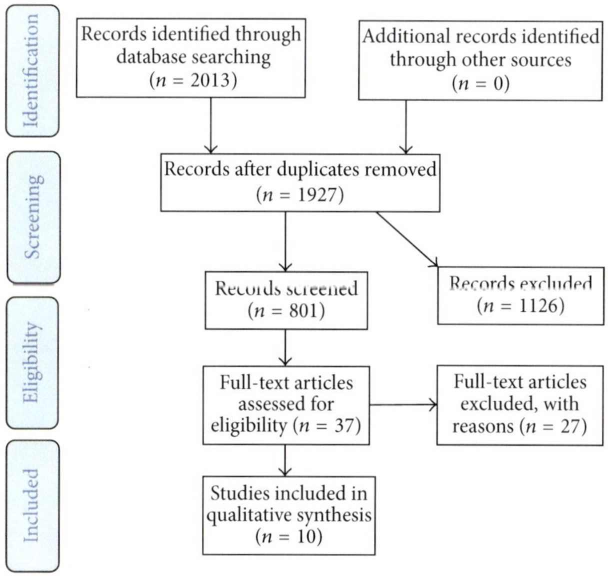

Figure 3: Flowchart.

3. Materials and Methods

Search terms included "rehabilitation", "disaster", "natural disaster", and "occupational therapy". Three independent searches were carried out using the following terminology: "disaster AND rehabilitation", "natural disaster AND rehabilitation", and "natural disaster AND occupational therapy". All included studies had the following criteria: published in English on MEDLINE from January 2005 to September 2015. All articles about rehabilitation and occupational therapy interventions in disaster areas were included. Studies that did not have these characteristics were excluded. Titles and abstracts were read, articles not meeting selection criteria were discarded, and those remaining were read in full to check for suitability, in accordance with the Preferred Reporting Items for Systematic and Meta-Analyses (PRISMA).

Data extraction was completed by one reviewer confirmed by a fellow author. Relevant articles meeting the inclusion criteria were reviewed with all relevant information, such as type of design, participants' characteristics, and significant findings of outcome.

4. Results

The database search yielded 10 papers which met inclusion criteria (Figure 3).

All articles referred only to postearthquake disaster management. Search results have been summarized in Table 1. Four interesting points emerged: the importance of having rehabilitation intervention in postdisaster situations, the necessity to include a rehabilitation team in the early phase of disaster response, the need to provide a method to address the difficult evacuation, and finding the safest method of mobilization.

4.1. Rehabilitation in Postdisaster. Zhang et al. [12] studied the survivors to understand the motor functions and ADL

Table 1: Data extraction.

References	Objectives	Study type	Participants' characteristics	Results	Conclusions
Reinhardt et al. [8], 2011, Global Health Action	To examine the role of health-related rehabilitation in natural disaster relief along three lines of inquiry: epidemiology of injury and disability, impact on health and rehabilitation systems, and the assessment and measurement of disability.	Qualitative literature review	N = 246 deaths and affected by year and region N = 568 deaths in earthquake N = 41 deaths and affected in Asia	Major impairments requiring health-related rehabilitation include amputations, traumatic brain injuries, spinal cord injuries (SCI), and long bone fractures. Studies show that persons with preexisting disabilities are more likely to die in a natural disaster.	Additional development of health-related rehabilitation following natural disaster is urgently required.
Hunt et al. [9], 2015, Global Health Action	To better understand the perceptions of responders and decision-makers regarding disability and efforts to address the needs of PWD following the 2010 earthquake.	Qualitative study	N = 24 persons involved in the national and international first aid associations; 11 women; 13 men	Participants identified PWD as being among the most vulnerable individuals following the earthquake. Though some forms of disability received considerable attention in aid efforts, the needs of other PWD did not. Several factors were identified as challenges for efforts to address the needs of PWD including lack of coordination and information sharing, the involvement of multiple aid sectors, perceptions that this should be the responsibility of specialized organizations, and the need to prioritize limited resources.	There have been several efforts to promote best practices and develop guidelines to better address the needs of PWD in disasters; significant obstacles remain to the implementation of disaster preparedness, relief, and reconstruction that is inclusive of PWD and responsive to their needs.
Khan et al. [3], 2015, Archives of Physical Medicine and Rehabilitation	To present an evidence-based overview of the effectiveness of medical rehabilitation intervention in natural disaster survivors and outcomes that are affected.	Systematic review	N = 10 studies (2 randomized controlled trials, 8 observational studies) N = 2013 participants; age 9–76, mostly women	There are some evidence for the rehabilitation short and long-term improvement in terms of functional activity, psychological symptom, and participation. More attention must be paid to the rescue of preexisting disabilities.	The findings highlight the need to incorporate medical rehabilitation into response planning and disaster management for future natural catastrophes. Access to rehabilitation and investment in sustainable infrastructure and education are crucial. More methodologically robust studies are needed to build evidence for rehabilitation programs, cost-effectiveness, and outcome measurement in such settings.

Table 1: Continued.

References	Objectives	Study type	Participants' characteristics	Results	Conclusions
Gosney et al. [5], 2013, Spinal Cord	To summarize epidemiological and scientific research on spinal cord injury (SCI) populations from three severe earthquakes (EQs) in rehabilitation resource-scarce settings; summarize SCI rehabilitation services by local and foreign providers; and provide implications including research gaps for a supporting global scientific research agenda.	Narrative literature review	$N = 11$ studies (4, 2005 Pakistan earthquake; 4, 2008 China earthquake; and 3, 2010 Haiti earthquake)	The range of long-term disabilities is more than death's range. Sometimes the rescue operation of SCI patients is not accurate; therefore the clinical picture is made worse.	A global disaster research agenda for SCI in EQs in rehabilitation resource-scarce settings is needed to strengthen the evidence base for improvement of clinical management and outcomes for SCI EQ survivors.
Liu et al. [10], 2012, Journal of Rehabilitation Medicine	To provide descriptive epidemiology and assess the activities of 10 rehabilitation-related organizations.	Descriptive	10 rehabilitation-related organizations	10-RRO provided relief activities at 3 shelters. Support activities included prevention of immobilization, daily life support, environmental improvement, and transition to temporary housing. The questionnaire survey revealed poor preparedness, satisfactory initial response and support activities, and problems of data collection and advocacy.	The disaster was characterized by minimal trauma and a great need for preventing immobilization. There is an urgent need to develop such a manual to improve preparedness and enhance capability of first aid team to cope with disasters.
Landry et al. [11], 2010, Disability and Rehabilitation	To underline the role of rehabilitation during and after Haiti earthquake	Report	Undefined	There is a remarkable increment of permanent disabilities caused also by attempt of rescues. For this reason there is a tremendous need of rehabilitation services.	The events have raised awareness of the importance of rehabilitation services and highlighted the need to incorporate rehabilitation into response planning for future humanitarian catastrophes.
Zhang et al. [12], 2011, Chinese Medical Journal	To value disability impact on motor function and ADL	Retrospective cohort study	$N = 395$ patients; 218 men, 55.2% fractures; 117 women, 44.8% fractures;	Most survivors 82% had decreased ROM and 23.5%. Muscle force 72.2% had also restricted ADL capacities. With time the ADL capacities of female patients increased compared to the male patients.	Fractures were the main issue among the injured. Many patients had decreased ROM, ADL capacities, and muscle force; this highlights that physician, involved in rehabilitation, should pay great attention to muscle force exercises, joint mobilization, and occupational therapy during the early phase after disaster.

Table 1: Continued.

References	Objectives	Study type	Participants' characteristics	Results	Conclusions
Rathore et al. [13], 2008, Archives of Physical Medicine and Rehabilitation	To sum up the interventions, the gaps, and the needs emerged the day after the 2005 earthquake in Pakistan.	Report	The ratio of males to females injured 1 : 1.3 Mean age 28, 16.5% less than 18 y; 89% paraplegia cases	Spinal trauma is a surgical emergency that requires specialized care in the initial immobilization and transport of a patient. Unfortunately, after the earthquake, there was usually such little care taken in transporting patients with a suspected or diagnosed SCI. Many physicians involved in the care of SCI patients were unaware of the ASIA system and its worksheet documentation. This resulted in errors in the diagnosis of complete and incomplete SCI.	There is a need to increase disaster preparedness and have a tangible disaster management plan in place and periodic disaster drills. Trauma management in disasters and the correct SCI evacuation, immobilization, and transport protocols should be taught during the training of emergency relief workers, ambulance officers, army medical staff, resident surgeons, and emergency physicians. Rescue units trained in methods to avoid and minimize spinal injuries should be established.
Rathore et al. [4], 2012, Archives of Physical Medicine and Rehabilitation	To stimulate development of research and practice in the emerging discipline of disaster rehabilitation within organizations that provide medical rehabilitation services during the postdisaster emergency response.	Report	Undefined	Medical rehabilitation is an urgent, essential emergency medical service in disasters and not restricted to the intermediate and long-term care settings. Emergency rehabilitation services should only be provided by trained, credentialed professionals to ensure practice accountability and proper standards of care. Nonqualified personnel, although well intentioned, should provide care only in the event of extreme emergency and under strict supervision.	Evidence on the effectiveness of disaster rehabilitation interventions is presented; indeed these services can reduce morbidity and improve functional results and survival.

capacity of patients with fractures sustained in the Wenchuan earthquake in 2008 and to provide a basis for rehabilitation and treatment. Fractures were the main issue in the seismic wounded; many of survivors had reductions in ROM, muscle force, and ADL capacities. Authors conclude that physicians involved in rehabilitation should pay greater attention to muscle force exercises, joint mobilization, and occupational therapy during the early phases after disaster.

Rauch et al. [14] described problems in functioning and associated rehabilitation needs in persons with spinal cord injury after the 2010 earthquake in Haiti by applying a newly developed tool based on the International Classification of Functioning, Disability and Health (ICF). This ICF-based needs' assessment provided useful information for rehabilitation planning in the context of natural disaster. Authors conclude that a multidisciplinary approach would be needed and in particular in low-resource countries it is crucial to enable local staff to perform assessments and provide education and training in rehabilitation management.

Reinhardt et al. [8] presented an evidence-based overview of the effectiveness of medical rehabilitation intervention in natural disaster survivors and outcomes that are affected. The findings suggest some evidence for the effectiveness of inpatient rehabilitation in reducing disability and improving participation and quality of life and in community-based rehabilitation program for participation. The findings also highlight the need to incorporate medical rehabilitation into response planning and disaster management for future natural catastrophes.

4.2. Rehabilitation during Early Phases of Response. Reinhardt et al. [8] have examined the role of health-related rehabilitation in disaster relief in terms of the epidemiology of injury and disability in natural disasters, the impact of natural disasters on health and rehabilitation systems, and the assessment of disability due to natural disasters. Authors also analyze the condition of persons with preexisting disabilities after a natural disaster: the loss of medications and assistive technologies can impair their quality of life. Furthermore the lack of trained support personnel can worsen the condition of these vulnerable persons. Authors conclude that significant systematic challenges to effective delivery of rehabilitation interventions during disasters include a lack of trained responders as well as a lack of medical recordkeeping, data collection, and established outcome measures.

Khan et al. [3] suggest that it is crucial to have support of a multidisciplinary team—including occupational therapist—in the early phase of a disaster. They also analyze the role of Physical and Rehabilitation Medicine and developed some recommendations including the necessity to develop scientific evidence for medical rehabilitation in the emergency disaster response, to develop a rehabilitation disaster relief expertise, and to strengthen an international rehabilitation emergency response capability where both International Society of Physical and Rehabilitation Medicine and other rehabilitative associations could cooperate.

Landry et al. [11] analyzed the situation that occurred after earthquake in Haiti in 2010 as an important inflection point for international humanitarian efforts that target rehabilitation. Authors analyzed problems related to organizing early intervention in a low-resources country based on treatment of disabling consequences and based on relieving the stress of local health care systems. In this article authors highlighted the need to incorporate rehabilitation into response planning for future humanitarian catastrophes.

4.3. The Issues of Persons with Preexisting Disabilities. Liu et al. [10] focused their intervention in particular to prevent immobilization syndrome and progressive functional deterioration among frail elderly survivors and persons with preexisting disabilities who were forced to stay in shelters that were not designed to encourage physical activity. Authors evaluate activities of 10 rehabilitation-related organizations, which include the occupational therapist. This first collaborative disaster relief endeavour by rehabilitation-related organizations and professionals has contributed to a strong foundation for future interdisciplinary and interorganizational collaborative activities.

Hunt et al. [9] contribute to better understanding of the perceptions of responders and decision-makers regarding disability and efforts to address the needs of persons with disabilities following the 2010 earthquake in Haiti. In fact, following disasters, persons with disabilities are especially vulnerable to harm, yet they have commonly been excluded from disaster planning, and their needs have been poorly addressed during disaster relief.

4.4. The Need of a Correct Mobilization and Transport for the Newly Acquired and Old Disabilities. Gosney et al. [5] in this narrative review collected data about spinal cord injury (SCI), one of the most frequently occurring disabilities after a hazard. Authors discuss the correct managing of SCI and underline the importance of correct mobilization of new acquired injury. This article strengthens the idea of the necessity of a multidisciplinary approach.

Rathore et al. [13] shed light on some crucial aspects that emerged during the first aid phases in the 2005 Pakistan earthquake by summarizing the services provided. Above all, the issue of evacuation and transport of the newly acquired SCI was addressed. Authors highlighted the lack of first response teams working in the emergency after disaster to correctly evacuate, safely mobilize, and transport people with SCI.

5. Discussion

Articles focusing on occupational therapy were not found. However, different experiences of occupational therapists were cited emphasizing their appropriateness due to professional training. After our analysis, it seems fitting that occupational therapist may be eligible into being a part of the response team in a natural disaster.

According to the American Occupational Therapy Association's (AOTA) position paper regarding the role of occupational therapy in disaster preparedness, response, and recovery, five stages of disaster relief were categorized:

(i) preimpact;
(ii) impact;
(iii) immediate postimpact;
(iv) recovery;
(v) reconstruction [15].

Considering preimpact and impact stages, occupational therapist may find his competencies more useful to organize in collaboration with multidisciplinary team such as an evacuation plan for people affected by preexisting disabilities and planning access to first aid facilities, which are not always accessible for people with mobility impairment.

Occupational therapists are also widely involved in immediate postimpact, recovery, and reconstruction stages. They can work both in subacute rehabilitation treatment facilities and promoting the reintegration of the individual into family and society. The immediate role of the occupational therapist in the postimpact phase is not well defined in the literature; evidence suggests the necessity to create a multidisciplinary network to better organize technical operations.

In Rathore et al.'s study "Rehabilitation during Early Phase of Response" focused on what physiatrists can do during early phases of intervention. Authors confirm the necessity to create a multidisciplinary international network to manage emergency operations.

In the "Rehabilitation in Post Disaster" section the authors highlight the importance of evaluation of any assistive technologies needed, such as wheelchairs. Furthermore mobilizing preexisting or newly acquired disabilities require professional skills and a trained therapist or volunteer in order to reduce the risk of wrong and hazardous movements.

In the "The Issues of Persons with Pre-Existing Disabilities" section the authors describe the importance of a communitarian approach to improve rehabilitation and prevent progressive functional deterioration of people with disabilities. Authors stressed the importance to define an operative framework within community health services.

Therefore, we believe that the occupational therapist can play a significant role in different situations.

6. Study Limitations

One of the most important limitations that our study encountered was the low number of scientific evidence and the lack of material on this topic in the literature. In fact there were no articles in which occupational therapy was the centre of the rehabilitation interventions. Furthermore, lots of studies were conducted in very poor areas, such as Haiti, Pakistan, and the countryside of China, where health and rehabilitation networks are not well developed.

7. Conclusions

In conclusion, this study had the objective of verifying evidence about occupational therapist intervention [16, 17] in a disaster area. We can state that occupational therapist could reduce complications' rate and worsening of medical case.

The ten articles included talked about the necessity of a rehabilitation team in providing measures to reduce damage in early postimpact phases. The occupational therapist could take an active role in emergency management, as follows:

(i) They are important members of any rehabilitation team and can provide vital service in the early phase of response.

(ii) They have expertise in caring for preexisting disabilities.

(iii) They have expertise in problem solving to correct mobilization and evacuation, while taking into consideration preexisting and newly acquired conditions.

Therefore, investing and introducing occupational therapists in first response teams could not only translate into a reduction of medical complications and a better quality of life for people with disabilities, but could also translate into potential economic benefits as cutting the cost for care additional services and assistance from National Health Systems.

Another aspect that we might consider is the possibility of using an occupation therapist as an instructor to provide necessary education to multidisciplinary team and as a volunteer who helps in emergency management.

Competing Interests

The authors declare that they have no competing interests.

References

[1] https://www.scribd.com/presentation/243634776/Simposium-Fisika-Nasional-Bali-Bali.

[2] D. Guha-Sapir, R. Below, and Ph. Hoyois, EM-DAT: The CRED/OFDA International Disaster Database, Université Catholique de Louvain, Brussels, Belgium, http://www.emdat.be.

[3] F. Khan, B. Amatya, J. Gosney, F. A. Rathore, and F. M. Burkle, "Medical rehabilitation in natural disasters: a review," *Archives of Physical Medicine and Rehabilitation*, vol. 96, no. 9, pp. 1709–1727, 2015.

[4] F. A. Rathore, J. E. Gosney, J. D. Reinhardt, A. J. Haig, J. Li, and J. A. Delisa, "Medical rehabilitation after natural disasters: why, when, and how?" *Archives of Physical Medicine and Rehabilitation*, vol. 93, no. 10, pp. 1875–1881, 2012.

[5] J. E. Gosney, J. D. Reinhardt, P. M. Von Groote, F. A. Rathore, and J. L. Melvin, "Medical rehabilitation of spinal cord injury following earthquakes in rehabilitation resource-scarce settings: implications for disaster research," *Spinal Cord*, vol. 51, no. 8, pp. 603–609, 2013.

[6] M. Liu, M. Kohzuki, A. Hamamura et al., "How did rehabilitation professionals act when faced with the Great East Japan earthquake and disaster? Descriptive epidemiology of disability and an interim report of the relief activities of the ten rehabilitation-related organizations," *Journal of Rehabilitation Medicine*, vol. 44, no. 5, pp. 421–428, 2012.

[7] M. R. Hunt, R. Chung, E. Durocher, and J. H. Henrys, "Haitian and international responders' and decision-makers' perspectives regarding disability and the response to the 2010 Haiti earthquake," *Global Health Action*, vol. 8, Article ID 27969, 2015.

[8] J. D. Reinhardt, J. Li, J. Gosney et al., "Disability and health-related rehabilitation in international disaster relief," *Global Health Action*, vol. 4, article 7191, 2011.

[9] M. R. Hunt, R. Chung, E. Durocher, and J. H. Henrys, "Haitian and international responders' and decisionmakers' perspectives regarding disability and the response to the 2010 Haiti earthquake," *Global Health Action*, vol. 8, no. 1, Article ID 27969, 2015.

[10] M. Liu, M. Kohzuki, A. Hamamura et al., "How did rehabilitation professionals act when faced with the Great East Japan Earth quake and Disaster? Descriptive epidemiology of disability and an interim report of the relief activities of the TEN Rehabilitation -related Organizations," *Journal of Rehabilitation Medicine*, vol. 44, no. 5, pp. 421–428, 2012.

[11] M. D. Landry, C. O'Connell, G. Tardif, and A. Burns, "Post-earthquake Haiti: the critical role for rehabilitation services following a humanitarian crisis," *Disability & Rehabilitation*, vol. 32, no. 19, pp. 1616–1618, 2010.

[12] J.-L. Zhang, H.-C. He, H.-D. Lin et al., "Motor function and activities of daily living capacity of patients with fractures sustained during the Wenchuan earthquake," *Chinese Medical Journal*, vol. 124, no. 10, pp. 1504–1507, 2011.

[13] F. A. Rathore, F. Farooq, S. Muzammil, P. W. New, N. Ahmad, and A. J. Haig, "Spinal cord injury management and rehabilitation: highlights and shortcomings from the 2005 earthquake in pakistan," *Archives of Physical Medicine and Rehabilitation*, vol. 89, no. 3, pp. 579–585, 2008.

[14] A. Rauch, M. Baumberger, F.-G. Moise, E. Von Elm, and J. D. Reinhardt, "Rehabilitation needs assessment in persons with spinal cord injury following the 2010 earthquake in Haiti: a pilot study using an ICF-based tool," *Journal of Rehabilitation Medicine*, vol. 43, no. 11, pp. 969–975, 2011.

[15] M. A. Pizzi, "Hurricane Sandy, disaster preparedness, and the recovery model," *American Journal of Occupational Therapy*, vol. 69, no. 4, pp. 6904250010p1–6904250010p10, 2015.

[16] G. Galeoto, R. De Santis, A. Marcolini, A. Cinelli, and R. Cecchi, "The informed consent in occupational therapy: proposal of forms," *Giornale Italiano di Medicina del Lavoro ed Ergonomia*, vol. 38, no. 2, pp. 107–115, 2016.

[17] G. Galeoto, R. Mollica, O. Astorino, and R. Cecchi, "Informed consent in physiotherapy: proposal of a form," *Giornale Italiano di Medicina del Lavoro ed Ergonomia*, vol. 37, no. 4, pp. 245–254, 2015.

27

Everyday Activities for Children with Mitochondrial Disorder: A Retrospective Chart Review

Marieke Lindenschot,[1,2,3,4] Imelda J. M. de Groot,[4] Saskia Koene,[5] Ton Satink,[2,3,6] Esther M. J. Steultjens,[2,3] and Maria W. G. Nijhuis-van der Sanden[1,4]

[1]*Department IQ Healthcare, Research Institute for Health Sciences, Radboud University Medical Center Nijmegen, Postbus 9101, 6500 HB Nijmegen, Netherlands*
[2]*Department of Occupational Therapy, HAN University of Applied Sciences, Postbus 6960, 6503 GL Nijmegen, Netherlands*
[3]*Research Group Neurorehabilitation, HAN University of Applied Sciences, Nijmegen, Netherlands*
[4]*Department of Rehabilitation, Donders Center for Neuroscience, Radboud University Medical Center Nijmegen, Postbus 9101, 6500 HB Nijmegen, Netherlands*
[5]*Department of Pediatrics, Radboud Center for Mitochondrial Medicine, Radboud University Medical Center Nijmegen, Geert Grooteplein Zuid 10, 6525 GA Nijmegen, Netherlands*
[6]*European Masters of Science in Occupational Therapy, Amsterdam University of Applied Sciences, Amsterdam, Netherlands*

Correspondence should be addressed to Marieke Lindenschot; marieke.lindenschot@radboudumc.nl

Academic Editor: Jodie A. Copley

Background. Engagement in everyday activities is important for the health and wellbeing of children. Children with mitochondrial disorders have impaired energy production leading to limitations in activity. It is unknown which activities these children perform and if the nature of activities of low-functioning children differs from average-functioning children. Therefore, this pilot study explored the activities reported in patient records of a heterogeneous group of children with genetically confirmed mitochondrial disorders. *Methods.* A retrospective qualitative directed content analysis by health care professionals reported activities (as part of their professional reasoning obligations) in hospital patient records of children with mitochondrial disorder. *Results.* Seventeen patient records, presenting notes on capacities and performed activities, showed an overview of everyday activities that covered the categories: self-care, house chores, therapy, school, computing, hobby, play, sports, and mobility/transport. The activity categories of low-functioning children did not differ from average-functioning children, although descriptions of specific activities differed between groups. *Conclusion.* This pilot exploration indicates that the types of activities that children with mitochondrial disorders perform are not necessarily linked to the child's impairments. However, differences in levels of independence, assistive device usage, and energy costs seem to exist. Future research should address the child's perspective on, and meaning of, activity performances.

1. Introduction

Performing everyday activities is viewed as an important factor for the wellbeing of an individual and is an important determinant of health [1–3]. If children are unable to be engaged in everyday activities, they do not have the opportunity to explore their environment and are less able to grow up as unique individuals [4]. Although children with disabilities might enjoy the same activities and have similar desires as their healthy developing peers [5, 6], they can experience limitations in activities, leading to restrictions in their participation in daily life.

Mitochondrial disorders, with an estimated prevalence of 23 in 100,000, are one of the most common inherited errors of metabolism [7]. Mitochondrial disorders can be caused by mutation of genes encoded by either nuclear DNA (nDNA) or mitochondrial DNA (mtDNA) [8]. Mutations have been identified in more than 230 different genes [8, 9], and the number of identified genes associated with mitochondrial disorder is continuously increasing [10]. This genetic heterogeneity is also reflected in the clinical phenotypes associated with mitochondrial disorder, with a large range of symptoms and impairments [11–13]. It was previously found that children (when we talk about children in this article, we mean children and adolescents in the age of 0–18 years) with mitochondrial disorders are less physically active and engage less in vigorous activities compared to healthy peers [14]. Children with a mitochondrial disorder experience these limitations in performing everyday activities due to motor and cognitive impairments including muscle weakness, balance problems, concentration problems, and intellectual disability [13]. These impairments have consequences for daily living activities and participation. The extent of perceived limitations in activities and participation of children with mitochondrial disorders varies from none to extremely high [13]. While some children remain in a mainstream school and achieve normal milestones, others barely interact with their environment [15].

Although literature states that children with mitochondrial disorder experience limitations in activities, a clear overview of their everyday activities is lacking. It is commonly expected that the nature of activities differs based on the global functioning of the child. Knowledge of these possible differences and similarities is important to choose or develop assessments for this population, to evaluate the outcome of treatment on participation, and to be able to tailor the assessments and treatment to the child's and parent's specific wishes. As healthcare professionals make clinical decisions based on information about the child's capacities and activities, we expect that information concerning the activities of the child is reported in patient records. Therefore, this pilot study is aimed at exploring which everyday activities of children with genetically confirmed mitochondrial disorders are reported in patient records by health care professionals and understanding the profile of activities these children participate in.

2. Methods

A retrospective chart review [16, 17] was performed. A directed content analysis [18] was used to explore which everyday activities were reported in patient records and to explore if they differed among the functional profiles of the children.

2.1. Participants. The participants of this study were children (0–18 years) with a genetically confirmed mitochondrial disorder who were periodically evaluated in the so-called "MitoRoute," a multidisciplinary, medical, and allied health care screening program at Radboud Center for Mitochondrial Medicine (RCMM), Radboud University Medical Center (Radboudumc), Nijmegen. During MitoRoute, the children were evaluated by a team consisting of several physicians of different disciplines and allied health professionals, including a physical therapist, occupational therapist, speech therapist, dietitian, social worker, and psychologist. The goal of this screening program was to establish a detailed overview of the consequences of the disorder for the child on different dimensions of the International Classification of Functioning, Disability and Health for Children and Youth (ICF-CY) [19], to prevent and detect possible complications and formulate treatment advice. The patient records of all children with a genetically proven mitochondrial disorder who were screened from May 2015 to May 2016 in the Radboudumc were included in this study.

2.2. Data Collection. Qualitative data concerning activities of children with mitochondrial disorders were extracted from clinical notes of (allied) health care professionals (MitoRoute) in the electronic patient records. The patient records contained unprompted written information relevant to the assessment and conversations performed by (allied) health care professionals, as they were not asked to collect data specific to this study.

2.3. Stratification. As motor function, cognitive abilities, and communication influence participation in activities [20, 21], these characteristics were used to construct functional capacity profiles of the children. To ensure the quality of the stratification into the profiles, a log was kept documenting thought processes and tracked decision-making. Member checking with health care professionals was used to verify the profiles. Functional capacities were stratified as the following: *Cognitive development* (based on the age-related norm-referenced test used for each child): 1 = extremely low cognitive functioning, 2 = low cognitive functioning, 3 = average cognitive functioning, and 4 = good cognitive functioning; *Ambulation* (Hoffer scale [22], with the normal ambulation level added by Schoenmakers et al. [23]): 1 = nonambulation, 2 = nonfunctional ambulation, 3 = household ambulation, 4 = community ambulation, and 5 = normal ambulation; and *Speech abilities* (Radboud dysarthria assessment [24]): 1 = no oral communication possible, 2 = communication with a known person, 3 = frequent repetitions (frequently repeating themselves to guarantee that they will be understood), 4 = incidental repetitions, 5 = effective despite small problems, and 6 = effective communication.

Other patient characteristics collected included gender, age, gross motor development (based on norm-referenced tests), performance in daily activities (based on Pediatric Evaluation of Disabilities Inventory (PEDI) [25]), and fatigue (measured with Pediatric Quality of Life Inventory Multidimensional Fatigue Scale (PedsQL-MFS) [26]). These characteristics were not used in defining the profiles but were used as descriptive outcomes linked to each profile.

2.4. Profiles Based on Functional Capacities. Three profiles could be defined based on the functional capacities of the children:

Global low functioning: children with an extremely low or low cognitive developmental level and limited motor functioning which lead to nonfunctional outdoor ambulation and nonfunctional communication.

Low cognitive functioning with a moderate to normal ambulation: children with extremely low or low cognitive developmental level and some limitations in motor functioning but able to have functional ambulation. Speech abilities in this profile differ among the children.

Global moderate functioning: children with average cognitive developmental level and some limitations in motor functioning but able to have functional ambulation. Speech abilities are sufficient to make themselves understandable.

2.5. Data Analysis. In this exploratory study, the method of directed content analysis [18] was used on the text fragments extracted from the patient records [27–29]. The text fragments were focused on information reported by the health care professionals regarding the experiences of children and parents in their daily life situations. Before starting the analysis of the patient records, two preliminary steps were conducted:

(1) Identify the key concept "activity" as initial coding category

(2) Operationalize the concept "activity" using theory

In step 2 of the data analysis, the term "activity" was defined based on the ICF-CY [19] and occupational therapy literature [30–32] as an activity that is the meaningful targeted performance of tasks and/or actions by an individual, like playing guitar, dressing yourself, eating, and cycling.

For the analysis of the patient records, the following steps were conducted by one of the researchers:

(1) Read text and highlight all text that appears to represent activity

(2) Code the highlighted text with codes fitting the concept activity

(3) Categorize the codes into groups of activities

(4) Organize the categories (the different groups of activities) into three occupational performance areas of Reed and Sanderson [33]: personal maintenance, productivity, and leisure

The procedure of the analysis and the result of steps 4 and 6 were peer reviewed by the fourth author (TS).

2.6. Ethical Considerations. The data used in this research were obtained during the medical care for which the child and parents gave approval to use anonymously for research (ethical board approval number 2013-287). Data were deidentified before analysis. The research was conducted conforming to the ethical principles of the Declaration of Helsinki [34].

3. Results

Patient records of seventeen children (five girls and twelve boys) were included. The age of the children varied from 4 to 18 years old. Eight children had a mutation on their nuclear DNA and nine children on mitochondrial DNA. Five children demonstrated a global low-functioning profile, five children demonstrated a low cognitive-functioning profile with a moderate to normal ambulation, and seven children demonstrated a global moderate-functioning profile. The clinical and genetic characteristics of the children are presented in Table 1. More clinically relevant priorities hindered scheduling of the fatigue assessment in two cases. Therefore, they were not available in the chart.

As mentioned before, the activities were organized in three occupational performance areas of Reed and Sanderson: personal maintenance, productivity, and leisure [33]. Personal maintenance activities permit a person to maintain individual life support needs, for example, getting dressed or taking a shower. Productivity activities assist society to facilitate each person to meet individual needs by the use of collective resources, for example, going to work or doing homework. Leisure activities permit the individual to express needs for creative outlet, for example, drawing or swimming [33]. The outcome of step 5 of the analysis was the activity categories: self-care, house chores, therapy, school, computing, hobby, play, sports, and mobility/transport. Some activity categories could be placed under two occupational performance areas as the meaning or value of the activity was not noted. For instance, mobility/transport activities could be performed as personal maintenance but also as leisure. The results, including any double placement, are presented in Figure 1.

3.1. Personal Maintenance. The area under personal maintenance included all the activities that children do to take care of themselves and organize their lives. It comprises the following categories: self-care, house chores, and mobility/transport. Across the three profiles, the (allied) health care professionals reported on all three different categories in personal maintenance. The patient records showed similarities across the profiles in self-care activities like showering, eating, taking rest, and getting dressed. In the category mobility/transport activities, cycling and taking the bus were commonly reported activities. Although in this category and the category house chores, the activities showed more differences among the profiles. The activities varied from doing the dishes to mowing the lawn.

The notes in the patient records indicate that there was a difference in the support or assistance that the children received when they performed the activity. For instance, the activity eating was mentioned as "*she can eat independently,*" "*with spreading butter and cutting he gets help,*" and "*he uses an eating device which makes him able to move the cutlery independently to his mouth.*" In several activities, receiving assistance or using assistive devices or adaptations were mentioned. For instance, getting dressed and showering were mentioned as "with help" or as "independent." Occasionally, no notes about the support or assistance were written.

3.2. Productivity. The area under productivity featured all the activities that children do to learn and work. It included the following categories: school activities and therapy activities. However, therapy activities can also be seen as personal maintenance. Across the three profiles the (allied) health care professionals documented notes that fit within both categories in productivity. Children within the global low-functioning profile all attended to special education, some

Table 1: Clinical and genetic characteristics of the children.

Gender (A)	Age (years)	Level of cognitive development (B)	Level of motor development (C)	Score on Hoffer scale (D)	Level of speech ability (E)	Level of functional abilities of daily activities (F)	Fatigue score (G)	Gene (H)	Mutation
Profile: global low functioning ($N = 5$)									
F	5	1	2	1	4	2	71	*OPA1*	c.910C>T
M	6	1	3	1	1	1	40	*FBXL*	c.1361A>C
M	12	1	2	2	3	2	49	*SDHA*	c.64-2A>G
M	18	1	2	1	3	3	?	*RARS2*	c.442A>G; c.1519G>A
M	18	1	2	3	3	2	49	*ATP6*	m.09176T>C
Profile: low cognitive functioning and moderate to normal ambulation ($N = 5$)									
M	13	2	4	4	6	4	58	*MT-TL1*	m.3243A>G
F	13	1	2	5	5	3	?	*RARS2*	c.442A>G; c.1519G>A
M	14	1	3	5	3	2	49	*MTFMT*	c.626C>T; c.766C>T
M	16	1	3	4	2	3	32	*ATP6*	m.8993T>G
F	17	1	3	5	6	4	54	*MT-TL1*	m.3243A>G
Profile: global moderate functioning ($N = 7$)									
M	4	3	3	4	5	3	65	*TAZ*	c.788_794del
M	4	3	4	4	3	3	72	*ATP6*	m.8993T>G
F	5	3	3	4	6	3	72	*NDUFS7*	c.364G>A
F	5	3	4	4	6	3	39	*MT-TL1*	m.3243A>G
M	7	3	2	4	6	3	66	*ATP6*	m.09185T>C
M	7	3	4	4	6	3	38	*mt-tRNASer*	m.7507A>G
M	13	3	3	4	5	4	58	*MT-TL1*	m.3243A>G
Total									
F: $N = 5$ M: $N = 12$	Range: 4–18	1: $N = 9$ 2: $N = 1$ 3: $N = 7$ 4: $N = 0$	1: $N = 0$ 2: $N = 6$ 3: $N = 7$ 4: $N = 4$ 5: $N = 0$	1: $N = 3$ 2: $N = 1$ 3: $N = 1$ 4: $N = 9$ 5: $N = 3$	1: $N = 1$ 2: $N = 1$ 3: $N = 5$ 4: $N = 1$ 5: $N = 3$ 6: $N = 6$	1: $N = 1$ 2: $N = 2$ 3: $N = 11$ 4: $N = 3$	Range: 32–72 2 unknown		

A: M = male, F = female; B: 1 = extremely low, 2 = low, 3 = average, 4 = good; C: 1 = spasticity, 2 = ataxia, 3 = extremely delayed, 4 = delayed, 5 = normal development; D: 1 = nonambulation, 2 = nonfunctional ambulation, 3 = household ambulation, 4 = community ambulation, 5 = normal ambulation; E: 1 = no oral communication possible, 2 = communication with a known person, 3 = frequent repetitions, 4 = incidental repetitions, 5 = effective despite small problems, 6 = effective communication; F: 1 = not self-independent, 2 = minimal self-independent, 3 = sufficient self-independent, 4 = fully self-independent; G: the higher the score, the better the (by fatigue impacted) health-related quality of life, unknown = missing data; H: OPA1 = optic atrophy 1; FBXL = F-box and leucine-rich repeat proteins; SDHA = succinate dehydrogenase complex, subunit A; RARS2 = arginyl-tRNA synthetase 2; ATP6 = ATP synthase 6; MT-TL1 = mitochondrial tRNA leucine; MTFMT = mitochondrial methionyl-tRNA formyltransferase; TAZ = taffazin; NDUFS7 = NADH-ubiquinone oxidoreductase Fe-S protein 7; mt-tRNASer = mitochondrial tRNA serine.

with training for future work positions: "*He goes to secondary special education, while doing two days of workplace training in an employment center for people with intellectual disabilities.*" Three children from the low cognitive level with a moderate to normal ambulation profile attended to special education, while two children attended to regular education. Two of the children with the global moderate-functioning profile attended to special education, while five attended to regular education. Sometimes, small adaptations were made: "*She goes to regular education, but when she is too tired she stays at home for the afternoon.*" This quote also illustrate that the energy level is used as a deciding factor in performing or avoiding the activity. Notes about the energy level as the deciding factor were present in all occupational performance areas. Although the type of education varied from special to regular education, the range of activities did not differ among the three profiles. Most children attended classes that included writing, spelling, and calculating, as well as physical and/or occupational therapy.

3.3. Leisure. The area under leisure featured all the activities that children do to play or occupy their free time. It included the following categories: computing, hobbies, play, and sports. In each of the three profiles, the (allied) health care

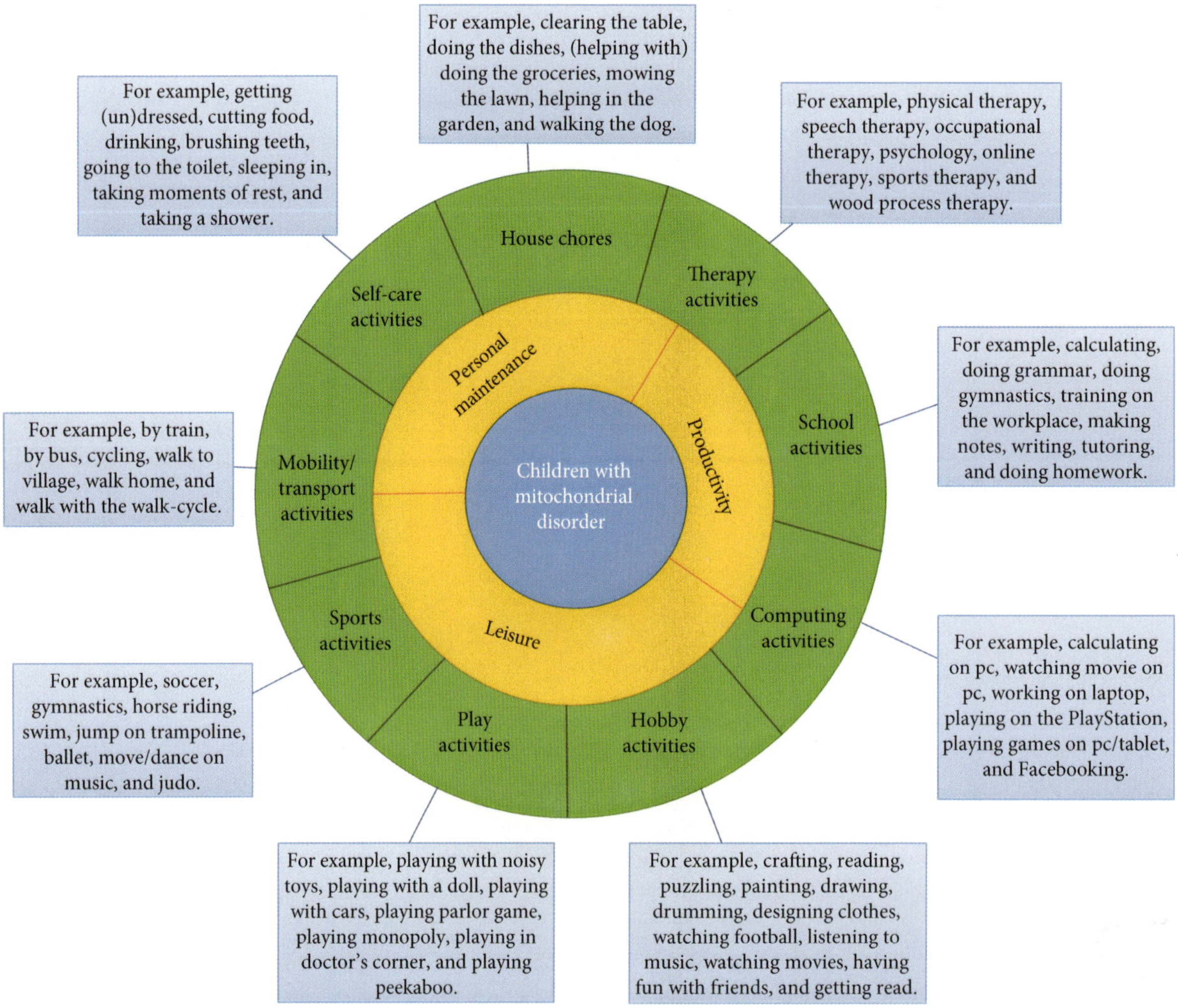

FIGURE 1: Activities, activity categories, and occupational performance areas of children with mitochondrial disorder.

professionals noted all four different categories in leisure. The physically passive activities were reported more in the global low-functioning profile than the other two profiles. For instance, it was mentioned that: "*After school he is tired and uses his laptop or tablet to play games, uses Facebook or watches movies.*" In the profiles of children with a better ambulation, there were more regular physically active activities, for instance, "*After finishing his homework he usually goes outside and jumps on the trampoline or plays soccer.*" The analysis showed that the children performed individual leisure activities, for example, horse riding, jumping on the trampoline, watching football, or going to Bible study. Some activities were more popular, including swimming, gymnastics, watching television, or a movie.

4. Discussion

This study provides a first overview of the activity categories of children with a mitochondrial disorder. Three occupational performance areas: personal maintenance, productivity, and leisure [33] comprised, as reported by allied health professionals in patient records, nine activity categories: self-care, house chores, therapy, school, computing, hobby, play, sports, and mobility/transport. Contrary to our expectations, we found that all activity categories were present in each global-functioning profile. This is congruent with the guiding principles for children's rehabilitation in the Netherlands, which stipulate that children with disabilities are full participants in everyday life [35].

The activities performed by children with mitochondrial disorders, as identified in this study, resemble the activities of typically developing children identified in the PACS Pediatric Activity Card Sort: the PACS [36], with one exception: "therapy activities". The PACS was developed based on typical activities of childhood that are relevant for all, not only for typically developing children. This means that this instrument has potential for use as an outcome measure for children with mitochondrial disorders. Although the current study did not compare the activities of children with mitochondrial disorders to healthy peers, the results appear to echo the findings of Shields et al. [6] and King et al. [37] who found that there were more similarities than differences in the participation of children with intellectual disabilities and their typically developing peers. The current findings and existing literature emphasize the fact that the type of activities a child engages in is not necessarily linked to the child's disabilities, but the nature of the performance differs.

Within and between the activities, we found diversity in the amount of support or assistance provided and the equipment used among the children to facilitate successful participation. For example, cycling was reported as performed differently, for example, on a regular bike, a walk-cycle or duo bicycle and with guidance or independently. Also, eating was an activity that was reported as performed independently, with help or with an eating device. It can be reasoned that the regular use of the PEDI [25] could have influenced the notes in the patient files as assistive devices or support is measured with this assessment. However, only the occupational therapist used the PEDI, the other (allied) health professionals did not, yet they also reported the amount of assistance or assistive devices. In addition to the notes on independence, there were also notes about energy levels as a deciding factor in performing or avoiding activities. This is not surprising, given that in the professional literature describing the care of children with mitochondrial disorder, fatigue is a frequently mentioned burden [13]. Although the study design did not allow for a comparison between the amount of assistance or adaptations to energy levels in performing activities, there are indications that differences exist in levels of independence, assistive devices, and energy costs across the children. When children have limited abilities or are more dependent, a higher burden is placed on parents to facilitate participation and autonomy [38, 39]. This suggests that future research should focus on the differences in levels of independence and assistive devices in relation to energy costs and caregiver burden.

We found clear activity categories that represent the different activities and could be organized into frequently used occupational performance areas [33] as described in the literature. The activity categories are also consistent with the (sub)domains of the ICF-CY [19]. We organized the activities in categories based on the typical purpose of the activities for children, which best fit the three occupational performance areas of Reed and Sanderson [33]. It was noticed that some activity categories could be linked to more occupational performance areas than others. For instance, computing activities are used to learn or work (productivity) but also for leisure. This supports the idea that the meaning of the activity can be viewed from different perspectives, can differ for each child and that activity categories are not solely linked to a certain occupational performance area [40]. To confirm to which activity categories an activity belongs, we need to gain insight in the perspectives of the children on the individual meaning each activity has for them. The categorization of activities by the children themselves is therefore suitable for use in future research.

Using patient records resulted in some limitations in interpreting the findings. As the written information was unprompted, not every (allied) health professional reported the same information. Another consequence of using patient records is that it was not always clear if the activities that were performed during therapy had a relationship to the activities that the children performed and experienced as meaningful in the daily life situation. For example, "*The child found the pencils and immediately started coloring.*" This note about a test situation in one of the patient records can imply that the child likes to color, but this is disputable. Outcomes of test situations cannot be seen as representative of the child's daily life [41]. In this research, we focused on activity performance, which describes what a person actually does in daily life, expressing the individual's involvement in a life situation [42]. Interviewing the children themselves would provide knowledge about their self reported activity performance and experience in daily life.

Another limitation of the study is the small sample size and stratification of the sample into three global-functioning profiles. However, the sample size overall is suitable for an exploratory study taking into account the low prevalence of the disease. In each profile, there were even smaller numbers of participants; however, this was necessary to address the difference in functioning levels of the children. Prediction of the activity profile based on the level of impairments in this population is difficult given the unpredictable nature of the condition. Nonetheless, our study showed a large diversity of functional capacities, which indicates that we covered the broad spectrum of impairments and limitations seen in this population [43]. Stratification into the functional capacity profiles enhanced the insight into activity categories of the total study population and each profile separately. Conversely, a selection bias might have occurred because solely reports of children within the specific MitoRoute were included. Pediatricians refer all children with mitochondrial disorder to be screened at the MitoRoute for different reasons (e.g., new diagnosis, two-yearly screening, or a deterioration in the clinical condition). Although not all parents and/or children with mitochondrial disorder agree to participate in the MitoRoute, it is not sure whether and how this will lead to selection bias. Despite this, we think that the findings may provide an overview of activity categories for possibly all children with mitochondrial disorders. Future research should include a representative sample, on all characteristics, of children with mitochondrial disorders.

The clinical implications of the large variation of reported activities found in this study could be that health care professionals need to consider all nine activity categories in their assessment and therapy. In addition, clinicians should consult children on the meaning they attach to an activity to decide on activity category to which it belongs. Furthermore, assessments and interventions should be tailored enough to encompass the diversity in activities performed as seen in the global functional capacity profiles of the children and the individual preferences in performance of activities.

5. Conclusions

This exploratory pilot retrospective chart review gives insight into the everyday activities performed by children with mitochondrial disorders as reported by professionals. Nine activity categories were identified that represent regular childhood activities. We found that, although the children varied in capacities and limitations, all activity categories were present in each global-functioning profile. There are indications that children perform activities differently in terms of the level of independence, assistive device usage, and energy costs. This study provides a foundation for a qualitative study on the activities of children with a mitochondrial disorder and whether allied health care professionals support their practice. Furthermore, it supports the need for personalized and strength-based care, which puts emphasis on involving the children's perspective in care.

Acknowledgments

The authors thank the professionals in the MitoRoute at the Radboudumc, Nijmegen, Netherlands, namely, (i) Kim van de Loo, MSc, and Dr. José Clusters, psychologists; (ii) Marjo van Gerven, speech therapist; (iii) Dr. Anjo Janssen, pediatric physical therapist; and (iv) Yvonne Veenhuizen, MSc, and Anita van der Molen, occupational therapists. The authors used their data to categorize the children into three profiles: global low functioning, low cognitive functioning with a moderate to normal ambulation, and global moderate functioning. For the ability to study all patient records, the authors would like to thank Professor Dr. J. A. M. Smeitink, head of the Radboud Centre for Mitochondrial Medicine. The authors also thank him for his critical review of the manuscript and the suggested improvements.

References

[1] M. Asbjørnslett and H. Hemmingsson, "Participation at school as experienced by teenagers with physical disabilities," *Scandinavian Journal of Occupational Therapy*, vol. 15, no. 3, pp. 153–161, 2008.

[2] R. M. Bendixen and C. M. Kreider, "Review of occupational therapy research in the practice area of children and youth," *The American Journal of Occupational Therapy*, vol. 65, no. 3, pp. 351–359, 2011.

[3] M. Law, C. Missiuna, N. Pollock, and D. Stewart, "Foundations for occupational therapy practice with children," in *Occupational Therapy for Children*, J. Case-Smith, Ed., pp. 53–87, Elsevier Mosby, St. Louis, MO, USA, 2005.

[4] G. King, M. Lawm, S. King, P. Rosenbaum, M. K. Kertoy, and N. L. Young, "A conceptual model of the factors affecting the recreation and leisure participation of children with disabilities," *Physical & Occupational Therapy In Pediatrics*, vol. 23, no. 1, pp. 63–90, 2003.

[5] T. Heah, T. Case, B. McGuire, and M. Law, "Successful participation: the lived experience among children with disabilities," *Canadian Journal of Occupational Therapy*, vol. 74, no. 1, pp. 38–47, 2007.

[6] N. Shields, M. King, M. Corbett, and C. Imms, "Is participation among children with intellectual disabilities in outside school activities similar to their typically developing peers? A systematic review," *Developmental Neurorehabilitation*, vol. 17, no. 1, pp. 64–71, 2014.

[7] G. S. Gorman, A. M. Schaefer, Y. Ng et al., "Prevalence of nuclear and mitochondrial DNA mutations related to adult mitochondrial disease," *Annals of Neurology*, vol. 77, no. 5, pp. 753–759, 2015.

[8] W. J. Koopman, P. H. Willems, and J. A. Smeitink, "Monogenic mitochondrial disorders," *The New England Journal of Medicine*, vol. 366, no. 12, pp. 1132–1141, 2012.

[9] A. Rötig, "Genetics of mitochondrial respiratory chain deficiencies," *Revue Neurologique*, vol. 170, no. 5, pp. 309–322, 2014.

[10] J. B. WJ Koopman, C. W. Fung, S. Koene, R. J. Rodenburg, P. H. Willems, and J. A. Smeitink, "Mitochondrial disorders in children: toward development of small-molecule treatment strategies," *EMBO Molecular Medicine*, vol. 8, no. 4, pp. 311–327, 2016.

[11] A. Dassler and P. J. Allen, "Mitochondrial disease in children and adolescents," *Pediatric Nursing*, vol. 40, p. 150, 2014.

[12] J. E. Kisler, R. G. Whittaker, and R. McFarland, "Mitochondrial diseases in childhood: a clinical approach to investigation and management," *Developmental Medicine & Child Neurology*, vol. 52, no. 5, pp. 422–433, 2010.

[13] S. Koene, S. B. Wortmann, M. C. de Vries et al., "Developing outcome measures for pediatric mitochondrial disorders: which complaints and limitations are most burdensome to patients and their parents?," *Mitochondrion*, vol. 13, no. 1, pp. 15–24, 2013.

[14] A. M. Martens, H. Gorter, R. G. Wassink, and H. Rietman, "Physical activity of children with a mitochondrial disease compared to children who are healthy," *Pediatric Physical Therapy*, vol. 26, no. 1, pp. 19–26, 2014.

[15] S. Koene, M. Jansen, C. M. Verhaak, R. L. A. De Vrueh, I. J. M. De Groot, and J. A. M. Smeitink, "Towards the harmonization of outcome measures in children with mitochondrial disorders," *Developmental Medicine & Child Neurology*, vol. 55, no. 8, pp. 698–706, 2013.

[16] D. R. Hess, "Retrospective studies and chart reviews," *Respiratory Care*, vol. 49, no. 10, pp. 1171–1174, 2004.

[17] M. Vassar and M. Holzmann, "The retrospective chart review: important methodological considerations," *Journal of Educational Evaluation for Health Professions*, vol. 10, p. 12, 2013.

[18] H. F. Hsieh and S. E. Shannon, "Three approaches to qualitative content analysis," *Qualitative Health Research*, vol. 15, no. 9, pp. 1277–1288, 2005.

[19] World Health Organization, *International Classification of Functioning, Disability, and Health: Children & Youth Version: ICF-CY.*, World Health Organization, 2007.

[20] M. KVN Braun and D. L. Yeargin-Allsopp, "Activity limitations among young adults with developmental disabilities: a population-based follow-up study," *Research in Developmental Disabilities*, vol. 30, no. 1, pp. 179–191, 2009.

[21] O. V. MK Bult, M. J. Jongmans, E. Lindeman, and M. Ketelaar, "What influences participation in leisure activities of children and youth with physical disabilities? A systematic review," *Research in Developmental Disabilities*, vol. 32, no. 5, pp. 1521–1529, 2011.

[22] E. MM Hoffer, R. Feiwell, J. Perry, and C. B. Perry, "Functional ambulation in patients with myelomeningocele," *The Journal of Bone & Joint Surgery*, vol. 55, no. 1, pp. 137–148, 1973.

[23] M. A. Schoenmakers, V. A. Gulmans, R. H. Gooskens, and P. J. Helders, "Spina bifida at the sacral level: more than minor gait disturbances," *Clinical Rehabilitation*, vol. 18, no. 2, pp. 178–185, 2004.

[24] S. Knuijt, J. G. Kalf, B. M. G. Van Engelen, B. J. M. De Swart, and A. C. H. Geurts, "The Radboud dysarthria assessment: development and clinimetric evaluation," *Folia Phoniatrica et Logopaedica*, vol. 69, no. 4, pp. 143–153, 2017.

[25] J. Wassenberg-Severijnen and J. Custers, *Handleiding PEDI-NL*, Pearson, 2005.

[26] J. W. Varni, *Scaling and Scoring of the Pediatric Quality of Life Inventory™ (PedsQL™)*, Mapi Research Trust, Lyon, 14 edition, 2014.

[27] H. Priest, P. Roberts, and L. Woods, "An overview of three different approaches to the interpretation of qualitative data. Part 1: theoretical issues," *Nurse Researcher*, vol. 10, no. 1, pp. 30–42, 2002.

[28] S. Elo and H. Kyngäs, "The qualitative content analysis process," *Journal of Advanced Nursing*, vol. 62, no. 1, pp. 107–115, 2008.

[29] M. Stanley, "Qualitative descriptive," in *Qualitative Research Methodologies for Occupational Science and Therapy*, S. Nayar and M. Stanley, Eds., Routledge, 2015.

[30] R. Hagedorn, *Foundations for Practice in Occupational Therapy*, Elsevier Health Sciences, 2001.

[31] M. le Granse and M. J. Hartingsveldt, *Grondslagen van de Ergotherapie*, Reed Business, 2012.

[32] A. A. Wilcock, *An Occupational Perspective of Health*, Slack Incorporated, 2006.

[33] K. L. Reed and S. N. Sanderson, *Concepts of Occupational Therapy*, Lippincott Williams & Wilkins, 1999.

[34] World Medical Association, "World Medical Association Declaration of Helsinki. Ethical principles for medical research involving human subjects," *Bulletin World Health Organization*, vol. 79, pp. 373-374, 2001.

[35] A. H. M. Mulders, M. J. Meihuizen-de Regt, and J. M. H. de Moor, "Kinderrevalidatie: een plaatsbepaling," in *Kinderrevalidatie*, M. J. Meihuizen-de Regt, J. M. H. Moor, and A. H. M. Mulders, Eds., pp. 1–48, Koninklijke Van Gorcum BV, Assen, 2009.

[36] A. Mandich, H. Polatajko, L. Miller, and C. Baum, *The Pediatric Activity Card Sort (PACS)*, Canadian Occupational Therapy Association, Ottawa, 2004.

[37] M. King, N. Shields, C. Imms, M. Black, and C. Ardern, "Participation of children with intellectual disability compared with typically developing children," *Research in Developmental Disabilities*, vol. 34, no. 5, pp. 1854–1862, 2013.

[38] B. Piškur, A. J. Beurskens, M. J. Jongmans et al., "Parents' actions, challenges, and needs while enabling participation of children with a physical disability: a scoping review," *BMC pediatrics*, vol. 12, no. 1, p. 177, 2012.

[39] B. Piškur, M. K. AJ Beurskens, M. J. Jongmans, B. M. Casparie, and R. J. Smeets, "Daily actions, challenges, and needs among Dutch parents while supporting the participation of their child with a physical disability at home, at school, and in the community: a qualitative diary study," *BMC Pediatrics*, vol. 17, no. 1, p. 12, 2017.

[40] D. Persson, L. Erlandsson, M. Eklund, and S. Iwarsson, "Value dimensions, meaning, and complexity in human occupation—a tentative structure for analysis," *Scandinavian Journal of Occupational Therapy*, vol. 8, no. 1, pp. 7–18, 2001.

[41] C. Morris, "Measuring participation in childhood disability: how does the capability approach improve our understanding?," *Developmental Medicine & Child Neurology*, vol. 51, no. 2, pp. 92–94, 2009.

[42] M. E. Michielsen, M. de Niet, G. M. Ribbers, H. J. Stam, and J. B. Bussmann, "Evidence of a logarithmic relationship between motor capacity and actual performance in daily life of the paretic arm following stroke," *Journal of Rehabilitation Medicine*, vol. 41, no. 5, pp. 327–331, 2009.

[43] S. Koene and J. Smeitink, "Mitochondrial medicine: entering the era of treatment," *Journal of Internal Medicine*, vol. 265, no. 2, pp. 193–209, 2009.

Role Participation: A Comparison across Age Groups in a Norwegian General Population Sample

Tore Bonsaksen [1,2]

[1]Department of Occupational Therapy, Prosthetics and Orthotics, Faculty of Health Sciences, OsloMet - Oslo Metropolitan University, Oslo, Norway
[2]Faculty of Health Studies, VID Specialized University, Sandnes, Norway

Correspondence should be addressed to Tore Bonsaksen; tore.bonsaksen@hioa.no

Academic Editor: Kathleen M. Matuska

Background. Life events, illness, and disability may alter a person's role participation, in which case occupational therapy may be an appropriate intervention. However, role participation data derived from the general population, which is required for meaningful comparison, is largely missing. This study is aimed at describing past, present, and anticipated role participation in a general population sample from Norway and at examining differences in current role participation between age groups. *Methods.* In 2015, a sample of 140 persons (age range 19–94 years, 65% females) from the Norwegian general population completed the Role Checklist at one occasion. The data were analyzed descriptively and with chi-square tests and one-way analysis of variance. *Results.* The most frequent role was a home maintainer (93.6%), and the least frequent was a religious participant (7.1%). Participants aged 65 years and above had fewer roles compared with their younger counterparts and had to a larger extent experienced role loss over the course of their lives. *Conclusions.* Role continuity was the most prevalent role pattern in the total sample, whereas role loss appeared to be the most prevalent role pattern among those in the oldest age group. Rehabilitation services in general and participation-focused occupational therapy in particular may profit from assessing role participation in clients and potentially target roles through intervention.

1. Introduction

A core aim for occupational therapy services is to promote participation in society by enabling the performance of meaningful, everyday-life occupation [1, 2]. Recently, researchers have suggested that participation may be understood primarily as participation within social roles [3–5]. This idea links the participation concept of the International Classification of Functioning, Disability and Health (ICF) [6] directly with the Model of Human Occupation (MOHO) theory [1], in which social roles are viewed as the main organizing principle of the person's occupational behavior. By performing the tasks and chores associated with social roles, one participates in society. Acting within social roles is *inter*acting—acting in relationship with others, directly or indirectly. The role content is constituted from the ongoing interaction between the person holding the role and their social environment. In other words, acting according to role expectations within the social context constitutes the theoretical definition of role participation [1].

Roles are partly prescribed—for example, one is born as someone's son or daughter. Over the life course, other social roles are acquired, as one takes on various social positions in relationship to others, for example, the role of a student or a teacher. The roles we enact at a given point in time influence what we do and how we do it. With practice, the person gradually identifies with their roles such that their role behaviors come naturally and without much consideration. At this point, the role is internalized within the person—it has become a part of the person's identity [1]. However, when reflecting on the value of roles, a study of Norwegian occupational therapy students showed that most of the performed roles, as reported on the employed Role Checklist, were also highly valued [7]. Subjective well-being among university students in Jordan was associated with having more roles and perceiving roles as more valuable [8], and similarly, participating in more valued roles was associated with higher quality of life among persons who had undergone liver transplantation [9].

Adverse life events, illness, and disability may limit the person's performance in social roles and may consequently change or restrict their social participation [1]. Several studies have been in support of this reasoning. For example, one study found more problems in academic, leisure, and work roles in adolescents with mental illness compared to healthy peers [10]. One year after the landfall of Hurricane Ike at the coast of Texas in September 2008, students in the area experienced that some previous roles were retained whereas others had been disrupted [11]. Scott's [9] study of liver transplant recipients also showed a pattern of disengagement with previously enacted roles, whereas Dickerson and Oakley's [12] study found a consistent pattern of more current roles among nondisabled community-living individuals compared with individuals who had physical or psychosocial disabilities.

However, not only do roles change as an effect of specific events but they also change over the natural life course, and occupational therapy may be relevant for remediating problematic role transitions [13]. In the words of Lee and Kielhofner [14], "Society expects and structures role transitions at various life stages such as entering and exiting the student role, beginning work, and retiring. People also choose to enter and leave roles" (p. 67). One perspective of role patterns across time, encompassing change as well as stability, was provided in a Canadian study of adults with severe mental health problems [15]. Using the Role Checklist [16] to examine roles in a time perspective, the researchers conceptualized role stability in terms of continuity (having the role in the past, present, and foreseen future) and absence (not having the role in the past, nor in the present or foreseen future). Role loss was conceptualized as having the role in the past, but not at present. Conversely, role gain was conceptualized as not having the role in the past, but having it at present. The concept "role change" was used to describe a situation where a role was not enacted at present but was expected in the future.

Conceptually, though, the above example of role change is more precisely one of the "expected role gains," which is merely one of several ways roles can change over time. Adding to this idea, we may therefore differentiate between two aspects of role change: expected role gain and expected role loss. A person heading towards retirement from work could exemplify how role change may involve both aspects. Retirement implies losing the role of a worker (role loss) but may also open up the possibility of taking up, for example, the role of a choir member or a volunteer for a charity organization (role gains).

Two contrasting theories of "successful aging" have traditionally been put forward: the activity theory and the disengagement theory [17, 18]. The latter view emphasizes accepting losses (e.g., of functional ability, activities, roles, and friends) and disengagement from active life, while the former emphasizes holding on—as far as possible—to the roles and activities of middle age. While both views seem valid, recent research evidence seems to favor the activity theory, essentially stating that having a good life in older years is not about giving in, but holding on. For example, Menec's [19] six-year longitudinal study of elderly persons demonstrated that in general, social and productive activities were positively related to higher levels of happiness, better functioning, and lower mortality. As activities are thought to be organized mainly according to roles [1], one could also suggest that having more roles might indicate greater satisfaction with life. Research has shown that currently held roles were often valued roles among students [7] and that participation in more valued roles was related to greater quality of life among liver transplant recipients [9]. However, the notion that having more roles is associated with greater life satisfaction, regardless of the person's valuation of these roles, is an assumption in need of further inquiry.

In summary, the available literature suggests that participating in more valued roles is a source of contentment and satisfaction with life. Moreover, it suggests that adverse life events, illness, and disability can potentially disrupt the individual's social roles. However, role participation is also affected by the normal progression through life. Thus, aging may often imply a need for adapting to new circumstances. Such adaptation may be a difficult process, and occupational therapy may be appropriate as a means to remediate disrupted participation in roles. However, existing studies have largely employed samples with highly specific characteristics, frequently related to a specific illness or disability (see, e.g., [9, 20, 21]). The one study providing comparisons with a general population sample [12] is both dated and concerned with the US context only. To be able to interpret role participation data from different clinical groups, one should preferably be able to compare with current data derived from the general population living in the relevant cultural context.

The present study is aimed at describing past, present, and anticipated role participation in a general population sample from Norway. Second, differences in current role participation between individuals in different age groups were examined. Lastly, building on the procedure described by Hachey and coworkers [15], we described the participants' role patterns.

2. Methods

The study employed a cross-sectional design, utilizing data from an assessment at one point in time. It serves as a Norway-specific substudy associated with a larger cross-cultural study of roles and their links with MOHO as a theoretical framework [3]. The data for the study was collected early in 2015.

2.1. Sample and Recruitment. The sample was a convenience sample of persons from the general population, recruited by personal contact made by nine occupational therapy students and occupational therapist colleagues in Oslo and in the surrounding metropolitan area. Age under 18 years was the only exclusion criterion. The participants were recruited with the aim of making the sample as diverse as possible, representing a blend of men and women and people in different age groups. The participants knew the recruiter in person, or they knew someone known to the researcher, for example, in cases where they were that person's friend or spouse ("snowballing recruitment"). To ensure a diverse sample composition, the recruiters were asked to include both men and women and to continue to include participants until the sample consisted of at least 20 persons in each of the predefined age groups. The age groups represented young persons (aged 18–24), adults (aged 25–44), middle-aged persons (aged 45–64), and elderly persons (aged 65 years and above). Unfortunately, however, the recruitment of participants to the oldest age group was not fully completed due to time restrictions on the part of the recruiters. On the other hand, more than 20 participants were recruited in the other age groups, increasing the statistical power of the analyses.

2.2. Measurement. Role participation was assessed with the Role Checklist [16]. The instrument is widely used—it is available in 13 languages and remains one of the most commonly used assessments in American occupational therapy practice [22]. It is a short self-report assessment that captures a person's perception of their participation in 10 defined roles. The roles are student, worker, volunteer, home maintainer, caregiver, friend, family member, hobbyist/amateur, religious participant, and participant in organizations. Part one of the Role Checklist, which was the only part employed in this substudy, instructs the person to indicate participation in any of the ten roles in the past (up until one week ago), present (today and the preceding week), and anticipated future (tomorrow and any time after tomorrow). The participant's responses to the part one of the Role Checklist are applied to determine the person's participation (or nonparticipation) in each of the listed roles in the past, present, and anticipated future. Scores pertaining to present role participation can also be summed, such that higher sum scores indicate participation in more roles. The roles assessed with the Role Checklist has been found to be consistent with the ICF framework [4], to be linked with the MOHO levels of both performance and participation [3], and to demonstrate concurrent validity with the more extensive Occupational Circumstances Assessment Interview and Rating Scale [5].

Previous translations of the Role Checklist into French [23] and Brazilian Portuguese [24] have both demonstrated good validity and reliability when used in their respective cultures. In addition, measurement properties have been shown to be equivalent when used in paper and electronic version [25], and later modifications of the checklist have similarly been tested with good results [26]. For this study, two independent Norwegian translations of the original instrument were produced and subsequently compared with one another. The comparisons are aimed at ensuring the clarity of concepts as well as the appropriate Norwegian phrasing and sentence structure. After reaching consensus on the forward translation, the instrument was translated back into English, and the back-translated version was checked against the original. Only small modifications were made after this process. Formal guidelines for the translation and adaptation of the Role Checklist have been provided at a later stage in the research process [27]. In addition to completing part one of the Role Checklist, the participants were asked about their age (in years) and gender.

2.3. Data Analysis. Descriptive statistics were used to examine the sample characteristics and their participation in roles. Differences between age groups with a view to the proportions currently participating in each role were examined by the χ^2 test. Differences between age groups with regard to the number of currently enacted roles were examined with one-way analysis of variance (ANOVA). In the ANOVA pairwise comparisons, Tukey's honest significant difference was used to adjust for inflating error levels.

Role patterns were described according to Hachey and coworkers [15]. Role loss was defined as having a role in the past, but not in the present. Role gain was defined as having a role at present, but not in the past. Continuous role was defined as having a role in the past, present, and expected future. Role absence was defined as not having the role in the past, not at present, and not in the expected future. By extending Hachey and coworkers' [15] procedure, expected role loss was defined as having a role at present, while expecting not to have the role in the future. Expected role gain was defined as not having a role at present, while expecting to have the role in the future. All analyses were performed with the software IBM SPSS for Windows [28], and the statistical significance was set at $p < 0.05$.

2.4. Ethics. All participants were verbally informed about the study by the recruitment collaborator. Written information about the study procedures was provided on the front page of the employed checklist. All participants volunteered to take part in the study, and informed consent was implied when we received the completed forms. As neither health-related information nor any person-identifying information was collected for the study, formal ethical approval was not required.

3. Results

3.1. Participants. One hundred and forty persons, 49 (35%) men and 91 (65%) women, opted to participate in the study. The age distribution showed that 45 (32.1%) of the participants were aged 18–24 years, 47 (33.6%) were aged 25–44 years, 31 (22.1%) were aged 45–64 years, and 17 (12.1%) were aged 65 years or older. The sample mean age was 40.2 years (SD = 18.8 years). The gender proportions did not differ significantly between the four age groups ($\chi^2 = 1.26$, $p = 0.74$).

3.2. Role Participation. Role participation in the past, present, and anticipated future is displayed in Figure 1. In the total sample, the most frequently endorsed role was home maintainer at present (93.6%), while the least frequently endorsed role was religious participant at present (7.1%). In the youngest age group (18–24 years), the most frequently endorsed role was home maintainer at present ($n = 45$, 100% within the age group), while the least frequently endorsed role was religious participant at present ($n = 3$, 6.7%). In the adult age group (25–44 years), the most frequently endorsed role was home maintainer at present ($n = 46$, 97.9%), while the least frequently endorsed role was religious participant at

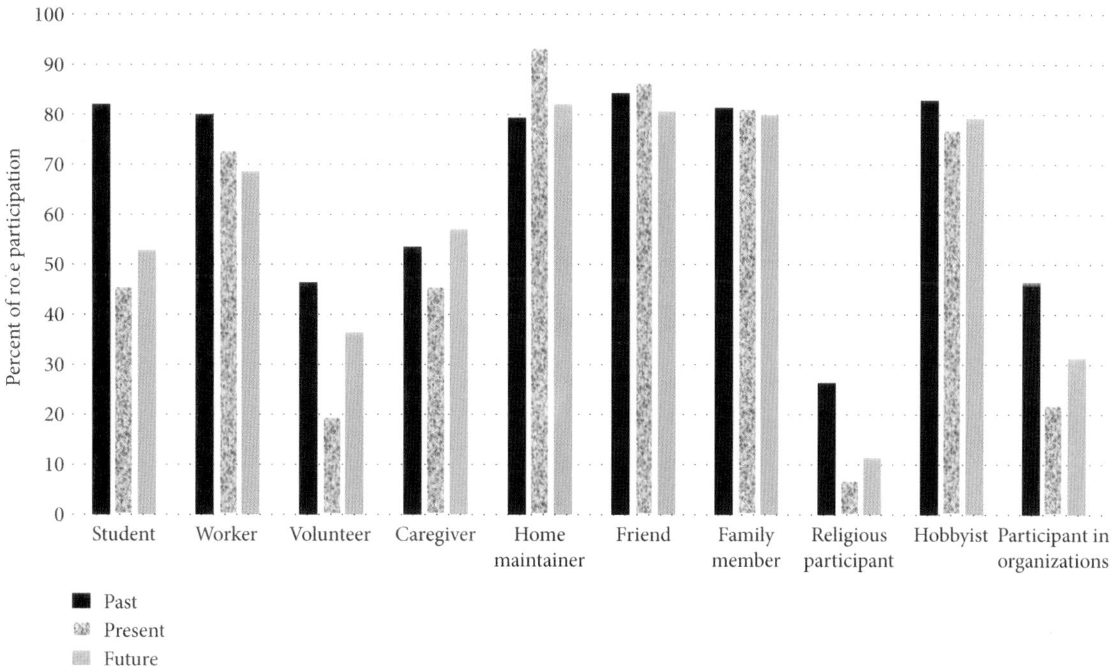

FIGURE 1: Role participation for past, present, and anticipated future roles in the sample ($n = 140$).

present ($n = 0$, 0%). Among the middle-aged participants (45–64 years), the most frequently endorsed role was home maintainer at present ($n = 31$, 100%), while the least frequently endorsed role was student at present ($n = 4$, 12.9%). Among the oldest participants (65 years and over), the most frequently endorsed roles were worker in the past and family member at present (both $n = 31$, 100%), while the least frequently endorsed roles were student at present ($n = 1$, 5.9%), student in the future ($n = 1$, 5.9%), and worker in the future ($n = 1$, 5.9%).

3.3. Current Role Participation according to Age Groups. Table 1 displays the age group comparisons related to currently enacted roles. Statistically significant differences between the age groups were found for the following roles: student, worker, volunteer, caregiver, home maintainer, friend, and religious participant. In addition, the mean number of currently enacted roles was different between participants in the four age groups. The pairwise comparisons revealed that those in the oldest age group participated in fewer roles compared to participants in all other age groups (all $p < 0.001$). Otherwise, no significant differences occurred.

3.4. Continuity and Change in Roles. Table 2 displays the participants' role patterns—that is, the continuity and change in roles across time—as interpreted from the participants' combinations of self-reported past, present, and anticipated future role participation. The roles most frequently lost were student and volunteer, whereas the roles most frequently gained were worker and home maintainer. Home maintainer and friend were the most frequent continuous roles, whereas religious participant and participant in organizations were the roles that most often showed an absent pattern. The roles most frequently expected to be lost were worker and home maintainer. Conversely, the roles most frequently expected to be gained were volunteer and caregiver. Of the predefined role patterns, most of the demonstrated patterns were examples of continuous roles (38.4%).

Considering that the participants in the oldest age group had significantly fewer roles compared to their younger counterparts (see Table 1), there was reason also to examine whether their role patterns across time deviated from the patterns shown for the total sample. The results from this additional analysis of continuity and change in roles for the participants in the oldest age group are displayed in Table 3. In comparison with the total sample, participants in the oldest age group had a higher proportion of the detected role patterns related to role loss and a smaller proportion of the role patterns related to continuous roles and expected role gains.

4. Discussion

The current study is aimed at examining participation in roles and patterns of role participation across time, in a general population sample from Norway. Several of the roles listed on the Role Checklist were currently held among a majority of the sample participants. In the high end of the scale, more than 90% of the sample participated in the role home maintainer. In the low end, fewer than 10% of the sample participated in the role religious participant. Participants over the age of 65 had fewer roles compared to their younger counterparts and showed a somewhat different pattern of continuity and change in role participation across time.

The roles listed in the Role Checklist [16] comprise different levels of necessity—some can be viewed as an integral and inescapable aspect of independent living, such as the most

TABLE 1: Frequency and proportion of individuals currently participating in roles according to age groups.

Current roles	Age groups 18–24 years n (%)	 25–44 years n (%)	 45–64 years n (%)	 ≥65 years n (%)	P
Student	43 (95.6)	16 (34.0)	4 (12.9)	1 (5.9)	<0.001
Worker	31 (68.9)	38 (80.9)	30 (96.8)	3 (17.6)	<0.001
Volunteer	8 (17.8)	8 (17.0)	11 (35.5)	0 (0.0)	0.02
Caregiver	9 (20.0)	30 (63.8)	19 (61.3)	6 (35.3)	<0.001
Home maintainer	43 (95.6)	46 (97.9)	31 (100.0)	11 (64.7)	<0.001
Friend	45 (100.0)	41 (87.2)	23 (74.2)	12 (70.6)	<0.01
Family member	33 (73.3)	39 (83.0)	26 (83.9)	18 (94.1)	0.27
Religious participant	3 (6.7)	0 (0.0)	5 (16.1)	2 (11.8)	<0.05
Hobbyist	34 (75.6)	37 (78.8)	24 (77.4)	13 (76.5)	0.99
Participant in organizations	7 (15.6)	11 (23.4)	9 (29.0)	4 (23.5)	0.56
	M (SD)	M (SD)	M (SD)	M (SD)	
Number of current roles	5.69 (1.56)	5.66 (1.20)	5.87 (1.65)	4.0 (1.37)	<0.001

Note. Differences by χ^2 tests for separate roles and by one-way ANOVA F-test for the number of current roles.

TABLE 2: Continuity and change in role participation across time in the total sample (n = 140).

Role	Loss n (%)	Gain n (%)	Continuous n (%)	Absence n (%)	Expected loss n (%)	Expected gain n (%)
Student	61 (43.6)	10 (7.1)	49 (35.0)	8 (5.7)	11 (7.9)	21 (15.0)
Worker	34 (24.3)	24 (17.1)	75 (53.6)	2 (1.4)	23 (16.4)	17 (12.1)
Volunteer	48 (34.3)	10 (7.1)	15 (10.7)	51 (36.4)	10 (7.1)	34 (24.3)
Caregiver	24 (17.1)	13 (9.3)	50 (35.7)	34 (24.3)	8 (5.7)	24 (17.1)
Home maintainer	3 (2.1)	23 (16.4)	107 (76.4)	3 (2.1)	19 (13.6)	3 (2.1)
Friend	15 (10.7)	18 (12.9)	103 (73.6)	3 (2.1)	17 (12.1)	9 (6.4)
Family member	18 (12.9)	18 (12.9)	94 (67.1)	4 (2.9)	18 (12.9)	16 (11.4)
Religious participant	27 (19.3)	0 (0.0)	10 (7.1)	100 (71.4)	0 (0.0)	6 (4.3)
Hobbyist	22 (15.7)	14 (10.0)	92 (65.7)	7 (5.0)	14 (10.0)	17 (12.1)
Participant in organizations	40 (28.6)	6 (4.3)	24 (17.1)	63 (45.0)	6 (4.3)	19 (13.6)
Total	292	136	619	275	126	166
Role patterns	18.1%	8.4%	38.4%	17.0%	7.8%	10.3%

Note. Role loss was defined as having a role in the past, but not in the present. Role gain was defined as having a role at present, but not in the past. Continuous role was defined as having a role in the past, present, and expected future. Role absence was defined as not having the role in the past, not at present, and not in the expected future. Expected role loss was defined as having a role at present, while expecting not to have the role in the future. Expected role gain was defined as not having a role at present, while expecting to have the role in the future.

frequently endorsed roles of worker and in particular home maintainer (see Figure 1). Other roles, such as the hobbyist and religious participant roles, are not connected to independent living. It is fully possible to lead both independent and fulfilling lives without these roles, and therefore, adopting these roles needs other sources of motivation. Empirical studies have shown that differently composed samples will have each own unique composition of the roles in which participants engage more and less frequently (compare, e.g., [7, 9, 12, 20, 29]). On the other hand, one should be able to assume that role participation in general has a relationship to basic human needs. As suggested by Deci and Ryan [30], such "human motivational universals" are comprised from basic needs for mastery, affiliation, and autonomy. In line with such a view, one may see the worker and home maintainer roles as linked with the need for autonomy, while roles like family member and religious participant link more strongly with the need for affiliation. However, affiliation needs may be expressed and met in different ways. People who live without a family may, for example, rely more on friends, neighbors, and interest groups as sources of companionship and support. This line of reasoning mirrors the recently introduced Model of Occupational Wholeness [31–33], suggesting that personal satisfaction with what we do is based on our tacit judgment of how our doing contributes to our satisfaction of needs. Taken together, this suggests that a majority of participants in any given sample will be expected to participate in some roles (worker, home maintainer, and friend), whereas the level of participation in other roles (e.g., hobbyist, religious participant, and

Table 3: Continuity and change in role participation across time among the participants in the oldest age group ($n = 17$).

Role	Loss n (%)	Gain n (%)	Continuous n (%)	Absence n (%)	Expected loss n (%)	Expected gain n (%)
Student	14 (82.4)	0 (0.0)	1 (5.9)	2 (11.8)	0 (0.0)	0 (0.0)
Worker	14 (82.4)	1 (5.9)	1 (5.9)	0 (0.0)	2 (11.8)	0 (0.0)
Volunteer	11 (64.7)	0 (0.0)	0 (0.0)	5 (29.4)	0 (0.0)	2 (11.8)
Caregiver	9 (52.9)	2 (11.8)	4 (23.5)	2 (11.8)	0 (0.0)	1 (5.9)
Home maintainer	3 (17.6)	3 (17.6)	7 (41.2)	3 (17.6)	3 (17.7)	0 (0.0)
Friend	3 (17.6)	2 (11.8)	10 (58.8)	2 (11.8)	2 (11.8)	0 (0.0)
Family member	1 (5.9)	3 (17.6)	13 (76.5)	0 (0.0)	2 (11.8)	0 (0.0)
Religious participant	3 (17.6)	0 (0.0)	2 (11.8)	12 (70.6)	0 (0.0)	0 (0.0)
Hobbyist	4 (23.5)	4 (23.5)	8 (47.1)	0 (0.0)	4 (23.5)	1 (5.9)
Participant in organizations	8 (47.1)	0 (0.0)	4 (23.5)	5 (29.4)	0 (0.0)	0 (0.0)
Total	70	15	50	31	13	4
Role patterns	38.3%	8.2%	27.3%	16.9%	7.1%	2.2%

Note. Role loss was defined as having a role in the past, but not in the present. Role gain was defined as having a role at present, but not in the past. Continuous role was defined as having a role in the past, present, and expected future. Role absence was defined as not having the role in the past, not at present, and not in the expected future. Expected role loss was defined as having a role at present, while expecting not to have the role in the future. Expected role gain was defined as not having a role at present, while expecting to have the role in the future.

participant in organizations) will depend more on the specific sample characteristics and the given cultural and environmental context [1, 34].

In line with the theoretical assumptions [1, 13, 17, 18], participants in the age group of 65 years and over participated in fewer roles than their counterparts of younger age (see Table 1). The participants in the oldest age group also experienced role loss more frequently compared to the younger participants (see Tables 2 and 3). Reduced role participation may be associated with reduced physical capacity and the onset of illness and functional limitations, which is more often the case in older years. In addition, reaching the normal retirement age (which in Norway is 67 years) directly implies loss of the worker role. Indirectly, it opens up the possibility that friends and family members of similar age may fall ill and eventually die. Consequently, roles like friend, family member, and caregiver may also be lost in the natural progression through life. Nonetheless, occupational therapists should be aware of the potential threats related to role loss. According to the MOHO [1], people organize their everyday lives according to roles. We do what we do much because we enact our roles as researchers, rock band guitarists, amateur kitchen chefs, and a multitude of others. Losing roles as an organizing principle for our everyday lives may further lead to a loss of meaning and purpose.

In most cases, people value the roles they have. In a previous Norwegian study, occupational therapy students demonstrated positive and statistically significant associations between currently enacted roles and their valuation of the same roles [7]. Further, participating in more valued roles appears to lead to more satisfaction, compared to having fewer roles. In support of this, researchers have demonstrated significant associations between participation in more valued roles and having higher quality of life [9] and more life satisfaction [35]. Thus, occupational therapists should pay attention to role loss. Such loss may indicate that the client may be at risk of experiencing reduced quality of life, and he or she may need help to remediate his or her role composition to restore life satisfaction.

In a study conducted in the midnineties, Dickerson and Oakley [12] compared an American nondisabled community sample with a matched sample of persons with physical or mental disabilities. They found that participants in the disabled sample not only had significantly fewer roles compared with the nondisabled sample but also had anticipated fewer future roles and tended to place lower value on several roles, compared to their nondisabled counterparts. The present study augments these previous results by indicating that role loss may not only be an effect of illness and disability but can also be an effect of the aging process itself, regardless of illness or disability (see Tables 2 and 3). At the same time, however, participants in the oldest age group did experience substantial role continuity across the past, present, and anticipated future. Moreover, building on Hachey and coworkers' [15] concept of "role change," we found that the possibility of *gaining* a role in the future was in fact expected by some of the older participants (Table 3). Two participants expected to gain the role of volunteer, one expected to become a caregiver, and one expected to enter the hobbyist role. Thus, in spite of reaching older age, role participation does not have to be all about losing roles, although this should also be expected.

4.1. Study Strengths and Limitations. The sample size, in particular for the oldest age group, was small. Thus, the reliability of the results for this age group is uncertain—there may not have been sufficient variability within the group, and this may have caused biased results. Further studies using larger sample subgroups are needed to shed light on the potential age differences in role participation. Participants were also recruited by convenience, such that we are unable to speak about how well they represent the Norwegian general population. The cross-sectional study design precludes us from establishing cause-effect relationships between the study variables. A trusted group of students and occupational therapist colleagues were used as collaborators in recruiting the participants and informing them about the study procedures. In addition, the employed Role Checklist is relatively straightforward to use, so there is good reason to trust the validity of the collected data. It provides, however, one particular set of roles with a particular set of definitions. Other ways of conceptualizing and measuring role participation may lead to different results. Thus, a limitation of the study is the use of a single measure to look at a complex phenomenon. Moreover, a weakness is the focus on role participation only, not taking into account the participants' valuation of the roles. In addition, potentially associated outcomes, like measures of health or quality of life, were not included. Thus, although previously demonstrated in a clinical sample [9], the study renders the question of whether role participation is related to significant outcomes in a general population sample. If indeed related to such outcomes, we should also ask whether role participation is important in and of itself or whether role participation only matters when the roles in question are personally valued. Future research may also include the Role Checklist in a variety of longitudinal rehabilitation studies to examine whether role participation outcomes are affected as a result of intervention, be they interprofessional or occupational therapy specific.

5. Conclusion

The most frequently endorsed current role in the sample was home maintainer, while the least frequently endorsed current role was religious participant. Compared with the total sample, the participants in the oldest age group participated less frequently in most listed roles, and they had a lower total number of current roles. The role patterns for the total sample indicated for the most part a continuity of roles, while the most frequent role pattern for the oldest group of participants was role loss. More health-related problems, but also the reaching retirement age itself, may lead to role loss as one moves towards older age. Rehabilitation services in general and participation-focused occupational therapy in particular may profit from assessing role participation in clients and potentially target roles through intervention.

References

[1] R. R. Taylor, *Kielhofner's Model of Human Occupation*, Lippincott Williams & Wilkins, Philadelphia, 5th edition, 2017.

[2] E. A. Townsend and H. J. Polatajko, *Enabling Occupation II: Advancing an Occupational Therapy Vision for Health, Well-Being, & Justice through Occupation*, Canadian Association of Occupational Therapists, Ottawa, 2007.

[3] T. Bonsaksen, U. Meidert, D. Schuman et al., "Does the Role Checklist measure occupational participation?," *The Open Journal of Occupational Therapy*, vol. 3, no. 3, p. 2, 2015.

[4] P. J. Scott, "Measuring participation outcomes following life-saving medical interventions: the Role Checklist version 2: quality of performance," *Disability and Rehabilitation*, vol. 36, no. 13, pp. 1108–1112, 2014.

[5] P. J. Scott, D. Cacich, M. Fulk, K. Michel, and K. Whiffen, "Establishing concurrent validity of the Role Checklist version 2 with the OCAIRS in measurement of participation: a pilot study," *Occupational Therapy International*, vol. 2017, Article ID 6493472, 6 pages, 2017.

[6] World Health Organization, *International Classification of Functioning, Disability and Health (ICF)*, WHO, Geneva, 2001.

[7] T. Bonsaksen and H. Kvarsnes, "Role performance and role valuation among occupational therapy students in Norway," *The Open Journal of Occupational Therapy*, vol. 4, no. 1, p. 7, 2016.

[8] F. Yazdani, M. Jibril, and G. Kielhofner, "A study of the relationship between variables from the Model of Human Occupation and subjective well-being among university students in Jordan," *Occupational Therapy In Health Care*, vol. 22, no. 2-3, pp. 125–138, 2008.

[9] P. J. Scott, "Participation in valued roles post-liver transplant," *British Journal of Occupational Therapy*, vol. 73, no. 11, pp. 517–523, 2010.

[10] R. Barris, G. Kielhofner, R. M. B. Martin, I. Gelinas, M. Klement, and B. Schultz, "Occupational function and dysfunction in three groups of adolescents," *The Occupational Therapy Journal of Research*, vol. 6, no. 5, pp. 301–317, 1986.

[11] T. M. Smith, A. Drefus, and G. Hersch, "Habits, routines, and roles of graduate students: effects of Hurricane Ike," *Occupational Therapy In Health Care*, vol. 25, no. 4, pp. 283–297, 2011.

[12] A. E. Dickerson and F. Oakley, "Comparing the roles of community-living persons and patient populations," *American Journal of Occupational Therapy*, vol. 49, no. 3, pp. 221–228, 1995.

[13] R. Wright and L. Sugarman, *Occupational Therapy and Life Course Development*, Wiley-Blackwell, Chichester, UK, 2009.

[14] S. W. Lee and G. Kielhofner, "Habituation: patterns of daily occupations," in *Kielhofner's Model of Human Occupation*, R. R. Taylor, Ed., pp. 57–73, Wolters Kluwer, Philadelphia, 2017.

[15] R. Hachey, G. Boyer, and C. Mercier, "Perceived and valued roles of adults with severe mental health problems," *Canadian Journal of Occupational Therapy*, vol. 68, no. 2, pp. 112–120, 2001.

[16] F. Oakley, G. Kielhofner, R. Barris, and R. K. Reichler, "The Role Checklist: development and empirical assessment of reliability," *The Occupational Therapy Journal of Research*, vol. 6, no. 3, pp. 157–170, 1986.

[17] R. J. Havighurst, "Successful aging," *The Gerontologist*, vol. 1, no. 1, pp. 8–13, 1961.

[18] R. Havighurst, "Successful aging," in *Processes of Aging*, R. Williams, C. Tibbitts, and W. Donahue, Eds., vol. 1, pp. 299–320, Atherton, New York, NY, USA, 1963.

[19] V. H. Menec, "The relation between everyday activities and successful aging: a 6-year longitudinal study," *The Journals of Gerontology Series B: Psychological Sciences and Social Sciences*, vol. 58, no. 2, pp. S74–S82, 2003.

[20] S. Corr and S. Wilmer, "Returning to work after a stroke: an important but neglected area," *British Journal of Occupational Therapy*, vol. 66, no. 5, pp. 186–192, 2003.

[21] J. M. Sepiol and J. Froehlich, "Use of the Role Checklist with the patient with multiple personality disorder," *American Journal of Occupational Therapy*, vol. 44, no. 11, pp. 1008–1012, 1990.

[22] S. W. Lee, R. Taylor, G. Kielhofner, and G. Fisher, "Theory use in practice: a national survey of therapists who use the Model of Human Occupation," *American Journal of Occupational Therapy*, vol. 62, no. 1, pp. 106–117, 2008.

[23] R. Hachey, J. Jumoorty, and C. Mercier, "Methodology for validating the translation of test measurements applied to occupational therapy," *Occupational Therapy International*, vol. 2, no. 3, 203 pages, 1995.

[24] J. R. Cordeiro, A. Camelier, F. Oakley, and J. R. Jardim, "Cross-cultural reproducibility of the Brazilian Portuguese version of the Role Checklist for persons with chronic obstructive pulmonary disease," *American Journal of Occupational Therapy*, vol. 61, no. 1, pp. 33–40, 2007.

[25] P. J. Scott, R. McFadden, K. Yates, S. Baker, and S. McSoley, "The Role Checklist v2: QP: establishment of reliability and validation of electronic administration," *British Journal of Occupational Therapy*, vol. 77, no. 2, pp. 96–102, 2014.

[26] M. Avrech Bar, V. Rubin, G. Gavrieal-Tyjchman, and T. Jarus, "The validity and reliability of the modified version of the Role Checklist (M-RCL)," *Scandinavian Journal of Occupational Therapy*, vol. 20, no. 6, pp. 454–462, 2013.

[27] L. R. Van Antwerp, L. Haglund, K. Fenger, and P. Scott, *Translation Guidelines: The Role Checklist*, Indiana University, Indianapolis, 2016.

[28] IBM Corporation, *SPSS for Windows, Version 24*, IBM Corporation, Armonk, NY, 2016.

[29] M. A. Watson and C. L. Ager, "The impact of role valuation and performance on life satisfaction in old age," *Physical & Occupational Therapy In Geriatrics*, vol. 10, no. 1, pp. 27–62, 1991.

[30] E. L. Deci, R. M. Ryan, P. J. Corr, and G. Matthews, Eds., "Self-determination theory: a consideration of human motivational universals," in *The Cambridge Handbook of Personality Psychology*, pp. 441–456, Cambridge University Press, Cambridge, 2009.

[31] F. Yazdani and T. Bonsaksen, "Introduction to the Model of Occupational Wholeness," *ErgoScience*, vol. 12, no. 1, pp. 32–36, 2017.

[32] T. Bonsaksen and F. Yazdani, "The Norwegian occupational wholeness questionnaire (N-OWQ): scale development and psychometric properties," *Scandinavian Journal of Occupational Therapy*, pp. 1–10, 2018.

[33] T. Bonsaksen and F. Yazdani, "Sociodemographic factors associated with the Norwegian occupational wholeness questionnaire scales," *ErgoScience*, vol. 13, no. 1, pp. 14–20, 2018.

[34] M. K. Duellman, R. Barris, and G. Kielhofner, "Organized activity and the adaptive status of nursing home residents," *American Journal of Occupational Therapy*, vol. 40, no. 9, pp. 618–622, 1986.

[35] M. S. Elliott and R. Barris, "Occupational role performance and life satisfaction in elderly persons," *The Occupational Therapy Journal of Research*, vol. 7, no. 4, pp. 215–224, 1987.

Permissions

All chapters in this book were first published in OTI, by Hindawi Publishing Corporation; hereby published with permission under the Creative Commons Attribution License or equivalent. Every chapter published in this book has been scrutinized by our experts. Their significance has been extensively debated. The topics covered herein carry significant findings which will fuel the growth of the discipline. They may even be implemented as practical applications or may be referred to as a beginning point for another development.

The contributors of this book come from diverse backgrounds, making this book a truly international effort. This book will bring forth new frontiers with its revolutionizing research information and detailed analysis of the nascent developments around the world.

We would like to thank all the contributing authors for lending their expertise to make the book truly unique. They have played a crucial role in the development of this book. Without their invaluable contributions this book wouldn't have been possible. They have made vital efforts to compile up to date information on the varied aspects of this subject to make this book a valuable addition to the collection of many professionals and students.

This book was conceptualized with the vision of imparting up-to-date information and advanced data in this field. To ensure the same, a matchless editorial board was set up. Every individual on the board went through rigorous rounds of assessment to prove their worth. After which they invested a large part of their time researching and compiling the most relevant data for our readers.

The editorial board has been involved in producing this book since its inception. They have spent rigorous hours researching and exploring the diverse topics which have resulted in the successful publishing of this book. They have passed on their knowledge of decades through this book. To expedite this challenging task, the publisher supported the team at every step. A small team of assistant editors was also appointed to further simplify the editing procedure and attain best results for the readers.

Apart from the editorial board, the designing team has also invested a significant amount of their time in understanding the subject and creating the most relevant covers. They scrutinized every image to scout for the most suitable representation of the subject and create an appropriate cover for the book.

The publishing team has been an ardent support to the editorial, designing and production team. Their endless efforts to recruit the best for this project, has resulted in the accomplishment of this book. They are a veteran in the field of academics and their pool of knowledge is as vast as their experience in printing. Their expertise and guidance has proved useful at every step. Their uncompromising quality standards have made this book an exceptional effort. Their encouragement from time to time has been an inspiration for everyone.

The publisher and the editorial board hope that this book will prove to be a valuable piece of knowledge for researchers, students, practitioners and scholars across the globe.

List of Contributors

Fatima Hendricks
OTASA, Vlaeberg, Cape Town 8018, South Africa

Susan Toth-Cohen
Department of Occupational Therapy, Thomas Jefferson University, 130 S. 9th Street, 632 Edison, Philadelphia, PA 19107, USA

Yu-Jin Cha
Department of Occupational Therapy, Semyung University, Jecheon, Republic of Korea

Wesam Barakat Darawsheh
Department of Occupational Therapy, School of Rehabilitation Sciences, The University of Jordan, Amman, Jordan

Martina Pellegrini, Veronica Bucciarelli and Stefania Fugazzaro
Department of Physical and Rehabilitation Medicine, Arcispedale Santa Maria Nuova-IRCCS, Azienda Unità Sanitaria Locale, 42100 Reggio Emilia, Italy

Debora Formisano
Scientific Directorate, Arcispedale Santa Maria Nuova-IRCCS, Azienda Unità Sanitaria Locale, 42100 Reggio Emilia, Italy

Margherita Schiavi
BSc in Occupational Therapy, Azienda Unità Sanitaria Locale, 42100 Reggio Emilia, Italy

Stefania Costi
Children Rehabilitation Special Unit, Arcispedale Santa Maria Nuova-IRCCS, Azienda Unità Sanitaria Locale, 42100 Reggio Emilia, Italy
Surgical, Medical and Dental Department of Morphological Sciences related to Transplant, Oncology and Regenerative Medicine, Università degli Studi di Modena e Reggio Emilia, 41100 Modena, Italy

Rosa Román-Oyola, Verónica Figueroa-Feliciano, Yoliannie Torres-Martínez, Jorge Torres-Vélez, Keyshla Encarnación-Pizarro, Samariz Fragoso-Pagán and Luis Torres-Colón
University of Puerto Rico, Medical Sciences Campus, School of Health Professions, Occupational Therapy Program, San Juan, PR 00936-5067, USA

DeokJu Kim
Department of OccupationalTherapy, Health Science College, Cheongju University, Cheongju, Republic of Korea

Alexandra Nugent, Nicola Hancock and Anne Honey
The University of Sydney, Cumberland Campus, 74 East St., Lidcombe, NSW2141, Australia

Chia-Ting Su
Department of Occupational Therapy, College of Medicine, Fu Jen Catholic University, New Taipei City, Taiwan

Ai-Lun Yang
Department of Sports Sciences, University of Taipei, Taipei, Taiwan

Chung-Ying Lin
Department of Rehabilitation Sciences, Faculty of Health and Social Sciences, The Hong Kong Polytechnic University, 11 Yuk Choi Road, Hung Hom, Hong Kong

Rachel A. Wortman, Theresa Vallone, Michele Karnes, Christine Walawander, Dion Daly and Bonnie Fox-Garrity
Department of Occupational Therapy, D'Youville College, 320 Porter Avenue, Buffalo, NY 14201, USA

Sean Reilly and Sinéad M. Hynes
Discipline of OccupationalTherapy, National University of Ireland Galway, Galway, Ireland

Ann-Charlotte Lindström
Närhälsan Rehabilitation Sörhaga, Alingsås, Sweden

Susanne Bernhardsson
Närhälsan Research and Development Primary Health Care, Region Västra Götaland, Gothenburg, Sweden
Institute of Neuroscience and Physiology, Department of Health and Rehabilitation, Unit of Physiotherapy, University of Gothenburg, The Sahlgrenska Academy, Gothenburg, Sweden

Lucy Jane Miller and Sarah A. Schoen
STAR Institute, 5420 S. Quebec Street, Suite 105, Greenwood Village, CO 80111, USA

Shelley Mulligan
Department of OccupationalTherapy, 4 LibraryWay, University of NewHampshire, Durham, NH03824, USA

Jillian Sullivan
Northeastern University, 312E Robinson Hall, 360 Huntington Ave., Boston, MA 02115, USA

Pragashnie Govender, December M. Mpanza, Tarryn Carey, Kwenzile Jiyane, Bicolé Andrews and Sam Mashele
Discipline of Occupational Therapy, School ofHealth Sciences, University of KwaZulu-Natal, Westville Campus, Westville, South Africa

Bárbara Iansã de Lima Barroso and Cláudia Regina Cabral Galvão
Graduate Student of the Graduate Program in Rehabilitation Sciences, Faculty of Medicine FMUSP, University of São Paulo, São Paulo, SP, Brazil

Luiz Bueno da Silva
Professor of the Postgraduate Program in Production Engineering, Federal University of Paraíba UFPB, João Pessoa, PB, Brazil

Selma Lancman
Professor of the Postgraduate Program in Rehabilitation Sciences. Faculty of Medicine FMUSP, University of São Paulo, São Paulo, SP, Brazil

Deborah Weissman-Miller, Rosalie J.Miller and Mary P. Shotwell
School of Occupational Therapy, Brenau University, 500Washington Street SE, Gainesville, GA 30501, USA

Rodolfo Morrison, Silvia Gómez, María Jesús Tapia and Laura Rueda
Department of OccupationalTherapy and Occupational Science, Faculty of Medicine, University of Chile, Santiago, Chile
Chilean Society of Occupational Science, Santiago, Chile

Enrique Henny
Chilean Society of Occupational Science, Santiago, Chile Tedes Center, Santiago, Chile

Masahiro Ogawa
Department of Human Health Sciences, Graduate School of Medicine, Kyoto University, Kyoto, Japan

Seiji Nishida
Faculty of Health andWelfare, Prefectural University of Hiroshima, Hiroshima, Japan

Haruna Shirai
School of Health Sciences, Bukkyo University, Kyoto, Japan

Sutinun Juntorn, Sarinya Sriphetcharawut and Peeraya Munkhetvit
Department of OccupationalTherapy, Faculty of Associated Medical Sciences, Chiang Mai University, Chiang Mai, Thailand

Mi Kyung Kim
Department of Occupational Therapy, Sanggye Paik Hospital, Seoul, Republic of Korea

Deok Ju Kim
Department of Occupational Therapy, Health Science College, Cheongju University, Cheongju, Republic of Korea

Svetlana Solgaard Nielsen
The Research Initiative of Activity Studies and Occupational Therapy, Research Unit of General Practice, Department of Public Health, The University of Southern Denmark, J.B. Winsløws Vej 9a, 5000 Odense C, Denmark

Jeanette Reffstrup Christensen
The Research Initiative of Activity Studies and Occupational Therapy, Research Unit of General Practice, Department of Public Health, The University of Southern Denmark, J.B. Winsløws Vej 9a, 5000 Odense C, Denmark
The Research Unit for Physical Activity and Health at Work, Department of Sports Science and Clinical Biomechanics, The University of Southern Denmark, Campusvej 55, 5230 Odense M, Denmark

A. Enemark Larsen and B. Rasmussen
Department of Occupational Therapy, Institute of Medwifery and Therapy, University College Copenhagen, Sigurdsgade 26, DK-2200 N Copenhagen, Denmark

J. R. Christensen
Department of Public Health, University of Southern Denmark, JB Winsløwsvej 9A, 5000 Odense, Denmark
Department of Sports Science and Clinical Biomechanics, University of Southern Denmark, Campusvej 55, 5230 Odense, Denmark

Eric Asaba
Department of Neurobiology, Care Sciences, and Society (NVS), Division of OccupationalTherapy, Karolinska Institutet, Alfred Nobels All´e 23, B4, Huddinge, Sweden
Unit for Research, Education, and Development (FoUU), Stockholms Sjukhem Foundation, Stockholm, Sweden
Department of Occupational Therapy, Tokyo Metropolitan University, Tokyo, Japan

Anders Kottorp
Department of Neurobiology, Care Sciences, and Society (NVS), Division of OccupationalTherapy, Karolinska Institutet, Alfred Nobels All´e 23, B4, Huddinge, Sweden

Faculty for Health and Society, Malmö University, Malm¨o, Sweden

Mio Nakamura
Department of Occupational Therapy, International University of Health andWelfare, Narita, Japan

Akie Asaba
Karolinska University Hospital, OccupationalTherapy and Physiotherapy Practice Areas, Huddinge, Sweden

Daiva Petruseviciene, Daiva Baltaduoniene and Egle Lendraitiene
Department of Rehabilitation, Medical Academy, Lithuanian University of Health Sciences, Kaunas, Lithuania

Deive Surmaitiene
Kulautuva Hospital of Rehabilitation, Hospital of Lithuanian University of Health Sciences Kauno Klinikos, Kaunas, Lithuania

Eris C. M. Ho
Occupational Therapy Department, Queen Elizabeth Hospital, Hospital Authority, Kowloon, Hong Kong

Andrew M. H. Siu
Department of Rehabilitation Sciences, The Hong Kong Polytechnic University, Kowloon, Hong Kong

M. Parente and G. Esposito
Sapienza Università di Roma, Rome, Italy

M. Tofani, R. De Santis, V. Santilli and G. Galeoto
Department of Anatomical, Histological, Forensic and Orthopaedic Sciences, Sapienza Universit`a di Roma, Piazzale Aldo Moro 5, 00185 Rome, Italy

Marieke Lindenschot
Department IQ Healthcare, Research Institute for Health Sciences, Radboud University Medical Center Nijmegen, Postbus 9101, 6500 HB Nijmegen, Netherlands
Department of Occupational Therapy, HAN University of Applied Sciences, Postbus 6960, 6503 GL Nijmegen, Netherlands
Research Group Neurorehabilitation, HAN University of Applied Sciences, Nijmegen, Netherlands
Department of Rehabilitation, Donders Center for Neuroscience, Radboud University Medical Center Nijmegen, Postbus 9101, 6500 HB Nijmegen, Netherlands

Maria W. G. Nijhuis-van der Sanden
Department IQ Healthcare, Research Institute for Health Sciences, Radboud University Medical Center Nijmegen, Postbus 9101, 6500 HB Nijmegen, Netherlands
Department of Rehabilitation, Donders Center for Neuroscience, Radboud University Medical Center Nijmegen, Postbus 9101, 6500 HB Nijmegen, Netherlands

Esther M. J. Steultjens
Department of Occupational Therapy, HAN University of Applied Sciences, Postbus 6960, 6503 GL Nijmegen, Netherlands
Research Group Neurorehabilitation, HAN University of Applied Sciences, Nijmegen, Netherlands

Ton Satink
Department of Occupational Therapy, HAN University of Applied Sciences, Postbus 6960, 6503 GL Nijmegen, Netherlands
Research Group Neurorehabilitation, HAN University of Applied Sciences, Nijmegen, Netherlands
European Masters of Science in Occupational Therapy, Amsterdam University of Applied Sciences, Amsterdam, Netherlands

Imelda J. M. de Groot
Department of Rehabilitation, Donders Center for Neuroscience, Radboud University Medical Center Nijmegen, Postbus 9101, 6500 HB Nijmegen, Netherlands

Saskia Koene
Department of Pediatrics, Radboud Center for Mitochondrial Medicine, Radboud University Medical Center Nijmegen, Geert Grooteplein Zuid 10, 6525 GA Nijmegen, Netherlands

Tore Bonsaksen
Department of Occupational Therapy, Prosthetics and Orthotics, Faculty of Health Sciences, OsloMet - Oslo Metropolitan University, Oslo, Norway
Faculty of Health Studies, VID Specialized University, Sandnes, Norway

Index